ADVANCING EVIDENCE-BASED PRACTICE IN NURSING AND HEALTHCARE

ADVANCING EVIDENCE-BASED PRACTICE IN NURSING AND HEALTHCARE

2nd EDITION

Mary Jo Vetter, DNP, RN, AGPCNP-BC, FAANP
Chief Clinical Officer
Parker Health Group
Highland Park, New Jersey

Kathleen Evanovich Zavotsky, PhD, RN, CCRN, CEN, ACNS-BC, FAEN, FCNS
System Senior Director, Nursing Research and Program Evaluation
Departments of Nursing
NYU Langone Health
New York, New York

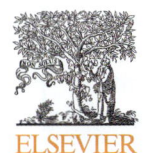

ELSEVIER

Elsevier
3251 Riverport Lane
St. Louis, Missouri 63043

ADVANCING EVIDENCE-BASED PRACTICE IN NURSING AND
HEALTHCARE, SECOND EDITION

ISBN: 978-0-323-93621-7

Copyright © 2026 by Elsevier Inc. All rights are reserved, including those for text and data mining, AI training, and similar technologies.

Publisher's note: Elsevier takes a neutral position with respect to territorial disputes or jurisdictional claims in its published content, including in maps and institutional affiliations.

No part of this publication may be reproduced or transmitted in any form or by any means, electronic or mechanical, including photocopying, recording, or any information storage and retrieval system, without permission in writing from the publisher. Details on how to seek permission, further information about the Publisher's permissions policies and our arrangements with organizations such as the Copyright Clearance Center and the Copyright Licensing Agency, can be found at our website: www.elsevier.com/permissions.

This book and the individual contributions contained in it are protected under copyright by the Publisher (other than as may be noted herein).

> **Notice**
>
> Practitioners and researchers must always rely on their own experience and knowledge in evaluating and using any information, methods, compounds or experiments described herein. Because of rapid advances in the medical sciences, in particular, independent verification of diagnoses and drug dosages should be made. To the fullest extent of the law, no responsibility is assumed by Elsevier, authors, editors or contributors for any injury and/or damage to persons or property as a matter of products liability, negligence or otherwise, or from any use or operation of any methods, products, instructions, or ideas contained in the material herein.

Previous editions copyrighted 2019.

Executive Content Strategist: Lee Henderson
Senior Content Development Manager: Laura Schmidt
Senior Content Development Specialist: Kristen Helm
Publishing Services Manager: Deepthi Unni
Project Manager: Nayagi Anandan
Designer: Patrick Ferguson

Printed in China by 1010 Printing International Ltd

Last digit is the print number: 9 8 7 6 5 4 3 2 1

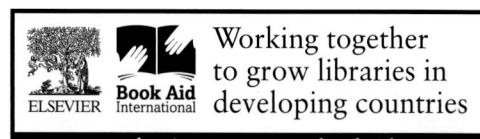

ABOUT THE AUTHORS

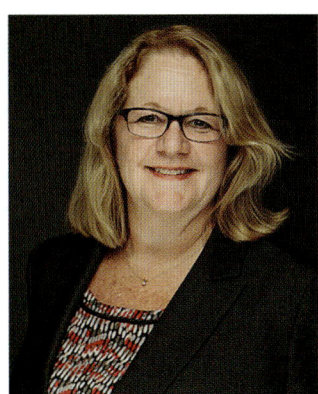

Mary Jo Vetter, DNP, RN, AGPCNP-BC, FAANP, is a nurse leader and clinician with over 45 years of experience in clinical and academic settings. She has maintained an active practice as a nurse and nurse practitioner with emphasis on care delivery in home and community-based settings. She has functioned in executive leadership roles in New Jersey and New York in health care organizations, providing ambulatory and primary care, certified home care, hospice, and long-term care with a primary focus on geriatric care innovation across the continuum of aging services. Mary Jo is a graduate of New Jersey City University where she received the bachelor's degree in nursing and Rutgers, the State University of New Jersey, attaining both the master's and doctorate in nursing. She has been a long-time supporter of evidence-based practice in nursing, advocating for uptake of associated competencies in diverse practice settings. She has enjoyed a multitude of joint appointments operationalizing meaningful and productive academic–practice partnerships and has published and presented nationally and internationally on topics related to innovation in geriatric nursing care and service delivery, the integration of design thinking in academic curricula to foster nurse entrepreneurship and intrapreneurship, and nurse-managed primary care management. She was inducted as a fellow of the American Association of Nurse Practitioners and has been actively involved in multiple professional and academic organizations. After serving as a clinical associate professor and director of the Doctor of Nursing Practice Program at New York University, Rory Meyers College of Nursing for 8 years, she recently joined Parker Health Group, a noted aging services organization, as Chief Clinical Officer.

ABOUT THE AUTHORS

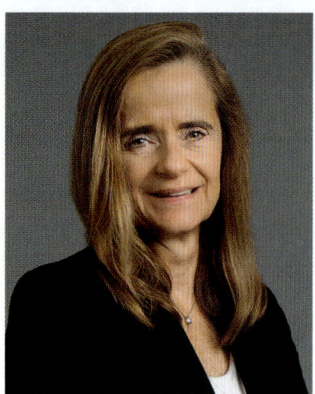

Kathleen Evanovich Zavotsky, PhD, RN, CCRN, CEN, ACNS-BC, FAEN, FCNS, is a nurse researcher/leader with more than 25 years of clinical, research, leadership, and education experience. She holds clinical certification as an emergency and critical care nurse, in which areas she has more than 40 years of clinical practice experience. She is a graduate of Rutgers, The State University of New Jersey for her bachelor's and master's degrees and a PhD in nursing from Seton Hall University. She is board-certified as an advanced practice nurse in adult gerontology and as a clinical nurse specialist since 1993. She is an award-recognized educator and national speaker on research, clinical, quality, and safety topics. She has published more than 60 scholarly publications in professional journals and book chapters. She has held various joint appointments at various universities and has mentored many PhD and doctor of nursing practice students through their doctoral work. She is the recipient of multiple private and federal grants for her collaborative research and scholarly work. Her research interests have been focused on patients' responses to wellness and illness, and the impacts of social determinants of health in the acute care setting, including the emergency department. She has also studied the scope of influence of workforce wellness in nurses working in acute care settings. Kathleen was inducted as a fellow in the Academy of Emergency Nursing by the Emergency Nurses Association and as a clinical nurse specialist fellow by the Clinical Nurse Specialist Institute. She has served on multiple local and national committees as both a member and a leader for both the Emergency Nurses Association and National Association of Clinical Nurse Specialists. She is currently the System Senior Director of Nursing Research and Program Evaluation at NYU Langone Health in New York City.

CONTRIBUTORS

Debra Albert, DNP, MBA, RN, NEA-BC
Chief Nursing Officer & Senior Vice President for Patient Care Services
NYU Langone Health
Lerner Director of Health Promotion
Adjunct Assistant Professor
Rory Meyers College of Nursing
New York University
New York, New York

Carlita Anglin, MSIS
Associate Curator
NYU Health Sciences Library
NYU Langone Health
New York, New York

Kathy Moore Baker, PhD, RN, NE-BC, FAAN
Chief Nursing Officer
Department of Patient Care Services
University of Virginia
Charlottesville, Virginia

Kathleen Begonia, PhD, RN, NI-BC, CCRN
Clinical Associate Professor
Department of Nursing
Mount Sinai Health System
New York, New York

Jenna Blind, DNP, RN, CPHQ
Director of Education, Professional Development, and Quality Improvement
Department of Home Health Care and Home Hospital
NYU Langone Health
Garden City, New York

Karyn L. Boyar, DNP, FNP-BC, CNE
Clinical Associate Professor
Rory Meyers College of Nursing
New York University
New York, New York

Mary Margaret Brennan, DNP, AGACNP-BC, FAANP
Clinical Associate Professor
Director
Adult-Gerontology Acute Care Nurse Practitioner Program
Director DNP Program
Rory Meyers College of Nursing
New York University
New York, New York

Dewi Brown-Deveaux, DNP, MS, BS, RN, ONC, FAAN
Senior Director of Nursing
Departments of Nursing
NYU Langone Health-Brooklyn
Brooklyn, New York

Brynne Campbell Rice, MLIS
Librarian for Health Sciences
Division of Libraries
New York University
New York, New York

Sean Clarke, PhD, RN, FAAN
Executive Vice Dean and Springer Professor in Nursing Leadership
Rory Meyers College of Nursing
New York University
New York, New York

Alexa Colgrove Curtis, PhD, MPH, APRN, FAANP
Associate Dean for Research and Innovation
Orvis School of Nursing
University of Nevada, Reno
Reno, Nevada

Daniel David, MS, PhD, RN
Assistant Professor
Rory Meyers College of Nursing
New York University
New York, New York

Pamela B. DeGuzman, PhD, MBA, RN, CNL
Nurse Scientist
Center for Nursing Excellence
University of Virginia Health
Associate Professor
School of Nursing
University of Virginia
Charlottesville, Virginia

Barbara Delmore, PhD, RN, CWCN, MAPWCA, IIWCC-NYU, FAAN
Senior Nurse Scientist
Departments of Nursing
NYU Langone Health
Clinical Assistant Professor
Hansjörg Wyss Department of Plastic Surgery
NYU Grossman School of Medicine
New York, New York

Kathleen DeMarco, PhD, NE-BC, CPHQ, RN
System Senior Director Nursing Wellness and Resilience
System Senior Director Lerner Health Promotion
Departments of Nursing
NYU Langone Health
New York, New York

Maja Djukic, PhD, RN, FAAN
Associate Professor
Department of Nursing
UTHealth Houston Cizik School of Nursing
Houston, Texas

Emerson E. Ea, PhD, DNP, APRN, FAAN
Chair and Professor, Department of Nursing
School of Professional Studies
New York City College of Technology
City University of New York
New York, New York

Elizabeth Anna Fair, BS, MBA
Adjunct Faculty
Colangelo College of Business
Application Support Specialist
Department of Information Technology
Grand Canyon Education
Phoenix, Arizona

Marie Foley, PhD, MA, BSN, RN, CNL, NJ-CSN
Director of Nursing Research
Department of Nursing
Atlantic Health System
Morristown, New Jersey

Mattia J. Gilmartin, PhD, RN, FAAN
Chief of Staff
Executive Faculty
Nurses Improving Care for Healthsystem Elders (NICHE)
Rory Meyers College of Nursing
New York University
New York, New York

Kimberly S. Glassman, PhD, RN, NEA-BC, FAONL, FAAN
Dean
Department of Nursing
Mount Sinai Phillips School of Nursing
New York, New York

Judith Haber, PhD, APRN, FAAN
Professor Emerita
Rory Meyers College of Nursing
New York University
New York, New York

Jin Jun, PhD, RN
Assistant Professor
College of Nursing
The Ohio State University
Columbus, Ohio

Stacen A. Keating, PhD, RN
Clinical Associate Professor
Rory Meyers College of Nursing
New York University
New York, New York

Courtney Keeler, PhD, MS
Associate Professor
School of Nursing and Health Professions
University of San Francisco
San Francisco, California

Martha Kent, EdD, RN, NEA-BC
System Senior Director, Nursing [Retired]
Departments of Nursing
NYU Langone Health
New York, New York

Carl A. Kirton, DNP, MBA, RN, ANP, FAAN
Editor-in-Chief
American Journal of Nursing
New York, New York
Adjunct Faculty
Rory Meyers College of Nursing
New York University
New York, New York
Adjunct Faculty
Department of Nursing
Temple University
Philadelphia, Pennsylvania

Robin Toft Klar, DNSc, FAAN
Clinical Associate Professor
Rory Meyers College of Nursing
New York University
New York, New York

Kathryn Lang, DNP, RN, NE-BC
Vice President
Department of Administration
Long Island Community Hospital
Patchogue, New York

Patricia Maria Lavin, DNP, RN, NEA-BC
Senior Director of Nursing Professional Development, Quality and Outcomes
Departments of Nursing
NYU Langone Orthopedic Hospital
New York, New York

Marilyn Lopez, DNP, RN, GNP-BC
Program Director, Nursing Geriatrics
Departments of Nursing
NYU Langone Health
New York, New York

Eileen P. Magri, PhD, RN, NEA-BC
Senior Director
Departments of Nursing
NYU Langone Health-Long Island
Mineola, New York

Diane Rita Maydick-Youngberg, EdD, ACNS-BC, CWOCN
Director of Nursing Education
Director Nursing Research
Director, Wound Ostomy Continence Nursing
Director, Nurse Residency Program
Departments of Nursing
NYU Langone Health-Brooklyn
Brooklyn, New York

Althea L. Mighten, EdD, DNP, APRN-BC, NPD-BC, MEDSURG-BC
Senior Director of Nursing for Innovation and Inquiry
Departments of Nursing
NYU Langone Health
New York, New York

Jeanmarie Moorehead, EdD, RN, NEA-BC
Senior Director of Operations
Department of Home Health Care, Home Hospital, and Hospice
NYU Langone Health
Garden City, New York

Amy Lynn Msowoya, DNP, FNP-C
Family Nurse Practitioner
Karibu Family Care
Peoria, Arizona

Hiyam M. Nadel, MBA, RN
Director
Center for Innovations in Care Delivery
Massachusetts General Hospital
Boston, Massachusetts

Alice M. Nash, PhD, RN, NPD-BC, NEA-BC
System Senior Director, Nursing Professional Development and Clinical Outcomes
Departments of Nursing
NYU Langone Health
New York, New York

CONTRIBUTORS

Chin Park, PhD, MBA, RN
Clinical Assistant Professor
Rory Meyers College of Nursing
New York University
New York, New York

Peter Rodney, DNP, MS, RN, CNOR, NEA-BC
Vice President of Nursing and Patient Care Services
Departments of Nursing
NYU Langone Health
New York, New York

Amy Witkoski Stimpfel, PhD, RN
Assistant Professor
Rory Meyers College of Nursing
New York University
New York, New York

Eileen Sullivan-Marx, PhD, RN, FAAN
Professor
Rory Meyers College of Nursing
New York University
New York, New York

Marita G. Titler, PhD, RN, FAAN
Professor Emeritus
School of Nursing
University of Michigan
Ann Arbor, Michigan

Mary Jo Vetter, DNP, RN, AGPCNP-BC, FAANP
Chief Clinical Officer
Parker Health Group
Highland Park, New Jersey

Kimberly Whalen, MS, RN, CCRN
Nurse Director
Department of Pediatric Critical Care
Massachusetts General Hospital
Plymouth, Massachusetts

Lisa A. Wolf, PhD, RN, CEN, FAEN, FAAN
Director, Emergency Nursing Research
Department of Research
Emergency Nurses Association
Schaumburg, Illinois
Associate Professor
Elaine Marieb College of Nursing
University of Massachusetts Amherst
Amherst, Massachusetts

Geri LoBiondo-Wood, PhD, RN, FAAN
Professor Emerita
Department of Research
University of Texas Health Science Center
Cizik School of Nursing
Houston, Texas

Kathleen Evanovich Zavotsky, PhD, RN, CCRN, CEN, ACNS-BC, FAEN, FCNS
System Senior Director, Nursing Research and Program Evaluation
Departments of Nursing
NYU Langone Health
New York, New York

Linda Zieman, DNP, MM, MSN, RN, CEN, NEA-BC
Senior Director of Nursing, Inpatient Services
Department of Nursing Administration
Hospital for Special Surgery
Adjunct Faculty Instructor
Rory Meyers College of Nursing
New York University
Adjunct Associate Professor
Lienhard College of Nursing
Pace University
New York, New York

INTRODUCTION

We would like to recognize the editors of the first edition, Dr. Geri LoBiondo-Wood, Dr. Judith Haber, and Dr. Marita Titler, for having the expertise and vision to create a textbook with such a strong foundation for evidence-based practice (EBP). The quality of the original version of the book has enabled practicing nurses and graduate students to have a greater understanding of the impact that EBP has on the quality of care overall. As healthcare continues to evolve, we have used the first edition to help us provide you with new and updated information for all nurses.

One of the changes on which we focused early on was highlighting the relationship, exchange of knowledge, and application of skills taught in the academic setting to impact outcomes in the practice setting. Through the process of academic–practice partnership (APP) we sought to broaden the utility of the textbook to meet the needs of both academia and practice by offering a pragmatic guide to EBP, quality improvement, and research that was relevant to nurses in graduate education and advanced clinical practice. This is especially important for organizations that are on the American Nurses Credentialing Center Magnet journey or those who have already received this designation. To meet established criteria, many have developed innovative programs such as residencies and fellowships that are dependent on EBP translation. Additionally, we were thoughtful to ensure that that the second edition reflects recent guidance and aspirations set forth in the new American Association of the Colleges of Nursing (AACN) *Essentials of Professional Education*, the AACN *Advancing Healthcare Transformation: A New Era for Academic Nursing* (2016), the *Future of Nursing 2020–2030: Charting a Path to Achieve Health Equity* published by the National Academies of Sciences, Engineering, and Medicine, and multiple other regulatory and quality standards across multiple practice settings. Our goal in revising and adding chapters was to demonstrate alignment between education-based domains and competencies and practice expectations regardless of practice setting. We also hoped to portray through this contemporary approach that this edition of the textbook will help guide both academic and practice organizations' programs as they continue to develop more sophisticated nursing science that keeps pace with and is relevant to the needs of health care organizations.

NYU Langone Health and Rory Meyers College of Nursing at New York University enjoyed a long, well-functioning relationship and history of collaboration in research and EBP, and that has led to an international reputation of nursing excellence. You will see elements of this partnership threaded throughout the chapters of the second edition. The textbook was a natural next step as we recognized the importance of synergy between what is taught in the classroom as it is translated to real-life, contemporary practice problems, such as nurse wellness, population health, and diversity, equity, inclusion, and belonging. Content was added to enhance the learning experience and guide scholarly work that reflects the current state of nursing science.

We welcomed the opportunity to serve as co-editors of the second edition as a way to memorialize the years of collaboration, recognizing that the next edition of the book will be different as healthcare, nursing practice, and academia evolve and mature to reflect current health care circumstances, and so we are already thinking updates for a third edition that will keep the textbook current and continue to meet the needs of nursing students and practicing clinicians.

Themes that guided contributors in revising existing chapters and writing new chapters were identified from both settings and shared, and teams of expert authors were purposefully partnered to complement and enhance each other's knowledge and experience.

Our vision was to directly apply concepts of EBP improvement to health care organizational priorities, strategies, and desired health system outcomes. Authors from both settings found the experience of collaboration extremely valuable and found that it enhanced their own practice and leadership. In response to a request for feedback from contributors about their thoughts regarding the importance of APP, we received several responses that are shared below:

"The current health care environment is particularly challenging for new graduate nurses transitioning to practice. Creating strong academic and practice partnerships is integral in preparing future nurses to be successful, applying knowledge acquired to the practice environment in all health care settings."

Dr. Eileen Magri, NYU Langone Health

"Lita and I both feel that this experience was emblematic of the power of academic and practice partnerships; our work was stronger as a synthesis of our different perspectives than it would have been if we had been writing from our unique stances alone. Since we went into this collaboration with the explicit intention of building bridges between academic and practice applications and checking each other's blind spots, we were really able to keep our focus on praxis, which provided a strong foundation from which to approach the chapter."

Brynne Campbell Rice/Carlita Anglin, Medical Librarians, New York University/ NYU Langone Health

"The academic–practice partnership supports a continuum of learning for professional nursing by creating a culture where frontline nurses are bedside change agents who improve outcomes associated with evidence-based care in alignment with organizational strategic goals. The continuum of learning through the academic and practice partnership empowers nurses throughout their academic and professional development to identify and bring forth opportunities for improving patient outcomes and the professional practice environment. It facilitates the development of a culture of excellence for all levels of nurses to promote quality improvement and practice innovation. The academic–practice partnership supports a learning environment where everyone identifies and solves problems, enabling the organization to experiment and improve patient, nursing, and organizational outcomes."

Dr. Patricia Maria Lavin, NYU Langone Health

"Thank you for your support on this massive undertaking. We both were willing to bring a new chapter, but not a new concept, to the book (i.e., population health). By taking an academic–practice partnership approach to this edition we, as coauthors of the population health chapter, learned so much more about the work toward population health from the clinical side and the connections in concepts and language between the clinical and academic sides. A synchrony that we would never have appreciated if we were not brought together for this new chapter and edition."

Dr. Robin Klar, New York University Rory Meyers College of Nursing

"At the outset, our team of four had great synergy and comradery. Getting to have meaningful discussions about population health from both the academic and practice side of things really enabled us to craft our chapter in a way that was comprehensive and creative—the product was something that would have been much different without our team's make-up and dedication to the topic. Because of our work together, I had many more offline conversations with our practice partners. This gave me the great fortune to engage our practice partners in my outpatient nursing elective. This in turn gave students a very real and rich exposure to a whole other side of nursing they were unfamiliar with previously!"

Dr. Stacen Keating, New York University Rory Meyers College of Nursing

Lastly, we must acknowledge every one of our contributors. Early in the process, each author shared our vision regarding the best way to meet the needs and address the complexities in healthcare by being inclusive of the various degree preparations present in both academia and practice. By doing this, we capitalized on each author's unique contribution and expertise. It was through this synergy that is evident in each chapter that you will see the commitment to advancing the nursing profession through evidence-based, person-centered, high-quality care. We are so very grateful that each contributor aligned with our vision and helped make this book come to fruition.

Looking forward into the future as co-editors we welcome your feedback about the second edition and seek to continuously improve our ability to support evidence-based quality improvement and nursing science efforts across the continuum of care!

In gratitude and partnership,

**Mary Jo Vetter
Kathleen Evanovich Zavotsky**

ACKNOWLEDGMENTS

This textbook represents the cumulative knowledge and expertise of so many dedicated contributors as well as the numerous nursing leaders who have nurtured evidence-based practice (EBP) as a foundational skill in the profession. While there are too many to name individually, I would like to personally acknowledge academic leaders who have mentored me in my EBP journey: Dr. Rona F. Levin, Dr. Bernadette Melnyk, Dr. Ellen Fineout-Overholt, and Dr. Judith Haber. Years before EBP was an essential competency in nursing practice and well-integrated in nursing education curricula, EBP mentors were essential in bringing EBP skill sets to the practice setting. The reciprocal learning that took place between academic and practice partners was nothing short of inspirational. Fortunately, when I first met these inspirational leaders, I was in a practice environment led by a visionary nurse executive, Joan Marren, who paved the way for the Visiting Nurse Service of New York to engage in the co-creation of a framework that combined EBP and quality improvement that guided nurses to access research evidence to inform improvement in care quality and outcomes. As a result, I quickly became an enthusiastic supporter of academic–practice partnerships and have subsequently served in roles in both settings, continually looking for opportunities to collaborate.

Upon my arrival at the Rory Meyers College of Nursing at New York University, the commitment to partnership between service and academia was exemplified by the leadership of Dean Eileen Sullivan-Marx and NYU Langone Health's chief nursing officer at that time, Dr. Kimberly Glassman. In my role as director of the Doctor of Nursing Practice (DNP) Program, I benefitted from the established relationship of these leaders as we operationalized a highly effective approach to the DNP Project. Students were able to directly apply the rigorous skills learned in the classroom to address a real clinical problem that was also an organizational priority for the health system. Our collaboration deepened when I met Dr. Kathy Zavotsky, a kindred spirit, with equal passion for advancing nursing science. Together, we role-modeled and promoted meaningful PhD/DNP collaboration and designed new and exciting ways to foster the partnership relationship. This book is one of the products of our work together.

At this time, I have returned to the practice setting as chief clinical officer of an aging services organization focused on meeting the current and future care needs of the geriatric population. My desire for academic practice partnership has endured because of the value such relationships offer in supporting clinical, quality, and person-centered outcomes.

I would like to thank all those who contributed to this textbook, the generations of nurse colleagues who have preceded me in their commitment to care excellence, and those who will continue to innovate care based on relevant evidence. We will continue to accelerate the integration and translation of research evidence in practice as the profession of nursing evolves to meet the needs of our collective, global society.

Finally, to my family and friends, I am eternally grateful for your sustained support and unconditional love. You energize me every day by demonstrating endless interest in my work and the people who weave the fabric of my professional life.

Mary Jo Vetter

First, I would like to thank the editors of the first edition, Dr. Geri LoBiondo-Wood, Dr. Judith Haber, and Dr. Marita Titler, for providing a foundation that was easy to build on. The thoughtfulness to the content has enabled us to add contemporary material that I believe will help enhance the benefits of this edition to the student, the practicing nurse, and beyond. It is an honor to continue the legacy that they have created.

Next, to my co-editor and friend Dr. Mary Jo Vetter. I knew from the moment that I met you and connected that we would continue to develop great nursing science for students and nurses at NYU Langone Health and beyond. I admire your commitment to the academic–practice partnership and the science of nursing, and I am so grateful to you for what you have taught me through this process and over the years. I am honored that you asked me to partner with you and so happy to call you a friend.

ACKNOWLEDGMENTS

I am also forever grateful to Dr. Debra Albert, System Chief Nursing Officer at NYU Langone Health, who has provided me with an opportunity of a lifetime; thank you for creating an environment that values the science of nursing. To be given the opportunity to work with the amazing nurses at NYU Langone Health and the caliber of faculty at New York University's Rory Meyers College of Nursing every day is truly an honor.

When I first agreed to serve as an editor, I asked a mentor of mine how do I know that chapters that my colleagues write are appropriate for a textbook. She told me that when I read the chapter and if I come away with at least one new thing that I learned, it was good! I can remember the first chapter that I received and how I was so moved by the effort and content that it exceeded my expectations. As the months continued and I received more and more chapters, it was like I was opening a present. The scholarly wisdom that each and every one of the contributors added to this book will undoubtably influence practice and academia well into the future. A sincere thank you to each and every one of you.

Taking on a challenge like editing this second edition takes courage, and I was so glad that my parents instilled that in me early on and that my beautiful brothers and sisters taught me how to use it. A big thanks to my husband, Jeffry, who reminds me every day that life is so much better with a little bit of humor. Lastly to my beautiful, fearless, and funny daughter Mary Kate who reminds me every day how precious life is.

Kathleen Evanovich Zavotsky

CONTENTS

PART I Introduction

1. **Leadership Implications for Evidence-Based Practice, Nursing Practice, and Healthcare,** 1
   Debra Albert and Eileen Sullivan-Marx
2. **Academic–Practice Partnership for the Future of Nursing and Healthcare,** 7
   Mary Jo Vetter and Kathleen Evanovich Zavotsky
3. **Overview of Evidence-Based Practice,** 19
   Kathleen Evanovich Zavotsky and Mary Jo Vetter
4. **Models to Support Evidence-Based Practice Outcomes,** 37
   Mary Jo Vetter and Kathleen Evanovich Zavotsky

PART II Processes of Developing Evidence-Based Practice and Questions in Various Clinical Settings

5. **Developing Compelling Clinical Questions,** 51
   Judith Haber and Martha Kent
6. **Searching the Literature for Evidence,** 59
   Brynne Campbell Rice and Carlita Anglin
7. **Principles of Assessing Research Quality,** 81
   Geri LoBiondo-Wood and Barbara Delmore
8. **Intervention Studies,** 91
   Lisa A. Wolf, Pamela B. DeGuzman, and Kathy Moore Baker
9. **Observational Studies,** 105
   Geri LoBiondo-Wood and Barbara Delmore
10. **Systematic Reviews and Clinical Practice Guidelines,** 117
    Amy Witkoski Stimpfel and Jin Jun
11. **Qualitative Studies,** 143
    Kathleen Evanovich Zavotsky and Marie Foley
12. **Sources of Data to Drive Evidence-Based Practice and Quality Improvement,** 159
    Patricia Maria Lavin and Mary Jo Vetter
13. **Understanding Statistics for Evidence-Based Practice,** 173
    Carl A. Kirton, Alexa Colgrove Curtis, and Courtney Keeler

PART III Implementation

14. **Evidence-Based Approaches for Improving Health Care Quality,** 199
    Maja Djukic, Mattia J. Gilmartin, and Marilyn Lopez
15. **Planning for Success,** 229
    Marita G. Titler, Eileen P. Magri
16. **Launching Implementation,** 243
    Marita G. Titler, Alice M. Nash
17. **Implementation Strategies for Stakeholders,** 253
    Mary Margaret Brennan and Linda Zieman
18. **Patient-Centered Evidence-Based Practices,** 277
    Amy Lynn Msowoya and Elizabeth Anna Fair

PART IV Evaluation and Dissemination

19. **Evaluation of Evidence-Based Practice,** 293
    Diane Rita Maydick-Youngberg and Daniel David
20. **Nursing Scholarship,** 309
    Alice M. Nash, Mary Jo Vetter, and Kathleen Evanovich Zavotsky
21. **Dissemination,** 317
    Carl A. Kirton and Althea L. Mighten

PART V Evidence-Based Practice Innovation in Healthcare

22. **Doctorally Prepared Nurses: Synergy for Professional Power,** 333
    Debra Albert, Kathleen Evanovich Zavotsky, and Mary Jo Vetter
23. **Innovation and New Models of Evidence-Based Care,** 343
    Hiyam M. Nadel, Karyn L. Boyar, and Kimberly Whalen
24. **Nursing Informatics,** 359
    Chin Park and Kathleen Begonia
25. **Population and Public Health,** 379
    Jenna Blind, Stacen A. Keating, Robin Toft Klar, and Jeanmarie Moorehead

26 **Health Policy,** 391
   Kimberly S. Glassman and Dewi Brown-Deveaux
27 **Nurse Wellness: An Evolving Concept and Its Connection to Health Care System Outcomes,** 401
   Kathleen DeMarco and Sean Clarke
28 **Harnessing the Power of Diversity, Equity, Inclusion, and Belonging to Advancing Health Care Systems Outcomes,** 417
   Emerson E. Ea, Kathryn Lang, Peter Rodney, and Kathleen Evanovich Zavotsky

Appendices

Appendix A, 431
Appendix B, 432
Appendix C, 433
Appendix D, 434
Glossary, 435
Index, 443

PART I Introduction

1

Leadership Implications for Evidence-Based Practice, Nursing Practice, and Healthcare

Debra Albert and Eileen Sullivan-Marx

LEARNING OUTCOMES

After reading this chapter, you should be able to do the following:

- Discuss the scope of leadership influence of evidence-based practice (EBP) implementation on nursing and healthcare.
  - Quality
  - Nurse wellness
  - American Nurses Credentialing Center (ANCC) Magnet
  - Education
- Review the leadership opportunities to sustain EBP in nursing practice and healthcare.
  - Advocate-EBP director
  - Quality-practice
  - Informatics/Quality and Safety Education for Nurses (QSEN)
- Discuss the opportunities for partnership between academia and practice in order to impact EBP, nursing, and healthcare.
  - Ensuring Doctor of Nursing Practice (DNP) project selection supports health care system needs/goals
  - Ambulatory care
  - Patient/family
  - Hospital at home
  - Education to reflect/mirror the practice
  - Specialty training
  - Sustainability
  - Benefits of partnership to both academia and service
- Review the call for action for DNP leaders to create the future for healthcare.

KEY TERMS

Academic–practice partnership   Healthcare   Leadership
Evidence-based practice

Overall, this chapter is geared toward equipping graduate-degree–prepared nurses and students (advanced practice nurses [APNs], clinical leaders) to serve as leaders in **healthcare** in various settings.

At the end of your graduate degree journey, you will be considered a leader in **evidence-based practice** (EBP). This is your opportunity to ensure that your education is filled with information you need to meet this challenge.

In addition to the didactic and clinical requirements necessary for the degree, you should take the time to develop and establish a mentor/mentee relationship with either one or more doctorally prepared nurses as well as other professional clinical leaders. As you begin to practice with your newly acquired credentials, you will soon find out that while the quality education you received is vitally important, the ability to execute in your practice is essential. Having a peer or nurse leader to guide and support you formally and informally should be part of your lifelong learning. Establishing and building mentor relationships is a process and a skill that can take time to develop. This process will certainly vary as you navigate roles in any health system, and as health policy, health care delivery, and professionals adapt, you will also need to adapt. Keeping in touch with faculty mentors and other professional advisors you have encountered in your graduate education is key to fostering solid mentorship and network support.

This chapter will help set the tone for you as a clinical leader through the valuable contribution from multidisciplinary leaders from both academia and clinical practice, writing together to present a partnership perspective on how practice, education, innovation, research, and leadership in nursing come together to drive EBP. The contributors in this textbook have very thoughtfully provided you with 28 chapters of contemporary, real-life information that is rooted in the latest art and science of nursing practice and will serve as a resource as you continue on your professional journey in our complex health care system.

SCOPE OF INFLUENCE

The scope of influence that you can have as a clinical leader is broad. As a nurse with an advanced degree, you will be called on to help ensure that nursing and healthcare provide value to our multiple constituencies and collaborators based on current evidence.

One of the most important things we can do as nurse leaders is ensure that our patients and staff are safe. As a nurse with an advanced degree, you will be called on to ensure that EBP is integrated in care delivery in all settings. While this seems like an easy, straightforward thing to do, there are often barriers to implementation in a complex system like healthcare. Utilizing a model/framework can help you ensure that EBP projects are executed successfully. EBP models can provide structure, and ensure that appropriate multidisciplinary stakeholders are involved and the project is metric driven and sustainable (see Chapters 4, 10, 12). The utilization of a model may be a new skill for many of the team members, and you will be called on to help with education and ensure proper utilization.

Those organizations that are American Nurses Credentialing Center (ANCC) Magnet designated, or on an ANCC Pathway to Excellence journey, must demonstrate that a culture of scientific inquiry is infused and based on contemporary nursing research and the latest evidence. Nurses with advanced degrees and clinical leaders are responsible for creating an inclusive practice environment to ensure that the appropriate people and processes are in place to help prepare for and sustain this highly coveted accreditation status.

LEADERSHIP OPPORTUNITIES

The **leadership** opportunities for nurses to influence EBP and healthcare are endless. Some priority should be given to serving as a role model and advocating for rigor in scholarly work/projects in order to ensure that the position remains highly respected. With an expansion of Doctor of Nursing Practice (DNP) programs in the last 15 years, producing leaders and practitioners to serve in various roles can potentially lead to role confusion for yourself and others in healthcare. One strategy that can be used to help prevent this role confusion could be to ensure that your practice is goal driven and in alignment with a health care organization as well as with nursing professional policy and practice as established by accrediting bodies, nursing specialty organizations, and emerging nursing science (see Chapters 6, 10, 25, 26).

Leading or partaking in initiatives that are rooted in addressing quality of care is probably one of the best ways to ensure that your hard-earned education is of value to a health care organization. Embedded throughout this textbook are everyday examples that can be integrated into your practice. The ability for nurses at all levels to understand the benefits of metric-driven quality care should be modeled and led by nurses with advanced degrees. Integrating models similar to the Quality and Safety Education for Nurses (QSEN) is a perfect opportunity for you to provide a structure and process to ensure nurses have the knowledge and skills necessary to improve patient care and healthcare in all settings.

Most frontline nurses do not understand the scope of influence that EBP and translational science can have on their patient care. Thus, you will be in a position to guide the development, implementation, and evaluation process for your own practice and that of the health system (see Chapters 22, 27). In addition, your leadership in clinical advancement can inform policy that impacts care nationally and internationally (see Chapters 25, 26).

Another important consideration in developing the reach of EBP through clinical leaders is establishing partnerships between academia and service, or an academic–practice partnership (APP) (see Chapter 2). Much of this work is guided by guidelines set by the American Association of Colleges of Nursing (AACN) and is dependent on developing relationships through a joint vision and goals for both the academic and practice partner. In addition, your practice may be linked with students, which is often the beginning of a larger APP initiative as you highlight success and/or innovation in your sphere of influence.

This partnership, while keeping in mind that each entity has its own purpose and mission, clearly shares a goal that includes developing nurses who are prepared for what the future of healthcare holds for each level of entry into practice. Specifically related to the advanced degree preparation, there are many opportunities for academia and practice to come together for curriculum development, clinical placement, and other scholarly work.

The APP should ensure that prelicensure curriculum is contemporary and reflective of the current state of healthcare. There is much opportunity to ensure that education reflects and mirrors practice—for example, ensuring that the curriculum integrates various critical practice areas that are important to healthcare such as the ambulatory setting, care coordination, chronic disease management programs, and other specialty training/immersion programs, such as perioperative and emergency department nursing. Contemporary curriculums enable us to leverage early career practice interest and professional curiosity, which can be carried on throughout a nurse's professional career. This may be a challenge for both the academic and practice partners who are rooted in traditional approaches. However, if the needs of our patients and the health care system are prioritized, creating innovative programs benefits all. Innovative APP programs could help provide opportunities for clinical leaders to be active participants in curriculum development, clinical placement, and program evaluation, leading to dissemination of the work to colleagues both internally and externally (see Chapters 2, 6, 12, 21, 23). Additionally, innovative APPs provide academic leaders the opportunity to influence the service practice environment and clinical care at the partner service organization. Moreover, successful and Magnet-certified APPs serve as standard bearers for smaller and emerging practices, particularly those that are community or long-term care based, to emulate them, particularly given the role that ANCC Magnet has in moving outcomes to excellence.

CALL TO ACTION

As a clinical leader you will be challenged to not only improve the health care system you serve but also act as a role model for nurses to build careers, strive for health equity, and promote nurse wellness, belonging, and joy (see Chapters 27, 28).

Walk the talk. Being able to take the time to reflect on your work is critical. Reflecting on the positive impact and perhaps missed opportunities will serve you well. Tapping into mentors' and colleagues' guidance and feedback is as valuable as receiving a formal evaluation from your direct leader. By taking the time to reflect on the work you have accomplished or set personal and professional goals, you can help ensure that you are staying true to the leadership role and your own personal values.

Lead with curiosity. The practice of nursing is infused with curiosity. Develop and sharpen the skill of a curious mind. Curiosity generally starts when you are a novice nurse, can be cultivated over time, and is vital to patient care. As a nurse in a leadership role, cultivating your own curiosity is as important as developing it in nurses and others in your sphere of influence. By developing this skill, you will be able to remain contemporary in your own practice and inspire others that you partner with to remain curious about the care delivered every day. Creating an environment of scientific and clinical curiosity is a key responsibility for any leader. In taking this work on, you empower nurses at all levels to have direct input into their practice and professional growth. Indeed, keeping professional curiosity as a core skill will ensure a career of constant growth (see Chapters 5, 6, 10).

Surround yourself with people who are smarter than you. Knowing your own strengths and weaknesses is important to any leadership role. As a leader in nursing, you will be challenged to work with nurses and other health care providers with a variety of backgrounds, in different care settings that might include your own private practice that serves a diverse patient population (see Chapters 25, 28). Being confident in what you have been prepared to do through your education and your clinical experience is critical. You will be challenged to bring groups together, and an honest self-assessment to determine what skills are needed to make the project successful is essential. Identifying exactly what you can contribute to the project and then selecting team members who can make up for your weaknesses and complement your strengths will be the key to a successful intervention or change initiative. The more diverse the team, the better the outcome.

Know your audience. As a leader you may be the only nurse who is participating on the team and will serve as the voice for nurses. Consider all team members as your peers and be true to what you contribute and that which is within your scope of practice, which is as an expert in EBP. Doing this will enable you to cultivate the right resources and support the collaborations necessary to help make complex projects in healthcare successful. Bring in other nurses when you find that you are the only nurse, and realize that you are there for the voice of a nurse. Do not be intimidated to bring forth your nursing knowledge as a driver to get to a solution with the group.

Emphasize strengths. Nursing leaders are called to evaluate people and processes, which can be highly complex and challenging to say the least. We are the only health profession with specific education, skill development, and accountability for bringing a team together for the patient and their family. Regardless of the target audience it is often most effective to emphasize the strengths of individuals and processes rather than to focus on the weaknesses. Teams function more efficiently when they tap into and build on strengths. Utilizing a glass-half-full lens is one of the most effective ways to drive change, both with the individuals you interact with and members of your interdisciplinary teams (see Chapter 22).

When you win, everyone else wins. Serving as an advocate for your team may come easy to some professionals, but advocating for yourself may be a bit more of a challenge. Recognize that serving as a voice for nurses and patients is a major responsibility as well as a distinct privilege. One of the most rewarding parts of your job will be to see nurses gain insight into their own practice and scope of influence on patient outcomes. It is important to let the full health professional team become aware of the unique contribution of nursing. As a clinical leader your most significant and lasting impact happens through others. We know that nurses are smart, passionate, and dedicated despite the challenges we face each and every day. Routinely we care for the marginalized and the most vulnerable people, and as a nurse leader taking the time to acknowledge those achievements is important. Remember to celebrate your and your team's accomplishments on a regular basis (see Chapters 27, 28).

CONCLUSION

You are going to be taking on a new, progressive role at a time in healthcare that has seen unprecedented changes. In the past 10 years we have experienced technological advances that impact patients and providers alike. We have endured a pandemic that pushed our nursing practice and the profession at large to new heights. We are experiencing the resulting challenges to our professional workforce and health care organizations. No doubt, the next 10 years will continue to bring on exciting challenges for leaders in both practice and academia. The only way for us to ensure that the nursing profession remains contemporary is to continue to develop the science through nursing research.

As a graduate-level–prepared clinical nursing leader, you are seen as an expert in translational science, which means you are dependent on rigorous and relevant research to be translated into practice. We do know that the number of nurses with a DNP degree compared to a PhD degree are outnumbered by approximately 2:1. The PhD role in nursing should be appreciated for what it was intended to do—developing new knowledge—which is complementary to the DNP role of applying that new knowledge to practice (see Chapter 22). Understanding and celebrating the synergistic relationship of these doctoral roles cannot be overemphasized. As nurses seek guidance on pursuing a terminal nursing degree, a clear understanding of each role and this interdependent, advantageous relationship is vital.

As a graduate-level–prepared clinical leader, you are in the position to make strong impressions and influence the choices that nurses make toward advancing their careers and formal education. As you serve as a model and guide nurses on their journey, offering external expert resources will help inform the process, such as the AACN site, which has an abundance of resources for them to explore (https://www.aacnnursing.org/students/nursing-education-pathways). Accessing information that is presented in a factual manner is very important for the individual or mentee to consider when deciding to advance their formal education, because it will take a good deal of time, money, and resources. This guidance may help them avoid making a wrong professional life-changing decision, which can lead to role disillusionment and disappointment. Also stay informed of higher education resources, opportunities to seek doctoral education, and what various schools of nursing offer on their websites, in interactive webinars, and through maintaining your professional network.

Your call to action as a clinical leader with an advanced degree is to lead the future of healthcare and nursing in all settings where people live, work, play, learn, and worship. While this may seem daunting, the knowledge and skills presented through the content, concepts, and examples in this textbook will help ensure that you are prepared to be a highly effective, visionary leader who is well positioned to guide the future of healthcare and nursing.

SUGGESTED READING

American Association of Colleges of Nursing. (2004). *AACN position statement on the practice doctorate in nursing.* https://www.aacnnursing.org/DNP/Position-Statement.

American Association of Colleges of Nursing. (2016). *Advancing healthcare transformation: A new era for academic nursing.* https://www.aacnnursing.org/Portals/0/PDFs/Publications/AACN-New-Era-Report.pdf.

American Association of Colleges of Nursing. (2020). *DNP fact sheet.* https://www.aacnnursing.org/News-Information/Fact-Sheets/DNP-Fact-Sheet.

American Association of Colleges of Nursing. (2006). *The essentials of doctoral education for advanced nursing practice.* https://www.aacnnursing.org/Portals/42/Publications/DNPEssentials.pdf.

American Association of Colleges of Nursing. (2021). *The essentials: Core competencies for professional nursing education.* https://aacnnursing.org/Portals/0/PDFs/Publications/Essentials-2021.pdf.

Bianchi, M., Bagnasco, A., Bressan, V., Barisone, M., Timmins, F., Rossi, S., et al. (2018). A review of the role of nurse leadership in promoting and sustaining evidence-based practice. *Journal of Nursing Management, 26*(8), 918–932. https://doi.org/10.1111/jonm.12638.

Castiglione, S. A. (2020). Implementation leadership: A concept analysis. *Journal of Nursing Management, 28*(1), 94–101. https://doi.org/10.1111/jonm.12899.

Crawford, C. L., Rondinelli, J., Zuniga, S., Valdez, R. M., Tze–Polo, L., & Titler, M. G. (2023). Barriers and facilitators influencing EBP readiness: Building organizational and nurse capacity. *Worldviews on Evidence-Based Nursing, 20*(1), 27–36. https://doi.org/10.1111/wvn.12618.

Harvey, G., Gifford, W., Cummings, G., Kelly, J., Kislov, R., Kitson, A., et al. (2019). Mobilising evidence to improve nursing practice: A qualitative study of leadership roles and processes in four countries. *International Journal of Nursing Studies, 90*, 21–30. https://doi.org/10.1016/j.ijnurstu.2018.09.017.

López–Medina, I. M., Sáchez–García, I., García–Fernández, F. P., & Pancorbo–Hidalgo, P. L. (2022). Nurses and ward managers' perceptions of leadership in the evidence–based practice: A qualitative study. *Journal of Nursing Management, 30*(1), 135–143. https://doi.org/10.1111/jonm.13469.

Lunden, A., Kvist, T., Teräs, M., & Häggman-Laitila, A. (2021). Readiness and leadership in evidence-based practice and knowledge management: A cross-sectional survey of nurses' perceptions. *Nordic Journal of Nursing Research, 41*(4), 187–196.

Melnyk, B. M., Hsieh, A. P., Messinger, J., Thomas, B., Connor, L., & Gallagher–Ford, L. (2023). Budgetary investment in evidence–based practice by chief nurses and stronger EBP cultures are associated with less turnover and better patient outcomes. *Worldviews on Evidence-Based Nursing, 20*(2), 162–171. https://doi.org/10.1111/wvn.12645.

National Academy of Medicine. (2021). *The future of nursing 2020–2030: Charting a path to achieve health equity.* https://nap.nationalacademies.org/catalog/25982/the-future-of-nursing-2020-2030-charting-a-path-to.

Reichenpfader, U., Carlfjord, S., & Nilsen, P. (2015). Leadership in evidence-based practice: A systematic review. *Leadership in Health Services, 28*(4), 298–316. https://doi.org/10.1108/lhs-08-2014-0061.

Shuman, C. J., Ehrhart, M. G., Torres, E. M., Veliz, P., Kath, L. M., Vanantwerp, K., et al. (2020). EBP implementation leadership of frontline nurse managers: Validation of the implementation leadership scale in acute care. *Worldviews on Evidence-Based Nursing, 17*(1), 82–91. https://doi.org/10.1111/wvn.12402.

Tucker, S. J., & Gallagher-Ford, L. (2019). EBP 2.0: From strategy to implementation. *American Journal of Nursing, 119*(4), 50–52. https://doi.org/10.1097/01.NAJ.0000554549.01028.af.

Warren, J. I., Mclaughlin, M., Bardsley, J., Eich, J., Esche, C. A., Kropkowski, L., & Risch, S. (2016). The strengths and challenges of implementing EBP in healthcare systems. *Worldviews on Evidence-Based Nursing, 13*(1), 15–24. https://doi.org/10.1111/wvn.12149.

Wonder, A. H., & Spurlock, D., Jr. (2020). A national study across levels of nursing education: Can nurses and nursing students accurately estimate their knowledge of evidence-based practice? *Nursing Education Perspectives, 41*(2), 77–82.

2

Academic–Practice Partnership for the Future of Nursing and Healthcare

Mary Jo Vetter and Kathleen Evanovich Zavotsky

LEARNING OUTCOMES

After reading this chapter, you should be able to do the following:
- Explore the historical and current status of academic–practice partnerships (APPs).
- Describe guiding principles of APPs.
- Explore ways that APPs are operationalized among academic and practice partners.
- Delineate the impact APPs have on evidence-based practice, healthcare quality, cost, and outcomes.
- Understand the potential impact APPs have on workforce development.
- Identify future implications in the evolution of APPs to impact transformational change in the nursing profession.

KEY TERMS

Academic–practice partnership
Clinical practice
Collaboration
Cost
Evidence-based practice
Education
Nursing workforce
Outcomes of care
Quality of care
Research

An **academic–practice partnership** (APP) is a **collaboration** between an academic institution and a healthcare organization. In nursing, an APP can empower innovative approaches in preparing the workforce of the future (Institute of Medicine [IOM], 2011; National Academies of Sciences, Engineering, and Medicine [NASEM], 2021). The goals of the partnership should be to enhance quality of healthcare delivery through the integration of **education**, **research**, and **clinical practice**. The academic institution provides opportunities for students and faculty to engage in learning experiences, while the healthcare organization benefits from access to the latest research, expertise, and educational programs that can positively impact the availability of a pipeline of highly trained professionals for employment. With students, faculty, clinical leaders, and staff working together to advance nursing knowledge, there is opportunity to simultaneously provide high quality care and workforce development.

Partnerships can be structured, executed, and governed in a variety of ways to meet the needs of both parties. Some are highly explicit and based on formal contracts that describe strategic plans, have bylaws and financial arrangements, and are overseen by clearly designated management resources to achieve mutual objectives; others are developed in an ad hoc manner in response to a particular situational need (De Geest et al., 2013).

> **TIP**
>
> Regardless of the formality in arrangements, the academic and practice setting should have a shared vision that builds on strengths, demonstrates collaboration, and supports relational change for the sake of improvement.

MUTUAL BENEFITS OF ACADEMIC–PRACTICE PARTNERSHIPS

There are mutual benefits to engaging in an APP. Sadeghnezhad and colleagues (2018) conducted an integrative review of global literature and identified broad areas of shared impact. By creating synergy in training and empowerment of nurses in both settings, educational capacity can be enhanced through reciprocal sharing of expertise and tangible resources to improve student and staff performance. APPs have the potential to both improve student transition to practice and staff knowledge and skill development to provide safe, high-quality services. Access to a supportive practice-based learning environment enables students to achieve professional competence through interaction with expert staff, which in turn influences curricular innovation to keep pace with health setting needs rendering new graduates ready for employment. Access to shared human and financial resources promote the identification and resolution of pressing practice issues through joint research and evidence-based practice (EBP) improvements to bridge the gap between theory and application of new knowledge to impact outcomes.

Additional benefits of APPs may include:

1. Improved patient care due to opportunities for health care professionals to have additional training and apply the latest evidence in practice
2. Enhanced education as a result of hands-on learning experiences and exposure to real-world health care challenges
3. Increased access to cutting-edge technology and care delivery models
4. Increased research capacity as partners engage in mutually valuable studies of new interventions to overcome practice challenges
5. Improved workforce development to enhance practice readiness of new graduates and address nursing shortages
6. Financial benefits that accrue to both partners through grant funding and other sources of savings and revenue generation, and shared resources
7. Strengthened community relationships to promote a collaborative and integrated health care system

Challenges in establishing and maintaining an APP include:

1. Aligning goals and objectives of the partnership to ensure both institutions realize the value proposition
2. Integration of systems, processes, and deliverables, especially when the organizations have different cultures and ways of operating
3. Managing finances to determine the division of costs and allocation of resources
4. Maintaining quality and safety while balancing the goals of education and research with the delivery of high-quality care
5. Ensuring faculty and staff of both institutions have the necessary skills, knowledge, and attitudes to work effectively in the partnership
6. Measuring and quantifying the success of the partnership
7. Sustaining an effective partnership over time with the commitment to addressing challenges that arise

> **TIP**
>
> An APP should meet the needs of both partners with ample opportunities provided to communicate in a transparent, respectful manner.

HISTORY

As health care demands become increasingly complex and nursing workforce shortages persist over time, nursing education and the delivery system recognized the limitations to working as independent entities and began to invest in a joint effort to address long-term challenges faced by the profession. A strategic response requires both academia and practice partners to develop sensitivity and respect for each other's different demands and priorities in order to mount coordinated action. Historically, academic and clinical practice settings engaged in various degrees of partnership and collaboration in the preparation of the nursing workforce. The nature of these relationships continually evolved to meet the needs of each partner driven by the nature of influencing forces that are in play at different points in time. Factors influencing the relationship include the current, prominent educational model, workforce demands, desired skills and characteristics of the nurse, and societal contributors influencing health care economics with increasing emphasis on cost and quality of care (Cronenwett, 2004). As evidence confirming the relationship between patient outcomes, staffing levels, educational preparation, and professional practice environments was confirmed through research studies, the need for meaningful collaboration between academia and practice became more urgent (Aiken et al., 2002; Aiken et al., 2003). Partnership was identified as a strategic response to enable and foster merging the collective intellectual capacity of both sectors to address issues such as nursing staff and faculty shortage, demanding workplace conditions, continual health care organization reprioritization, public recognition opportunities, and the need to improve health care delivery by integrating nursing research and EBPs in the workplace (American Nurses Credentialing Center, 2023; O'Neill & Kraul, 2004; Horns et al., 2007).

Over time, with perseverance and a commitment to innovation, academic and practice partners have continued to define the elements of an effective partnership. In 2012, the American Association of Colleges of Nursing (AACN) and the American Organization of Nurse Leaders (AONL) (2012) published guiding principles developed by a task force convened to address the recommendations of the *Future of Nursing: Leading Change, Advancing Health* report (IOM, 2011). The report charged the profession with creating systems for nurses to achieve educational and career advancement, preparing nurses of the future to practice and lead, and providing mechanisms for lifelong learning. The task force defined the APP as an intentional, formal relationship based on mutual goals, respect, and shared knowledge that can function to advance nursing practice to improve population health. The AACN/AONL APP Steering Committee developed a set of guiding principles, templates, and resources to support the growth of meaningful partnerships including a tool kit and outcome matrix (https://www.aacnnursing.org/Academic-Practice-Partnerships/The-Guiding-Principles). The guiding principles advocate for strong commitment and reciprocal support to achieve innovation in professional education and practice (Table 2.1).

With shifting health system priorities and movement toward value-based reimbursement strategies that include assumption of responsibility for health outcomes at the population level, ensuring safe transitions of care across the health care continuum while simultaneously ensuring a high level of efficiency and effectiveness, further alignment of APP priorities was needed. The *Advancing Healthcare Transformation: A New Era for Academic Nursing* report (AACN & Manatt Health, 2016) outlined opportunities for academic nursing to enhance partnership with academic health centers (AHCs) to advance care in integrated health systems, further improve health outcomes, and foster new models for care innovation. Findings from interviews and surveys of academic and health system executive leaders from around the United States captured perspectives of a diverse set of individuals and yielded key recommendations to achieve deeper understanding and commitment to work collaboratively to achieve health care transformation. Major conclusions were that academic nursing was not well positioned as a partner in healthcare transformation. Often, there is minimal faculty participation in health system governance, marginal participation of faculty in clinical practice, and siloed nursing research initiatives that are not mutually beneficial to care delivery. Institutional leaders recognized the missed opportunity for alignment of efforts and endorsed the need to redefine relationships and set a dynamic vision for academic nursing in health care settings despite the challenge of having insufficient financial resources to facilitate success. A summary of the six action-oriented recommendations made in the report are found in Table 2.2 (Fig. 2.1).

ACADEMIC–PRACTICE PARTNERSHIP CHARACTERISTICS

When APPs have intentionally planned, clear objectives and a structured framework for developing and implementing partnership endeavors, evaluation of the effectiveness of the relationship is possible. Clearly defined goals and implementation activities enable identification of specific, measurable outcomes, time frame for achievement, opportunities to modify partnership strategies, and regular follow-up to evaluate the success of the partnership. Utilizing a standard method of quantifying outcomes of the partnership enhances the ability to communicate the impact of the collaboration. It is important to keep key stakeholders abreast of partnership outcomes as they have the power to sustain and evolve the relationship informed by lessons learned.

TABLE 2.1	AACN/AONL Guiding Principles for Academic–Practice Partnerships (2012)
Guiding Principle	**Strategies**
Collaborative relationships are established and maintained	• Formal relationships established at the senior leadership level and practiced throughout the organization • Shared vision and expectations are clearly articulated • Mutual goals are set and evaluated at set points in time
Mutual respect and trust are cornerstones of the relationship	• Shared conflict engagement competencies • Joint accountability and recognition for contributions • Frequent and meaningful engagement • Mutual investment and commitment • Transparency
Knowledge is shared among partners through a variety of mechanisms	• Commitment to lifelong learning • Shared knowledge of current best practices • Shared knowledge management systems • Joint preparation for national certification, accreditation, and regulatory reviews • Interprofessional education • Joint research • Joint committee appointments • Joint development of competencies
Shared commitment to maximize the potential of each nurse to reach the highest level within their scope of practice	• Culture of trust and respect • Shared responsibility to prepare and enable nurses to lead change and advance health • Shared governance that fosters innovation and advanced problem solving • Shared decision making • Consideration and evaluation of shared opportunities • Participation on regional and national committees to develop policy and strategies for implementation • Joint meetings between regional/national constituents of AONL and AACN
Commitment is shared by partners to work together to determine an evidence-based transition program for students and new graduates that is sustainable and cost effective	• Collaborative development, implementation, and evaluation of residency programs • Leveraging competencies from practice to education and vice versa • Mutual/shared commitment to lifelong learning for self and others
Commitment is shared by partners to develop, implement, and evaluate organizational processes and structures that support and recognize educational achievements	• Lifelong learning for all levels of nursing, certification, and continuing education • Seamless academic progression • Joint funding and in-kind resources for all nurses to achieve a higher level of nursing • Joint faculty appointments between academic and clinical institutions • Support for increasing diversity in the workforce at the staff and faculty levels • Support for achieving an 80% baccalaureate prepared RN workforce and doubling the number of nurses with doctoral degrees
Commitment is shared by partners to support opportunities for nurses to lead and develop collaborative models that redesign practice environments to improve health outcomes	• Joint interprofessional leadership programs • Joint funding to design, implement, and sustain innovative patient-centered delivery systems • Collaborative engagement to examine and mitigate non-value–added practice complexity • Seamless transition from the classroom to bedside • Joint mentoring programs/opportunities

CHAPTER 2 Academic–Practice Partnership for the Future of Nursing and Healthcare

TABLE 2.1 AACN/AONL Guiding Principles for Academic–Practice Partnerships (2012)—cont'd

Guiding Principle	Strategies
Commitment is shared by partners to establish infrastructures to collect and analyze data on the current and future needs of the RN workforce	• Identification of useful workforce data • Joint collection and analysis of workforce and education data • Joint business case development • Assurance of transparency of data

AACN, American Association of Colleges of Nursing; *AONL*, American Organization of Nurse Leaders; *RN*, registered nurse.
From AACN/AONL, 2012.

TABLE 2.2 AACN Manatt Report (2016)

Recommendations	Strategies
Embrace a new vision for academic nursing	Be a full partner in health care delivery, education, and research that is integrated and funded across all professions and missions in the academic health system • Participate in health system governance • Expand academic nursing leadership in clinical practice and care delivery • Grow and evolve academic nursing research in partnership with the medical school, health system, and other professional schools • Collaborate on workforce plans and training program in partnership with the health system • Integrate academic nursing into population health initiatives • System-wide commitment to leadership development to prepare and support future nursing leaders
Enhance the clinical practice of academic nursing	• Implement initiatives that more fully bring nursing faculty into the clinical practice of the health system • Connect clinical service more closely to the academic mission of the school
Partner in preparing the nurses of the future	• Build a pipeline of nurses (BSN, MSN, DNP, PhD) to meet the clinical requirements of the academic health system • Create leadership development programs for faculty and practicing nurses that are jointly managed
Partner in the implementation of accountable care	• Engage in joint clinical planning to develop linkages between acute and postacute care services • Expand nurse-led community programs led by faculty and in partnership with health system leaders and clinicians
Invest in nursing research programs and better integrate research into clinical practice	• Create mechanisms to coordinate research projects and activities across academic nursing and AHCs • Develop joint research programs • Integrate nurse researchers into developing informatics programs • Strengthen training programs for nurse clinical trial coordinators and clinical research nurses • Provide leadership in establishing links to other professional schools • Expand faculty development to include PhD investigators across multiple disciplines in targeted research areas
Implement an advocacy agenda in support of a new era for academic nursing	• Seek growth in funding for the training of nurse scientists • Advocate for scope of practice changes to have all nurses perform at the full potential of their license

AACN, American Association of Colleges of Nursing; *AHC*, academic health center; *BSN*, bachelor of nursing science; *DNP*, doctorate of nursing practice; *MSN*, master's of nursing science; *PhD*, doctorate of philosophy.
From AACN & Manatt Health, 2016.

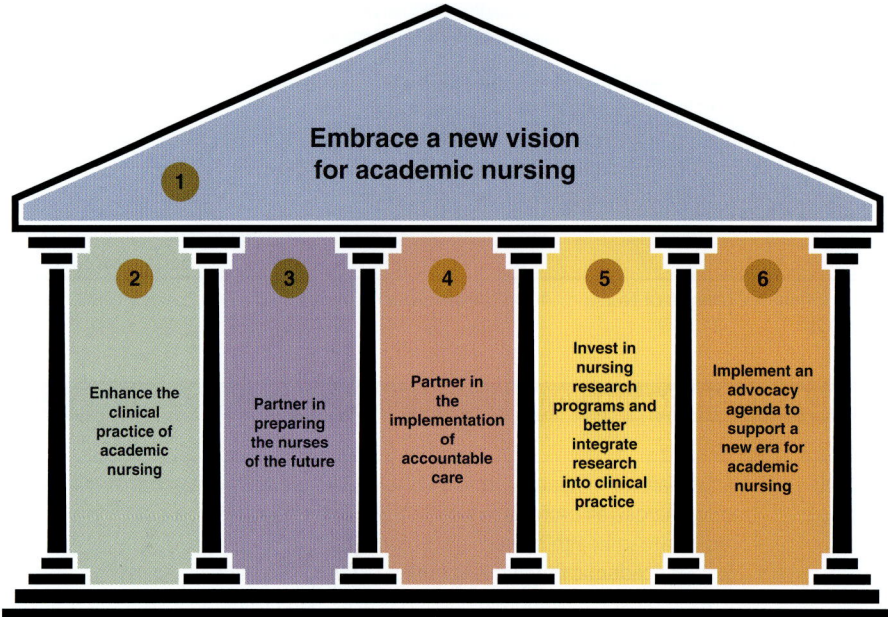

Fig. 2.1 Six Action-Oriented Recommendations for Academic Nursing. (From AACN & Manatt Health, 2016.)

Outcome data enable the ability to make necessary adjustments in academic and care delivery processes to demonstrate the progress and highlight the value of the APP (Polancich et al., 2021; Beal et al., 2012).

Several outcomes associated with APPs may make engaging in these relationships more attractive and worth the investment of time and effort. Academic program redesign is more effective when partners create innovation education models to advance the profession. APP programs have reported increased recruitment of students, faculty, and staff nurses as well as improved retention. Students relate increased readiness for practice and more high-quality clinical experiences for both students and preceptors. Partnerships have promoted cultural shifts by increasing percentage of bachelor of nursing science-prepared nurses and adoption of EBP and research that lead to improved patient outcomes while decreasing costs associated with onboarding newly licensed registered nurses (RNs) (Robertson et al., 2021).

OPERATIONALIZING ACADEMIC–PRACTICE PARTNERSHIPS

Practice settings operationalize APPs in various ways with targeted goals that include growth in professional practice and improved quality of care and patient outcomes. Common activities focus on joint support of EBP, nursing research, dissemination, clinical redesign, innovative clinical experiences, and strategies to recruit and retain nurses (Dols et al., 2019). APPs should support evidence-based transition to practice programs, lifelong learning, and nursing leadership development (Beal et al., 2012). Typically, students and faculty representing all levels of academic education work with clinical leaders and interprofessional staff across an organization on initiatives that are strategic priorities for both partners.

A common method utilized to achieve the shared objectives in an APP is a joint appointment where an academic nurse educator or practice leader has a role with responsibilities in both settings. Salary expenses for an individual may or may not be shared by the partners, but goals for the role should be mutually beneficial. The person provides consultation and collaborates closely with key individuals or departments on agreed-upon focus areas that may support attainment or recertification of American Nurses Credentialing Center (ANCC) Magnet designation, meet organizational quality improvement or accreditation goals, promote academic curriculum development or revision, and support scholarship among partners (Hinic et al., 2017).

Academicians in a practice setting may:
1. Support research by partnering to offer clinical or methodological expertise in the formulation of research questions, planning research study design and data analyses, and guiding Institutional Review Board application submission
2. Support EBP and quality improvement efforts by supporting literature review and synthesis, designing practice change approaches, and defining outcomes, measures, targets, and goals reflective of strategic priorities of the organization
3. Explore avenues and support efforts geared toward funding of practice-based initiatives
4. Assist in dissemination of organizational work through publication, presentation, and social media outlets
5. Support staff education directly or indirectly by targeted accessing of academic resources
6. Participate in shared governance committees, task forces, and other scholarly efforts
7. Foster attainment of current clinical knowledge and advanced educational degrees among nursing staff and administration

Practice leaders in an academic setting may:
1. Function as adjunct faculty to support academic education at all levels in courses, simulation centers, and academic advising
2. Support curriculum revision to align with the realities of the current practice
3. Contribute to curriculum revision to meet goals in the practice setting
4. Identify opportunities for collaboration with practice partners to enhance nursing science
5. Function as a role model, liaison, and coach for new graduates and graduate students

> **TIP**
>
> Take the time to understand the nature of an APP that already exists or try to work with partners to establish a new relationship based on available guiding principles. Impact of the APP may be observed immediately or take longer to develop the shared value proposition.

APPs have been effective in meeting the need for innovative clinical placement models that allow students to develop knowledge, skills, and attitudes to manage patient care safely and effectively. The Dedicated Education Unit (DEU) is a health care unit where education, in addition to patient care, is a primary function. Students are responsible for their learning and peer teaching. RNs are responsible for overall patient care and mentoring students and faculty ensure that students have relevant learning opportunities and evaluate student progress. An effective APP is a key ingredient for a successful DEU where relationships are based on formal agreements founded on a united commitment to enhance both student learning and quality clinical outcomes. The APP relationship in the DEU is built on mutual respect, trust, and goodwill, and equal voice in building optimal practice environments where students, faculty, and nurses are valued partners who contribute to both education and practice processes and outcomes. The presence of a formal shared or professional governance structure and mutual vision for the partnership promotes a culture of learning that is sustained by strong structural foundations, ongoing dialogue, and continuous evaluation to produce practice-ready graduates. An effective DEU possesses a culture of educational excellence and is supported by responsive leadership where there is clarity of roles and responsibilities that builds capacity for both nursing staff and faculty to ensure high-quality outcomes (Marcellus et al., 2021). Compared to traditional models of education, the DEU enhances clinical learning and allows educational and service institutions to integrate needed resources to create an environment capable of achieving the best quality patient care while sustaining nurses' professional growth and promoting a positive experience for students (Pedregosa et al., 2021). The financial impact of a DEU has been analyzed from the perspective of both partners and found to offer advantages to participating health care institutions and schools of nursing (Greene & Turner, 2014). Calculating the return on investment on a DEU, which is often preferred by students, can positively impact the perception of value for both partners.

APPs foster high-quality doctoral education programs in nursing and are vital to positioning nurses to lead innovation in healthcare. Both research and practice doctoral education students benefit from immersion in a practice setting to generate new knowledge or apply existing evidence to inform best practice. Students' dissertation or doctorate of nursing practice project work can be customized to meet the needs of a health care organization while ensuring development of essential competencies related to research, critical appraisal, and translation of evidence to create sustainable, data-driven practice change (Prado-Inzerillo et al., 2023). Graduates of doctoral programs have the potential to infuse the practice setting with learned skills and systems-level competencies that enable flexible system responses to address both anticipated and unanticipated demands. Health systems benefit from jointly created innovative, evidence-based models of care that have the ability to increase access, improve outcomes, and decrease cost. Nurses collaborating to design innovations are at the forefront of patient care and are well positioned to address new and emerging trends in order to affect positive change despite barriers and challenges (Howard et al., 2021).

APPs may focus exclusively on developing research and EBP capacity (Horns et al., 2007; Davis et al., 2019). These partnerships set goals to support generation of new knowledge that is specific to the needs of the practice settings to improve patient and health system outcomes. Collaboration and mentoring activities effectively engage faculty and staff nurses in identifying strategic priorities for research studies to directly inform changes in practice standards. Nursing science fellowships involving a structured didactic curriculum, ongoing mentorship, and ad hoc consulting are an effective way to ensure completion of the full cycle of knowledge generation, translation, and sustainability of practice improvements. Partners should jointly design and implement initiatives, measure outcomes, analyze generated data, and disseminate findings internally and externally (Phillips et al., 2019).

APPs can focus on addressing shortages of nurses and advanced practice staff when educators are also in short supply. Academic programs can be codesigned and delivered to meet the workforce needs of the practice partner for RNs serving a specific specialized population, advanced practice nurses where critical shortages of providers exist, and nursing educators when enrollment targets in the academic setting is limited by faculty shortages. Varying arrangements for tuition remission, dual funding of compensation packages, workload expectations, and hiring, recruitment, and retention strategies can be funded by the partners or governmental grants (Horns et al., 2007; Paton et al., 2022; Rowen et al., 2023). In circumstances where academic educator shortages exist, APPs can be mutually beneficial when academic time, which is typically devoted to teaching, curriculum development, and other faculty role obligations, is dedicated to practice setting priorities. Clinician–educator roles allow for current bedside practice to be brought to the educational setting, reducing the theory–practice gap, enhancing academic credibility, and integrating best evidence in clinical practice. Reciprocal value accrues to the practice partner when role transition for novice clinicians is facilitated, greater inquiry into practice issues occur promoting integration of research evidence in practice, and partners jointly advocate for the future of nursing (Pfister et al., 2021).

Partners have also collaborated to expand the role of nurses throughout the continuum of healthcare to improve the nations' health while decreasing costs. In a rapidly changing health care environment, nursing education and practice reforms are necessary to meet current and future population health demands (NASEM, 2021). An exemplar APP is working together to scale up nursing competency in care coordination and patient-centered care in both students and practicing nurses by providing educational content, supporting quality and performance improvement projects, and assessing impact of the collaboration on patient, education, and practice outcomes (Nahm et al., 2022). Care coordination across the lifespan is an essential competency that further expands the role of nurses in providing effective, efficient, equitable, accessible care using collaborative practice models (AACN, 2021).

As care delivery moves increasingly toward the outpatient settings in response to shifts in evolving care delivery models designed to meet patient needs while reducing costs, enhancing the patient experience, and promoting population health, the American Academy of Ambulatory Care Nursing recognized the opportunity to define best practices to facilitate successful APPs outside of the acute care setting. With an increased need for competent ambulatory care nurses, evidence-based guidelines were created and published to promote setting-specific pre-and postlicensure clinical experiences that support independent and collaborative practice in health promotion, chronic illness management, and transitional care. Ongoing professional development of faculty and preceptors to support an ambulatory care nursing workforce was identified as a key factor for long-term success of the APP (DeBiase et al., 2022; Witwer et al., 2022; DiGiuli, et al., 2022).

The COVID-19 pandemic forced nursing programs, health care systems, and community-based organizations to quickly adapt to meet the needs of students, patients, populations, and communities while addressing safety concerns and preserving limited health care resources. The resulting amplification of the value and need for APPs served to increase awareness and support for these relationships in a rapidly evolving, sometimes uncertain environment. The pandemic impacted APPs by decreasing or temporarily suspending student placements, shifting clinical experiences to virtual care delivery modes, increasing collaboration with new, nontraditional partners, and highlighting the need to be prepared for additional public health crises. APPs were leveraged by new and existing partners to mobilize collaborative efforts to meet predominant health care needs such as staffing mass vaccination clinics, contributing to community coalition efforts, and engaging in virtual public health education and outreach efforts to support social connection and resource navigation. The diversification of APPs to practice arenas previously not considered refocused academic and practice partners and emphasized the need to align academic educational content with service delivery needs in order to contribute meaningfully in the development of the workforce (Bejster et al., 2022). Nurses were rapidly responding to demands to care for patients and families without sufficient evidence to guide best practice, which led to the rapid deployment of research initiatives to inform evidence-based care. In response to the impact of the pandemic on nursing education and practice, the National Council of State Boards of Nursing (NCSBN) convened nurses from around the country to explore the multitude of issues identified and develop possible solutions. A national model of APP was recommended with the goal of creating clinical education opportunities to support care delivery during a crisis. Building on the guiding principles set forth by AACN and AONL in 2012, the committee recommended the APP as the appropriate mechanism to define roles and responsibilities of health care organizations and schools of nursing. The APP provides a solid foundation for a bidirectional relationship where communication is vital in achieving clarity about issues such as who provides personal protective equipment and whether compensation is offered for engaging in certain clinical activities such as screening, outreach, vaccination, and public health education activities. The NCSBN endorsed the creation of APPs outside of large academic medical centers in community-based settings as long as faculty are well prepared in codesigning valuable experiences that are in compliance with scope of practice parameters and both partners understand and are involved in establishing the APP agreement. The important role of state boards of nursing in defining APPs in the future was emphasized to ensure state regulatory compliance with appropriate educational oversight (Spector et al., 2021).

> **TIP**
>
> An APP should change to address the evolving demands of the academic and practice partner. Goals of the relationship and desired outcomes should be evaluated and revised periodically.

SYNTHESIS

APPs have evolved along with the profession of nursing. As healthcare becomes more complex with increased emphasis on quality, cost, and the health and well-being of patients and providers, it is essential that APPs remain dynamic and responsive to the unique requirements of participating partners. Expert guidance and tools are available to establish and maintain a productive APP. Clinical leaders should be transparent in expressing the desired characteristics, available resources, goals, and outcomes that benefit both partners.

KEY POINTS

- An APP can be structured in a variety of ways with common goals that build on strengths, demonstrate collaboration, and support relational change for the sake of improvement in the quality of health care delivery through the integration of education, research, and clinical practice.

- Mutual benefits are derived from APPs by creating value through synergy between partners in both settings who engage in reciprocal sharing of expertise and tangible resources to improve student and staff performance.

- Challenges to effective APPs must be proactively addressed through open, transparent communication, shared decision making, and goal setting.
- APPs foster innovation in care delivery, education, and leadership, positioning the nursing profession for the future of healthcare.

REFERENCES

Aiken, L. H., Clarke, S. P., Cheung, R. B., Sloane, D. M., & Silber, J. H. (2003). Educational levels of hospital nurses and surgical patient mortality. *Journal of the American Medical Association*, 290, 1617–1623.

Aiken, L. H., Clarke, S. P., Sloane, D. M., Sochalski, J., & Silber, J. H. (2002). Hospital nurse staffing and patient mortality, nurse burnout and job dissatisfaction. *Journal of the American Medical Association*, 288, 1987–1993.

American Association of Colleges of Nursing (AACN). (2021). *The essentials: Core competencies for professional nursing education*. AACN. https://www.aacnnursing.org/Portals/42/AcademicNursing/pdf/Essentials-2021.pdf.

American Association of Colleges of Nursing (AACN), & American Organization for Nursing Leadership (AONL). (2012). *Guiding principles for academic-practice partnerships*. AACN/AONL. https://www.aacnnursing.org/Academic-Practice-Partnerships/The-Guiding-Principles.

American Association of Colleges of Nursing (AACN), & Manatt Health. (2016). *Advancing healthcare transformation: A New Era for academic nursing*. https://www.manatt.com/Insights/White-Papers/2016/Advancing-Healthcare-Transformation-A-New-Era-for-Academic-Nursing.

American Nurses Credentialing Center. (2022a). *2023 magnet application manual*. American Nurses Credentialing Center, Silver Springs, MD.

American Nurses Credentialing Center. (2022b). *Magnet Recognition Program Application Manual*. Silver Spring, MD.

Beal, J. A., Alt-White, A., Erickson, J., Everett, L. Q., Fleshner, I., Karshmer, J., et al. (2012). Academic practice partnerships: A national dialogue. *Journal of Professional Nursing*, 28(6), 327–332. https://doi.org/10.1016/j.profnurs.2012.09.001.

Bejster, M., Geis, A., Cygan, H., Ferry-Rooney, R., Kalensky, M., & Moss, A. (2022). Effects of the COVID-19 pandemic on academic–practice partnerships: Implications for nursing education. *Journal of Nursing Education*, 61(9), 533–536.

Cronenwett, L. (2004). A present-day academic perspective on the Carolina Nursing experience, building on the past, shaping the future. *Journal of Professional Nursing*, 20(5), 300–304.

Davis, K. F., Harris, M., & Boland, M. (2019). Ten years and counting: A successful academic–practice partnership to develop nursing research capacity. *Journal of Professional Nursing*, 35, 473–479. https://doi.org/10.1016/j.profnurs.2019.04.013.

De Geest, S., Dobbels, F., Schonfeld, S., Duerinckx, N., Sveinbjarnardottir, E. K., & Denhaerynck, K. (2013). Academic service partnerships: What do we learn from around the globe? A systematic literature review. *Nursing Outlook*, 61(6), 447–457. https://doi.org/10.1016/j.outlook.2013.02.001.

DeBiase, V., Coburn, C., More, L., & Parsons, L. (2022). Changing landscapes: Academic–practice partnerships in evolving ambulatory care settings—Part 1. *Nursing Economics*, 40(20), 98–103.

DiGiulio, M., Alemar, D., Hamlin, A., Jones-Bell, L., & More, L. (2022). Developing the American Academy of Ambulatory Care nursing academic–practice guidelines: Academic–practice partnership in action. *Nursing Economics*, 40(4).

Dols, J. D., Hole, M. M., & Allen, D. (2019). Building a practice-focused academic–practice partnership. *Journal of Nursing Administration*, 49(7–8), 377–383. https://doi.org/10.1097/NNA.0000000000000771.

Greene, M., & Turner, J. (2014). The financial impact of a clinical academic partnership. *Nursing Economics*, 32(1), 45–48.

Hinic, K., Kowalski, M., & Silverstein, W. (2017). Professor in residence: An innovative academic–practice partnership. *Journal of Continuing Education in Nursing*, 48(12), 552–556.

Horns, P., Czaplijski, T., Engelke, M., Marshburn, D., McAuliffe, M., & Baker, S. (2007). Leadings through collaboration: A regional academic service partnership that works. *Nursing Outlook*, 55(2), 74–78. https://doi.org/10.1016/j.outlook.2013.02.001.

Howard, P., Williams, T., Melander, S., Tharp-Barrie, K., MacCallum, T., Pendleton, M., et al. (2021). Sustained impact of an academic–practice partnership. *Journal of Professional Nursing*, 37, 995–1003. https://doi.org/10.1016/j.profnurs.2021.07.018.

Institute of Medicine (IOM)Committee on the Robert Wood Johnson Foundation Initiative on the Future of Nursing. (2011). *The future of nursing: Leading change, advancing health*. National Academies Press. PMID: 24983041.

Marcellus, L., Jantzen, D., Sawchuck, D., & Gordon, C. (2021). Characteristics and processes of the dedicated education unit practice education model for undergraduate nursing students: A scoping review. *Joanna Briggs Institute*

Evidence Synthesis, 19(11), 2993–3039. https://doi.org/10.11124/JBIES-20-00462.

Nahm, E., Mills, M., Raymond, G., Costa, L., Chen, L., Nair, P., et al. (2022). Development of an academic–practice partnership model to anchor care coordination and population health. *Nursing Outlook, 70*, 193–203. https://doi.org/10.1016/j.outlook.2021.09.005.

National Academies of Sciences, Engineering, and Medicine (NASEM). (2021). *The future of nursing 2020-2030: Charting a path to achieve health equity*. National Academies Press. https://doi.org/10.17226/25982.

O'Neill, E., & Krauel, P. (2004). Building partnerships in nursing. *Journal of Professional Nursing, 20*(5), 295–299.

Paton, E., Wicks, M., Rhodes, L., Key, C., & Day, S. (2022). Journey to a new era: An innovative academic–practice partnership. *Journal of Professional Nursing, 40*, 84–88. https://doi.org/10.1016/j.profnurs.2022.03.006.

Pedregosa, S., Fabrellas, N., Risco, E., Periera, M., Dmoch-Gajzlerska, E., Senuzun, F., et al. (2021). Effective academic–practice partnership in nursing students' clinical placement: A systematic review. *Nurse Education Today, 95*, 1–14. https://doi.org/10.1016/j.nedt.2020.104582.

Pfister, J., Kuester, J., McDermott, K., Talbert, L., & Schindler, C. (2021). Living the Manatt report: Advancing the future of nursing through joint academic appointments. *Journal of Professional Nursing, 37*, 422–425. https://doi.org/10.1016/j.profnurs.2020.05.004.

Phillips, J., Phillips, C., Kaufman, K., Gainey, M., & Schnur, P. (2019). Academic–practice partnerships: A win–win. *Journal of Continuing Education in Nursing, 50*(6), 282–288. https://doi.org/10.3928/00220124-20190516-09.

Polancich, S., Miltner, R., Poe, T., Harper, D., Moneyham, L., & Shirey, M. (2021). Innovations in evaluating nursing academic practice partnerships. *The Journal of Nursing Administration, 51*(6), 347–353.

Prado-Inzerillo, M., Rivera, R., & Fitzpatrick, J. (2023). Academic–practice partnership for doctor of nursing practice in a large medical center. *Nurse Leader, 21*(3), 366–369. https://doi.org/10.1016/j.mnl.2023.02.004.

Robertson, B., McDermott, C., Star, S., & Clevenger, C. (2021). The academic–practice partnership: Educating future nurses. *Nursing Administration Quarterly, 45*(4), 1–11.

Rowen, L., Howett, M., Embert, C., Baeson, N., Bosah, B., Chen, L., et al. (2023). Academy of clinical essentials: A revolutionary nurse staffing and education model. *The Journal of Nursing Administration, 53*(1), 27–33. https://doi.org/10.1097/NNA.0000000000001238.

Sadeghnezhad, M., Nabavi, F., Najafi, F., Kareshki, H., & Esmaily, H. (2018). Mutual benefits in academic–service partnership: An integrative review. *Nurse Education Today, 68*, 78–85.

Spector, N., Buck, M., & Phipps, S. (2021). A new framework for practice-academic partnerships during the pandemic—and into the future. *AJN, 121*(12), 39–44.

Witwer, S., Fritz, E., Antol, S., & Biliskis, S. (2022). In search of the evidence: Informing academic–practice partnerships in ambulatory care. *Nursing Eoconomics, 40*(3).

3

Overview of Evidence-Based Practice

Kathleen Evanovich Zavotsky and Mary Jo Vetter

LEARNING OUTCOMES

After reading this chapter, you should be able to do the following:
- Describe the historical perspective of evidence-based practice (EBP).
- Compare and contrast the benefits of research, EBP, translation/implementation science, and quality improvement in healthcare.
- Describe Donabedian's Framework for Quality Improvement.
- Describe the strategies and work of public and private agencies that guide the national agenda for EBP in healthcare.
- Describe the steps of EBP.
- Discuss benefits of including consumers on EBP teams.
- Describe actions that can be used to promote EBPs in healthcare.

KEY TERMS

Care bundles
Conduct of research
Evidence-based practice
Implementation science
Outcomes
Processes of care
Quality improvement
Translation science

Since the early 2000s, the advancement of knowledge about effective interventions to achieve improved outcomes has exploded. As nurses and nursing leaders you will assume responsibility for ensuring that evidence from nursing science and the science of other disciplines is used in practice. Whether as faculty, clinical nurses, or nurse leaders in health care organizations, you will be preparing the nursing workforce to be members of interprofessional and intraprofessional health care teams that use the best available evidence to achieve optimal patient outcomes across various settings. Among the greatest challenges you will face as nurses and nursing leaders is engaging your colleagues in committing to using an evidence-based approach to guide practice. In your role, you will lead or be interprofessional and intraprofessional team members, asking relevant clinical questions, accessing and assessing the best information, implementing evidence-based practice (EBP), and evaluating the effect on expected outcomes. Meeting this challenge is integral to improving healthcare, which is guided by the Institute for Healthcare Improvement's (IHI's) Quadruple Aim framework that seeks to optimize health system performance by simultaneously focusing on improving the patient care experience, improving the experiences of those in the workforce who provide healthcare, enhancing population health, and reducing health care cost (Nundy et al., 2022). The four elements of the Quadruple Aim of Healthcare include addressing social determinants of health (SDOH). SDOH is defined as conditions in the environments where people are born, live, learn, work, play, and age that affect a wide range of health, functioning, and quality of life outcomes and risks. According to Healthy People 2030 (U.S. Department of Health and Human Services, & Office of Disease Prevention and Health Promotion, n.d.), SDOH can be grouped into five domains: economic stability, education access and quality, health care access and quality, neighborhood and built environment, and social and community context (IHI, 2023).

The application of evidence to improve quality of care and patient outcomes is essential to health care improvement. The United States faces the threat of explosive growth in chronic illness incidence, an aging population, persistent challenges to improve and address SDOH and patient safety, and rising health care expenditures that are projected to reach 5.8% by 2024 (Keehan et al., 2015; World Health Organization [WHO], 2022). Although U.S. spending in health exceeds that of all other developed nations, key measures of health lag behind, particularly for preventable chronic conditions and associated functional decline (Squires & Anderson, 2015). Several reports of the National Academy of Medicine describe multiple opportunities for implementation of evidence in healthcare to improve population health and health care delivery (Institute of Medicine [IOM], 2009, 2011, 2012a, 2012b, 2013, 2015, 2021). Despite the availability of evidence-based recommendations for practice, challenges continue in integrating this approach to care delivered across the lifespan (Agency for Healthcare Research and Quality [AHRQ], 2022). There is a need to continue to develop EBP recommendations and applications to improve patient care and address population health issues. This EBP gap is linked to poor health outcomes such as obesity, food insecurities, substance abuse, health care-acquired infections, falls with injury, and pressure injuries (Brownson et al., 2017; Centers for Disease Control and Prevention [CDC], 2024). This chapter provides an overview of EBP in order to lay the groundwork for you to participate in EBP promotion in healthcare.

> **TIP**
>
> Evidence-based practice is a team activity! The Interprofessional Education Collaborative (IPEC) Competencies (https://www.ipecollaborative.org/ipec-core-competencies) can provide a framework for you to use when thinking about how successful EBP teams operate. The IPEC Competencies provide an understanding of the roles and responsibilities of intra- and interdepartmental team members, valuing, and respecting what each team member has to offer, and communicating effectively in order to build highly functioning teams.

HISTORICAL OVERVIEW

Nursing has a rich history of using research in practice, pioneered by Florence Nightingale, who used data to change practices that helped reduce mortality rates in hospitals and communities (Nightingale, 1858, 1859, 1863a, 1863b). Beginning in the 1970s, nursing science has grown, and findings have become available to guide practice. EBP (called *research utilization*) was advanced by demonstration projects and programs such as the following:

- Conduct and Utilization of Research in Nursing project (Horsley, 1983)
- Western Interstate Commission for Higher Education in Nursing regional program on nursing research development (Krueger, 1978; Krueger et al., 1978; Lindeman & Krueger, 1977)
- Nursing Child Assessment Satellite Training project (King et al., 1981)
- Moving New Knowledge into Practice project (Cronenwett, 1995; Funk et al., 1989)
- Orange County Research Utilization in Nursing project (Rutledge & Donaldson, 1995)

These seminal projects laid the groundwork for application of research findings in practice to improve patient care, known today as *evidence-based practice*. The nursing profession has made great strides in ensuring that EBP is integrated into undergraduate curriculums (Abu-Baker et al., 2021) as well as graduate programs including serving as a foundation for meeting the requirement for a doctorate in nursing practice (DNP) (Moore et al., 2019). The introduction of EBP principles through formal education has allowed us to serve as leaders in the field of translational science (Kalhor et al., 2017; Bianchi et al., 2018; Alqahtani et al., 2022). As a result of the work conducted by Titler (2010) and more recently Melnyk and colleagues (2017), the scientific body of knowledge translation and the application of evidence in nursing and healthcare are continuing to grow. Advancements in implementation science can expedite and sustain the successful integration of evidence in practice to improve care delivery, provide a framework for addressing SDOH, and improve patient outcomes (Tucker, 2021).

> **TIP**
>
> The new knowledge created from nursing research will help address health care challenges in practice, promote policy development, and advance health equity into the future (National Institute of Nursing Research (NINR), 2022).

DEFINITION OF TERMS

Various terms are used in the field of EBP (Table 3.1). It is essential that you start or advance your involvement in EBP by improving your understanding of the differences between the conduct of research and EBP. As detailed in Table 3.2, you will note that EBP and the conduct of research have distinct purposes, questions, approaches, and evaluation methods. **Conduct of research** is the systematic investigation of a phenomenon to answer research questions or hypotheses that generate new knowledge and advance the state of the science. For example, as an investigator, you may be testing the impact that a stress reduction program has on patients following an acute stroke. Patients' length of stay poststroke has been reduced dramatically thereby impacting their transition to home. This change has led to many unanswered questions about how we can better address this high-risk patient population's needs. Researching the effects that a stress-reducing program has on them may indeed help address their critical needs that include medication compliance and overall self-care management. Because the state of the science is questionable, this topic may benefit from a randomized control trial. As a randomized control trial, your study aims to advance science by using a more rigorous design in which participants in your study will meet specific inclusion criteria, and be randomized to the experimental or comparison arm (see Chapter 8). Measures of health literacy, self-care management and perhaps medication compliance using reliable and valid tools at baseline, after the completion of the intervention, and at specified follow-up time points will demonstrate the effect of the intervention. Upon study completion, you will disseminate your findings internally and externally at scholarly conferences and in peer-reviewed publications (see Chapter 21).

Evidence-based practice is the conscientious and judicious use of current best evidence in conjunction with clinical expertise, patient values, and circumstances to guide health care decisions (Straus et al., 2011; Titler, 2014). Best evidence, as guided by the EBP hierarchy, includes findings from randomized control trials, evidence from other scientific designs such as descriptive and qualitative research, and information from case reports and scientific principles (Chapter 4, Figure 4.1) When enough reliable research evidence is available, practice should be guided by research findings in conjunction with clinical expertise and patient values. In some cases, however, a sufficient research base may not be available, and health care decision making is derived principally from other evidence sources such as scientific principles, case reports, expert opinions, and outcomes of quality improvement (QI) projects. For example, there is a strong evidence base for nurses to perform a structured handoff. The results of structured handoffs during changes of shift and changes in condition or location have proven to positively impact patient outcomes, including the overall patient experience (Kim et al., 2020; Rhudy et al., 2022) When thinking about use of this intervention in your practice, you will need to consider the following:

- The components of the intervention
- Whether you or other staff have the expertise to deliver this intervention
- The perceptions of the populations of patients you care for
- In what circumstances you will offer this intervention (e.g., change of shift, transfer from another unit/facility)
- The specific workflow of the unit or department you are offering this intervention to

In making these decisions, you will need to carefully weigh the research regarding the following:

- Multiple elements required in a structured handoff
- Unit, setting, and format in which it has been utilized (medical surgical, emergency department, intensive care unit)
- Specialized training required for the intervention
- Inclusion and exclusion criteria of the caregivers included in previous studies

> **TIP**
>
> When planning for implementation of EBPs, remember that it is not just the importance or value of the EBP topic as perceived by users and stakeholders (e.g., ease of use, valued part of practice) that will influence their adoption. It is the interaction among the importance of the EBP topic, the intended users' perception, and how it impacts their practice and workflow that determines the rate and extent of adoption.

Quality improvement (QI) is both a philosophy of organizational functioning and a set of analysis tools and change techniques to reduce variations in the quality

TABLE 3.1 Terms Used in EBP and Implementation Science

Term	Description
Translational research	A dynamic continuum from basic research through application of research findings in practice, communities, and public health settings to improve health and health outcomes; progresses across five phases: preclinical and animal studies (T0/basic science research); proof of concept/Phase 1 clinical trials (T1/testing efficacy and safety with small group of humans); Phase 2 and Phase 3 clinical trials (T3/testing the efficacy and safety with larger group of humans; compare to common treatments); Phase 4 clinical trials and clinical outcomes research (T4/translation to practice); Phase 5 population-level outcomes research (T5/translation to community) The translational phases along this continuum are sometimes referred to as "bench-to-bedside" and "bedside-to-community" (IOM, 2013)
Conduct of research	Systematic investigation of a phenomenon to answer research questions or hypotheses that advances the state of the science
Implementation science (also called translation science)	Field of science that focuses on testing implementation interventions to improve uptake and use of evidence to improve patient outcomes and population health, and explicate what implementation strategies work for whom, in what settings, and why (Eccles & Mittman, 2006; Titler, 2010, 2014)
Dissemination research	Targeted distribution of information and intervention materials to a specific public health or clinical practice audience with the intent to spread, scale up, and sustain knowledge use and evidence-based interventions (National Institutes of Health, 2013)
Comparative effectiveness research	Generation and synthesis of evidence that compares benefits and harms of alternative methods to prevent, diagnose, treat, and monitor a clinical condition, or to improve the delivery of care Purpose: to assist consumers, clinicians, purchasers, and policy makers to make informed decisions that will improve healthcare at both the individual and population levels This definition implies the direct comparison of two or more effective interventions in patients who are typical of day-to-day clinical care (IOM, 2009)
Knowledge translation	A term primarily used in Canadian implementation research and defined by the Canadian Institute for Health Research (www.cihr-irsc.ca/e/) as "a dynamic and iterative process that includes synthesis, dissemination, exchange, and ethically sound application of knowledge to improve the health of Canadians, provide more effective health services and products, and strengthen the health care system"
Knowledge transfer	"The process of getting knowledge from producers to potential users" (Graham et al., 2006) Knowledge transfer has been criticized for its "unidirectional notion and its lack of concern with the implementation of transferred knowledge" (Graham et al., 2006)
Evidence-based practice	Conscientious and judicious use of current best evidence in conjunction with clinical expertise and patient values to guide health care decisions (Straus et al., 2011; Titler, 2014)
Quality improvement	A set of statistical analysis tools and change techniques used to reduce variations in the quality of care provided by health care organizations (Nelson et al., 2007)
Evidence-based policy	Policy developed through a continuous process that uses the best available quantitative and qualitative evidence to improve public health outcomes (Brownson et al., 2009)
Evidence-informed decision making	Process of combining a range of sources of evidence to inform a decision In practice, this occurs within a political context that requires consideration of a range of other factors including research evidence, community views, budget constraints, and expert opinion (Armstrong et al., 2013)
Policy dissemination and implementation research	Research focused on generating knowledge to effectively spread research evidence among policy makers and integrate evidence-based interventions into policy designs (Purtle et al., 2016)

TABLE 3.2 Comparison of EBP and Conduct of Research

Components	Conduct of Research	EBP[a]
Purpose	Knowledge/science generation Example: Test an intervention to improve cognitive performance of older adults with HF.	Application of research findings and/or other evidence in local practice and/or communities Example: Implement evidence-based fall prevention bundles of care targeted to patient-specific fall risk factors for hospitalized older adults.
Synthesis of the science/knowledge	Identify gaps in the science Example: Despite high prevalence and severe consequences of memory loss in HF, there are no research-based therapies to improve memory in HF patients. Few studies have tested interventions to improve cognition in HF. Prior studies have been small sample sizes and lacked control groups.	Synthesize the evidence and set forth EBP recommendations Example: Because falls are complex and risks for falls are multifactorial, beneficial effects of fall reduction interventions increase when interventions target patient-specific fall risk factors. Fall prevention interventions should be customized to the individual's identified fall risk factors. Example: For those with mobility risk factors (e.g., gait instability, lower limb weakness, required assistance getting out of bed), the following EBPs are recommended: • Ambulate 3–4 times per day with assistance as needed unless contraindicated. • Refer to physical therapy for assessment and gait and strength training. • Minimize use of immobilizing equipment (e.g., indwelling urinary catheters, restraints). • Ensure proper assist equipment (e.g., walker, cane) is readily available and in proper working condition. • Utilize a standardized mobility assessment tool.
Question	Research questions or hypotheses that advance the state of the science Example: Compared with active control and usual-care control groups, do HF patients who receive BrainHQ have greater improvement in delayed recall memory, instrumental activities of daily living, and health-related quality of life?	Clinical question or purpose of the EBP project derived from the PICOT Example: Does implementing EB fall prevention interventions that target patient-specific risk factors decrease falls and fall injuries of hospitalized older adults? The purpose of this EBP project is to implement EB fall prevention interventions targeted to hospitalized older adults' fall-specific risk factors for those cared for in noncritical care settings to decrease falls and fall injuries.
Approach	Research design that is aligned with the research questions/hypotheses (e.g., observational; RCT; step-wedge design) Example: A three-arm RCT comparing BrainHQ with computerized general cognitive stimulation with crossword puzzles (active control) and usual care with no computerized cognitive stimulation (usual care).	Nonresearch design: Track measures (see Evaluation in this table) for a specified period of time preimplementation, during implementation, and postimplementation. Example: Falls and types of fall injuries for 6 months before implementation, midway through implementation (3 months), and after implementation (6 months).

Continued

TABLE 3.2	Comparison of EBP and Conduct of Research—cont'd	
Components	**Conduct of Research**	**EBP[a]**
Evaluation	Standardized dependent measures with known reliability and validity Example: Hopkins Verbal Learning Test—Revised delayed recall measure; instrumental activities of daily living; Everyday Problems Test; Minnesota Living with Heart Failure Questionnaire.	QI metrics that address both processes of care and patient outcomes. Use standardized QI measures when available Example: *Outcome indicator*—fall rates defined as an unplanned descent to the floor, calculated, at the unit level, by the number of inpatient falls multiplied by 1,000 and divided by the total number of inpatient days *Process indicator*—If a specific fall risk factor was present, was the EB fall prevention bundle of care implemented that targeted the patient-specific fall risk factor? Number of patient days a specific risk factor is present, such as gait instability (1,285 patient days); number of times an EB fall prevention care bundle was implemented that targeted the patient-specific fall risk factor per 100 patient days; rates of correct intervention per 100 patient days (e.g., 31/100 patient days; 88/100 patient days).

[a]Examples from Titler et al., 2016.
BrainHQ, A computerized cognitive training program; *EB*, evidence-based; *EBP*, evidence-based practice; *HF*, heart failure; *PICOT*, problem/patients/populations, intervention, comparison, outcome, time; *QI*, quality improvement; *RCT*, randomized control trial.

of care provided by health care organizations (Nelson et al., 2007). QI emphasizes the continuous improvement of workflow that can involve the patient experience, teamwork, and the organization's safety initiatives. Other defining features include setting organizational or departmental performance goals and expectations that can be guided by outside organizations' standards that help qualify for public recognition such as *U.S. News and World Reports*, American Nurses Credentialing Center (ANCC) Magnet Designation, and the Joint Commission. The appropriate use of data is critical in order to help make evidenced-based decisions, and to assist in standardization of care and work processes that help in the reduction of variations in care (see Chapter 13). For example, members of your health care organization's QI council are concerned about an increase in fall rates over the past six months that are higher than those of peer organizations in National Database of Nursing Quality Indicators (NDNQI) reports. You are charged with addressing this concern. You will use principles of QI and organizational quality data in conjunction with the latest evidence to guide your approach.

W. Edwards Deming is the father of modern QI, which started in the 1940s. Deming's QI approach is centered on process management (Best & Neuhauser, 2005). The principles for QI set forth by Deming include the following: (1) QI must be data driven; (2) improving the **process of care** is necessary to improve **outcomes**; (3) about 20% of the health care processes account for nearly 80% of the inefficiencies and wide variations in process of care (Pareto principle); and (4) managing processes of care means engaging clinicians who understand the care delivery process and are equipped to figure out improving processes of care over time (Haughom, 2016). A common QI framework used with EBP is *Structure-Process-Outcome* (Donabedian, 1966). *Structure* includes the physical and organizational components of care delivery such as facilities, equipment, and staffing. *Process* of care is the services and treatments patients receive (e.g., early removal of Foley catheters). *Outcomes* are the effect that the processes of care have on patients and populations, such as catheter-associated urinary tract infection (CAUTI) rates. This framework will be helpful as you plan EBP initiatives (see Chapter 5), implementation strategies (see Chapter 17), and evaluation (see Chapter 19).

QI and EBP have similarities and differences. As depicted in Fig. 3.1, EBP is a type of QI that focuses

CHAPTER 3 Overview of Evidence-Based Practice

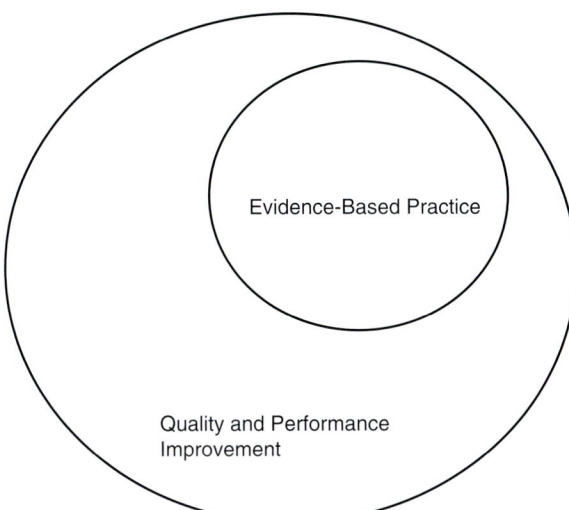

Fig. 3.1 Relationship Between EBP and Quality Improvement.

on implementing evidence-based processes of care to improve patient outcomes and population health. Not all QI, however, is based on scientific findings; it may use organization-specific data to guide actions for improving care processes. For example, if QI data in your organization show a wide variation in outpatient clinic wait times, organizational QI data about care processes (e.g., number of scheduled patients in specific time blocks) may be used to determine actions to decrease variation across clinics and shorten clinic wait times. This is a QI project, but not an EBP project. Both are important for quality of care. In comparison, your QI data may reveal high rates of CAUTI. Review of the evidence reveals a set of EBP recommendations or bundles of care that can be implemented to lower CAUTI rates in the identified patient population. Bundles of care or care bundles are a set of three to five evidence-based interventions that, when used together, can consistently help improve quality of care (Lavallée et al., 2017). The bundles of care in this example are guided by the most current evidence from research and other evidence sources (e.g., limit bladder catheter insertion, catheter care, early removal of bladder catheters) to decrease CAUTI. QI data (e.g., CAUTI rates) are tracked over time with expectations that your rates will decline if the bundles of care are followed. The Donabedian framework of QI is useful in considering the types of metrics to use in evaluating the impact of EBPs (Donabedian, 1966).

Translation science, also more recently known as **implementation science**, is a type of research science that focuses on testing implementation of interventions to improve uptake and use of evidence to improve patient outcomes and population health, as well as to clarify what implementation strategies work for whom, in what settings, and why (National Institutes of Health [NIH], 2017; Tucker, 2021). An emerging body of knowledge in translation science provides a scientific base for guiding the selection of implementation strategies to promote adoption of EBPs in real-world settings (Dobbins et al., 2009; Titler, 2010; Titler et al., 2016). Thus, EBP and translation science, although related, are not interchangeable terms. EBP is the actual application of evidence in practice (the "doing of" EBP), whereas translation science is the study of implementation interventions, factors, and contextual variables that affect knowledge uptake and use in practices and communities. Translation science is research; various research designs and methods are used to address research hypotheses. Having knowledge of translational science can help clinicians better adopt evidence-based care. This can also help guide nurses through the EBP process and reduce the knowledge-to-action gaps (Tucker, 2021).

> **TIP**
>
> EBP is the actual application of evidence in practice (the "doing of" EBP), whereas translation science is the study of implementation interventions, factors, and contextual variables that affect knowledge uptake and use in practices and communities.

THE NATIONAL AGENDA FOR EVIDENCE-BASED PRACTICE

As current and future leaders, it is important for you to recognize that the national agenda for EBP is clearly in the forefront of healthcare. Multiple federal and national agencies are dedicated to promoting quality, safety, and population health through the application of evidence. EBP is now a national standard, as demonstrated by the agendas of several agencies including the following:
- Agency for Healthcare Quality and Research (AHRQ)
- American Nurses Credentialing Center (ANCC) Magnet Recognition Program
- Centers for Medicare and Medicaid Services (CMS)

- Home Health Care Consumer Assessment of Healthcare Providers and Systems (HHCAHPS)
- Hospital Consumer Assessment of Healthcare Providers and Systems (HCAHPS)
- Joint Commission for Accreditation of Healthcare Organizations
- Centers for Disease Control and Prevention (CDC)
- U.S. Preventive Services Task Force
- National Database of Nursing Quality Indicators (NDNQI)
- National Quality Forum (NQF)
- Institute for Healthcare Improvement (IHI)

Table 3.3 provides a general description of each agency's evidence-based initiatives and examples of evidence-based standards, recommendations, or programs. Private and public agency websites noted in Table 3.3 are rich resources for locating evidence-based information on a variety of health care topics.

As systems-level change agents, you will need to be knowledgeable about the CMS's value-based programs

TABLE 3.3 National Agency EBP Initiatives

Agency	General Description: Evidence-Based Initiatives
Centers for Medicare and Medicaid Services (http://www.CMS.gov)	Value-based programs: incentive payments for the quality of care provided to people with Medicare coverage • Hospital Value-Based Purchasing • Hospital Readmission Reduction • Value Modifier (Physician Value-Based Modifier) • Hospital-Acquired Conditions
Joint Commission for Accreditation of Healthcare Organizations (https://www.jointcommission.org)	Sets standards of care for accreditation of health care organizations. Standards informed by scientific literature and expert consensus and reviewed by the Board of Commissioners.
Centers for Disease Control and Prevention (CDC) (https://www.cdc.gov)	Works to protect the United States from health, safety, and security threats, both foreign and in the United States. Fights disease and supports communities and citizens in doing the same. As the nation's health protection agency, the CDC saves lives and protects people from health threats. To accomplish the mission, the CDC conducts critical science and provides health information that protects our nation against expensive and dangerous health threats, and responds when these arise.
Agency for Healthcare Quality and Research (https://www.AHRQ.gov)	Lead federal agency charged with improving the safety and quality of America's health care system. Ensures that the evidence is understood and used in an effort to achieve the goals of better care, smarter spending of health care dollars, and healthier people. Funds health services research
U.S. Preventive Services Task Force (https://www.uspreventiveservicestaskforce.org)	Independent, volunteer panel of national experts in prevention and evidence-based healthcare. The Task Force works to improve the health of all Americans by making evidence-based recommendations about clinical preventive services such as screenings, counseling services, and preventive medications. Task Force members come from the fields of preventive medicine and primary care, including internal medicine, family medicine, pediatrics, behavioral health, obstetrics and gynecology, and nursing. Their recommendations are based on a rigorous review of existing peer-reviewed evidence and are intended to help clinicians and patients decide together whether a preventive service is right for a patient's needs.

CHAPTER 3 Overview of Evidence-Based Practice

TABLE 3.3 National Agency EBP Initiatives—cont'd

Agency	General Description: Evidence-Based Initiatives
National Quality Forum (NQF) (http://www.qualityforum.org)	The NQF is a not-for-profit, nonpartisan, membership-based organization that works to catalyze health care improvements. NQF measures and standards serve as a critically important foundation for initiatives to enhance health care value, make patient care safer, and achieve better outcomes. NQF-defined measures or health care practices are evidence-based approaches to improving care. The federal government, states, and private-sector organizations use NQF's endorsed measures, which must meet rigorous criteria, to evaluate performance and share information with patients and families.
National Database of Nursing Quality Indicators (https://www.pressganey.com/platform/ndnqi/)	Used by leaders and nurses on the front lines of care, across ambulatory and inpatient care settings, to assist with measures of nursing quality within health care organizations to help improve patient outcomes.
Hospital Consumer Assessment of Healthcare Providers and Systems (HCAHPS) (https://www.hcahpsonline.org/)	The intent of the HCAHPS initiative is to provide a standardized survey instrument and data collection methodology for measuring patients' perspectives on hospital care.
Institute for Healthcare Improvement (IHI) (http://www.IHI.org)	The IHI takes a unique approach to working with health systems, countries, and organizations on improving quality, safety, and value in healthcare. IHI focuses on the science of improvement, an applied science that emphasizes innovation, rapid-cycle testing in the field, and spread to generate learning about what changes, in which contexts, produce improvements. It is characterized by the combination of expert subject knowledge with improvement methods and tools. It is multidisciplinary—drawing on clinical science, systems theory, psychology, statistics, and other fields. Quadruple Aim of Healthcare
Home Health Care Consumer Assessment of Healthcare Providers and Systems (HHCAHPS) (https://homehealthcahps.org)	The intent of the HHCAHPS initiative is to provide a standardized survey instrument and data collection methodology for measuring patients' perspectives on hospital care.
American Nurses Credentialing Center (ANCC) Magnet Recognition Program (https://www.nursingworld.org)	The Magnet Recognition Program designates organizations worldwide where nursing leaders successfully align their nursing strategic goals to improve the organization's patient outcomes. The Magnet Recognition Program provides a roadmap to nursing excellence, which benefits the whole of an organization. To nurses, Magnet Recognition means education and development through every career stage, which leads to greater autonomy at the bedside. To patients, it means the very best care, delivered by nurses who are supported to be the very best that they can be.

(VBPs), which illustrate the national importance of evidence-based healthcare. These VBPs reward health care systems with incentive payments for the quality of care provided to people with Medicare coverage and support the four-part aim of better care for individuals, better health for populations and providers, and lower cost. The VBPs include items such as (1) using incentives to improve care, (2) tying payment to value through new payment models, (3) changing how care is delivered through better coordination across health care settings, and (4) more attention to population health (CMS, 2021).

The seven current VBPs are the following:
1. Hospital Value-Based Purchasing Program
2. Hospital Readmission Reduction Program
3. Value Modifier Program (also called the Physician Value-Based Modifier)
4. Hospital Acquired Conditions Program
5. End Stage Renal Disease
6. Skilled Nursing Facility VBP
7. Home Health VBP

Driven by the CMS's VBPs, hospitals are paid for acute care services based on the quality of care rather than quantity of the services provided. *Quality measures are based on evidence.* For example, the inpatient quality measures for those with heart failure (HF) include discharge instructions to include weight monitoring, activity, diet, provider follow-up, and monitoring and addressing signs and symptoms for worsening HF. These are important evidence-based components for self-care management of HF after hospital discharge. A second example, CAUTI, is a quality measure because research demonstrates that following the care bundle that includes proper insertion and early removal of urinary catheters can reduce CAUTIs. Similarly, unplanned hospital readmission for those with HF is based on research demonstrating that effective coordination of care can lower the risk of readmission for patients with HF. Care coordination, home-based interventions, remote monitoring devices, and exercise-based rehabilitation therapy among patients with HF all contribute to reducing the risk of hospitalization (CMS, 2021; see Chapter 25).

There are many funding opportunities that are offered by both government and private organizations that support translational and implementation science programs and projects. This is done to ensure that the best evidence interventions are explored and integrated into practice. The National Institutes of Health (NIH) is one example of an organization that provides funds for research in translation and implementation science. While applying for a federal grant can seem daunting, it is an opportunity for the academic and practice partners to come together to pursue a common interest (Brown, 2021). For example, hospital-at-home programs that are utilizing a nurse-driven model that is dependent on technology would benefit from academic and practice partners' collaboration. Both the academic and the practice partner would have something to contribute while at the same time benefit from developing a grant proposal to help guide this innovative practice model.

The benefits for practice would include improved patient care, scholarly recognition, and the opportunity to work with experienced funded, faculty. The academic partner would gain access to a study population to pursue their research interests while at the same time advancing the body of knowledge available to inform continued evolution of the evidence-based model of care.

STEPS OF EVIDENCE-BASED PRACTICE

Multiple models of EBP, QI, and translation/implementation science are available for you to use as an organizing framework for your agency's EBP initiatives (see Chapter 4). Choosing a model is critical as it helps ensure that practitioners are guided through a structured process and can help make the project useful to practice. For the process or the model to be meaningful it should take into consideration clinical expertise/experience of team members, available research evidence, and value to patients. Choosing an EBP model should be driven by the organization, design of the project, the knowledge of the team members, as well as a professional preference or previous experience. The steps of EBP are overviewed in Table 3.4 with linkages to other chapters that provide detailed information about completing each step.

> **TIP**
>
> Adoption of EBPs is influenced by the nature of the topic (e.g., the type and strength of evidence, complexity) and the manner in which it is communicated to members (nurses) of a social system (organization, setting).

THE EVIDENCE-BASED PRACTICE TEAM

The composition of your EBP team, also referred to as stakeholders, will vary depending on the question being asked, the patient population, and the anticipated resources needed. You want to think about potential EBP teams as interprofessional, comprising a broad array of appropriate health professionals in order to help you with the planning and implementation of the project. The stakeholders can include, but are not limited to, clinical nurses, nurse practitioners, clinical nurse specialists and midwives, physicians, physician assistants,

TABLE 3.4 Overview of EBP Steps and Chapter Linkages

EBP Step	Description	Factors to Consider	Book Chapter(s)
Select an EBP Topic Topic selection is often driven by problem- and/or knowledge-focused triggers. Example: increasing early mobility in the critical care unit	Problem-focused: QI and risk surveillance data, financial data, recurrent clinical problems. Knowledge-focused: research publications, scientific papers at research conferences, EBP guidelines	Be sure to include clinicians who will implement the potential practice changes in selecting the topic. Do clinicians view the topic as contributing significantly to the quality of care? Consider QI data in topic selection.	Chapter 5: Developing Compelling Clinical Questions Chapter 14: Evidence-Based Approaches for Improving Healthcare Quality Chapter 15: Planning for Success
Form a Team Example: physical therapists, clinical nurses, advanced practice nurses, physicians	The composition of the team is directed by the topic selected and should include those in the delivery of the EBPs. Consider other key stakeholders who may not be team members but can facilitate the work of the team (Box 3.1).	An important early task for the team is to use PICOT in formulation of the clinical question. This helps set boundaries for the project and assists in evidence retrieval.	Chapter 5: Developing Compelling Clinical Questions Chapter 15: Planning for Success
Evidence Retrieval Search for evidence sources on your topic	Use search engines. Retrieve relevant research and related literature, including clinical studies, meta-analyses, systematic reviews, and EBP guidelines.	Keep track of your search strategies. Include websites such as AHRQ, CDC, etc.	Chapter 6: Searching the Literature for Evidence
Critical Appraisal of the Evidence Requires critique of all types of evidence (e.g., research, systematic reviews, EBP guidelines)	Should be a shared responsibility with one individual providing the leadership (e.g., advance practice nurse). A group approach distributes the workload, helps those responsible for implementing the EBPs to understand the scientific base, arms nurses with citations and research-based language to use in advocating for practice changes with and across disciplines, and provides novices an environment to learn, critique, and application of research findings.	Critical appraisal tools are available for specific research designs, EBP guidelines, systematic reviews, etc. Understanding statistical methods is important to determining whether study findings are congruent with research design and study aims.	Chapter 4: Models and Evidence-Based Practice Chapter 6: Searching the Literature for Evidence Chapter 7: Principles of Assessing Research Quality Chapter 8: Intervention Studies Chapter 9: Observational Studies Chapter 10: Systematic Reviews and Clinical Practice Guidelines Chapter 11: Qualitative Studies Chapter 13: Understanding Statistics for Evidence-Based Practice

Continued

TABLE 3.4 Overview of EBP Steps and Chapter Linkages—cont'd

EBP Step	Description	Factors to Consider	Book Chapter(s)
Evidence Synthesis Synthesis is integrating and linking different types and sources of evidence into a comprehensive whole, thereby providing a foundation for making EBP recommendations	Evidence synthesis uses tools and techniques to combine multiple sources of evidence. In general, there are two types of synthesis: narrative synthesis (e.g., systematic reviews) and quantitative synthesis (e.g., meta-analysis).	Various tools and strategies are helpful in synthesizing the evidence. Considerations for inclusion of evidence in a synthesis are overall scientific merit, similarity of subjects to patient populations, and relevance to the clinical question/topic.	Chapter 6: Searching the Literature for Evidence Chapter 10: Systematic Reviews and Clinical Practice Guidelines
Set Forth Evidence-Based Practice Recommendations Summarize recommendations about assessments, actions, interventions/treatments derived from the evidence synthesis with an evidence grade assigned to each	Recommendations for practice are set forth based on the synthesis of the evidence. The strength of evidence for each practice recommendation needs to be clearly documented.	Use a standard grading schema.	Chapter 4: Models and Evidence-Based Practice Chapter 6: Searching the Literature for Evidence Chapter 15: Planning for Success
Decision to Change Practice Based on critical appraisal and synthesis of evidence, decisions are made about practice changes	Critical appraisal and synthesis may result in validating that current practices are aligned with the evidence or result in minor or major practice changes.	Consider the following: • Consistent results from several well-designed studies • Findings are consistent across systematic reviews, EBP guidelines, and critiqued research • Benefits of applying the EBPs outweigh potential risks	Chapter 15: Planning for Success
Convert EBP Recommendations into Local Standards, Policies, or Procedures	A written EBP standard (e.g., policy, procedure, guideline) for the organization or setting is necessary so that individuals in the setting know (1) that the practices are based on evidence and (2) the type of evidence (e.g., RCT, expert opinion) used in development of the practice.	Have EBP standard reviewed by key stakeholders for feedback. Focus groups are a useful way to provide discussion about the EBP and to identify key areas that may be potentially troublesome during the implementation phase.	Chapter 4: Models and Evidence-Based Practice Chapter 15: Planning for Success

TABLE 3.4 Overview of EBP Steps and Chapter Linkages—cont'd

EBP Step	Description	Factors to Consider	Book Chapter(s)
Implement the Practice Change			
Multiple implementation strategies are needed	Use the Translating Research into Practice model to guide selection of implementation strategies. Trying the EBPs on a small scale first is recommended to determine whether process and outcome improvements occur as expected (Piloting).	Select implementation strategies that address each of the following areas: <ul><li>Nature of the EBP topic (e.g., complexity)</li><li>Methods for communicating the EBPs</li><li>Users of the EBPs social context/setting for implementation</li></ul>	Chapter 15: Planning for Success Chapter 16: Launching Implementation Chapter 17: Implementation Strategies for Stakeholders Chapter 18: Patient-Centered Evidence-Based Practices
Evaluation			
Collection and analysis of data aligned with use of new EBPs; used to determine the overall impact and sustainability of the EBPs	Evaluation criteria are derived from the evidence sources and should include process and outcome indicators.	Use QI data when available. Focus on collecting essential data. Evaluation includes planned feedback to staff making the practice change.	Chapter 12 Sources of Data to Drive Evidence-Based Practice and Quality Improvement Chapter 13: Understanding Statistics for Evidence-Based Practice Chapter 14: Evidence-Based Approaches for Improving Healthcare Quality Chapter 19: Evaluation of Evidence Based-Practice
Dissemination			
Plan for ways to share the results of the EBP implementation with internal and external audiences.	Make presentations to key stakeholder groups. Write executive summaries. Give presentations at regional and national conferences.	Consider use of active dissemination strategies. Know your dissemination options. Use social media and blogs.	Chapter 21: Dissemination

EBP, evidence-based practice; *PICOT*, problem/patients/populations, intervention, comparison, outcome, time; *QI*, quality improvement; *RCT*, randomized control trial.

social workers, pharmacists, academic partners, occupational and physical therapists, and administrative staff. You might broaden your thinking about other potential members as your project continues to evolve to include those who have important contributions to make, such as QI specialists, infection prevention staff, finance personnel, health science librarians, or IT support staff. Depending on your patient population and practice setting, point-of-care providers such as care coordinators, patient navigators, chaplains, medical assistants, and community health workers may also offer important contributions to your EBP team.

ENGAGING CONSUMERS IN EVIDENCE-BASED PRACTICE

Although not traditionally included as part of the EBP team, engaging patients, family members, and consumers

> **BOX 3.1 Questions to Consider in Identification of Key Stakeholders**
>
> - How are decisions made in the practice areas where the evidence-based practice (EBP) will be implemented?
> - Is there an opportunity and benefit to engage and create an academic–practice partner in the project?
> - What types of system changes will be needed?
> - Who is involved in decision making?
> - Who is likely to lead and champion implementation of the EBP?
> - Who can influence the decision to proceed with implementation?
> - What type of cooperation is needed from the stakeholders for the project to be successful?
> - What other stakeholders are needed to ensure the project is sustainable over time?

as team members is receiving more attention in the form of patient family advisory councils (PFACs). According to the American Hospital Association (AHA, 2022), PFACs are an excellent way to help health care institutions and providers better understand the perspective of patients and families. They can also help caregivers better identify the needs of their patient population and bring patients' and clinicians' views closer together. PFACs can help organizations implement best practices by bringing an approach from a completely different perspective while at the same time providing a forum for patients and families to engage with leaders to share their very valuable insights to our EBP projects.

When considering either a layperson or a member of a PFAC to serve on your EBP team, it is best to see if there is interest, previous experience, and a willingness to participate. For example, a team that is focusing on improving pediatric outpatient central line education may want to see if any member of the PFAC has had previous experience with this procedure or has been recently discharged from the hospital and is willing to participate. Having a layperson participate may help reduce the amount of community acquired central line acquired blood stream infections.

There are several rationales for including consumers in EBP teams. First, they can lend their expertise as consumers of healthcare and provide input on practices important to them. Second, involving consumers may increase their understanding of why certain EBPs are used in specific circumstances and why they are important. Third, consumers may be helpful in championing the use of EBPs. Fourth, consumers may provide insights into evaluation components of EBPs such as specific health outcomes and the overall patient experience (see Chapter 18).

CALL TO ACTION

Application of evidence in practice is now a national health care agenda. Each of us are called to act within our practice organizations to lead EBP improvements, to participate in organizational initiatives to improve care through implementation of the latest evidence, and to critically question current practices with an eye toward improving care through evidence application.

The new *Essentials: Core Competencies for Professional Nursing Education* (AACN, 2021) are a product of collaboration between education and practice representatives that serve as a foundation for continued discussion of both entry-to-practice and advanced-level competencies required in rapidly changing health care environments. EBP is identified as one of several concepts of importance that serve as a core component of knowledge and skills needed across multiple situations and contexts within nursing practice. As the next generation of nursing leaders, you must acquire the essential competencies to carry out the work of EBP. Advanced practice nurses are expected to do the following:

- Select an EBP model to help guide the project
- Lead interprofessional EBP teams
- Critically appraise and synthesize the evidence for use in practice
- Articulate to a variety of audiences the evidence base for practice decisions, including the credibility of sources of information and the relevance to the practice problem confronted
- Set forth EBPs for the local setting, based on evidence synthesis
- Use effective implementation strategies, such as care bundles
- Apply the principles and tools of QI
- Direct EBP evaluation
- Disseminate the impact of EBPs to internal and external audiences
- Identify key stakeholders, including both practice and academic partners

All advanced-level nurses prepared at the master's or doctoral level are expected to be experts in EBP and must be able to do the following:

- Be knowledgeable about the latest evidence for your patient populations
- Develop, implement, and evaluate the effect of EBP programs at the organization and system levels that are based on the organization's and departmental strategic goals and priorities
- Design, direct, and evaluate QI methodologies to promote safe, timely, effective, efficient, equitable, and patient-centered care
- Explicate the return on investment of EBP
- Negotiate system changes that foster practice climates for EBP
- Role model knowledge and skills of EBP

Evidence is now available for a variety of topics to inform leadership and administrative decision making (e.g., staff turnover, staff performance and engagement, optimizing staffing patterns and models of care). Therefore, the leaders of your health care system have an accountability to promote an organizational culture that makes evidence-informed leadership decisions and creates EBP environments to promote high-quality, safe patient care. These leadership decisions should be based on principles outlined by the American Organization of Nurse Leaders (AONL, 2022) and should include the following:

- Creating and enacting an organizational mission, vision, and strategic plan that incorporates EBP
- Developing and implementing performance expectations for all staff that include EBP work
- Integrating the work of EBP into the governance structure of the health system
- Role modeling the value of EBPs through administrative behaviors
- Establishing explicit expectations that nurse leaders create microsystems that value and support scholarship and clinical inquiry
- Bridging the gap through encouragement of collaboration between academic and practice partnerships

It is our hope that you will accept this call to action. Whether as clinical nurses, educators, clinical nurse specialists, administrators, leaders, or nurse practitioners, we must possess the knowledge and skills to ensure healthcare is accessible, of the highest quality, and based on the latest evidence. The chapters in this text are designed to give you the necessary knowledge and skills regarding EBP for you to succeed in making a difference through the utilization of all resources available to you.

SYNTHESIS

The nursing profession has a robust history of using research evidence to improve patient care. As a nurse and a nursing leader, you will be challenged to engage your colleagues and key stakeholders in using an evidence-based approach as the foundation of their practice. Building effective teams is key to undertaking EBP and QI projects. The IPEC Competencies will be valuable for you to use as you collaborate to achieve successful EBP project outcomes. Understanding the roles and responsibilities of colleagues from different professions, including consumers, will increase the degree to which you respect and value their contributions. You will lead or be a member of intraprofessional and interprofessional teams where you will need to cultivate EBP champions who are committed to developing clinical questions, searching the literature for the best available evidence, critically appraising the evidence, and using it to inform clinical decision making about implementing and evaluating tests of change. Meeting this challenge is essential for achieving the Quadruple Aim of improving population health, reducing the per capita cost of healthcare, and enhancing the experience of care and provider well-being. QI initiatives strive to address the components of the Quadruple Aim. QI models like Donabedian's Structure-Process-Outcome framework are often used with EBP initiatives. EBP is a type of QI. Utilizing an EBP model is critical in order to help guide clinicians in completing EBP initiatives and ensure sustainability. Clinical, academic, and administrative leaders are called to action to lead organization- and system-level change using EBP and QI to advance the quality of cost-effective and satisfying healthcare based on the best available evidence.

KEY POINTS

- The application of evidence to improve quality of care and patient outcomes is central to healthcare.
- Nursing has a rich history of using research in practice, pioneered by Florence Nightingale.
- The national agenda for EBP is clearly in the forefront of healthcare.
- EBP and conduct of research have distinct purposes, questions, approaches, and evaluative measures.

- A model commonly used to guide QI is Donabedian's Structure-Process-Outcome framework, which addresses improving quality of care in these three fundamental components of health care.
- EBP is a type of QI that focuses on implementing evidence-based processes of care to improve patient outcomes and population health. Not all QI, however, is evidence based.
- An emerging body of knowledge in translation science provides an empirical base for guiding the selection of implementation strategies to promote adoption of EBPs in real-world settings.
- EBP and translation science are not interchangeable terms.
- Utilizing a model to guide EBP projects will help provide a structure for nurses to comprehensively address issues in healthcare.
- Consideration should be given to including on the EBP team a layperson or a member of a PFAC who has experience or a vested interest in a selected topic. Involving consumers may increase their understanding of why certain EBPs are used in what circumstances and why they are important.
- Each of us is called to act within our practice organizations to lead EBP improvements, participate in organizational initiatives to improve care through implementation of the latest evidence, and critically question current practices with an eye toward improving care through evidence application.
- Performance expectations regarding knowledge and competency of EBP are explicated for advanced-level nurses prepared in graduate programs.
- The academic practice partnership should also be explored when integrating EBP into health care organizations, it can add depth and breadth to a project that is mutually beneficial.

REFERENCES

Abu-Baker, N. N., AbuAlrub, S., Obeidat, R. F., & Assmairan, K. (2021). Evidence-based practice beliefs and implementations: A cross-sectional study among undergraduate nursing students. *BMC Nursing, 20*(1), 13.

Agency for Healthcare Research and Quality (AHRQ). (2015). *2014 national healthcare quality and disparities report* (AHRQ Publication No. 15–0007) U.S. Department of Health and Human Services. http://www.ahrq.gov/research/findings/nhqrdr/nhqdr14/index.html.

Agency for Healthcare Research and Quality (AHRQ). (2016a). *About the comparative health systems performance (CHSP) initiative*. https://www.ahrq.gov/chsp/about-chsp/index.html.

Agency for Healthcare Research and Quality (AHRQ). (2016b). *AHRQ research: Examples of AHRQ's research and evidence that makes health care safer and improves quality*. https://www.ahrq.gov/research/ahrq-research.html.

Agency for Healthcare Research and Quality (AHRQ). (2022). *AHRQ's Evidence-Based Practice Center Program: 25 years of supporting healthcare with evidence*. https://www.ahrq.gov/news/epcs-25years.html.

Alqahtani, N., Oh, K. M., Kitsantas, P., et al. (2022). Organizational factors associated with evidence-based practice knowledge, attitudes, and implementation among nurses in Saudi Arabia. *International Journal of Environmental Research and Public Health, 19*(14), 8407.

American Association of Colleges of Nursing (AACN). (2021). *The essentials: Core competencies for professional nursing education*. American Association of Colleges of Nursing. https://www.aacnnursing.org/Portals/42/AcademicNursing/pdf/Essentials-2021.pdf.

American Hospital Association. (2022). *Patient and family advisory councils blueprint: A start-up map and strategy guide*. https://www.aha.org/system/files/media/file/2022/01/alliance-pfac-blueprint-2022.pdf.

American Organization of Nurse Leaders (AONL), & American Organization of Nurse Executives (AONE). (2022). *AONL nurse leader core competencies*. AONE, AONL.

Armstrong, R., Waters, E., Dobbins, M., et al. (2013). Knowledge transition strategies to improve the use of evidence in public health decision making in local government: Intervention design and implementation plan. *Implementation Science, 8*(1), 121–131.

Best, M., & Neuhauser, D. (2005). W. Edwards Deming: Father of quality management, patient and composer. *Quality and Safety in Health Care, 14*(4), 310–312.

Bianchi, M., Bagnasco, A., Bressan, V., Barisone, M., Timmins, F., Rossi, S., … Sasso, L. (2018). A review of the role of nurse leadership in promoting and sustaining evidence-based practice. *Journal of Nursing Management, 26*(8), 918–932. https://doi.org/10.1111/jonm.12638.

Brown, B. (2021). Research-practice partnerships in education: Benefits for researchers and practitioners. *Alberta Journal of Educational Research, 67*(4), 421–441.

Brownson, R. C., Allen, P., Jacob, R. R., et al. (2017). Controlling chronic diseases through evidence-based decision making: A group-randomized trial. *Preventing Chronic Disease, 14.* :170326. https://doi.org/10.5888/pcd14.170326.

Brownson, R. C., Chriqui, J. F., & Stamatakis, K. A. (2009). Understanding the evidence-based public health policy. *American Journal of Public Health, 99*(9), 1576–1583.

Centers for Medicare and Medicaid Services (CMS). (2021). *CMS quality strategy 2016.* https://www.cms.gov/Medicare/Quality-Initiatives-Patient-Assessment-Instruments/QualityInitiativesGenInfo/Downloads/CMS-Quality-Strategy-Overview.pdf.

Cronenwett, L. R. (1995). Effective methods for disseminating research findings to nurses in practice. *Nursing Clinics of North America, 30*(3), 429–438.

Dobbins, M., Hanna, S. E., Ciliska, D., et al. (2009). A randomized controlled trial evaluating the impact of knowledge translation and exchange strategies. *Implementation Science, 4*(1), 61–77.

Donabedian, A. (1966). Evaluating the quality of medical care. *The Milbank Memorial Fund Quarterly, 44*(3), 166–206.

Eccles, M. P., & Mittman, B. S. (2006). Welcome to implementation science. *Implementation Science, 1*(1), 1–3.

Funk, S. G., Tornquist, E. M., & Champagne, M. T. (1989). A model for improving the dissemination of nursing research. *Western Journal of Nursing Research, 11*(3), 361–367.

Graham, I. D., Logan, J., Harrison, M. B., et al. (2006). Lost in knowledge translation: time for a map? *Journal of Continuing Education in the Health Professions, 26*(1), 13–24.

Haughom, J. (2016). *Five Deming principles that help healthcare process improvement.* Health Catalyst. https://www.healthcatalyst.com/wp-content/uploads/2014/11/Five-Deming-Principles-That-Help-Healthcare-Process-Improvement.pdf.

Horsley, J. (1983). *Using research to improve nursing practice: A guide.* WB Saunders Company.

Institute for Healthcare Improvement (IHI). (2023). www.ihi.org.

Institute of Medicine (IOM). (2009). *Initial national priorities for comparative effectiveness research.* The National Academies Press.

Institute of Medicine (IOM). (2011). *Clinical practice guidelines we can trust.* The National Academies Press.

Institute of Medicine (IOM). (2012a). *Living well with chronic illness: A call for public health action.* The National Academies Press.

Institute of Medicine (IOM). (2012b). *For the public's health: Investing in a healthier future.* The National Academies Press.

Institute of Medicine (IOM). (2013). *The CTSA program at NIH: Opportunities for advancing clinical and translational research.* The National Academies Press.

Institute of Medicine (IOM). (2015). *The current state of obesity solutions in the United States: Workshop in brief.* The National Academies Press.

Kalhor, R., Azmal, M., Khosravizadeh, O., Asgari, M. S., & Gharaghieh, F. (2017). Nurses' perception of evidence-based knowledge, attitude and practice: A quantitative study in teaching hospitals. *Evidence-Based Health Policy, Management and Economics, 1*(2), 103–111.

Keehan, S. P., Cuckler, G. A., Sisko, A. M., et al. (2015). National health expenditure projections, 2014–24: Spending growth faster than recent trends. *Health Affairs, 34*(8), 1407–1417.

Kim, J. H., Lee, J. L., & Kim, E. M. (2020). Patient safety culture and handoff evaluation of nurses in small and medium-sized hospitals. *International Journal of Nursing Sciences, 8*(1), 58–64. https://doi.org/10.1016/j.ijnss.2020.12.007.

King, D., Barnard, K. E., & Hoehn, R. (1981). Disseminating the results of nursing research. *Nursing Outlook, 29*(3), 164–169.

Krueger, J. C. (1978). Utilization of nursing research: The planning process. *Journal of Nursing Administration, 8*(1), 6–9.

Krueger, J. C., Nelson, A. H., & Wolanin, M. O. (1978). *Nursing research: Development, collaboration, and utilization.* Aspen.

Lavallée, J.F., Gray, T.A., Dumville, J., Russell, W., & Cullum, N. (2017). The effects of care bundles on patient outcomes: A systematic review and meta-analysis. Implementation Science, 12(1), 142. https://doi.org/10.1186/s13012-017-0670-0.

Lindeman, C. A., & Krueger, J. C. (1977). Increasing the quality, quantity, and use of nursing research. *Nursing Outlook, 25*(7), 450–454.

Melnyk, B. M., Fineout-Overholt, E., Giggleman, M., & Choy, K. (2017). A test of the ARCC model improves implementation of evidence-based practice, healthcare culture, and patient outcomes. *Worldviews on Evidence-Based Nursing, 14*(1), 5–9. https://doi.org/10.1111/wvn.12188.

Moore, E. R., Watters, R., & Wallston, K. A. (2019). Effect of evidence-based practice (EBP) courses on MSN and DNP students' use of EBP. *Worldviews on Evidence-Based Nursing, 16*(4), 319–326. https://doi.org/10.1111/wvn.12369.

National Academies of Sciences, Engineering, and Medicine. 2021. *The future of nursing 2020–2030: Charting a path to achieve health equity.* Washington, DC: The National Academies Press. https://doi.org/10.17226/25982.

National Institute of Nursing Research (NINR). (2022). *The NINR strategic plan: Advancing science, improving lives.* National Institutes of Health. NIH publication #16-NR-7783. National Institute of Nursing Research.

National Institutes of Health (NIH). (2017). *Dissemination and implementation research in health.* http:/grants.nih.gov/grants/guide/pa-files. 9/18/2017.

National Institutes of Health (NIH). (2013). https://grants.nih.gov/grants/guide/pa-files/PAR-13-055.html.

Nelson, E. C., Batalden, P. R., & Godfrey, M. M. (2007). *Quality by decision: A clinical microsystem approach.* Jossey-Bass.

Nightingale, F. (1858). *Notes on matters affecting the health, efficiency, and hospital administration of the British Army.* Harrison & Sons.

Nightingale, F. (1859). *A contribution to the sanitary history of the British Army during the late war with Russia.* John W. Parker & Sons.

Nightingale, F. (1863a). *Notes on hospitals.* Longman, Green, Roberts, & Green.

Nightingale, F. (1863b). *Observation on the evidence contained in the statistical reports submitted by her to the Royal Commission on the sanitary state of the army in India.* Stanford: Edward.

Nundy, S., Cooper, L., & Mate, K. (2022). The quintuple aim for health care improvement: A new imperative to advance health equity. *Journal of the American Medical Association, 327*(6), 521–522. https://doi.org/10.1001/jama.2021.25181.

Purtle, J., Peters, R., & Brownson, R. C. (2016). A review of policy dissemination and implementation research funded by the National Institutes of Health, 2007–2014. *Implementation Science, 11*(1), 1–8.

Rhudy, L. M., Johnson, M. R., Krecke, C. A., Keigley, D. S., Kraft, S. J., Maxson, P. M., … Warfield, K. T. (2022). Standardized change-of-shift handoff: Nurses' perspectives and implications for evidence-based practice. *American Journal of Critical Care, 31*(3), 181–188. https://doi.org/10.4037/ajcc2022629.

Rutledge, D. N., & Donaldson, N. E. (1995). Building organizational capacity to engage in research utilization. *Journal of Nursing Administration, 25*(10), 12–16.

Squires, D., & Anderson, C. (2015). U.S. health care from a global perspective: Spending, use of services, prices, and health in 13 countries. *Issue Brief (Commonwealth Fund), 15*, 1–15.

Straus, E., Richardson, R. B., Glasziou, P., Richardson, W. S., & Haynes, R. B. (2011). *Evidence-based medicine: How to practice and teach* (4th ed.). Elsevier.

Titler, M. G. (2010). Translation science and context. *Research and Theory for Nursing Practice, 24*(1), 35–55.

Titler, M. G. (2014). Overview of evidence-based practice and translation science. *Nursing Clinics of North America, 49*(3), 269–274.

Titler, M. G., Conlon, P., Reynolds, M. A., et al. (2016). The effect of a translating research into practice intervention to promote use of evidence-based fall prevention interventions in hospitalized adults: A prospective pre-post implementation study in the U.S. *Applied Nursing Research, 31*, 52–59.

Tucker, S., McNett, M., Mazurek Melnyk, B., Hanrahan, K., Hunter, S. C., Kim, B., Cullen, L., & Kitson, A. (2021). Implementation Science: Application of evidence-based practice models to improve healthcare quality. *Worldviews on Evidence-Based Nursing, 18*(2), 76–84. https://doi.org/10.1111/wvn.12495.

U.S. Department of Health and Human Services, & Office of Disease Prevention and Health Promotion. (n.d.). *Healthy People 2030.* https://health.gov/healthypeople/objectives-and-data/social-determinants-health.

World Health Organization (WHO). (2022). *Ageing and health.* https://www.who.int/news-room/fact-sheets/detail/ageing-and-health.

4

Models to Support Evidence-Based Practice Outcomes

Mary Jo Vetter and Kathleen Evanovich Zavotsky

LEARNING OUTCOMES

After reading this chapter, you should be able to do the following:
- Describe the value of selecting and using an appropriate model to guide evidence-based practice (EBP).
- Identify elements that are commonly found in a variety of models.
- Discuss similarities and differences in EBP, quality improvement, implementation science, and research methods.
- Compare selected models and their value in supporting clinical improvement initiatives.
- Identify expert recommendations for implementing practice change that have a positive impact and improve sustainability of the change.

KEY TERMS

Combined model
Critical appraisal
Evidence-based practice model
GRADE (Grading of Recommendations Assessment, Development, and Evaluation) criteria
Implementation science model
Quality improvement model
Research
Research evidence pyramid
Table of evidence

Nurses need to routinely question their practice and remain continuously responsive to using alternatives to current standards of care delivery, education, leadership, and health policy practices. The complexity of the health care delivery system makes it challenging to seek and use best evidence to guide practice in an environment where quality, safety, and satisfaction are key drivers of success. There is a tremendous growth in new knowledge that is available to inform practice, making it difficult to remain abreast of the latest scientific advances. Impacting the research–practice gap to ensure the incorporation of new evidence in practice in a timely manner requires concerted efforts by clinicians and health systems. As a leader you will be called to engage in a variety of strategies to resolve barriers and promote facilitation of evidence-based practice (EBP) by helping to create an organizational culture and work environment that enables nurses and other health care providers to make a difference every day.

Evidence-based models and frameworks provide a guide for clinical leaders and their teams as they facilitate the identification of clinical issues in need of attention and provide guidance on approaches to complete evidence-based initiatives that improve outcomes. Models are used to organize strategies and plans for change and clarify understanding of extraneous variables that may influence adoption of EBPs. An EBP model can offer clarification regarding internal and external factors that influence the adoption of practice change. There are many models that have been developed to organize and assist professionals in asking clinical questions, evaluating new evidence, and making sustainable change in practice. EBP models are often applied to help break down the complex processes associated with translating evidence into practice. Use of an EBP model helps avoid failure of knowledge translation efforts that result in costly investment of time and resources. You may choose a specific EBP model based on individual or team preference to guide an initiative as well its characteristics and contextual fit with the needs of the practice setting. Often, health care organizations deliberately select an EBP model to be used consistently by staff at all levels of the health system to facilitate consistency in the approach to clinical problem solving. While an EBP model may be adopted for use by a health care setting because of its value and ease of use, there may be varying degrees of adoption and understanding by all nurses that require ongoing reinforcement and mentoring. Although models vary in detail, explicit criteria, and methods to engage in EBP, there are elements that are common to most models:

1. Identification of a clinical problem or question of practice
2. Search for the best evidence that is applicable to the practice setting
3. Engagement of the appropriate stakeholders
4. Critical appraisal and synthesis of strength, quality, quantity, and consistency of evidence
5. Recommendations for action (no change, change, further investigation) based on the appraisal of evidence
6. Implementation of recommendations
7. Evaluation of the recommendation in relationship to desired outcomes
8. Dissemination

PROBLEM IDENTIFICATION AND NATURE OF THE EVIDENCE

The need for EBP change may be identified at the individual or system level through risk management or quality improvement (QI) initiatives, efforts to achieve organizational strategic priorities, reviewing and embracing external benchmarks, and becoming aware of new evidence-based clinical knowledge. Once a focus area for EBP change is identified and a clinical question (see Chapter 5) is posed, EBP models guide the selection of strategies to utilize the best evidence to answer the question or intervene to solve a clinical problem. The type, quality, and quantity of available evidence will influence the rate, extent, and adherence to practice change in a health care setting. Clinicians are influenced by the relative advantage the evidence offers to benefit patient or health care system outcomes. The evidence should ideally be perceived as adaptable and compatible with their own practice values and not difficult to use because of its complexity. When the evidence has been tested, it enables clinicians to observe positive and negative results to determine if the evidence should be implemented based on potential risks and benefits. Individual clinicians, within the context of their organizational setting, exhibit various levels of motivation for change based on the absorptive capacity of the organization, which is influenced by the culture of organizational leadership, allocation of required resources, and perceptions of the change as a practice priority. Patterns of communication and facilitation promote adoption when they are tailored to local needs and include engaging change champions, peer opinion leaders, and social networks to overcome barriers to integrating evidence. Ideally, a team of interprofessional individuals come together and assume responsibility for the development, implementation, and evaluation of an EBP change. The inclusion of interested stakeholders who will be directly or indirectly affected by the change should be included to facilitate implementation and remove barriers to adoption.

FINDING, LEVELING, AND GRADING THE EVIDENCE

Evaluating and grading the strength, quality, and consistency of research evidence retrieved through a systematic search of the literature (see Chapter 6) requires a multilevel approach. The first step is to identify the level of evidence according to the design of the study by using an evidence hierarchy such as the one in Fig. 4.1. Before critically appraising research, it is useful to first read background literature about the phenomena of interest, related theories, health policies, and existing guidelines to incorporate a broad view of the topic and related concepts. It is helpful to critique articles in the following order:

1. Clinical and theory articles to understand the state of the practice and theoretical perspectives and concepts that may be encountered in critiquing studies
2. Meta-analyses, systematic reviews, and integrative reviews to understand the state of the science

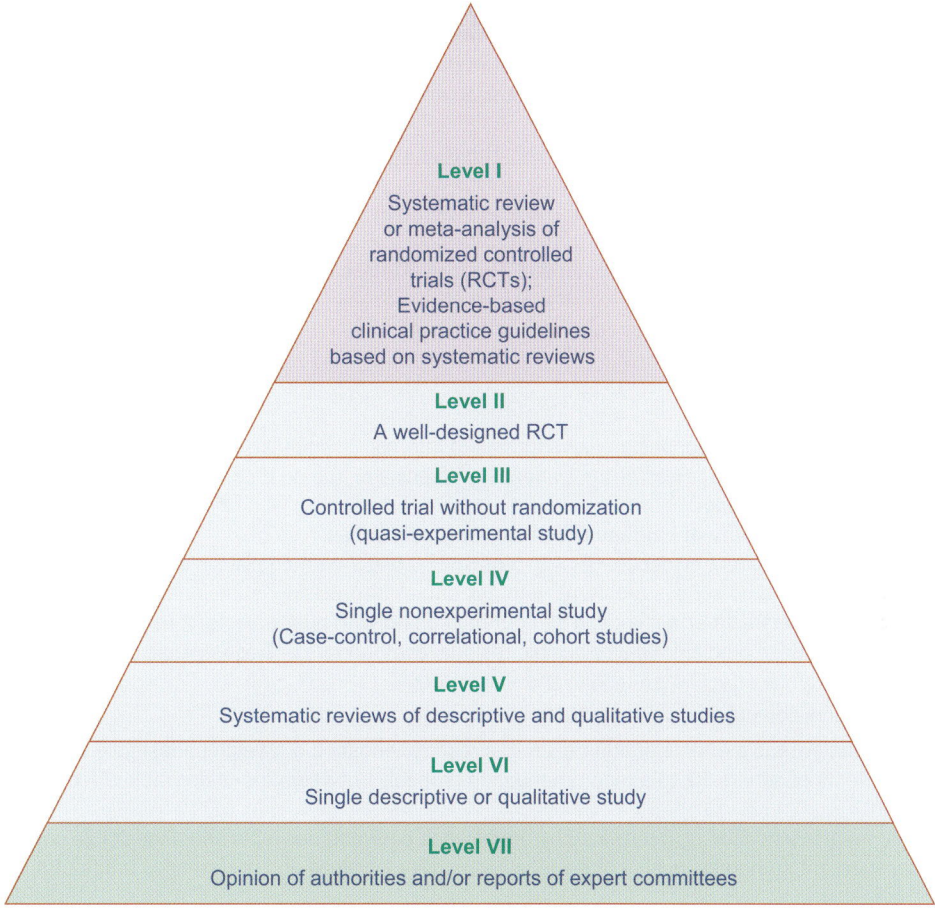

Fig. 4.1 Evidence Hierarchy.

3. EBP guidelines and evidence and case reports
4. Research articles

To truly understand the strength of the evidence, however, all components of studies reviewed need to be assessed for quality. A specific schema, the **GRADE (Grading of Recommendations Assessment, Development, and Evaluation)** system, provides a structure and criteria for grading the quality and strength of evidence and formulating recommendations based on the evidence. Table 4.1 illustrates the GRADE system's schemas for assessing the quality of studies. Information posted on the GRADE website (http://www.gradeworkinggroup.org) is also important to assist in understanding the challenges of and approaches to assessing the quality of evidence and strength of recommendations. Important domains and elements to include in grading the strength of the evidence are defined in Table 4.2.

In grading evidence, two areas are essential to address: (1) the quality of the evidence (e.g., the individual studies, systematic reviews, meta-analyses) and the strengths and weaknesses of the individual studies; and (2) the overall strength of the synthesized body of evidence. Important domains and elements of any system used to rate the quality of individual studies are featured in Tables 4.1 and 4.2. Before the body of evidence can be evaluated, the team needs to critically appraise the scientific merit of the studies and other evidence sources found in the literature search (see Chapter 6). A **research evidence pyramid** is a visual representation used in EBP to rank the strength of the various research study designs when being used to make decisions about using evidence to drive practice. Those at the top of the pyramid are considered the highest level of evidence with expert opinion being at the base. It is important to

TABLE 4.1 Quality of the Evidence (Balshem et al., 2011; Guyatt et al., 2011)

High: Very confident that the true effect lies close to that of the estimate of the effect. Scientific evidence provided by well-designed, well-conducted, controlled trials (randomized and nonrandomized) with statistically significant results that consistently support the recommendation.

Moderate: Moderately confident in the effect estimate. The true effect is likely to be close to the estimate of the effect, but there is a possibility that it is substantially different.

Low: Confidence in the effect estimate is limited. The true effect may be substantially different from the estimate of the effect.

Very Low: Very little confidence in the effect estimate. The true effect is likely to be substantially different from the estimate of effect.

Note: The type of evidence is first ranked as follows:
Randomized trial = high
Observational study = low
Any other evidence = very low

Quality may be downgraded due to: design flaws/threats to internal validity (risk of bias), important inconsistency of results, uncertainty about the directness of the evidence, imprecise or sparse data, and high probability of publication bias can lower the evidence grade.

Factors that may increase quality of evidence of observational studies:
(1) large magnitude of effect (direct evidence, RR = 2–5 or RR = 0.5–0.2 with no plausible confounders); very large with RR > 5 or RR < 0.2 and no serious problems with risk of bias or precision (sufficiently narrow confidence intervals); more likely to rate up if effect is rapid and out of keeping with prior trajectory; usually supported by indirect evidence; (2) dose–response gradient; (3) all plausible residual confounders or biases would reduce a demonstrated effect or suggest a spurious effect when results show no effect.

Strength of Recommendations (Andrews et al., 2013)

Strong: Confident that desirable effects of adherence to a recommendation outweigh undesirable effects.

Weak: Desirable effects of adherence to a recommendation probably outweigh the undesirable effects, but developers are less confident.

Note: Strength of recommendation is determined by the balance between desirable and undesirable consequences of alternative management strategies, quality of evidence, variability in values and preferences (trade-offs), and resource use.

RR, Relative risk.
From the GRADE Working Group (http://www.gradeworkinggroup.org).

TABLE 4.2 Domains and Elements for Grading the Strength of Evidence

Quality	The aggregate of quality ratings for individual studies, predicated on the extent to which bias was minimized
Quantity	Magnitude of effect, numbers of studies, and sample size or power
Consistency	For any given topic, the extent to which similar findings are reported using similar and different study designs, including relevance, benefits, and harm

cite the research pyramid when it is being used to evaluate research studies. Although all pyramids apply the general concept of being a hierarchy, they may vary in terms of the specific designs that are included and can be adapted to meet the needs of a specific initiative, discipline, or organization.

Several highly respected EBP centers, such as the Centre for Evidence-Based Medicine, provide internationally recognized critical appraisal tools that assist with evaluating the scientific merits of different types of research designs. Table 4.3 provides a list of commonly used critical appraisal tools. Application of these critical appraisal tools to various design types and levels of evidence are described in Chapters 7–11.

CRITICAL APPRAISAL AND SYNTHESIS OF EVIDENCE

Critical appraisal is the process of critiquing individual studies to identify their strengths and weaknesses. The next step in the critical appraisal process is to synthesize

TABLE 4.3 Evidence-Based Resources

Resource	Purpose
Centre for Evidence-Based Medicine	Provides education and the dissemination of evidence-based resources for promoting evidence-based practices in health care decision making through research and education
Grading of Recommendations Assessment, Development, and Evaluation (GRADE)	Provides consensus resources on rating quality of evidence and strength of practice recommendations, system of rating quality of evidence and grading strength of recommendations in systematic reviews, health technology assessments, and clinical practice guidelines addressing alternative management options
Critical Appraisal Skills Programme	Provides critical appraisal skills training, workshops, and tools used to evaluate research for trustworthiness and relevance; offers eight critical appraisal tools designed to be used for assessing research

the overall strengths and weaknesses of the group of studies as a body of literature. The steps of critical appraisal require a working knowledge of the types of research designs and their components. When critiquing studies and evidence based guidelines (see Chapters 7–11), the critical appraisal process should be a shared responsibility. It is helpful, however, to have one individual provide leadership for the EBP or QI project team and design strategies for completing critical appraisals of pertinent studies. A group approach to critical appraisal is recommended because it:

- Distributes the workload
- Provides a unique perspective
- Helps those responsible for implementing the changes to understand the scientific base for the practice change
- Arms nurses with citations and research-based language to use in advocating for changes with health system leadership, peers, and other disciplines
- Provides novices with an environment to learn critical appraisal and application of research findings

> **TIP**
>
> Partnering with doctorally prepared nurses and other members of the academic–practice partnership (APP) can also add to the depths and breadth of the appraisal. Encourage staff participation in the appraisal process by enlisting intra- and interdisciplinary members to work in teams to complete the steps of the critical appraisal processes.

Once individual studies are critiqued, the literature should to be synthesized; that is, the overall strengths and weaknesses of the studies as a whole need to be considered. A decision is made regarding use of each study in the synthesis of the evidence for application in practice. Factors that should be considered as inclusion of studies in the synthesis of findings are the:

- Overall scientific merit
- Type of subjects enrolled in the study (e.g., age, gender, pathology) and the similarity to the patient population to which the findings will be applied
- Relevance of the study to the clinical question topic

When synthesizing study findings, it is important to develop a synthesis summary or evidence table that includes the overall strengths and weaknesses of the studies (see Chapter 6). The synthesis summary table should include the critical information from each study, as well as other evidence sources. Essential information to include in a **table of evidence** is as follows (Table 4.4):

- Research questions/hypotheses
- Independent and dependent variables studied
- Description of the study sample and setting
- Type of research design
- Methods used to measure each variable and outcome
- Study findings
- Strengths and weaknesses of each study
- Level of evidence and grade

Some methods that you can use to make the critical appraisal process fun and interesting include the following:

- Use a journal club to discuss critiques completed by each member of the group.

TABLE 4.4 Summary Table of Evidence for Research Critiques

Citation	Research Questions/ Hypothesis	Design	Independent Variables and Measures	Dependent Variables and Measures	Sample Size Population n	Results	Strengths	Weaknesses/ Limitations/ Bias	Level of Evidence and Grade Recommendation

Use of a summary table helps identify information across studies regarding findings and the types of patients to which study findings can be applied.

- Pair a novice and expert to complete critiques.
- Elicit assistance from both undergraduate and graduate students who may be interested in the topic and want experience doing critiques, and are interested in the topic and process.
- APP opportunities.
- Use structured critical appraisal tools to guide you (see Chapter 6).

> **TIP**
> A table of evidence is key because it serves to identify commonalities and differences across studies regarding study findings and the types of patients to which findings can be applied. A well-done table also provides a synthesis of the overall strengths and weakness of the studies as a group.

PROPOSING EVIDENCE-BASED PRACTICE RECOMMENDATIONS FOR ACTION

On the basis of the critical appraisal of the literature, practice recommendations are made. The type and strength of evidence used to support the practice needs to be clearly delineated in the evidence table. Fig. 4.1 and Tables 4.1 and 4.2 are useful tools to assist with this activity.

After the studies are critiqued and synthesized, the next step is to decide whether the findings are appropriate for implementation in practice. Criteria to consider include the following:
- Relevance of evidence for the respective practice area
- Consistency of findings across studies and/or guidelines
- A significant number of studies and/or EBP guidelines with population characteristics similar to those to which the findings will be used
- Consistency among evidence from research and other nonresearch evidence
- Feasibility for use in practice
- The risk/benefit ratio (risk of harm vs. the potential benefit for the patient/population of interest)
- Cost–benefit analysis

Synthesis of study findings and other evidence may result in supporting current practice, making minor practice modifications, undertaking major practice changes, or developing a new area of practice. When critique results and synthesis of evidence support practice or justify a practice change, a written EBP standard (e.g., policy, standard of practice protocol, guideline) is warranted. This is necessary so care providers (1) know that the practices are based on evidence and (2) understand the type of evidence (e.g., randomized controlled trial, expert opinion) used in development of the practice.

It is imperative that once an EBP standard is written, key stakeholders have an opportunity to review it and provide feedback to the team responsible for developing it. Focus groups are a useful way to provide discussion about the EBP and to identify key areas that may be potentially troublesome during the implementation phase.

> **TIP**
> A consistent approach to developing EBP standards and referencing the research and related literature is key.

IMPLEMENTATION AND DISSEMINATION OF THE PRACTICE CHANGE

If a practice change is warranted, it is useful to pilot the practice change to ensure that the change is consistent with the patients, environment, and staff. Piloting the change allows staff the opportunity to provide feedback in real time on the practice and modify it if necessary. Changes extend beyond writing a policy or procedure that is evidence based; it requires interaction among direct care providers to champion and foster evidence adoption, leadership support, and health system changes.

Evidence-based change involves a series of action steps in a complex, nonlinear process. Implementing the change requires shifting the perceptions of users and stakeholders, understanding that the amount of time it takes time to integrate the change depends on the nature of the practice change. Merely increasing staff knowledge about an EBP and passive dissemination strategies are not likely to work, particularly in complex health care settings. Use of expert recommendations for implementing change enhances the plan designed by EBP leaders to promote and sustain meaningful practice change.

EVALUATION OF THE PRACTICE CHANGE

Evaluation of a practice change provides an opportunity to collect and analyze data regarding use of the new EBP and then to modify the practice as necessary. It is important that the evidence-based change is evaluated, both at the pilot testing phase and when the practice is spread to additional settings or sites of care. The importance of the evaluation cannot be overemphasized; it provides information for performance gap assessment, audit, and feedback and provides information necessary to determine whether the EBP should be retained, modified, or eliminated (see Chapter 19).

Evaluation should include both process and outcome measures (Titler et al., 2016). The process component focuses on how the practice change is being implemented. It is important to know whether staff members are using and implementing the practice as noted in the EBP guideline. Evaluation of the process should also note (1) barriers that staff encounter in carrying out the practice, (2) differences in opinions among health care providers, and (3) difficulty in carrying out the steps of the practice as originally designed. Outcome data are an equally important part of evaluation. The purpose of outcome evaluation using baseline and outcome measures is to assist in assessing whether the patient, staff, quality, and health system outcomes expected are achieved.

EVIDENCE-BASED PRACTICE/QUALITY IMPROVEMENT/IMPLEMENTATION SCIENCE/RESEARCH

EBP, QI, and research are unique processes (see Chapter 3). Each of these processes has unique components that, although independent, complement each other. The unique yet complementary components of each requires an understanding of how these processes mesh with clinical expertise, patient values, and context. Whereas research supports or generates knowledge, EBP uses currently available research knowledge to improve health care delivery. The key similarity among these three processes is that each begins with a question. Keep in mind that it is the question that drives the methodology. The difference among the three is that a research study actively tests a research question with a design and specific methodology (i.e., sample, instruments, procedures, and data analysis) appropriate to the research question or hypothesis and contributes to new, generalizable knowledge. EBP uses research findings as the basis of practice, and QI may or may not use research findings to improve quality of care (see Chapters 17–19). The EBP process uses a clinical question (see Chapter 5) to search the published literature for completed studies to bring about improvements in care. To successfully use EBP processes, clinicians must be knowledgeable consumers of research who can evaluate the strengths and weaknesses of research evidence and use existing standards to determine the merit and readiness of research for use in clinical practice (American Association of Colleges of Nursing, 2021). In contrast, **translation or implementation science**, as discussed in Chapter 3, focuses on testing the implementation of interventions to improve uptake and use of evidence to improve patient outcomes and population health, as well as to clarify what implementation strategies work for whom, in what settings, and why (Titler, 2014).

EVIDENCE-BASED PRACTICE MODELS

A cross-sectional research study of leaders at American Nurses Credentialing Center (ANCC) Magnet-designated facilities found that 90% of those surveyed used an EBP model most frequently for education and training, nurse residency programs, and EBP and research fellowships (Speroni et al., 2020). The study found that EBP models promoted the translation of evidence through policy and procedure committee processes, shared governance structures, and EBP processes supported by nursing leadership that involved sharing and disseminating findings by engaged nurses. The top three models most frequently cited by survey participants included the Iowa Model of Evidence-Based Practice to Promote Quality Care, the Johns Hopkins Nursing Evidence-Based Practice Model, and the Advancing Research and Clinical Practice Through Close Collaboration Model. Numerous other models have been used to guide EBP depending on the fit of the model to the characteristics and needs of the organization. A summary of select EBP models can be found in Table 4.5.

QUALITY IMPROVEMENT MODELS

Nursing leaders are expected to identify quality and safety needs within the health system, utilize and interpret data to identify trends, develop interventions that directly address data trends, and implement and sustain practice change. QI efforts purposefully mobilize interprofessional teams within the health care system to work together in a systematic way using evidence-based strategies and tactics to improve the care they provide. As an applied science, QI stresses innovation, rapid-cycle testing in the practice arena, and spread of identified best practices to generate learning about what changes actually produce the intended improvement in similar contexts. A critical feature of QI is the use of data-driven processes to design, test, implement, and evaluate change at the local level and then scale the change to impact system-level improvement. Informed by the experience and knowledge of individuals involved in making the practice change, QI facilitates reflective practice to ensure sustained and meaningful improvement.

QI models facilitate the assessment of causal linkages between health care structures and care processes and the impact these links have on outcomes. Coupled with strong evidence, a variety of QI models can support improved health care outcomes. Common QI models include the Model for Improvement and Lean Six Sigma.

Model for Improvement

The Model for Improvement (MFI) created by Associates in Process Improvement (http://www.apiweb.org/) is an evidence-based, effective, and reliable framework used to bring about process or system change. It is simple, which makes it easy for anyone to use, reduces risk by starting with small tests of change, and is useful to help plan, develop, and implement change (Institute for Healthcare Improvement, 2023). The MFI is a two-part problem-solving model. Part 1 asks three fundamental questions to test changes in the practice setting:

1. What are we trying to accomplish? To answer this question, an aim statement for the project must be developed that is specific, measurable, attainable, realistic, and time limited.
2. How do we know that a change is an improvement? To answer this question, measures must be developed to assess for progress toward the aim.
3. What change can we make that will result in an improvement? To answer this question, change ideas must be generated that will lead to accomplishing the aim.

Part 2 uses Plan-Do-Study-Act (PDSA) cycles to implement change on a small scale and can be conducted in rapid succession:

Plan—Question what will happen and develop an action plan describing the solutions

Do—Implement possible solutions

Study—Evaluate the results to build new knowledge

Act—Adopt results, abandon results, or run through the cycle again, possibly under different conditions with varying materials, people, or rules

Lean Six Sigma

Lean Six Sigma is a powerful methodology for improving organizational performance and enabling a system's ability to be more efficient, effective, and competitive. The model combines principles from Lean Manufacturing and Six Sigma with goals of eliminating waste and improving quality and satisfaction. Data-driven methods are utilized to identify and eliminate errors and inefficiencies in processes leading to improved customer satisfaction, increased productivity, and reduced costs. Lean principles focus on reducing variability, and

TABLE 4.5 Examples of Evidence-Based Practice Models

Model Name	Major Constructs/Concepts
The Iowa Model–Revised (Titler et al., 2001; Iowa Model Collaborative, 2017)	Original model validated and revised to meet current trends in healthcare. Uses branching logic to guide users to identify triggering issues and opportunities for EBP and make decision about the priority status of the initiative, form a team, then assemble, appraise, and synthesize evidence. If sufficient evidence, proceed with design and pilot of the EBP change; if not, conduct research. If appropriate for system-wide adoption, integrate and sustain the practice change and disseminate results.
Advancing Research Through Close Clinical Collaboration Model (Fineholt et al., 2005)	Developed to promote EBP, establish a network of clinicians who support EBP, disseminate best evidence through research and conference. The model follows the steps of EBP: Ask a question, obtain best evidence, appraise the evidence, decide to implement change or not, and evaluate outcomes.
Johns Hopkins Nursing EBP Model (Newhouse et al., 2005)	Uses the PET Process for EBP: P = Practice question, E = Evidence, and T = Translation. The three phases have related steps to accomplish the process.
Ottawa Model of Research Use (Graham & Logan, 2004)	Three phases: (1) Assess barriers and supports while considering the evidence-based innovation, adopters' characteristics, and environment's structure and social context. (2) Monitor intervention and degree of use, considering implementation such as diffusion, dissemination and transfer of strategies, and innovation adoption. (3) Evaluate and monitor patient, practitioner, and system outcomes.
Knowledge to Action Model (Graham & Tetroe, 2007)	Has eight cycles that lead to knowledge translation: Problem identification, adaptation of the knowledge use to the local context, assessment of barriers to knowledge use, selection, tailoring and implementing interventions to promote knowledge use, monitoring knowledge use, evaluating outcomes of use, and sustaining knowledge use.
ACE Star Model of Knowledge Transformation (Stevens, 2013)	Involves steps of discovery of new knowledge through traditional research, creating a rigorous evidence summary, translation of the evidence in a practice guideline, integration of the change to influence individual and organizational change, and evaluation of the impact of the EBP on quality of care
Dobbins's Framework for Dissemination and Utilization of Research (Dobbins et al., 2002)	The model has five stages of innovation: knowledge, persuasion, decision, implementation, and confirmation. Within each stage are factors to consider for transferring research to practice.
Stetler Model (Stetler, 2001)	Focuses on critical thinking and use of internal and external data to promote EBP with steps of **preparation** for change through literature search, **validation** and critique of the evidence, **comparative evaluation and decision making** about what evidence to use, **translation and application** using a change plan, and **evaluation** of whether goals of using evidence are met.

EBP, Evidence-based practice; *A*, ask relevant questions to identify evidence; *C*, collect evidence through systematic searches; *E*, evaluate the quality and relevance of the evidence.

non-value–added activities. The model is used to remove defects from the system related to overproduction, waiting, confusion, unnecessary motion/travel, excess inventory, and overprocessing. Lean defines steps in a process as valuable if perceived so by the patient/customer. Six Sigma aims to eliminate or reduce variation and defects in processes. Together, Lean Six Sigma provides a comprehensive approach to process improvement that can be applied in a wide range of organizational settings.

Health care settings have been successful in using this model for the many years (Graban, 2016). The steps in the model are represented by the pneumonic DMAIC and include:

1. **Define** the problem or opportunity for improvement
2. **Measure** the current process and identify key metrics to track progress
3. **Analyze** the data to identify root causes of the problem

4. **Improve** the process by implementing solutions and verifying their effectiveness
5. **Control** the process by monitoring performance and ensuring sustainability over time

Lean Six Sigma typically involves using a range of tools and techniques such as a project charter, data collection tools, process flow diagrams, fishbone diagrams, run charts, Pareto charts, control charts, and histograms (see Chapter 14).

IMPLEMENTATION SCIENCE (IS) MODELS

Clinicians often use EBP and QI models to provide guidance into *what* needs to be implemented to improve practice, but these frameworks do not address *how* to successfully implement practice change. In response to the need to support clinicians in defining strategies for how to translate, adopt, and sustain evidence-based change as routine clinical practices, the field of implementation science (IS) developed over the last decade. Support for use of evidence-based implementation strategies is evident in the website sponsored by the National Institutes of Health Fogarty International Center of Advancing Science for Global Health (https://www.fic.nih.gov/About/center-global-health-studies/neuroscience-implementation-toolkit/Pages/methodologies-frameworks.aspx). Defined as the study of methods to promote systematic uptake of research findings and other EBPs to improve quality and effectiveness of health services, IS guides the exploration of factors impacting sustainability of practice change and offers specific implementation strategies to promote EBP translation in real-world settings (Reynolds & Granger, 2023). System factors to be explored include organizational context and system influences such as culture, leadership, communication and networks, resources, evaluation, monitoring, and feedback. Clinician-oriented factors include knowledge, skills, and confidence in promoting a practice change based on strong, high-quality evidence that offer advantages to the clinical setting in terms of fit, feasibility, and cost. Patient and family-related factors involve whether an EBP is acceptable in terms of their values, preferences, experiences, and health-related goals (Tucker et al., 2021).

Common IS frameworks used in healthcare include the Consolidated Framework for Implementation Research (CFIR) and the Promoting Action on Research Implementation in Health Services (PARIHS).

Consolidated Framework for Implementation Research

The CFIR (https://cfirguide.org/) is used to identify factors that may impact implementation of EBPs by cataloging potential barriers and opportunities associated with making an organizational change. Five domains that influence success of the change in practice are considered throughout the evidence translation process steps of planning, engaging, executing, reflecting, and evaluating. The characteristics of the new intervention itself, including the strength and quality of the supporting evidence and its cost, complexity, and adaptability to local needs, are important to understand. Both the outer setting and the inner setting of the organization are also considered. The outer setting is concerned with the degree an organization prioritizes patient needs, the status of organizational networking with outside entities, peer pressure to implement a change to have a competitive edge, and external policy, regulatory, or payment incentives. The inner setting encompasses the characteristics of individuals involved in the change, organizational communication networks, culture, implementation climate, and readiness to implement the change. The CFIR model also considers the characteristics of the individuals actually implementing the change, including their knowledge and beliefs about the innovation, level of confidence and self-efficacy in executing it, and their degree of commitment to the organizational effort. Once factors that have the potential to impact implementation of EBP have been identified, strategies can be defined to maximize adoption of the EBP in practice (see Chapter 17).

PROMOTING ACTION ON RESEARCH IMPLEMENTATION IN HEALTH SERVICES

The PARIHS model is a conceptual framework that represents the dynamic interplay of factors that influence successful implementation of EBPs. Three elements are examined to identify the barriers and enablers of implementation outcomes:

1. Evidence—refers to the strength and quality of the evidence supporting the practice, including research, clinical experience, patient experience, and local information; strong evidence is necessary but not sufficient for successful implementation

2. Context—refers to the environmental context in which a practice is being implemented and includes organizational culture, leadership, resources, and stakeholder engagement
3. Facilitation—refers to the strategies used by internal and/or external resources to support implementation and involves the use of techniques such as education, training, and ongoing support to promote adoption and sustainability of the change

The PARIHS framework was initially published in 1998, updated based on a conceptual analysis in 2002, and further refined in 2015 resulting in the integrated or i-PARIHS model. The updated version of the model recognizes that implementing research evidence into practice is complex, unpredictable, and nonlinear, requiring a flexible approach. Facilitation is identified as the active ingredient that integrates action around innovation and the recipients within their local, organizational, and wider health system content (Hunter et al., 2020; Bergstrom et al., 2020). Facilitation allows for flexible application of the i-PARIHS framework by encouraging the iterative tailoring of implementation strategies to a dynamic context. To support and promote more widespread use of the i-PARIHS framework among novice and experienced users, the Mobilizing Implementation of i-PARIHS Facilitation Planning Tool (https://www.flinders.edu.au/caring-futures-institute/do/mi-parihs) was developed and offers a suite of practical and pragmatic i-PARIHS resources (Hunter et al., 2023).

COMBINED MODELS

Often, clinicians find that there is not one singular model that meets the needs of all practice settings in an organization or is suited to every evidence-based improvement initiative. In these circumstances, site-developed models that combine EBP, QI, and IS strategies are valuable in improving care and outcomes. Examples of site-developed models include the I3 Model for Advancing Quality Patient Care (Hagle et al., 2020) and the Evidence-Based Practice Improvement Model (Levin et al., 2010).

I3 Model

After using a selected EBP model, an ANCC Magnet-designated organization questioned the use of a singular model when nurses were expected to participate in research, EBP, QI, and innovation. A review of other available models revealed that none met their need for a contextually relevant model to guide professional performance in all domains. After an extensive literature review, a workgroup developed a new model that incorporates multiple competencies and guides nurses involved in all domains of inquiry. The I3 Model (Hagle et al., 2020) represents Inquiry, Improvement, and Innovation and offers a step-by-step process to determine what type of project best answers their clinical question. Each process begins with a focused question such as "Why are we doing it this way?" or "Is there a new way?" The next step supports identifying the clinical issue, developing a goal/aim, and defining the problem. A subsequent step involves obtaining stakeholder buy-in. A common thread for each process is to obtain predata or best evidence and empowers clinicians to incorporate the voice of the customer. Unique steps in each of the three processes guide users to completion of the project. The model has been disseminated throughout the health system, incorporated into interprofessional education curricula for staff and managers, and provides a consistent mechanism of communication when beginning the project, reporting and disseminating outcomes, and participating in innovative solutions (Hagle et al., 2020).

Evidence-Based Practice Improvement Model

The Evidence-Based Practice Improvement Model (Levin et al., 2010) merged two paradigms of EBP and QI in an organization that had heavily invested in QI infrastructure that did not incorporate EBP principles in the process of practice change. Organizational perception was that there was value in both methodologies and leveraging the assets of each would best serve the practice setting. Supported by contributors in an academic–practice partnership, a new model was created to guide interprofessional teams to focus on improving outcomes using the best evidence. The model guides the user to describe the problem with validating evidence from internal and external sources, then formulate a focused clinical question that is further refined through systematically searching the literature as defined by traditional EBP approaches. The QI component of the model then directs attention to development of an aim statement that is expressed in measurable terms followed by engagement in small tests of change using PDSA cycles. Until the predetermined aim is met, continuous refinement of the evidence-based intervention occurs before disseminating best practice. The model has been utilized extensively in practice and academia because of its simplicity and practicality in solving clinical problems.

SYNTHESIS

The steps of EBP require not only knowledge of the process but also consideration of the context in which a change is recommended. Health care organizations are continually changing to keep pace with guidance from all types of payers and care systems. Change in any system or level of care is never an easy process regardless of whether there is buy-in from staff and support of leadership. Finding solutions requires not only the ability to search the literature but to engage critical stakeholders while having a keen awareness of the larger system factors that influence adoption of practice change.

Selecting and using an appropriate model to guide the process of practice change improves efficiency and effectiveness of the effort and utilizes organizational resources in a cost-effective manner. Using expert recommendations for implementing change improves sustainability and impact of the EBP improvement. Successful small tests of change can be scaled up for population-level implementation in the broader health system or community-based organization.

KEY POINTS

- EBP models and frameworks provide guidance to individuals and interprofessional teams to organize strategies and plans for practice change that address issues that may influence adoption of EBPs.
- EBP, QI, IS, and research have unique, independent, but complementary features.
- An evidence hierarchy/pyramid provides a schema for rating the strength of specific types of research designs.
- A clinical question guides the search for the best available evidence.
- Critical appraisal using standardized critical appraisal tools identifies the strengths and weaknesses of each individual research study.
- Synthesis refers to assessing the overall strengths and weaknesses of a group of studies.
- Evaluating the outcomes of an EBP project occurs prior to making recommendations about applicability to practice.
- Recommendations for applying evidence to practice depend on the strength and quality of the evidence to support current practice, making minor changes in practice, undertaking major practice changes, or developing a new area of practice.
- Evidence provides the foundation for developing or revising practice standards, protocols, and polices.
- Piloting an EBP practice change is an important step that allows staff to provide feedback and modify as appropriate.
- Numerous models and frameworks are available to guide practice change and are chosen to address the nature of the clinical problem and fit the contextual needs of a health care setting.

REFERENCES

American Association of Colleges of Nursing. (2021). *The essentials: Core competencies for professional nursing education*. American Association of Colleges of Nursing.

Andrews, J., Guyatt, G., Oxman, A. D., Alderson, P., Dahm, P., Falck-Ytter, Y., Nasser, M., Meerpohl, J., Post, P. N., Kunz, R., Brozek, J., Vist, G., Rind, D., Akl, E. A., & Schünemann, H. J. (2013). GRADE guidelines: 14. Going from evidence to recommendations: The significance and presentation of recommendations. *Journal of Clinical Epidemiology*, 66(7), 719–725. https://doi.org/10.1016/j.jclinepi.2012.03.013. Epub 2013 Jan 9. PMID: 23312392.

Balshem, H., Helfand, M., Schünemann, H. J., Oxman, A. D., Kunz, R., Brozek, J., Vist, G. E., Falck-Ytter, Y., Meerpohl, J., Norris, S., & Guyatt, G. H. (2011). GRADE guidelines: 3. Rating the quality of evidence. *Journal of Clinical Epidemiology*, 64(4), 401–406. https://doi.org/10.1016/j.jclinepi.2010.07.015. Epub 2011 Jan 5. PMID: 21208779.

Bergstrom, A., Ehrenberg, A., Eldh, A., Graham, I., Gustaffson, K., Harvey, G., Hunter, S., KItson, A., Rycroft-Malone, J., & Wallin, L. (2020). The use of the PARIHS framework in implementation research and practice—a citation analysis of the literature. *Implementation Science*, 15, 68.

Dobbins, M., Ciliska, D., Cockerill, R., Barnsley, J., & DiCenso, A. (2002). A framework for the dissemination and utilization of research for health-care policy and practice. *The Online Journal of Knowledge Synthesis for Nursing, 9*, document no.7.

Fineholt-Overholt, E., Melynk, B. M., & Schultz, A. (2005). Transforming health care from the inside out: Advancing evidence-based practice in the 21st century. *Journal of Professional Nursing, 21*(6), 335–344.

Graban, M. (2016). *Lean hospitals: Improving quality, safety, and employee engagement.* CRC Press Taylor and Francis Group.

Graham, I. D., & Logan, J. (2004). Innovations in knowledge transfer and continuity of care. *Canadian Journal of Nursing Research, 36*(2), 89–103. PMID: 15369167.

Graham, I. D., Tetroe, J., & KT Theories Research Group. (2007). Some theoretical underpinnings of knowledge translation. *Academic Emergency Medicine, 14*(11), 936–941. https://doi.org/10.1197/j.aem.2007.07.004. PMID: 17967955.

Guyatt, G., Oxman, A. D., Akl, E. A., Kunz, R., Vist, G., Brozek, J., Norris, S., Falck-Ytter, Y., Glasziou, P., DeBeer, H., Jaeschke, R., Rind, D., Meerpohl, J., Dahm, P., Schünemann, H. J. (2011). GRADE guidelines: 1. Introduction-GRADE evidence profiles and summary of findings tables. *Journal of Clinical Epidemiology, 64*(4), 383–394. https://doi.org/10.1016/j.jclinepi.2010.04.026. Epub 2010 Dec 31. PMID: 21195583.

Hagle, M., Dwyer, D., Gettrust, L., Lusk, D., Peterson, K., & Tennies, S. (2020). Development of a model for research, evidence-based practice, quality improvement, and innovation. *Journal of Nursing Care Quality, 35*(2), 102–107.

Hunter, S. C., Kim, B., & Kitson, A. (2023). Mobilising implementation of i-PARIHS (Mi-PARIHS): Development of a facilitation planning tool to accompany the integrated promoting action on research implementation in health services framework. *Implementation Science Communications, 4*, 2.

Hunter, S. C., Kim, B., Mudge, A., Hall, l., Young, A., McRae, P., & Kitson, A. (2020). Experiences of using the i-PARIHS framework: A co-designed case study of four multi-site implementation projects. *BMC Health Services Research, 20*, 573.

Institute for Healthcare Improvement. (2023). *How to improve.* https://www.ihi.org/resources/Pages/HowtoImprove/default.aspx.

Iowa Model Collaborative. (2017). Iowa Model of evidence-based practice: Revisions and validation. *Worldviews on Evidence-Based Nursing, 14*(3), 175–182.

Levin, R., Keefer, J., Vetter, M. J., Lauder, B., & Sobolewski, S. (2010). Evidence-based practice improvement: Merging 2 paradigms. *Journal of Nursing Care Quality, 25*(2), 117–126.

Newhouse, R. P., Dearholt, S. L., Poe, S. S., Pugh, L. C., & White, K. M. (2005). Evidence-based practice: A practical approach to implementation. *Journal of Nursing Administration, 35*(1), 35–40.

Reynolds, S., & Granger, B. (2023). Implementation toolkit for clinicians. *Dimensions of Critical Care Nursing, 42*(1), 33–41.

Speroni, K., McLaughlin, M., & Freisen, M. (2020). Use of evidence-based models and research findings in magnet-designated hospitals across the United States: National survey results. *Worldviews on Evidence-Based Nursing, 17*(2), 98–107.

Stetler, C. B. (2001). Updating the Stetler Model of research utilization to facilitate evidence-based practice. *Nursing Outlook, 49*(6), 272–279. https://doi.org/10.1067/mno.2001.120517. PMID: 11753294.

Stevens, K. R. (2013). The impact of evidence-based practice in nursing and the next big ideas. *The Online Journal of Issues in Nursing, 18*(2). https://doi.org/10.3912/OJIN.Vol18No02Man04. manuscript 4.

Titler, M. G., Conlon, P., Reynolds, M. A., Ripley, R., Tsodikov, A., Wilson, D. S., & Montie, M. (2016). The effect of translating research into practice interventions to promote use of evidence-based fall preventions in hospitalized adults: A prospective pre-post implementation study in the US. *Applied Nursing Research, 31*, 52–59.

Titler, M. G., Kleiber, C., Steelman, V., Goode, C., Rakel, B., Budreau, G., Everett, L. Q., Buckwalter, K. C., Tripp-Reimer, T., & Goode, C. H. (2001). The Iowa Model of evidence-based practice to promote quality care. *Critical Care Nursing Clinics of North America, 13*(4), 497–509.

Titler, M. G. (2014). Overview of evidence-based practice and translation science. *Nursing Clinics of North America, 49*(3), 269–274.

Tucker, S., McNett, M., Mezurek-Melnyk, B., Hanrahan, K., Hunter, S., Kim, B., Cullen, L., & Kitson, S. (2021). Implementation science: Application of evidence-based practice models to improve healthcare quality. *Worldviews on Evidence-Based Nursing, 18*(2), 76–84.

PART II Processes of Developing Evidence-Based Practice and Questions in Various Clinical Settings

5

Developing Compelling Clinical Questions

Judith Haber and Martha Kent

LEARNING OUTCOMES

After reading this chapter, you should be able to do the following:
- Discuss the purpose of developing a clinical question.
- Compare the differences between a clinical question and a research question or hypothesis in relation to evidence-based practice.
- Apply the PICOT framework to the formulation of clinical questions.
- Evaluate how the clinical question guides the search for evidence.

KEY TERMS

Clinical question
Hypothesis
PICOT
Research question

Whether you are a nurse practitioner, clinical nurse specialist, clinical nurse leader, nurse educator, nurse manager, or a member of the quality improvement team at your health care organization, you are a clinical leader. Evidence-based practice (EBP) is a key component of the expertise you offer to your patients and staff. It provides the foundation for developing clinical questions that launch your search for health information that provides the best available evidence to inform healthcare and clinical decisions. High-quality, cost-effective care that provides a satisfying experience for patient, provider, and staff challenges health professionals to provide patient care that is informed by the latest and best evidence (Berwick et al., 2008). Increasingly, the external health care environment—including, but not limited to, patients, employers, certifying organizations, regulatory boards, insurers, and professional organizations—expects that evidence-based information guides clinical practice.

An essential component of the American Nurses Credentialing Center (ANCC) Magnet Recognition model is providing evidence for new knowledge, innovation, and improvement. Magnet-recognized organizations have an ethical and professional responsibility to contribute to patient care, the organization, and the profession in terms of new knowledge, innovations, and improvements. Magnet-designated organizations must demonstrate integration of EBP and research into clinical and operational processes. (ANCC, 2021).

The American Association of Colleges of Nursing (AACN) *Essentials: Core Competencies for Professional Nursing Practice* (2021) identify that a feature of advanced-level nursing practice is the ability to apply and critically evaluate advanced knowledge in a defined area of nursing practice. This includes competencies related to appropriate application of quality improvement (QI), research, and evaluation methods for EBP.

Clinical practice is kept up to date by searching for, retrieving, and critically appraising QI reports, research studies, systematic reviews, and EBP guidelines that apply to practice issues encountered in clinical settings. Clinicians strive to navigate the wealth of clinical information available to health professionals; finding the right information, at the right time, using the right search strategy (see Chapter 6) is a challenge!

Your search for information—that is, the best available evidence—is converted into focused clinical questions that are the foundation of EBP and QI. The evidence, coupled with clinical judgment, as well as patient preferences and contextual factors, combine to inform the most effective clinical decision making about practice (see Chapter 3). The purpose of this chapter is to highlight the importance of clinical questions, that is, how to develop and use them in searching for the best available evidence to find answers that inform clinical practice.

WHAT IS A CLINICAL QUESTION?

Clinical questions form the basis for searching the literature to identify supporting evidence from research to inform development or revision of clinical standards, protocols, and policies that guide professional nursing and interprofessional best practice. Clinical questions have five basic components:
- **P**opulation and problem
- **I**ntervention
- **C**omparison
- **O**utcome
- **T**ime

These components, known as PICOT, provide an effective format for developing focused and searchable clinical questions. PICOT is a tool to help you formulate the clinical question. Box 5.1 presents components of the PICOT question. PICOT question formats linked with types of clinical questions are illustrated in Box 5.2. PICOT questions linked with types of designs are highlighted in Table 5.1. The significance of the clinical question becomes apparent as research evidence from the search is critically appraised. Research evidence, clinical judgment, and patient preferences are used to validate, develop, or revise best practices.

BOX 5.1 PICOT Question Components

- Patient/Population/Problem
  - Diagnosis
  - Age
  - Gender
  - Ethnicity/race
  - Marital status
  - Social determinants of health
- Intervention or Clinical Issue of Interest
  - Risk behavior (e.g., unprotected sex)
  - Therapy/intervention
  - Exposure to disease
  - Prognosis
- Comparison Intervention or Clinical Issue of Interest
  - No-risk behavior (e.g., protected sex)
  - Alternative therapy/intervention, placebo, no intervention at all
  - No disease
  - Alternative prognosis
- Outcome
  - Risk of disease or condition
  - Expected/predicted outcome expected from therapy/intervention (e.g., decreased catheter-associated urinary infections)
  - Accuracy of diagnosis (e.g., sensitivity and specificity)
  - Rate of occurrence of adverse outcome (e.g., mortality)
- Time
  - Length of time to achieve the stated outcome
  - Optional element of the PICO(T) question

Identifying the **P**—patient population, problem, or setting—may seem obvious to you as a clinician or to your team. However, it is often stated too generally and may be misleading in terms of using the correct search terms when designing your evidence search. Using Box 5.1 will be helpful to you in focusing identification of the target population or setting. For example, limiting the population to a specific diagnostic subgroup of adults with hospital-acquired pneumonia (HAP) is appropriate when there is a rationale for doing so and the population is linked to the other components of the PICOT question and search terms. When the setting is the focus of interest, the setting becomes the key focus of your search.

The **I**, the issue of interest, commonly the intervention, should reflect greater diversity than the traditional definition of an intervention. For example, it may include a treatment stratified oral hygiene protocol based on

> **BOX 5.2 PICOT Question Formats**
>
> **Therapy/Intervention**
> In _____ (population), what is the effect of _____ (intervention), compared with _____ (comparison intervention), on _____ (outcome)?
>
> **Diagnosis/Assessment**
> For _____ (population), does _____ (tool or procedure) yield more accurate or more appropriate diagnostic/assessment information than _____ (comparison tool/procedure) about _____ (outcome)?
>
> **Prognosis**
> For _____ (population), does _____ (disease/condition), relative to _____ (comparison disease or condition) increase the risk for or influence _____ (outcome)?
>
> **Causation/Harm/Etiology**
> Does _____ (exposure or characteristic) increase the risk for _____ (outcome) compared with _____ (comparison exposure or condition) in _____ (population)?
>
> **Meaning or Process**
> What is it like for _____ (population) to experience _____ (condition, illness, circumstances?)
> Or:
> What is the process through which _____ (population) cope with, adapt to, or live with _____ (circumstance)?

effect of a preventive stratified oral hygiene protocol compared with no standardized oral hygiene care. The **C**—the comparison intervention—may be the current standard of care or no intervention at all. For example, in this clinical setting there was no standard of care for prevention of HAP. But QI data from a pilot implemented at one hospital revealed that a significant reduction in the incidence and prevalence of HAP, especially nonventilator HAP (NVHAP), was possible using a stratified standardized oral hygiene protocol based on self-care capacity for completing oral hygiene (Baker et al., 2022; Giuliano, 2021; Munro & Baker, 2018; Scannapieco et al., 2022).

Other clinicians may be focused on prognosis as an issue of interest. For example, there are data to support that the NVHAP mortality rate is 15% to 30%. Will a pilot QI initiative provide an evidence-based answer about whether implementing a stratified oral hygiene protocol will be associated with a significant reduction in mortality?

The **O**—outcome—specifies the focus of the answer to the PICOT question that will be revealed by the targeted search for and critical appraisal and synthesis of the evidence. There was a dearth of evidence from QI initiatives or research studies related to nursing interventions for NVHAP that were effective in decreasing the incidence and prevalence of this common hospital-acquired infection. Sometimes, a PICOT question will specify more than one outcome as a result of a single intervention. In this situation, outcome measures for each will need to be identified.

The **T** specifies what the projected time frame will be for answering the PICOT question and obtaining outcome data. For example, the projected time frame for the pilot NVHAP QI initiative was one year.

> **TIP**
>
> A well-developed PICOT question guides a focused search for scientific evidence about assessing, diagnosing, treating, or providing patients with information about the prognosis for their specific health condition.

level of self-care capacity, a diagnostic test chest x-ray or complete blood count (CBC), exposure to bacteria in oral cavity, risk factor of tooth decay or periodontal disease, or prognostic factor comorbidities (e.g., chronic obstructive pulmonary disease/affecting survival rates). Greater specificity for the **I** and the **C** will be associated with a more focused search strategy. When the **I** is a new intervention, you may have to do some background searching and reading before specifically identifying the **I** as well as the comparison. The comparison is usually the current standard of care, a placebo, or another intervention or combination of interventions. For example, the **I** may be examining the

WHY ARE CLINICAL QUESTIONS IMPORTANT?

Busy clinicians, like you, can be overwhelmed by the volume of literature you have to access, sift through, and evaluate to identify the best practice supported by the strongest evidence that is applicable to your population and practice issue or problem. Moreover, no two patients

TABLE 5.1 Classifying Types of Clinical Questions and Kind of Study Providing Best Evidence

Clinical Question	Type of Question	Kind of Study Design Providing Best Evidence
How can the problem be prevented?	Prevention	Randomized clinical trial/systematic review
Will detecting the problem early, before symptoms, make a difference in my health?	Screening	Randomized clinical trial/systematic review Cohort studies
How good is this test for detecting my problem?	Diagnosis	Cohort studies
What is the likely outcome of this problem?	Prognosis	Cohort studies
What proportion of the population is newly diagnosed with this problem each year?	Incidence	Cohort studies
What proportion of the population is currently living with the problem?	Prevalence	Case-control/cohort studies
What causes the problem?	Etiology	Randomized clinical trials/systematic review
What should be done to treat this problem?	Therapy	Randomized clinical trials/case-control studies
Will there be any negative effects from an intervention?	Harm	

are exactly alike, and colleagues may have differing opinions on the best approach to resolving a patient problem. When your team members ponder the clinical question they want to develop, it may be helpful to think about the purpose or objective of the evidence-based project they want to implement. The purpose of an EBP project includes what the clinical team aims to achieve with the initiative. When a purpose statement is used, it suggests the planned approach that will be used to guide the project. When the purpose of an EBP is to ask a clinical question that compares the effectiveness of two interventions, the search for evidence will be linked to intervention or therapy studies that focus on testing the effectiveness of interventions queried in the PICOT question. For example, if the purpose of an evidence-based project aims to answer whether, in a population of preoperative patients, the practice of oral care immediately prior to the procedure compared with no oral care will have a significant effect on outcomes by decreasing the incidence of ventilator-associated pneumonia, the search for the best available evidence will focus on studies that are Level I systematic reviews, Level II randomized clinical trials, or Level III quasi-experimental designs (see Chapter 8).

Clinical questions are important as they provide a structured format focused on finding an answer to a clinical question that may originate when there is a gap in knowledge or from a clinical problem for which there is not an evidence-based answer.

Formulating the PICOT question facilitates searching the literature efficiently to locate and retrieve the right information in a timely manner so that the best available information can be shared with your colleagues and patients (Chapters 6 and 19). Integrating a proactive evidence-seeking approach into your clinical practice style is essential to remaining at the cutting edge of clinical practice to provide high-quality, cost-effective care and satisfying patient and staff experiences.

> **TIP**
>
> Teamwork is involved in developing a clinical PICOT question. Team members may have differing perspectives about the focus of the clinical question. They need to respect and consider the value of each member's contribution to finalizing the PICOT question and making sure it aligns with the aims of the EBP or QI project.

SOURCES OF CLINICAL QUESTIONS

Clinical questions originate from multiple sources, including the patient and family. There are many models that have been developed to organize and assist professionals in asking clinical questions, evaluating new evidence, and making sustainable change in practice. Although models vary in detail, explicit criteria, and methods to engage in EBP, there are elements that should be addressed for the PICOT question:

1. Identification of a clinical problem or question of practice

2. Search for the best evidence that is applicable to the practice setting
3. Critical appraisal and synthesis of strength, quality, quantity, and consistency of evidence
4. Recommendations for action (no change, change, further investigation) based on the appraisal of evidence
5. Implementation of recommendations
6. Evaluation of the recommendation in relationship to desired outcomes
7. Dissemination (see Chapter 3).

TYPES OF CLINICAL/PICOT QUESTIONS

A well-developed PICOT question has the following advantages:
- It helps clarify the clinical problem and the information required to solve it.
- It helps define the type of evidence needed from which type of study.
- It helps provide terms to make searching for evidence more effective.

Classifying PICOT questions according to the type of question being asked is one approach, as illustrated in Table 5.1. As Box 5.2 indicates, there are different clinical question formats depending on the type of clinical question being asked. For example, the clinical question about whether implementing a standardized stratified oral hygiene protocol compared to normal oral hygiene would affect the incidence of NVHAP suggests thinking about which therapy is most effective for treating this patient or patient population. Generally, the kind of studies that potentially provide the best evidence for answering this kind of therapy clinical question are randomized controlled trials (RCTs) (see Chapter 8) as illustrated in Table 5.1. Box 5.3 provides a case study illustrating a PICOT question and how research evidence was used to promote practice change. Using the PICOT format ensures that you will be able to search for and find the answer to your clinical questions effectively or have an evidence-based rationale for modifying your clinical question.

> **TIP**
>
> Once you have developed a focused clinical question using the PICOT format, you will search the literature for the best available evidence to answer your clinical question.

CLINICAL QUESTIONS DIFFER FROM RESEARCH QUESTIONS AND HYPOTHESES

Clinical questions differ from research questions and hypotheses in their approach. They may sound alike, but their purposes differ. Both research questions and hypotheses are key preliminary steps in conducting research studies and guide the design and implementation of a research study. Both are used by researchers to test the relationships between and among variables. **Research questions** are written as questions that address a gap or conflict in the literature. They test a measureable relationship between the independent and dependent variable that is examined in the study. The remainder of the study should flow from the research question. The research question is answered by the findings of the study. A properly written research question will be clear and concise. It should contain the topic being studied (purpose), the variable(s), and the population. **Hypotheses** are used in research studies to predict the outcome(s) of the study. A hypothesis is predictive in nature and typically used when significant knowledge already exists on the subject, which allows the prediction to be made. Both research questions and hypotheses are commonly used in quantitative research. Guided by their *clinical questions*, clinicians search for and use evidence provided by the findings of research studies to answer clinical questions. Once found and retrieved, the evidence is critically appraised, and, based on the strength, quality, and consistency of the evidence, it is used to answer the clinical question by determining whether the evidence is applicable to clinical practice and to provide a basis for implementation of EBPs.

> **TIP**
>
> Information from online resources that will help you formulate searchable, answerable questions include the following:
> - Centre for Evidence-Based Medicine University of Toronto: https://guides.library.utoronto.ca/evidence-basedmedicine
> - Agency for Healthcare Research and Quality (AHRQ): https://www.ahrq.gov
> - About EBP - Resources for Evidence-Based Practice - Guides at McMaster University Health Sciences Library (libguides.com) https://hslmcmaster.libguides.com

BOX 5.3   Case Study 1: PICOT Question

In a population of hospitalized adults at risk for nonventilator hospital-acquired pneumonia (NVHAP), what is the effect of a stratified oral hygiene intervention in comparison to usual care on reducing the incidence and prevalence of NVHAP by 20% in 6 months?

Erica and Nathan are co-chairs of the Quality Improvement (QI) Council at Hospital XYZ. The QI Council reviewed the hospital-acquired infection data for the past year and observed that the NVHAP rate has risen and is associated with an increased length of stay, complexity of care, and cost. One of the QI Council members recently read a journal article about a QI initiative implemented in the Veteran's Health Care System using a leveled oral hygiene protocol based on self-care capacity administered by nurses and nursing assistants that had a dramatic effect on reducing the incidence of NVHAP. Council members agreed to review the literature to locate QI and research studies for evidence of effective interventions to address this clinical problem. They developed a PICOT question to guide their search. They prioritized searching for therapy, cohort, or case-control studies, systematic reviews, or clinical practice guidelines that provide the best available evidence for developing an effective QI plan. Their search revealed that although one of the most common hospital-acquired infections, most hospitals do not routinely conduct NVHAP surveillance or implement NVHAP prevention measures because it is not a standardized national quality indicator (Baker et al., 2022; Scannapieco et al., 2022; Munro & Baker, 2018). Because NVHAP frequently originates from bacteria in the mouth then travels to the lungs, several studies reported focusing on NVHAP prevention oral hygiene protocols. Poor oral health is a modifiable risk factor for NVHAP and, frequently, a missed care opportunity in hospital settings with up to 82% of patients not receiving oral care assistance during their hospital stay (Munro & Baker, 2018) and with a 15% to 30% mortality rate. Strong QI and research evidence was reported by Munro and colleagues (2018), who successfully piloted, scaled, and spread local research on NVHAP prevention as best practice at all 155 sites in the Veterans Affairs (VA) Medical Centers nationwide following staff development NVHAP implementation programs. Each NVHAP case costs an estimated $40,000, thus preventing 100 cases may save up to $400 million and 700 to 900 hospital days. Data from the pilot revealed a 92% reduction in NVHAP incidence in 1 year. Based on the evidence, the QI Council decided that this would be an important QI initiative that could be piloted on two acute care units implementing a leveled oral hygiene protocol on one unit and compare the NVHAP outcomes with usual care on the comparison unit. The QI Council brainstormed about the logistics of a pilot implementation plan, including the financial and other resources that would be needed. They knew it would have to be approved by several departments. They planned to contact the nurse practitioner and nurse researcher who led the VA's NVHAP program for permission to adapt the VA model for use at their hospital. They scheduled a meeting with the staff development team to discuss training and coaching the staff regarding implementation. Erica and Nathan prepared a proposal to present at the next Nursing Leadership Council that included the implementation process, engaged stakeholders, tools, strategies, resources, and outcomes for the initiative. It was essential to obtain "buy-in" from nursing and hospital leadership for the NVHAP QI initiative.

SYNTHESIS

Clinicians are increasingly concerned about ensuring that the care they provide is evidence based. In your leadership role, you will be asked to provide evidence to support the quality and cost effectiveness of the care provided for your patient population or program. Individual research studies, systematic reviews, and clinical guidelines are evidence-based products you will use to support your practice. Formulating clinical questions is fundamental to and the first step in the EBP process. Clinical questions convert situations and problems into answerable questions that you will use to guide your search for the best available evidence, coupled with clinical expertise and patient preferences that you will use to make a difference and act as a role model for colleagues. As you become confident as an EBP clinical leader, another aspect of your role will be to mentor other nurse practitioners, nurses, and colleagues from other professions to develop their clinical question and other EBP competencies.

TIP

The QI data at your hospital indicate that the prevalence of skin injuries during prolonged prone positioning during operative procedures has increased by 10% in the last two quarters. As a member of the Perioperative Quality Improvement Committee you will collaborate with your committee colleagues and stakeholders from other professions to develop an interprofessional action plan based on the literature search conducted using key terms in the clinical question.

KEY POINTS

- Clinical questions form the basis of the search of the literature for supporting evidence from research to inform development or revision of clinical standards, protocols, policies, and guidelines that guide clinical practice.
- Clinical questions are important as they provide a structured format focused on providing an answer to a clinical problem or gap in knowledge.
- Clinical questions have five basic components that specify the population or problem (P), intervention (I), comparison (C), outcome (O), and time (T), all of which are known as PICOT, a tool to help formulate a clinical question.
- There are different types of clinical questions that focus on finding answers to issues related to therapy, prognosis, diagnosis, prevention, screening, harm, incidence, and prevalence.
- Specific types of clinical questions are associated with research study designs that provide the best available evidence.
- Clinical questions differ from research questions and hypotheses. Research questions and hypotheses guide the direction of research studies that generate evidence, whereas clinical questions use the evidence generated by research studies to inform clinical decision making.

REFERENCES

American Association of Colleges of Nursing (AACN). (2021). *The essentials: Core competencies for professional nursing education*. AACN.

American Nurses Credentialing Center (ANCC). (2021). *2023 Magnet recognition program application manual*. ANCC.

Baker, D., Giuliano, K., Thakkar-Samtani, M., Scannapieco, F., Glick, M., Restrepo, M., et al. (2022). The association between accessing dental services and nonventilator hospital-acquired pneumonia among 2019 Medicaid beneficiaries. *Infection Control & Hospital Epidemiology*, 1–3. https://doi.org/10.1017/ice.2022.163.

Berwick, D. M., Nolan, T. W., & Whittington, J. (2008). The triple aim: Care, health, and cost. *Health Affairs*, 27(3), 759–769.

Giuliano, K. (2021). Oral care a prevention for nonventilator hospital acquired pneumonia. *American Journal of Nursing*, 21(15), 24–33.

Munro, S., & Baker, D. (2018). Reducing missed oral care opportunities to prevent non-ventilator associated hospital acquired pneumonia at the VA. *Applied Nursing Research*, 44, 48–53.

Munro, S., Haile-Mariam, A., Greenwell, C., Demirci, S., Farooqi, O., & Vasudeva, S. (2018). Implementation and dissemination of a Department of Veterans Affairs oral care initiative to prevent hospital acquired pneumonia among non-ventilated patients. *Nursing Administration Quarterly*, 42(4), 363–372.

Scannapieco, F., Giuliano, K., & Baker, D. (2022). Oral health status and the etiology and prevention of nonventilator hospital-associated pneumonia. *Periodontology 2000*, 89(1), 51–58. https://doi.org/10.1111/prd.12423.

6

Searching the Literature for Evidence

Brynne Campbell Rice and Carlita Anglin

LEARNING OUTCOMES

After reading this chapter, you should be able to do the following:
- Differentiate between different types of information sources, including secondary information sources and primary sources.
- Recognize the range, scope, strengths, and limitations of bibliographic databases and other digital repositories as discovery tools for different types of information sources.
- Identify core search concepts based on a clinical question of interest and locate subject headings and keywords that map to these concepts.
- Describe the process of screening, abstracting, critiquing, and organizing research evidence.
- Feel confident approaching the literature search process.
- Identify actionable, practical strategies for finding high-quality information that can inform clinical practice within a rapidly changing professional environment.

KEY TERMS

Bibliographic record
Cited reference searching
False hit
Field tag
Gray literature
Keyword
Literature database
Literature search flow diagram
Meta-analysis
Metadata
Primary source
Preprint
Point-of-care (point-of-service) tool
Saturation
Scoping search
Search query
Secondary source
Sensitive search
Snowballing
Specific search
Subject heading
Systematic review

Finding high-quality biomedical research information is often a process much like nursing practice itself. Although there are ideal frameworks and models to follow, the actual process is frequently adaptive, responsive, iterative, social, context dependent, and ever changing. All nurses, particularly clinical leaders and decision makers, must be knowledgeable about how to be critical information consumers and how to disseminate knowledge to others effectively. The health information landscape for both nursing practice and academic purposes is influenced by the broader digital environment and, more than ever, requires informed, thoughtful engagement.

The purpose of this chapter is to provide friendly strategies to help readers apply and adapt searching frameworks for their own purposes. This chapter will introduce different sources of evidence, research support tools, and structured search processes that yield results that are timely, thorough, relevant, reliable, and

59

PRODUCTION AND COMMUNICATION OF EVIDENCE IN NURSING

Original evidence in the life and health sciences is typically generated using empirical research methods such as randomized control trials (RCTs), laboratory experiments, observational studies, or qualitative research studies. In these methods, researchers seek to understand the world through direct or indirect observation, collecting, analyzing, and interpreting data. Chapters 8, 9, and 11 offer more in-depth information about the research methods used by health researchers to generate new knowledge. Additionally, nurse scientists and researchers might engage in thought work, producing scholarship in which they propose new theories or philosophies that are meant to explain and logically organize abstract ideas, concepts, or phenomena. Through original research, theoretical work, and professional experiences, nursing scholars and leaders develop informed perspectives and viewpoints that are worth disseminating broadly. Expert opinion is an important category of evidence, particularly when empirical or theoretical research is lacking. In nursing, original research and arguments shared directly by the scholar or researcher who generated them, are typically considered **primary sources** of evidence.

Another important consideration within nursing science is a category of evidence known as **secondary sources**, evidence that is synthesized and summarized for the reader. Secondary sources are interpretations of primary research. Practice guidelines and standards, white papers, reviews, systematic reviews, **meta-analyses**, evidence summaries, or even books are examples of how original research is synthesized and transformed into secondary evidence. Many scholarly and practice-focused knowledge products present secondary evidence to guide readers quickly through complex topics and contextualize the current state of a problem (Table 6.1 for more information about primary and secondary sources in nursing).

HIERARCHY AND EVIDENCE TYPES

Health care outcomes are determined by rigorously and thoughtfully produced research that is evaluated and put into practice by clinicians and health care leaders. The strength or appropriateness of a particular type of evidence to address a specific health care question or problem depends on the nature of the question (see Chapter 5, Table 5.1), as well as the methodology for how that evidence was generated. For clinical decision making, the strongest evidence is produced by reproducible, quantitative methods, which are considered more objectively rigorous and unbiased. In contrast, expert opinions, case reports, and commentaries are considered relatively weak. Within healthcare, evidence strength is typically expressed as a pyramid hierarchy comprised of levels of evidence that become more rigorous, building up from the foundation (see Chapter 4, Fig. 4.1). Systematic reviews, meta-analyses, and meta-syntheses sit highest on the evidence hierarchy because they methodically synthesize multiple sources of evidence. A **systematic review** is a form of meta-research in which researchers follow a prospectively structured protocol in order to locate all relevant studies on a given question, evaluate the evidence strength, and then summarize in a state-of-the-science conclusion. A **meta-analysis** is a type of systematic review in which data from multiple studies are analyzed in aggregate to reach a quantitative conclusion about the group of studies examined (see Chapter 10 for an in-depth discussion of systematic reviews).

> **TIP**
>
> Beginning a search for information by seeking the highest levels of evidence first (e.g., systematic reviews of RCTs or meta-analyses) can be a great time saver. Many health literature databases will allow you to selectively filter your results to see systematic reviews or meta-analyses.

COMMUNICATION OF EVIDENCE

Communicating advances in health care evidence and practice changes is central to nursing science. When evidence is shared, interpreted, challenged, evaluated, and synthesized by a community of scholar-scientists, that evidence can inform the practice of healthcare, improve practice, and operationalize new knowledge. For that reason, the American Nurses Credentialing Center (ANCC) Magnet Recognition Program and formalized models of evidence-based practice (EBP) nursing require research

TABLE 6.1 Primary and Secondary Sources in Nursing

	Primary	Secondary
Authorship	The researcher(s) who conducted the study or proposed the theory/idea	Not necessarily the scholar who originally conducted the research, but people with some expertise in the field
Content/Process	• Results of empirical research 　• Experimental methods 　• Observational methods 　• Qualitative methods • Results of theoretical research • Results of scholarly discourse/opinion	• Results of aggregation, evaluation, interpretation, and synthesis of primary evidence
Sources	• Peer-reviewed research articles 　• Scholars report their method for data collection and analysis, and their results • Conference presentations/posters/abstracts 　• Scholars briefly describe their method for data collection and analysis, and their results • Data sets and statistics 　• Scholars share the data they have collected, in its raw form, or processed using statistical methods • Scholarly commentary/editorials 　• Scholars share their expert opinions or ideas about important topics in the field	Articles in evidence summary journals • Also called abstract journals, these contain expert commentary and critical appraisal of published studies (e.g., *Evidence-Based Nursing*) Evidence summaries/syntheses • Aggregate and appraise evidence related to clinical topics of interest (e.g., resources from Joanna Briggs EBP Institute Database) Review articles • Collect, summarize, and sometimes appraise primary evidence on a given research question (e.g., systematic reviews from the Cochrane Database of Systematic Reviews) Practice guidelines • Authored by professional agencies or societies, guidelines, often based on systematic reviews Government reports and topic summaries • Contain official guidance and overviews from health-related government bodies
Uses	• Staying current on the most recent emergent information and conversations in the field • Providing the evidence base to be appraised and synthesized for an EBP/quality improvement project	• Building knowledge base to understand nuances of clinical questions • Building capacity to understand and critique primary literature • In a clinical setting, evidence summaries and practice guidelines can guide decision making

findings to be disseminated. Most frequently, original research is disseminated broadly through written research papers, which are submitted for publication in discipline-specific, peer-reviewed journals.

While peer-reviewed journals are the mode of a great deal of scholarly communication, evidence may also be shared outside traditionally published journals. Findings are both internally and externally communicated at conferences (as published conference abstracts, posters, or papers), or may be shared through dissertations or theses, non–peer-reviewed reports, white papers, and personal communications. These types of sources, which often exist outside of traditional publication channels, are referred to as **gray literature**. Gray literature is unevaluated and not peer reviewed, and covers a wide range of sources, including patents, pamphlets, trial registrations, podcasts, websites, research studies in progress, or organizational reports.

DISCOVERING EVIDENCE

The landscape of evidence in the health sciences is constantly growing and evolving, more quickly now than ever. The generation of data has proliferated alongside rapid advances in technologies for personal health and for broader social and health care systems-level data.

Literature Databases

Although health care research information is widely available electronically, researchers and nurses in practice should develop contemporary skills to navigate new complexities.

Scholarly literature is described and organized in centralized **literature databases**. These databases are searchable collections of **bibliographic records** that describe the information sources. Databases vary in the scope of the subjects and types of information sources they cover. Most literature databases are composed of records describing articles from scholarly journals, but some databases may also include records for other types of sources, like dissertations, conference abstracts, or articles from newspapers/magazines. Some multidisciplinary databases include literature from a wide range of academic subjects, while others offer deep coverage of the literature of a few specific disciplines (e.g., health or psychology). With a few notable exceptions that are freely available online (e.g., PubMed), most literature databases are commercial products that are purchased through libraries at universities, academic medical centers, hospitals, and public library systems. See Table 6.2 for descriptions, access, and scope of databases in the health sciences.

Indexing and Metadata

When a new article is published in an academic journal, the article goes through indexing, a process of creating a structured record of the article. That record includes

TABLE 6.2 Recommended Literature Databases

Core Health Sciences Databases
List is not meant to be exhaustive; consult your librarian for more institution-specific recommendations

CINAHL (Cumulative Index to Nursing and Allied Health Literature)
Access via EBSCO (https://www.ebsco.com/products/research-databases/cinahl-database); requires institutional subscription

Content Coverage	Types of Sources	Features
Covers nursing, biomedicine, health sciences librarianship, alternative/complementary medicine, consumer health, and 17 allied health disciplines	Scholarly, peer-reviewed journal articles Health care books Nursing dissertations Conference proceedings	Filters for: • Research subject characteristic (age, sex, human), date, publication type, "research" article Preformulated "Clinical Queries" for: • Therapy, Prognosis, Qualitative, Review, Causation Subject Thesaurus: CINAHL Subject Headings

MEDLINE
pubmed.ncbi.nlm.nih.gov/
https://www.wolterskluwer.com/en/solutions/ovid/ovid-medline-901
PubMed offers free, public access to citations and abstracts; links to full-text coverage for some content in PubMed Central or open-access journals
Subscription access via Ovid

Content Coverage	Types of Sources	Features
The premier source for coverage of clinical biomedical topics; also includes coverage of health administration, public health, technology, and other nonclinical aspects of healthcare	Scholarly, peer-reviewed journal articles A small number of newspapers, magazines, and newsletters	Filters for: • Research subject characteristic (age, sex, species), date, and article type Preformulated "Clinical Queries" for: • Etiology, Prognosis, Therapy, Clinical Prediction Subject Thesaurus: NLM Medical Subject Headings (MeSH) www.ncbi.nlm.nih.gov/mesh/

TABLE 6.2   Recommended Literature Databases—cont'd

PsycInfo
Access via Ovid, EBSCO, or ProQuest or directly from American Psychological Association PsycNET (www.apa.org/pubs/databases/psycinfo); requires subscription

Content Coverage	Types of Materials	Features
Coverage centers on psychology and related disciplines, including medicine, psychiatry, nursing, sociology, pharmacology, physiology, and linguistics	Journal articles Books and book chapters Selected dissertations	Filters for: • Population characteristics (age, sex), methodology, tests and measures, publication type Preformulated "Clinical Queries" for: • Reviews, Therapy, Qualitative Subject Thesaurus: Thesaurus of Psychological Index Terms

EMBASE
Access via Ovid or Elsevier (www.elsevier.com/solutions/embase-biomedical-research); requires subscription

Content Coverage	Types of Materials	Features
Biomedical and pharmaceutical database indexing journals from more than 90 countries with selective coverage for nursing, psychology, and alternative medicine	Journal articles Conference abstracts (biomedical, drug and medical device)	Filters for: • Publication type, experimental subjects, subject age and sex (Ovid only) Preformulated "Clinical Queries" for: • Reviews, Therapy, Diagnosis, Prognosis, Causation, Economics, Qualitative Subject Thesaurus: Emtree

Recommended Multidisciplinary Databases

Web of Science
Access via Clarivate (clarivate.com/webofsciencegroup/solutions/web-of-science/); requires subscription

Content Coverage	Types of Materials	Features
Includes Core Collection, which covers Science Citation, Social Sciences Citation Index, and the Arts & Humanities Citation Index, among others	Scholarly journal articles Conference proceedings	Filters for: • Document types, funding agencies and Web of Science discipline categories, publication date Tools for: • Article and author metrics, cited reference searching Subject Thesaurus: None

ProQuest Central
Access via ProQuest (https://about.proquest.com/en/products-services/ProQuest_Central/); requires subscription

Content Coverage	Types of Materials	Features
Discovery tool that allows searching across multiple databases and disciplines, including business, health and medical, social sciences, arts and humanities, education, science and technology, and more	Scholarly journal articles Newspaper and magazine articles Dissertations Books	Filters for: • Source and document type, peer-reviewed literature, and subject Tools for: • Cited reference search, related articles Subject Thesaurus: Multiple

Modified from Campbell & Jacobs, 2021.

important descriptive information about the article, or *metadata*, that can help researchers locate it efficiently (much like descriptive online "tags"). Most literature databases contain records with common metadata fields like article title, author, journal title, and publication date, but in specialized health sciences databases, records may include descriptive information such as publication type/methodology, or population characteristics (e.g., species, age, sex). Fig. 6.1 illustrates the structure of a bibliographic record from PubMed, noting the metadata that is included.

Researchers and clinicians can leverage a database's specialized vocabulary known as *subject headings* to yield more precise search results. Subject headings (such as Medical Subject Headings (MeSH) within the MEDLINE database or APA Index Terms in PsycInfo) are the preferred terms that are used to express a concept consistently within a database. Journal articles are assigned

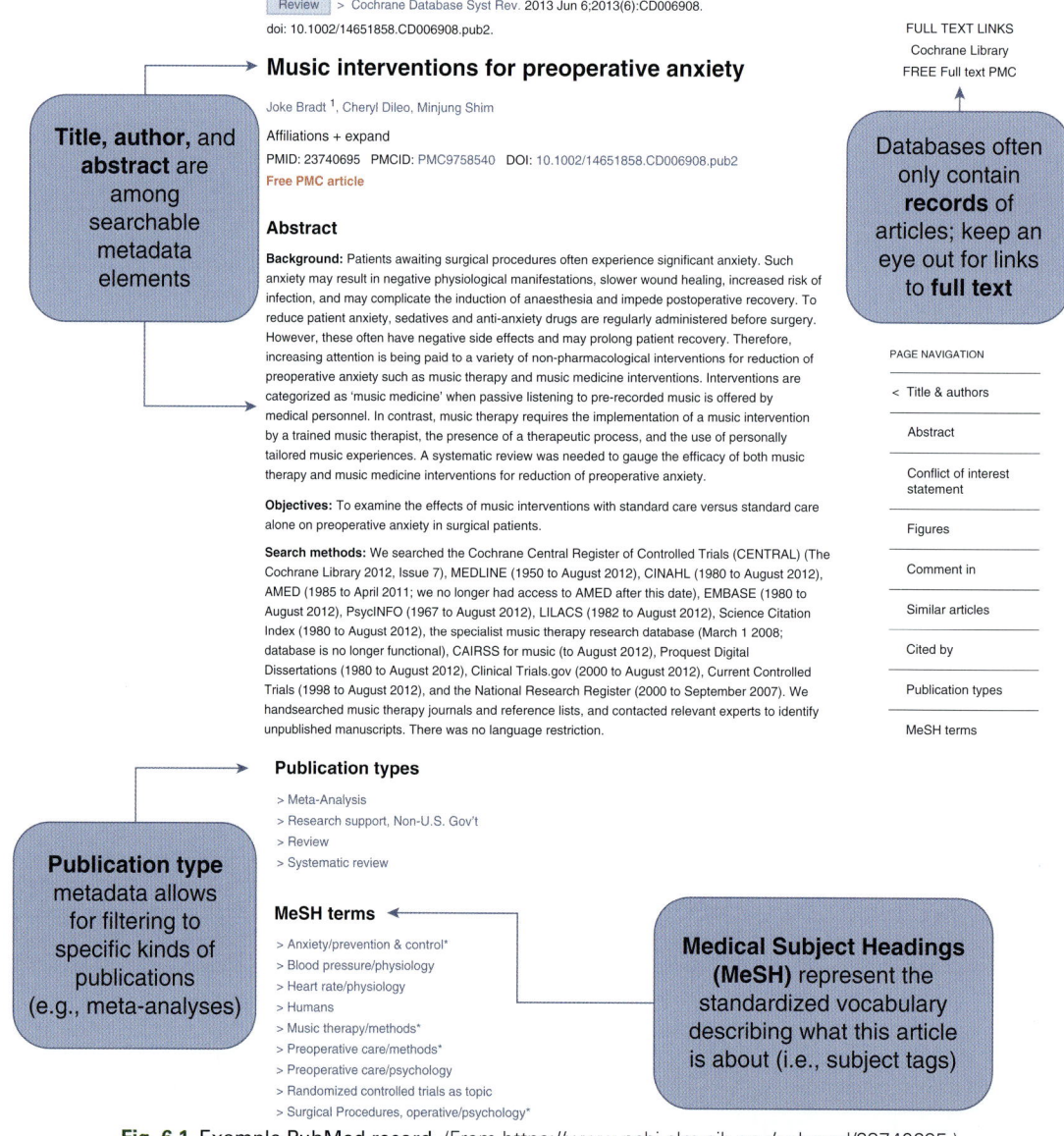

Fig. 6.1 Example PubMed record. (From https://www.ncbi.nlm.nih.gov/pubmed/23740695.)

subject heading tags to ensure researchers will be able to retrieve articles precisely among nuanced scientific concepts. Researchers and nurse clinicians in specialty areas benefit from learning the subject heading terminology in their field in order to make searching more precise and efficient.

Other Tools and Repositories

Beyond the core literature databases for locating health evidence, other types of tools and repositories can lead to valuable discoveries. For specific tools and sources, see Table 6.3.

Institutional and Preprint Repositories

Many research organizations host institutional repositories, which are online collections designed to preserve and share scholarly intellectual output. Scholars can choose to deposit their work into these collections in order to share information about their projects, often including a full manuscript and any associated materials. This material is stably hosted online, and discoverable via web search engines like Google and GoogleScholar. As such, digital repositories are a way for researchers to improve the visibility, accessibility, and utilization of their scholarly output. As an author of a scholarly work, you should consider depositing your finished projects in a repository. There is likely a repository associated with your university, and there may even be a repository specifically for doctor of nursing practice (DNP) projects at your institution. The American Association of Colleges of Nursing (AACN) has recommended that DNP programs employ digital repositories as a way to disseminate students' final DNP projects (AACN, 2015)

As part of a literature search, looking in digital repositories can be a useful way to discover evidence that might be harder to find in traditional literature databases, especially if a search focuses on a known scholar or research area. Moreover, in a health system, identifying other current and past efforts is useful for reducing duplication of effort and networking with colleagues whose areas of interest may align with your own.

Some repositories are not associated with specific institutions, but instead with certain scholarly disciplines. For example, the Sigma Repository is a nursing-specific scholarly archive, and the Social Sciences Research Network (SSRN) is a digital library covering the social sciences. Many of these repositories contain **preprints**, or preliminary versions of scholarly papers that allow authors to share their work rapidly before peer review and formal publication in a journal. There are also repositories that are devoted to preprints (like medRxiv and bioRxiv) where you can find the most recently emerging research, bearing in mind the research reports hosted there may not be peer reviewed.

Data Sets, Health Care Statistics, and Trial Registries

Health data and statistics are collected by government, private, and nonprofit organizations and can be challenging to track down. Some data sources will provide raw data sets (e.g., survey responses) researchers can analyze and interpret, while other sources communicate numeric statistics or facts (e.g.,

TABLE 6.3 Beyond Literature Databases: Other Sources for Discovering Evidence

Institutional and Preprint Repositories
- Sigma Repository (sigma.nursingrepository.org)
- Social Sciences Research Network (SSRN) (www.ssrn.com)
- OpenDOAR (v2.sherpa.ac.uk/opendoar/)
- OSF Preprints (osf.io/preprints/)
- MedRxiv (www.medrxiv.org)
- ASAPbio (asapbio.org/preprint-servers)

Sources for Data and Statistics
- National Center for Health Statistics (www.cdc.gov/nchs/)
- Centers for Medicare and Medicaid Services (www.cms.hhs.gov/)
- World Bank Health Data (data.worldbank.org/topic/health)

Trial Registries
- ClinicalTrials.gov
- World Health Organization ICTRP Search Portal (https://trialsearch.who.int/)

Point-of-Care/Point-of-Service Tools
- UpToDate (Wolters Kluwer)
- Lexicomp (Wolters Kluwer)
- Dynamic Health (EBSCO)

Evidence Awareness Tools and Alert Services
- EvidenceAlerts (www.evidencealerts.com)
- KT+ (KnowledgeTranslation+) (plus.mcmaster.ca/kt/)
- JournalTOCs (www.journaltocs.ac.uk/)
- Trip (Turning Research Into Practice) Database (www.tripdatabase.com)
- Read by QxMD (https://read.qxmd.com/)

rates of prevalence or mortality). Statistical data are often collected within a specific geographic scope to align with city, state, national, or global-level data profiles (e.g., state health departments, the National Center for Health Statistics [https://www.cdc.gov/nchs], or the World Health Organization [https://www.who.int]). The Centers for Medicare and Medicaid Services (CMS) (https://www.cms.gov), in particular, has rich public data sets that complement many nursing research projects.

Additionally, in order to understand the research landscape on a particular topic, particularly on an emerging issue that may lack published studies, it can be helpful to locate in-progress or planned studies. Trial registries like Clinicaltrials.gov and the World Health Organization's International Clinical Trials Registry Platform (ICTRP) contain prospective registrations for studies, and can thus offer insight into research currently being conducted on a topic of interest. The Cochrane Library, well-known for their systematic reviews, also offers a database called CENTRAL, which includes trial registrations from sources like ICTRP and Clinicaltrials.gov.

Point-of-Care Tools

Point-of-care tools (also referred to as point-of-service tools) or **clinical decision support systems** provide synthesized and summarized evidence for common clinical problems, diseases, drugs, and therapies. Clinical decision support tools can increase provider adherence to guidelines and support patient safety goals particularly around medication dosing and interactions. These tools are frequently integrated into clinical workflows or electronic health record systems and are typically subscription based through hospitals and academic health centers. Summarized high-quality evidence, preappraised synopses, care sheets, and patient-level handouts can be invaluable for advanced practice nurses at the "point of service," as well as for graduate student research. Examples of these tools include UpToDate, Nursing Reference Center Plus, Dynamic Health, Lippincott Procedures and Advisor, DynaMed, Lexicomp, Micromedex, and others. These tools are usually offered in desktop, mobile, and clinical workflow formats.

Evidence Awareness Tools, Aggregators, and Alert Services

Current awareness tools are useful to nurses in academic, research, and health care settings. These tools help you keep up with new content as it is published and allow you to focus on a research interest or practice area. Developing skills using these tools and integrating them into your workflow will impact your professional engagement and knowledge of health care trends. Given the dynamic nature of nursing science, nurse scholars can save time by using contemporary current awareness tools to stay up to date. There are a number of knowledge products, tools, and aggregators from which to choose. For example, curated collections of clinically relevant evidence (e.g., KT+, EvidenceAlerts, Read by QxMD) allow users to set email alerts for topics of interest (see Table 6.3). Another approach is to set up "table of contents" alerts from scholarly or clinical journals directly in order to be notified about newly published journal content. Most scholarly literature databases also have features to save searches and receive alerts when new content is published. Researchers, clinicians, and scholars may also socialize articles to share with colleagues through reference management tools (e.g., Zotero, Mendeley) as well as through other channels.

DEFINING YOUR EVIDENCE NEED

Getting started on a literature review can be overwhelming in a project's early stage until the problem comes into focus. In the initial phases of a literature search, it can be helpful to take a step back and reflect on the question very broadly in order to make strategic decisions about where to search, what to look for, and how comprehensively to address the question.

Clinical Questions and Eligibility Criteria

Clinical questions (including Patient, Intervention, Comparison, Outcome, Timing [PICOT] questions) are typically best addressed by evidence from health research studies.

At the beginning of the literature search process, it is useful to consider what kinds of information sources would be eligible to provide evidence for your question. The eligibility criteria, sometimes called inclusion/exclusion criteria, is a set of defined characteristics that a study or article must have in order to provide worthwhile evidence to address a structured clinical question. These characteristics might relate to:

- The focus of the studies themselves (e.g., details about the population, problem, intervention, or issue

being investigated, or geographic details about where the study was conducted)
- The methodology that was used to generate the evidence (e.g., what study designs could provide useful evidence relative to that question)
- The way the evidence was shared (e.g., details about the publication, like peer-reviewed status, or date or language of publication)

For an example of a PICOT question and eligibility criteria, see Table 6.4. Having well-conceptualized eligibility criteria facilitates the process of screening through the literature search results in order to identify relevant evidence. Some databases even allow you to structure your search query in PICOT format (e.g., the Trip database).

> **TIP**
> When considering eligibility criteria for studies, think critically about the importance of information currency. Could older studies be applicable, or does the question at hand require the most up-to-date evidence? It may be helpful to consider how science and practice related to your topic of interest has (or has not) evolved over time, or if there are landmark events that would affect the research on a particular topic (e.g., changes in legislation or policy, the commercial release of a new technology, a disruptive global public health crisis, etc.). When seeking evidence, it is typical to only consider studies from within the last five years, unless there is a good rationale for including older studies.

TABLE 6.4 Example PICOT Question and Eligibility Criteria

PICOT Question

In surgical patients, what is the effect of music therapy on anxiety during the preoperative period, compared to standard care?

Eligibility Criteria

	Include:	Exclude:
Study Focus (PICOT)	**Population:** adult (18+) patients undergoing any kind of surgical procedure in any setting (inpatient or outpatient) **Intervention:** music therapy conducted during the preoperative period **Comparison:** standard care, or another relaxation technique such as meditation, pharmacological therapy, no therapy **Outcome:** preoperative anxiety (as measured by STAI, VAS, NRS) and/or physiological manifestations of anxiety (e.g., heart rate, blood pressure) **Time:** during the period of time between when a patient enters the health care setting for surgery, and the beginning of the surgery	**Population:** dental surgical patients; patients undergoing nonsurgical procedures; pediatric patients **Intervention:** nonmusic, sound interventions (e.g., guided meditation), music interventions only implemented during or after the surgical procedure **Outcome:** anxiety measured with scale lacking established validity/reliability **Time:** the time before the patient enters the health care facility for the surgery
Study and Publication Characteristics	• Studies published in peer-reviewed journals • Quantitative research, of any empirical methodology, including quasi-experimental • Studies published in English • Studies published from 2018 to 2023	• Non–peer-reviewed study reports • Pilot studies • Theoretical literature, modeling studies • Descriptive research • Qualitative research • Editorials, opinions, commentaries • Conference proceedings/abstracts • Narrative reviews, integrative reviews, reviews of qualitative studies

NRS, Numerical Rating Scale; *STAI*, State-Trait Anxiety Inventory; *VAS*, visual analog scale.

Background Questions

Good PICOT questions, with clearly defined eligibility criteria, are informed by foundational background knowledge. Researchers can strengthen their projects by asking important background questions that provide a broader context in which the question is situated. Background questions illuminate the breadth and depth of the topic. Developing understanding of a new topic may include:

- Investigating the current "state of the science"
- Tracing the development of a theory
- Seeking statistics regarding the prevalence or incidence of a problem or disease on a global, regional, and local level
- Investigating the broader social forces behind a health care phenomenon
- Identifying issues around a parallel problem in a different industry
- Identifying highly cited works and thought leaders
- Seeking the history of a disease or an intervention across diverse populations or settings
- Conducting reconnaissance on the breadth and depth of the literature on a general topic
- Locating conceptual or operational definitions for your problem, population, intervention, or outcome of interest

Information gleaned from background questions can be used to refine PICOT questions and eligibility criteria. Background questions are often best addressed by secondary sources like review articles, guidelines, evidence summaries, recent textbooks, care sheets, preappraised overviews, or governmental and organizational reports. Researchers develop nuanced understanding of their problem through background questions. Scoping searches, identifying broad existing evidence or a research gap, are an important beginning step to developing a well-crafted literature search.

> **TIP**
>
> While it is not appropriate to rely exclusively on web-scale search tools for literature searching, search engines like Google or GoogleScholar are very useful for identifying formative background evidence as part of an initial scoping search.

TECHNIQUES FOR SEARCHING DATABASES

Approaching a Search: Considering Sensitivity and Specificity

Within clinical practice, sensitivity and specificity are terms that describe diagnostic tests, or the confidence in results of test results. The concepts of sensitivity and specificity translate to the literature search process by describing the narrowness or breadth of a search. For example, a clinical leader might be looking for a single, high-quality source to inform a clinical decision, or perhaps they might have a very discrete and well-defined question (e.g., the diagnostic criteria for a condition, or the appropriate dosage for a drug). In these instances, it would be appropriate to conduct a specific search, or one that is relatively narrow and targeted in order to retrieve only highly relevant sources.

Conversely, an exhaustive literature review (particularly a systematic-style or comprehensive literature review) calls for a more sensitive search, because the objective is to capture all the available evidence on a topic (Bramer et al., 2018). Sensitive searches require broad, expansive approaches to attempt to locate all references relevant to the topic of interest, followed by a more extensive process of manually screening through the results.

Both these approaches to searching have advantages and drawbacks. When you search in a very narrow (specific) way, you do not necessarily have to spend a lot of time screening through irrelevant sources and may locate high-quality sources quickly. But you also run the risk of missing useful sources if they do not exactly match the specific way that you searched. When you search in a very broad (sensitive) way, you can be more confident that you are not missing anything relevant, but you will also have to spend more time screening through irrelevant sources, or **false hits** (results that are retrieved by your search because they technically fit your search criteria, but are not actually relevant to your needs). Very often, searching for literature involves balancing both specificity and sensitivity—whether you prioritize sensitivity or specificity will be determined by the overall purpose that is driving you to search the literature in the first place.

> **TIP**
>
> When you have an information need that will inform immediate patient care, it is often necessary to search in a very specific way, seeking a presynthesized evidence source like an evidence summary; point-of-care tools can be useful sources for this kind of search.

Getting Started: Identifying Core Search Concepts and Descriptive Vocabulary

Core Concepts and Finding Search Terms

An effective literature search begins by clarifying a question's core concepts and brainstorming vocabulary that describes the concepts and related issues. Researchers typically design an initial search around two or three primary concepts that are central to the research question being investigated. For example, consider the PICOT question, "In surgical patients, what is the effect of music therapy on anxiety during the preoperative period, compared to standard care?" Within this PICOT question, there are essentially three core concepts that could be used to organize a search for literature: *preoperative surgical patients*, *music therapy*, and *anxiety*. An effective database search will find the overlap between those three concepts. Alternatively, researchers might explore a combination of two concepts broadly at first (anxiety and music therapy) and then focus the search if needed.

Generally speaking, it is good practice to develop database searches building on relevant terms from the *Patient/Problem/Participant/Population* and *Intervention* concepts. After screening through each potentially relevant record and full text, one can determine if an article meets all PICOT and eligibility criteria. Searching for too many concepts simultaneously can be too limiting, yielding no relevant results. Recall that databases are typically collections of records that describe articles, not the articles themselves. Therefore, the most effective literature search strategies will reflect ways of finding the search concepts through the record's metadata fields (e.g., title, abstract, author-supplied keywords, or subject headings).

After the core search concepts are established, the next step is to brainstorm related **keywords**. Keywords are free text words or phrases that describe an idea in multiple ways. A quick preliminary search, or scoping search, is a good way to identify keywords, understand trends, and get a sense of the scale of a particular topic. After a few scoping searches, notice the most relevant articles; what language describes the key concepts of interest? It can be helpful to reverse-engineer a search by examining a few relevant articles for terminology clues around the problem, and then using the terms found in those articles and their database records to build a better search.

> **TIP**
>
> Creating a detailed concept table (see Fig. 6.2A) helps track search terms and document the search strategy, which is important content to include in the methods section when you are writing up the findings from a literature review.

Selecting useful keywords and synonyms is an iterative process, and is driven by a researcher's understanding of the topic and the language used in the literature. With that said, there are some general best practices for choosing keywords to include in a search strategy: avoiding value-laden terms that might introduce bias, considering both antonyms and synonyms for search concepts, and including abbreviations, acronyms, or variant spellings (see Fig. 6.3 for tips related to selecting search keywords).

Identifying Subject Headings

In addition to identifying relevant keywords for core concepts of a literature search, a strong and comprehensive search will also employ controlled vocabulary subject headings. Subject heading terms are database-specific and vary among different databases (see Table 6.2). As relevant literature emerges through keyword searches, researchers may note what subject headings are tagged for those relevant article records. Relevant articles retrieved outside of academic databases (e.g., through GoogleScholar, or by following a citation in a reference list) are also useful; looking up those citations in a health literature database will show which subject headings or indexing terms are used. Another way to identify subject headings directly is to explore a database's thesaurus

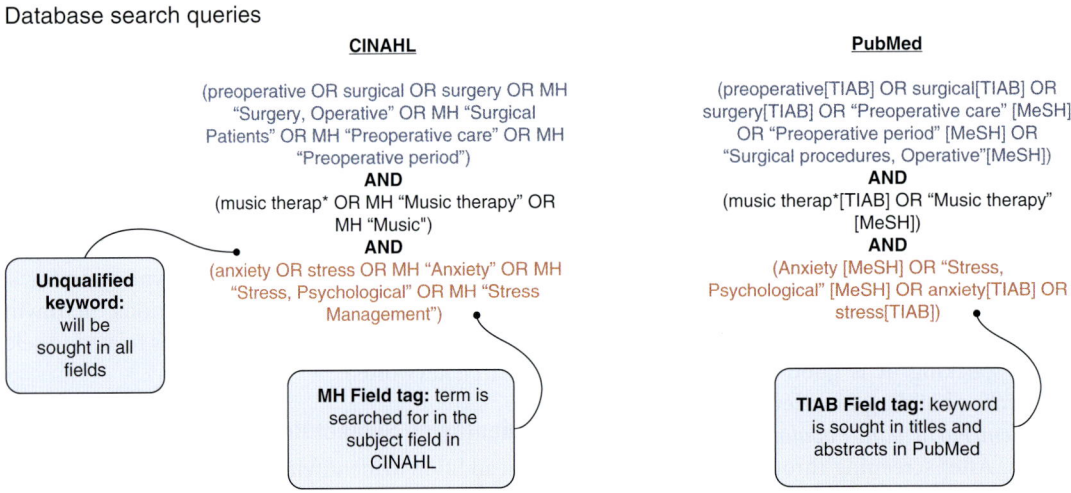

Fig. 6.2 Alignment Between (A) PICOT Question, Search Criteria, and (B) Database Search Queries.

(e.g., MeSH) to understand how subjects are described and organized in that database. A subject heading's "scope note" for the term clarifies how that heading is defined and used.

Structuring a Search Query

Literature search projects often begin with experimentation and then come into focus after researchers identify key terminology and published works. Building on the initial scoping phase, a number of techniques can bring structure, reproducibility, and efficiency to the search. Using Boolean operators, specific punctuation, and field tags will build a more explicit, structured search. The series of terms, Boolean operators, field tags, and punctuation used in a database search, is called a search string or **search query**. In an ideal project, there will be alignment between the clinical question, the selected search concepts, and the structured search query strings (Fig. 6.2B).

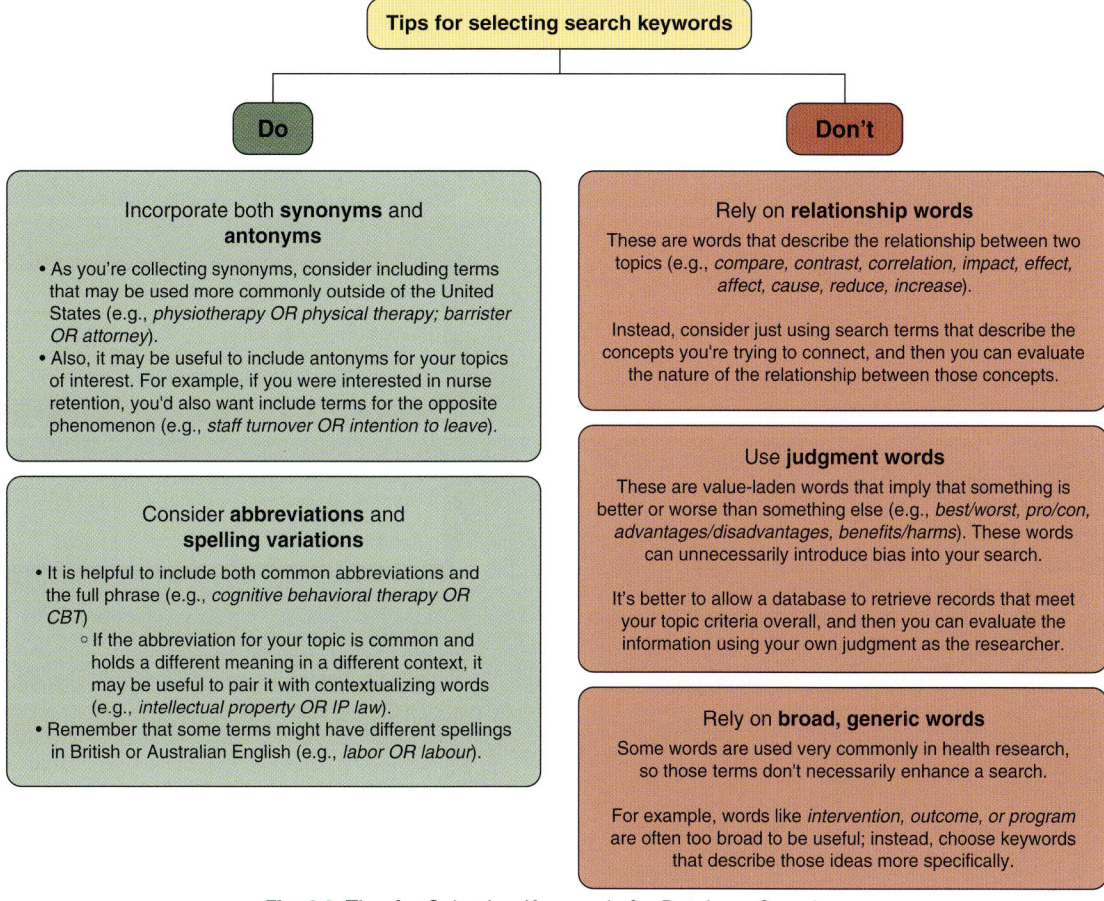

Fig. 6.3 Tips for Selecting Keywords for Database Searches.

> **TIP**
>
> Developing complex database searches is a skill that improves with practice and coaching, and it gets easier over time. Ask for advice from a librarian or knowledgeable colleague who can provide feedback and suggestions about your approach.

Boolean Operators and Punctuation

Combining Boolean operators (also called connectors), nesting, and certain punctuation marks provide search processing instructions within a database search platform (Fig. 6.4). The operator OR strings together the synonymous keyword terms and subject headings that describe a single concept of interest (e.g., *surgery OR surgical procedure*). Two or more different core search concepts are then connected with the AND operator (for instance, the P and I concept from a PICOT question like *music therapy AND anxiety*). While there is some variety among databases, there are a few techniques that are common, like phrase searching using quotation marks and using wildcard characters (e.g., an asterisk) to account for unknown characters or variant word endings.

Field Tags and Unqualified Searching

Field tags, also known as field codes or search tags, are short codes that can be added to search terms to specify which field of the database record the term should appear in. For example, in PubMed, a search for *"Health Status Disparities"(MeSH)* uses the field code (MeSH) to only retrieve records where the phrase "Health Status Disparities" is listed in the subject (MeSH) field of the record.

If no field tags are used in a search, the database search engine will typically look for the search terms in multiple fields of the record (e.g., in the title, the abstract, the

Boolean Operators and Punctuation to Structure Search Queries

AND
Retrieve results that include all terms

Tips: Use AND to narrow a search: the more terms/concept sets connected with AND, the smaller the results pool will be

Search query	Results
diabetes AND exercise	29,000
diabetes AND exercise AND metformin	900

OR
Retrieve results that include any of the linked terms

Tips: Use OR to expand a search: the more alternate terms/synonyms that are connected with OR, the larger the results pool will be

Search query	Results
exercise	19,500
exercise OR physical activity	25,000
exercise OR physical activity OR fitness	27,000

Proximity/Adjacency
AJNn / Nn / NEAR/n / W/n

Retrieve results when the search terms occur within a certain number of words (n) of each other.

Tips: Different database platforms use different proximity operators; check database-specific guidance

Search query*	Results
health AND inequalities	16,000
health N3 inequalities	7,700

*In CINAHL (EBSCO) *health N3 inequalities* finds results that have a maximum of three words between health and Inequalities. Results might contain phrases like: "inequalities in health," "health care inequalities," "Inequalities related to health"

Parentheses ( )
Designate priority or order of operations in retrieval of terms

Tips: Keep sets of synonyms (OR'd together) grouped within parentheses

Search query	Results
diabetes AND (exercise OR physical activity)	29,000
diabetes AND exercise OR physical activity	690.000

Without parentheses, the database just reads the query from left to right, so you retrieve records about diabetes and exercise together, or anything about physical activity

Truncation/Wildcards *
Retrieve results that contain root word, with variable ending

Tips: The shorter the root, the more results will be returned, with a greater possibility of irrelevant results. Try to use the longest root possible that will still capture all the desired variations.

Search query	Results
hesitant	700

↳ Returns results with only that form of the word

| hesitan* | 2,100 |

↳ Returns results for "hesitant", but also "hesitance", "hesitate", "hesitancy" etc.

Phrase searching " "
Search for exact, specific phrases

Tips: Use quotation marks around phrases that have a clearly defined, conceptual meaning and do not have variation in grammatical construction

Search query	Results
metabolic syndrome	83,000

↳ Returns results with the words "metabolic" and "syndrome" anywhere in the record

| "metabolic syndrome" | 2,100 |

↳ Only returns results that contain the words "metabolic syndrome" together as a phrase

Fig. 6.4 Boolean Operators and Punctuation to Structure Search Queries.

journal title, the author-supplied keywords, or the subject field). This type of search is known as an unqualified search; different database platforms have different settings for how they treat unqualified searches. In order to be explicit and intentional about what kinds of records are retrieved in your database searches, you can use all these structural elements together to build search queries for each database (Fig. 6.2b).

Refining and Revising a Search
Filters
Database filters, also referred to as limits or limiters, are search tools within a database interface that allow you to restrict your search to only retrieve records that contain specific metadata. For example, a publication date limiter will restrict the search to records if the resource was published within a particular date range. Different database platforms offer different filtering capabilities, depending on the metadata that is present in the database's records. For instance, health-focused databases (like MEDLINE, CINAHL, EMBASE, JBI EBP Database, Trip, and PsycInfo) include metadata that describe the characteristics of the participants in a study. Thus, in these databases it is possible to limit a search by elements like participants' age, sex, or species.

Applying database filters helps focus a search. For example, if you know you are targeting higher levels of evidence only, you could use a database filter for methodology or publication type to see if a meta-analysis has been published on your topic. The extent of filtering you employ will be determined by what kind of search you are performing (intentionally broad, or very specific) and the purpose of your search. Because the metadata in database records can occasionally be incorrect or incomplete, if you are attempting a comprehensive search, it is better to filter sparingly.

Additional Strategies for Narrowing or Broadening
Constructing an effective database search is a highly iterative process. You are likely to strategically refine and edit your search based on the relevance and number of results you retrieve. There are a number of strategies you can employ to revise your database searches (see Fig. 6.5). In addition to applying database filters, if you find that you need to focus your search, you can also revise the structure of your search query to narrow your results. Some suggested techniques include: adding an additional concept with AND, experimenting with quotation marks for phrase searching, using a field tag to restrict your terms to just certain database fields, or selecting a more specific subject heading.

If your initial searches are too narrow, see if there are any search terms that would benefit from wildcard punctuation (e.g., plural or variant terms), and make certain that you have identified all the appropriate synonyms for your concepts and included them in the search query with OR. This practice is particularly important when you are trying to build a broader, more sensitive search.

Finally, **snowballing** can be a useful phase in searching for literature, especially when you are attempting to be comprehensive with the way that you search. For a "snowballing" search, you can follow up on citations in the reference list of a highly relevant article, as well as perform **cited reference searching** to see what other literature has cited that article since it was published. There are several databases and search platforms that allow you to perform cited reference searching, including Web of Science, GoogleScholar, CINAHL, and PubMed.

When Are You Finished?
A literature search for a nursing science project may not always have a clear endpoint. Although some types of searches will have very clear, unambiguous parameters (e.g., articles limited to a defined date range, a search to address a discrete and answerable question), most do not. Instead, researchers can have confidence in their search results by following a methodical framework in multiple databases that are appropriate for the question.

If your search has been revised, restructured, and refined and yet the same citations are retrieved or nothing new is found, you have likely reached a point of **saturation**. Although a question can be complex and possibly endlessly revisable, a scholarly project is really a snapshot in time as defined by you as the nurse project leader. Your work will be evaluated on the rigor of your methodology and the transparency of process, which ensures the science can be reproducible and verified. Contemporary nursing science must be held to a high standard and communicate the significance of the new knowledge developed, so that it can be translated into practice.

DOCUMENTING, SCREENING, AND ORGANIZING RESULTS
Saving Search Strategies
Most of the core health sciences databases offer you the option of creating an account to save your own searches.

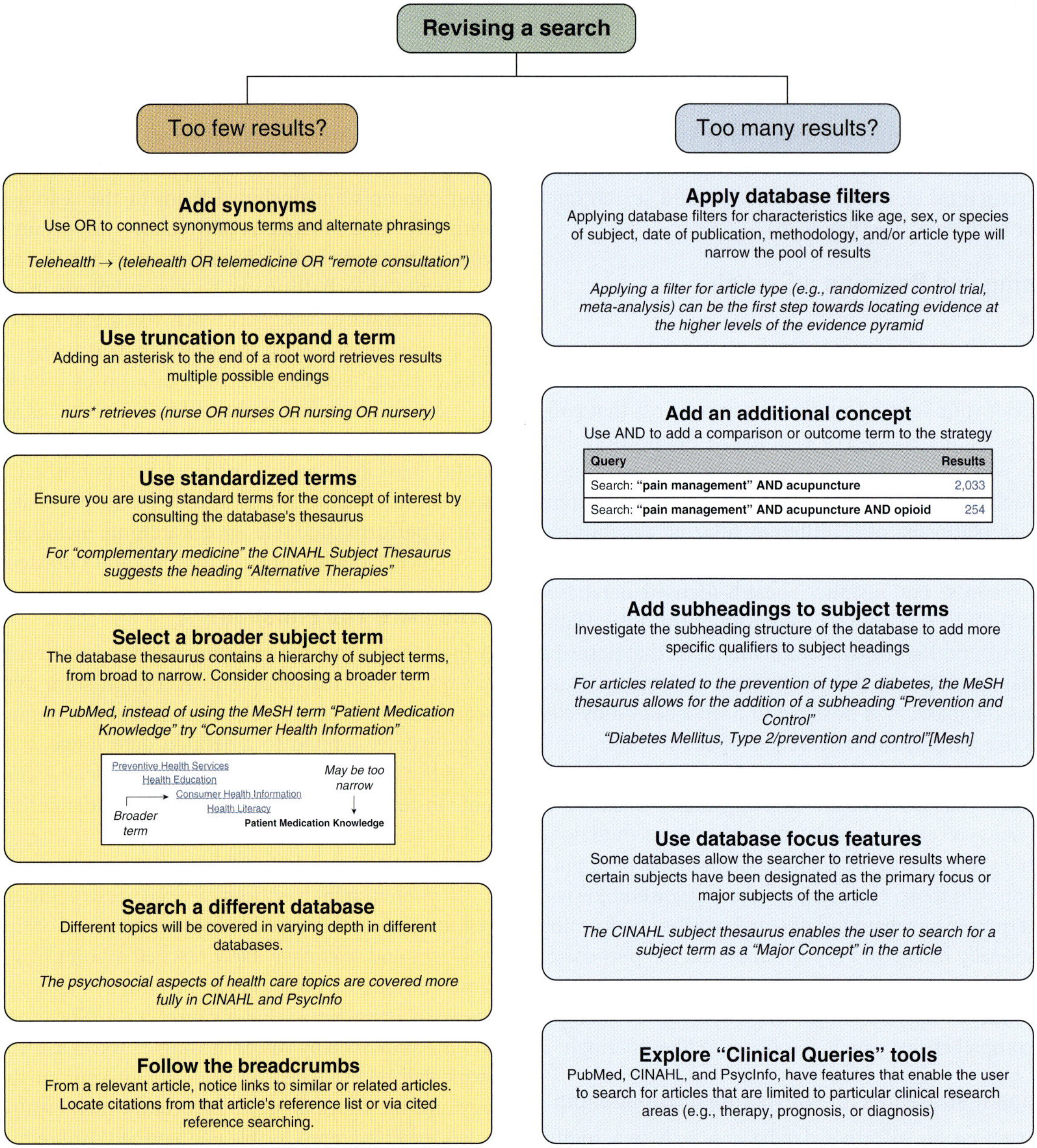

Revising a search

Too few results?

Add synonyms
Use OR to connect synonymous terms and alternate phrasings

Telehealth → (telehealth OR telemedicine OR "remote consultation")

Use truncation to expand a term
Adding an asterisk to the end of a root word retrieves results multiple possible endings

nurs* retrieves (nurse OR nurses OR nursing OR nursery)

Use standardized terms
Ensure you are using standard terms for the concept of interest by consulting the database's thesaurus

For "complementary medicine" the CINAHL Subject Thesaurus suggests the heading "Alternative Therapies"

Select a broader subject term
The database thesaurus contains a hierarchy of subject terms, from broad to narrow. Consider choosing a broader term

In PubMed, instead of using the MeSH term "Patient Medication Knowledge" try "Consumer Health Information"

```
Preventive Health Services          May be too
   Health Education                    narrow
     Consumer Health Information
        Health Literacy
Broader                      Patient Medication Knowledge
 term
```

Search a different database
Different topics will be covered in varying depth in different databases.

The psychosocial aspects of health care topics are covered more fully in CINAHL and PsycInfo

Follow the breadcrumbs
From a relevant article, notice links to similar or related articles. Locate citations from that article's reference list or via cited reference searching.

Too many results?

Apply database filters
Applying database filters for characteristics like age, sex, or species of subject, date of publication, methodology, and/or article type will narrow the pool of results

Applying a filter for article type (e.g., randomized control trial, meta-analysis) can be the first step towards locating evidence at the higher levels of the evidence pyramid

Add an additional concept
Use AND to add a comparison or outcome term to the strategy

Query	Results
Search: "pain management" AND acupuncture	2,033
Search: "pain management" AND acupuncture AND opioid	254

Add subheadings to subject terms
Investigate the subheading structure of the database to add more specific qualifiers to subject headings

For articles related to the prevention of type 2 diabetes, the MeSH thesaurus allows for the addition of a subheading "Prevention and Control"
"Diabetes Mellitus, Type 2/prevention and control"[Mesh]

Use database focus features
Some databases allow the searcher to retrieve results where certain subjects have been designated as the primary focus or major subjects of the article

The CINAHL subject thesaurus enables the user to search for a subject term as a "Major Concept" in the article

Explore "Clinical Queries" tools
PubMed, CINAHL, and PsycInfo, have features that enable the user to search for articles that are limited to particular clinical research areas (e.g., therapy, prognosis, or diagnosis)

Fig. 6.5 Strategies for Refining Database Searches. (Modified from Campbell & Jacobs, 2021.)

Additionally, you may find it useful to copy your search queries into an external document, especially if you need to report how you structured your search in a reproducible way as part of a literature review manuscript. When you need to report your search strategy in a way that is reproducible, be sure that you note:

- The name and platform of the database you searched (e.g., CINAHL via EBSCO or PsycInfo via PsycNET)
- The search terms you used
- How those terms were combined with Boolean operators (ANDs/ORs)

- The database-specific syntax you used
  - If you searched specific fields using field tags (e.g., the subject field, using the tag MH), be sure to report that (and if you did not specify the field, it is likely you searched for terms in "all fields," or whatever the database platform default is)
- Database-specific punctuation you used
- What filters were applied, if any
- The date you performed the search

Managing and Screening Records

In addition to documenting the search queries that you use in each database, it can be important to save relevant records throughout the search process. With a database account, you will typically be able to save useful records into a "folder" or "clipboard" of some kind, but a better practice is to use citation management software.

Citation management software, or citation managers, are applications (either web based, or downloaded as programs onto your computer) that allow you to create your own central library of bibliographic records, collected from disparate sources like literature databases, web pages, and library catalogs. Citation managers allow you to organize relevant literature into different folders or collections, take notes, and attach the PDF of the article to the bibliographic record. Additionally, most citation managers will integrate with word processors (e.g., Microsoft Word or GoogleDocs), enabling you to insert in-text citations and reference lists in the citation style of your choosing. Some citation managers require a personal or institutional subscription (e.g., EndNote, RefWorks, Paperpile), while others are free, with additional storage available to purchase, like Mendeley and Zotero.

> **TIP**
>
> Citation management software is invaluable for helping you stay efficient and organized as you locate literature, but as with any new tool, it may take a bit of time to learn the functions of the program. As such, it is a good idea to pick a citation manager early in your scholarly career in order to allow yourself sufficient time to get accustomed to how it works and how to integrate it into your workflow.

If you are working on an evidence synthesis project, where you will need to carefully document the number of records you screen through and your inclusion decisions, it may also be helpful to be aware of literature review screening tools like Covidence, DistillerSR, and Rayyan. These are specialized software applications that are designed to help teams move through the screening and data management processes necessary for systematic-style reviews.

Citation managers and systematic screening tools are particularly important if you plan to report the results of your literature searching with a search flow diagram. These **literature search flow diagrams** (sometimes called PRISMA diagrams because of their use as part of the Preferred Reporting Items for Systematic Reviews and Meta-Analyses) are graphical depictions of the literature identification process for systematic and systematic-style review. Creating this diagram provides a snapshot of the sources searched, the numbers of citations screened after duplicates were removed, and the application of eligibility criteria to select the included studies; such diagrams are often a requirement for publishing the results of a systematic review or an integrative review. Creating a search flow diagram requires careful record keeping, and almost always requires the use of a citation manager or systematic screening tool.

> **TIP**
>
> When you are working on a team to review the literature, consider using a citation management tool that offers collaboration features, like shared reference libraries. Additionally, tools like Covidence are designed to support team-based workflows for screening literature for systematic and systematic-style reviews.

APPRAISING AND SYNTHESIZING THE EVIDENCE

Critical Appraisal

Not all evidence is created equal. While identifying research that has been published in peer-reviewed journals may be a valuable initial step in identifying high-quality research, do not assume that just because a study's written report has passed peer review the study itself was conducted in an unbiased way, or contains results that are clinically significant. As such, critical appraisal is a crucial part of the evidence gathering process. When you have gathered a body of research evidence that addresses your clinical question of interest, you will need to appraise these articles to determine the quantity, quality, consistency, and strength of the existing evidence. You should pay attention to key elements like how well the research method fits the research question, how the authors controlled for bias, and how the results may be clinically significant and applicable to practice. Critical appraisal criteria for specific study designs are found in Chapters 7 to 11.

> **TIP**
>
> Journal clubs are important in both academic and practice settings for nurse clinicians and scientists to discuss newly published works. Discussing and critically analyzing recent research evidence with your peers and colleagues is an excellent way to develop fluency in appraising and interpreting evidence, reflect on applicability to practice, and stay up to date on the most recent developments in your field.

Extracting Data from Studies and Synthesizing Findings

Beyond critically appraising studies as sources of evidence, it is helpful to systematically extract the data from a study that will help answer a clinical question. It is common to extract information from each included study that pertains to the elements of a PICOT question. For instance, for a question of therapy effectiveness, for each study you might record information about the population that was studied, as well as the details of the intervention and what outcomes were measured.

When pertinent data have been extracted from each study, a synthesis of the overall strengths and weaknesses of the studies as a group should be developed. The purpose of synthesizing a body of critically appraised evidence is to establish the state of the science for answering your PICOT question and provide an evidence-based foundation on which to base practice and standards of care.

Recommendations to validate current practice or to adopt a sustained change in practice require a careful evaluation and synthesis of the evidence, one that challenges you as clinicians, educators, and administrators to inform your decision making with the best available evidence (Berkman et al., 2013; Albarqouni, 2018).

Table 6.5 illustrates the features of data from studies that may be included in a synthesis evidence table.

Nurses who are searching for and synthesizing evidence often ask, "How many studies do I need to include in my synthesis?" While there is rarely a one-size-fits-all answer, ideally, synthesis of a group of studies provides a sufficient quantity of high-quality, consistent evidence to make one of the following recommendations: (1) validate current practice, (2) make a minor change in practice, or (3) make major change in practice. The synthesis also may reveal evidence that is inadequate or too weak to support a recommendation for a practice change.

There is a debate (Suri, 2013) about the practice of including only high-quality studies, such as systematic reviews (see Chapter 10) and randomized clinical trials (see Chapter 8) to answer a PICOT question and include in an evidence synthesis. On one hand, you and your team always search for studies that provide the highest level and strongest evidence. On the other hand, the state of the science may be that there is a paucity of high-quality studies. Observational studies, those that use a cohort or case-control design, may be those that offer the strongest evidence (see Chapter 9). As such, inconsistent findings and/or studies with multiple threats to internal and external validity may represent the "best available evidence." In that case, an evidence synthesis is particularly important because you will use it to inform your decision making about clinical issues as well as allocation of financial and human resources.

> **TIP**
>
> Remember that the PICOT question drives what information is included and considered in the synthesis of individual studies. Project partners in nursing often share responsibility for developing and reviewing a table of evidence in order to advance projects in the practice setting. A table of evidence can be used in different ways, but it is often an abbreviated framework for reviewing literature related to a clinical question.

It is common to present the results of evidence synthesis in a tabular format (sometimes called a synthesis table, or table of evidence). When developing a synthesis table, consider the following recommendations:

- Decide which study components make sense to include in the synthesis table
- Include verbatim information from each study (you can avoid synthesis bias by not paraphrasing or interpreting what was stated by the researcher)
- Develop an organization strategy for the table (e.g., listing studies in chronological order, according to their level of evidence, or by study methodology)
- Include all of the critically appraised studies in the evidence table
- Compare and contrast similar components across studies to determine the overall strength or weakness of that component (e.g., compare sampling strategies or type of design)

The synthesis table, as presented in Table 6.5, enables you and your team to view, at a glance, the critical appraisal data from each study, as well as the comparison information that keeps you focused on comparing and contrasting the overall strengths and weaknesses of the studies as a group. When your project team completes the synthesis and considers the set of studies as a whole, you will draft a narrative evidence synthesis summary that includes your recommendation about applicability for adoption in practice.

The evidence synthesis summary should consider issues like:
- Design
- Level of evidence
- Clinical significance versus statistical significance
- Fidelity
- Effect size
- Effect on patient outcomes
- Implementation cost
- Ethical issues, if any, related to proposed practice change

For example, in the PICOT question regarding use of a music intervention to decrease adult patients' preoperative anxiety, the evidence synthesis, as illustrated in Table 6.5, highlights that the evidence provided by the studies were of low to moderate quality, had a number of moderate threats to internal validity indicating evidence of bias, and had limitations in external validity, limiting generalizability. For example, the studies provided no evidence of blinding, had inconsistent evidence of power analysis and intervention fidelity, and used different music modalities. However, all of the studies consistently reported a significant decrease in preoperative anxiety. The evidence synthesis concluded that no negative effects were noted, and as such, listening to music may help reduce anxiety in patients waiting for surgery. The recommendation was that preoperative patients can be offered this inexpensive music intervention and should be able to choose the type of music to listen to while waiting to go to surgery.

> **TIP**
>
> When developing an evidence synthesis aimed at answering a clinical question, you need to carefully consider the consistencies as well as the inconsistencies across studies. You will become skilled at identifying what gaps have been filled, what gaps still exist, and what researchers need to focus on to improve the evidence base to answer a specific clinical question.

SYNTHESIS

Overall, a focused search of the literature includes an iterative process of evidence-based practice that supports the process of asking, gathering, assessing, evaluating, and synthesizing research evidence. Your search of the literature should follow a road map for translating background queries and focused clinical questions into a search for evidence, using the suggested core databases and gray literature resources to locate the best available evidence. Critically appraising individual studies and synthesizing the overall strengths and weaknesses of a group of studies requires practice. Repeated, continual engagement in evidence searching, appraising, and synthesizing will help you gain competence with the multiple tools, platforms, and knowledge practices involved in these processes. Navigating the complexity of the literature, while avoiding bias, is a challenge for lifelong learning, and is a valuable skill that informs clinical decision making and supports high-quality, cost-effective, and satisfying evidence-based care.

TABLE 6.5 Evidence Synthesis Data Summary Table

Study Citation	Study Design and Level of Evidence	Risk of Bias	Study Sample	Data Collection[a]	Intervention	Outcomes	Strength, Quality of Findings
(Thompson et al., 2014)	Quasi-experimental Level III	No blinding No random assignment	N = 137 men and women Evidence of fidelity	Pre/posttest using VAS	Music or no music before invasive or noninvasive surgery; no premedication	Significant decrease in preop anxiety	Low No harm
(Bradt et al., 2013)	Systematic review/meta-analysis Level I	High risk for bias—no blinding Some studies had no random assignment Some had no evidence of fidelity	26 RCTs and quasi-experimental studies met the inclusion criteria	State Scale of STAI or VAS	Music or no music before surgery; no premedication	Significant decrease in preop anxiety across studies	Low r/t high risk for bias across studies
(Ni et al., 2012)	RCT Level II	No blinding No evidence of fidelity	N = 183 adult men and women randomly assigned to intervention or control group using computer-generated program	State scale of STAI	Music or no music before ambulatory day surgery; no premedication	Significant decrease in preop anxiety	Low No harm
(Lee et al., 2011)	RCT Level II	No blinding No evidence of fidelity	N = 111 men and women randomly assigned to an intervention or control group using a table of random numbers	VAS	Music or no music before surgery; no premedication	Significant decrease in preop anxiety	Low No harm

RCT, Randomized control trial; STAI, State-Trait Anxiety Inventory; VAS, visual analog scale; r/t, related to.
[a]Including outcome measures.

KEY POINTS

- Research evidence is discovered by searching the published and unpublished literature.
- When searching the literature, you will often need to seek primary and secondary sources.
- Evidence is hierarchical; evidence hierarchies provide a first step to evaluate the strength of research evidence.
- Background sources of evidence include reports, evidence summaries, clinical practice guidelines, abstracts, point-of-care tools, and review articles.
- Tools for organizing, citing, and sharing evidence are important for promoting collaboration on EBP and quality improvement projects.
- Identifying a clinical question can be informed by formulating broad background questions and using secondary sources and point of care tools.
- Core databases like CINAHL, PubMed (MEDLINE), PsycInfo, and EMBASE are essential in searching for primary and secondary sources that provide evidence for developing and answering a clinical PICOT question.
- Searching electronic databases is an iterative process, beginning with selecting a database, conducting an initial search with key terms, and expanding the search using synonyms and subject headings.
- Selecting and critically appraising relevant articles and documents is essential for determining gaps and revising, expanding, or narrowing the search strategy.
- Citation management tools are platforms for downloading citations to build a personal data/article repository that assists you in writing, citing, and formatting written papers.
- Literature search flow diagrams provide a graphical format for depicting the process of completing a literature review in a systematic way, including identifying records from databases, applying eligibility criteria, and identifying studies for inclusion in the review.
- Synthesis of evidence in the service of a PICOT question requires the researcher to identify the overall strengths and weakness of the body of evidence obtained from a literature search, including a process of critical appraisal of a study's methodology.
- Synthesis of the evidence provides the basis for making recommendations about applicability of findings for practice.

REFERENCES

Albarqouni, L., Hoffmann, T., Straus, S., Olsen, N. R., Young, T., Ilic, D., et al. (2018). Core competencies in evidence-based practice for health professionals: Consensus statement based on a systematic review and Delphi survey. *JAMA Network Open*, 1(2):e180281. https://doi.org/10.1001/jamanetworkopen.2018.0281.

American Association of Colleges of Nursing (AACN. (2015). *The Doctor of nursing practice: Current issues and clarifying recommendations*. https://www.aacnnursing.org/Portals/42/DNP/DNP-Implementation.pdf.

Berkman, N. D., Lohr, K. N., Ansari, M., McDonagh, M., Balk, E., Whitlock, E., Reston, J., et al. (2013). *Grading the strength of a body of evidence when assessing health care interventions for the effective health care program of the agency for healthcare research and quality: An update (AHRQ Publication 13(14)-EHC130-EF)*. Agency for Healthcare Research and Quality. https://effectivehealthcare.ahrq.gov/products/methods-guidance-grading-evidence/methods.

Bradt, J., Dileo, C., & Shim, M. (2013). Music interventions for preoperative anxiety. *Cochrane Database of Systematic Reviews*, 6. https://doi.org/10.1002/14651858.CD006908.pub2.

Bramer, W. M., de Jonge, G. B., Rethlefsen, M. L., Mast, F., & Kleijnen, J. (2018). A systematic approach to searching: An efficient and complete method to develop literature searches. *Journal of the Medical Library Association*, 106(4), 531–541. https://doi.org/10.5195/jmla.2018.283.

Campbell, B. A., & Jacobs, S. K. (2021). Gathering and appraising the literature. In G. LoBiondo-Wood, & J. Haber (Eds.), *Nursing research: Methods and critical appraisal for evidence-based practice* (10th ed.) (pp. 47–70). Elsevier.

Lee, K.-C., Chao, Y.-H., Yiin, J.-J., Chiang, P.-Y., & Chao, Y.-F. (2011). Effectiveness of different music-playing devices for reducing preoperative anxiety: A clinical control study. *International Journal of Nursing Studies*, 48(10), 1180–1187. https://doi.org/10.1016/j.ijnurstu.2011.04.001.

Ni, C.-H., Tsai, W.-H., Lee, L.-M., Kao, C.-C., & Chen, Y.-C. (2012). Minimising preoperative anxiety with music for day surgery patients—a randomised clinical trial.

Journal of Clinical Nursing, 21(5–6), 620–625. https://doi.org/10.1111/j.1365-2702.2010.03466.x.

Suri, H. (2013). *Towards methodologically inclusive research syntheses: Expanding possibilities*. Routledge.

Thompson, M., Moe, K., & Lewis, C. P. (2014). The effects of music on diminishing anxiety among preoperative patients. *Journal of Radiology Nursing, 33*(4), 199–202. https://doi.org/10.1016/j.jradnu.2014.10.005.

Principles of Assessing Research Quality

Geri LoBiondo-Wood and Barbara Delmore

LEARNING OUTCOMES

After reading this chapter, you should be able to do the following:
- Analyze how a study's design type affects evaluation and interpretation of the findings.
- Compare and contrast elements that affect the evaluation and fidelity of a study's findings.
- Identify threats to internal validity.
- Analyze how threats to internal validity can affect interpretation of a study's findings.
- Identify external validity threats.
- Analyze conditions that affect external validity and interpretation of a study's findings.
- Identify links between study design and evidence-based practice.

KEY TERMS

Bias
Constancy
Control
Control group
Dependent variable
Experimental group
External validity
Extraneous variable
Generalizability
History
Homogeneity
Independent variable
Instrumentation
Internal validity
Intervening variable
Intervention fidelity
Maturation
Measurement effect
Mortality
Randomization
Reactivity
Selection bias
Testing

After the development of a PICOT question and search of the literature, the next phase of a practice change involves critically appraising the identified studies. How a researcher structures, implements, or designs a study affects the study's results, appraisal, and, ultimately, application of the results to practice. Understanding the implications and usefulness of a study for evidence-based practice (EBP) requires understanding key research design issues. This chapter provides an overview of key issues related to assessing the strength and quality of quantitative research designs. Chapters 8 through 11 present specific design types and important critical appraisal principles for assessing scientific quality and practice applicability of quantitative designs related to threats to control and internal and external validity. Evaluation of research findings requires an evaluation of individual studies as well as a synthesis evaluation of the collective group of studies investigating the same topic (see Chapter 6).

ISSUES RELATING TO MAXIMIZING APPLICABILITY OF FINDINGS TO PRACTICE

Let's suppose that you have developed an intervention-focused PICOT question, and during your search of the literature, you locate and retrieve several randomized controlled trials (RCTs). You may think, "Eureka! My search is complete; now I can answer my clinical question." Actually, this is not the case. You will need to evaluate each study to assess its overall scientific quality, including the design, sample type and size, measurement instruments, data collection, and data analysis methods. You will also need to evaluate the studies as a collective group by synthesizing the overall strengths, quality, and consistency of the evidence provided by the studies retrieved (see Chapter 6). When thinking about your synthesis, keep in mind that you may have a collection of studies that include different design types and methods to answer the same PICOT question. The overall goal is to critically appraise each component of the individual studies found in your search, synthesize the findings across studies, and then determine applicability of the findings to practice. This chapter presents quantitative design elements that affect the application of findings to practice.

Elements of quantitative research designs include the following:

- Assessing how the research team conceptualized and tested the hypothesis or research question
- Assessing how the research team maintained control in the study
- Assessing threats to internal and external validity

The design, coupled with the methods and analysis, provides control for the study. **Control** is defined as the measures that the researcher uses to hold the conditions of the study consistent, thereby minimizing possible **bias** (any influencing factor that may change a study's results) in selection of participants, **randomization** or assignment to **experimental groups** and **control groups**, and error in the measurement of the **dependent variable**(s) (outcome variable). Control measures help control threats to the study's internal and external validity and applicability of findings to practice. Internal validity is the degree to which one can infer that the intervention (independent variable), rather than another condition or variable, resulted in the outcome (dependent variable) or observed effects. External validity is the degree to which findings can be generalized to other populations or environments. As you review studies for application to practice, you will need to make judgments about the quality of the studies. Be aware that it may not be possible to avoid validity threats, both internal and external. You will need to assess how the threats were minimized, how seriously they affect the credibility of the findings, and how the researchers, in the discussion of the findings of the article, account for any internal or external validity issues that may have occurred. Control is weighted and assessed according to the level of the designs (see the discussion on evidence hierarchy in Chapter 3).

An example that demonstrates how the design can address a research question and maintain control is illustrated in the study by Yap and colleagues (2022). Yap and colleagues (2022) conducted an embedded, pragmatic cluster RCT addressing repositioning protocols in nine nursing homes. The study's aim was to determine if the standard 2-hour repositioning schedule to prevent pressure injuries could be extended to 3 or 4 hours without compromising patients. A wearable device helped prompt staff for when to reposition the patient. There were three arms in this study and each arm consisted of a repositioning interval (2, 3, or 4 hours). Nursing homes were assigned to an arm using randomized sequencing so that three nursing homes were in each arm. Each repositioning interval (arm) was executed in a chronological sequence so that each arm could be safely implemented over 4 weeks. The interventions were clearly defined. The authors also discuss how **intervention fidelity**—faithfulness or constancy of the intervention as planned—was maintained during the delivery of the intervention and data collection. First, each nursing home included in the study met a standard care delivery policy for preventing pressure injuries. Second, within the nursing homes, only residents who met the inclusion criteria participated. Third, nursing home staff received extensive education regarding pressure injury prevention practices and on using the wearable device. Finally, diligent skin assessments were conducted on the residents and recorded during the 4 weeks of the intervention. By establishing nursing home and participant eligibility (inclusion criteria), methods for randomization of a nursing home to an arm, and clearly describing and designing the intervention, the researchers demonstrated that they had a well-developed plan and were able to consistently maintain the study protocol. A variety of considerations, including the chosen design type, affect a study's successful completion and utility for EBP. These considerations include the following:

- Objectively conceptualized research question or hypothesis addressing gaps in the science
- Homogeneous sample

- Data collection constancy
- Intervention fidelity
- Internal validity
- External validity

Statistical principles are associated with the mechanisms of control, but it is more important that you have a clear conceptual understanding of these mechanisms. As you will recall from Chapter 3, a study's design type is linked to a level of evidence. As you appraise the design, you must also take into account other aspects of a study's design and implementation. These aspects are reviewed in this chapter. How the elements of control are applied depends on the type of design (see Chapters 8–11).

AN OBJECTIVELY CONCEPTUALIZED RESEARCH QUESTION

Objectivity in a study begins with a review of the scientific literature. Researchers assess the depth and breadth of available knowledge about a question that, in turn, affects the design chosen. For example, the research question "What is the optimal length of a teaching program to promote adherence to oral cancer medication?" may suggest an experimental design (RCT; see Chapter 8), whereas the question "What are the symptoms and coping strategies of children with cancer?" suggests an observational design (see Chapter 9).

> **TIP**
>
> When reading a study, the literature review that incorporates all aspects of the question allows you to judge the objectivity of the research question and assess whether the design matches the question.
> A thorough review of the literature also identifies gaps that indicate a need for research.

HOMOGENEOUS SAMPLE

The characteristics of a study's participants/sample such as age, sex, and health history are common **extraneous variables** or variables that may confound a study's outcome. Extraneous variables may also be referred to as *confounding variables*. For example, in the study by Yap and colleagues (2022), the researchers ensured **homogeneity** of the sample by including nursing homes and residents that met specific criteria (inclusion criteria). This step limits the **generalizability** or application of the outcomes only to similar populations when applying the outcomes (see Chapter 8). As you read studies, you will often find that researchers limit their statements about generalizability of the findings to like samples.

As a control for these and similar problems, the researcher's participants should demonstrate homogeneity or similarity with respect to minimizing extraneous variables relevant to the particular study (see Chapter 8). Extraneous variables are not fixed but must be reviewed and decided on according to the study's purpose. By having a sample of homogeneous participants, based on inclusion and exclusion criteria, a researcher has a straightforward approach to maximizing control.

DATA COLLECTION CONSTANCY

A critical component of control is **constancy** in data collection. The concept of constancy refers to the methods used to maintain sameness in data collection. That is, data should be collected in the same way from each participant under the same conditions. This means that environmental conditions, timing of data collection, data collection instruments, and data collection procedures used to collect data are the same for each participant. The degree to which researchers maintain constancy in data collection is known as **fidelity**. In observational studies or nonexperimental studies, constancy of data collection is achieved through the use of a homogeneous sample and consistent data collection procedures. If a study includes an intervention, data collection constancy and implementation (or delivery of an intervention as planned) help ensure intervention fidelity.

INTERVENTION FIDELITY

Researchers choose a design that is consistent with the research question or hypothesis and maximizes the degree of control, fidelity, or uniformity of the study methods. Control is maximized by a well-planned study that considers each step of the research process and the potential threats to internal and external validity. Intervention studies are used to test whether a treatment or intervention affects patient outcomes. The use of a control group in intervention studies is related to the aim of the study (see Chapter 8). Observational studies do not test an intervention or manipulate the **independent** variable but rather are fixed such as in a retrospective case-control design (Thiese, 2014).

In studies that test an intervention, manipulation of the independent variable is used as a means of control. This refers to the administration of a program, treatment, or intervention to only one group within the study and not to the other participants in the study. The first group is known as the experimental group or intervention group, and the other group is known as the control group. In a control group, the variables under study are held at a constant or comparison level.

Researchers choose a design that is consistent with the research question and maximizes the degree of control, **fidelity,** or uniformity of the study methods. Control is maximized by a well-planned study that considers each step of the research process and the potential threats to internal and external validity. Control is accomplished by ruling out other variables, termed **intervening variables,** that compete with the independent variables as an explanation for a study's outcome. An intervening variable is a variable that may occur during a study that contributes to the change of the dependent variable or outcome. For example, in a study that aims to test an intervention to improve cancer patients' adherence to a medication trial, an intervening variable may be an antianxiety medication given to some patients during the medication trial. An **extraneous**, mediating, or intervening variable is one that interferes with interpretation of the dependent variable. An example would be the effect of the stage of cancer and depression during different phases of cancer treatment.

In a study that tests interventions (Interventions Studies; see Chapter 8), intervention fidelity (also referred to as treatment fidelity) is a key concept. Fidelity means trustworthiness or faithfulness. Intervention fidelity means that the researcher standardized the intervention and demonstrates how the intervention was administered to each participant in the same manner under the same conditions. A study designed to address issues related to a study's fidelity maximizes results, decreases bias, and controls preexisting conditions that may affect outcomes. The elements of control and fidelity differ based on the design type and the variables tested. Thus, when various research designs are critically appraised, the issue of control is always raised but with varying levels of flexibility. The issues discussed here will become clearer as you review the various design types discussed in Chapters 8 and 9.

Means of controlling for intervention fidelity include the following:
- Use of a homogeneous sample
- Use of consistent data collection procedures
- Training and supervision of interventionists
- Manipulation of the independent variable and intervention fidelity
- Randomization

> **TIP**
>
> As you review studies, assess whether the study included an intervention and whether there is a clear description of the intervention and how it was controlled. If the details are not clear, the intervention may have been administered differently among the participants, affecting the interpretation and strength of the results.

CRITICAL APPRAISAL CRITERIA

When reviewing studies, assess whether the researchers clearly identified controls that enhance generalizability from the sample to the specific population.

The elements of *intervention fidelity* (Yap et al., 2022; French et al., 2015; Gearing et al., 2011; Nelson et al., 2012; Preyde & Burnham, 2011) are as follows:
- Design: Allows an adequate testing of the hypothesis(es) in relation to the underlying theory and clinical processes
- Training: Training and supervision of the data collectors and/or interventionists to ensure that the intervention is delivered as planned and in a consistent manner
- Delivery: Assessing whether the intervention is delivered as intended, including that the "dose" (as measured by the number, frequency, and length of contact) is well-described for all participants, the dose is the same in each group, and there is a plan for possible problems
- Receipt: Verifying the treatment was delivered and understood by the participant
- Enactment: Assessing whether the intervention the participant performs is completed as intended

This type of control strengthens the investigators' ability to draw conclusions, discuss limitations, and cite the need for further research. When interventions are implemented, researchers should describe the training and supervision of interventionists completed to ensure fidelity. All study designs should demonstrate constancy (fidelity) to the methods of data collection. Studies that test an intervention require particular attention to intervention fidelity.

> **TIP**
>
> The lack of manipulation of the independent variable does not mean a weaker study. The type of question, amount of theoretical development, and research that has preceded the study affect the researcher's design choice. If the question is amenable to a design that manipulates the independent variable, it increases the power of a researcher to draw conclusions; that is, if all of the considerations of control are equally addressed.

INTERNAL VALIDITY

Internal validity assesses whether the change in the dependent variable or study outcome was related to the *independent variable*. When conducting a study, researchers consider the potential impact of internal validity threats on findings as one or more sources of bias. Clinicians must evaluate whether the study's findings are valid before implementation in practice. To establish internal validity, the researcher rules out other factors or threats as rival explanations of the relationship between the variables—essentially, sources of bias. There are a number of threats to internal validity. You should note that the threats to internal validity are mainly assessed in intervention studies but can also compromise outcomes of all quantitative studies. The overall strength and quality of a study's findings should be considered to some degree in all studies. How these threats may affect specific designs is addressed in Chapters 8 through 10. Threats to internal validity include **history**, **maturation**, **testing**, **instrumentation**, **mortality**, and participant **selection bias**. Table 7.1 provides definitions and examples of internal validity threats. Generally, researchers will discuss the threats to validity that they encountered in the discussion or limitations section of a research article.

> **TIP**
>
> More than one threat can be found in a study, depending on the study design. Finding a threat to internal validity in a study does not invalidate a study's results but should be acknowledged in the study's "Results" or "Discussion" or "Limitations" section.

> **TIP**
>
> Avoiding threats to internal validity can be difficult. This reality does not render studies that have threats useless, however. Take them into consideration and weigh the total evidence of a study for not only its statistical meaningfulness but also its clinical meaningfulness.

EXTERNAL VALIDITY

External validity is an assessment of the generalizability of a study's findings to additional populations and environmental conditions. External validity questions under what conditions and with what types of participants the same results can be expected to occur.

The factors that may affect external validity are related to selection of participants, study conditions, and type of observations. These factors are termed *selection effects*, *reactive effects*, and *testing effects*. You will notice the similarity in the names of the factors of selection and testing to those pertaining to threats to internal validity. When assessing a study's internal validity threats, you assess for their potential as they relate to the testing of *independent* and *dependent* variables within a study. External validity threats are assessed in terms of the *generalizability* or use of the study findings in other populations and settings. The threats to internal and external validity can interact with each other. It is important to remember that the interaction of these threats varies with the design and methods of the study. Problems of internal validity are generally easier to control. Generalizability issues are more difficult because it means that the researcher is assuming that other populations are similar to the one being tested. As more controls are designed into a study, internal validity improves, but generalizability is likely to decline.

> **TIP**
>
> Generalizability depends on who actually participates in a study. Not everyone who is approached actually participates, and not everyone who agrees to participate completes a study. As you review studies, think about how well the particpants reflect the population of interest.

Selection Effects

Selection refers to the generalizability of the results to other populations. An example of selection effects occurs when the researcher cannot attain the ideal sample population. At times, the numbers of

TABLE 7.1 Internal Validity Threats—Definitions and Examples

Threat	Definition	Example
History	In addition to the independent variable, another specific event that may have an effect on the dependent variable may occur either inside (during the study) or outside the experimental setting.	A study tested a partial weight-bearing activity intervention for athletes recovering from lower leg injuries at two sites. During the study's final month, a new, partial weight-bearing treadmill, the Super G, was introduced to some of the patients at one site only, leaving the researchers to question the outcomes from the center that instituted the added intervention. Data from the one hospital (cohort) were not included in the analysis.
Maturation	Can occur in studies that test an intervention or variables over time and refers to the developmental, biological, physiological, or psychological processes within an individual as a function of time and are external to a study's event, differences between the two testing periods rather than the experimental treatment.	Donovan and colleagues (2017) conducted a longitudinal study (12 years) to examine the reciprocal relationships of loneliness and cognitive function in older adults. They hypothesized that loneliness and poor cognition would have a bidirectional relationship and significant association independent of demographic factors, social network, health conditions, and depression. They found that loneliness predicted accelerated cognitive decline over 12 years but acknowledged that data was not available to classify the level of baseline cognitive status (normal cognition, mild cognitive impairment, dementia) and, therefore, the subsequent changes over time. The lack of baseline may have altered the relevance of loneliness as a risk factor across progressive stages of cognitive impairment. Another example: Suppose one wishes to evaluate the effect of an intervention in a group of older adult participants in a dementia center over a period of time. The investigator would record the participants' abilities before and after the intervention. Between the pretest and posttest, the participants' health and dementia status can change. The growth or change may be unrelated to the study and may explain differences between the two testing periods.
Testing	Taking the same test repeatedly could influence participants' responses the next time the test is completed. The effect of taking a pretest on the participant's posttest score is known as testing. The pretest may sensitize an individual and improve the posttest score. Individuals generally score higher when taking a test on a second occasion, regardless of the treatment. The differences between posttest and pretest scores may not be a result of the independent variable but rather of the experience gained through the testing.	Thomas et al. (2017) discussed how parent self-report of skill attainment in seeking services for their children may have influenced responses on actual skill attainment level.

TABLE 7.1 Internal Validity Threats—Definitions and Examples—cont'd

Threat	Definition	Example
Instrumentation	Changes in the measurement of the variables or observational techniques may account for changes in the measurement obtained.	In a study designed to test a sleep promotion protocol on intensive care unit patients regarding overnight in-room disturbances Knauert et al. (2019) acknowledged that "because this study did not include objective sleep measurement, such as polysomnography, our outcomes were limited to environmental measures" (p. 5). Another example: Researchers may wish to study several types of cardiac monitoring to compare the accuracy of the different monitor types. To prevent instrumentation threat, a researcher must check the calibration of the monitors according to the manufacturer's specifications before and after data collection.
Mortality	The loss of study participants from the first data collection point (pretest) to the second data collection point (posttest). If the participants who remain in the study are not similar to those who dropped out, results could be affected. Participant loss may be from the sample as a whole, or, in a study that has both an experimental and a control group, there may be differential loss of participants. Differential loss of participants means that more of the participants in one group dropped out than in the other group.	In a community intervention study designed to achieve healthy eating standards, evaluation of 2-year changes in outcomes in types of food and beverages served revealed that over the study period, 30% of the participants dropped out of the study.
Selection bias	If the precautions are not used to gain a representative sample, selection bias could result from how the participants were chosen. To avoid selection bias, participants can be randomly assigned to groups. In a nonexperimental study, even with clearly defined inclusion and exclusion criteria, selection bias is difficult to avoid completely.	Yap and colleagues (2022) controlled for selection bias within the sample by including participants who met the inclusion criteria and may be at risk to develop a pressure injury. However, patients at severe risk for a pressure injury formation were excluded based on their increased resource needs beyond the study's scope. This exclusion may have caused a selection bias.

available participants may be low or not accessible. Therefore the type of sampling method used and how participants are assigned to research conditions affect the generalizability to other groups: the external validity.

Examples of selection effects are reported when researchers note the following:

"This trial excluded nursing home residents with severe pressure injury risk because their care delivery is highly individualized using specialized surfaces and repositioning intervals. Evidence regarding median time to pressure injury development varies; for example, recent acute care evidence shows a 2- to 5-day median time to pressure injury

development when using high-density foam mattresses and 4-hour repositioning."

Yap et al., 2022, p. 325

These remarks caution you about potentially generalizing beyond the type of sample in a study, but also point out the usefulness of the findings for practice and future research aimed at building the research in this area.

Reactive Effects

Reactivity is defined as the participants' responses to being studied. Participants may respond to the investigator not because of the study procedures but merely as an independent response to being studied. This is also known as the Hawthorne effect, which is named after Western Electric Corporation's Hawthorne plant, where a study of working conditions was conducted. The researchers developed several working conditions (i.e., turning up the lights, piping in music loudly or softly, and changing work hours). They found that no matter what was done, the workers' productivity increased. They concluded that production increased as a result of the workers' realization that they were being studied rather than because of the experimental conditions.

In the study by Yap and colleagues (2022), the investigators could not blind the intervention from the nursing home staff because it was essential for conducting the study. A Hawthorne effect may have occurred because the patient monitoring device made staff continually aware of the resident's need for repositioning.

Measurement Effects

Administration of a pretest in a study affects the generalizability of the findings to other populations and is known as **measurement effects**. Pretesting can affect the posttest responses in a study (internal validity) and affects the generalizability outside the study (external validity). For example, suppose a researcher wants to conduct a study with the aim of changing attitudes toward breast cancer screening behaviors. To accomplish this, an education program is incorporated on the risk factors for breast cancer. To test whether the education program changes attitudes toward screening behaviors, tests are given before and after the teaching intervention. The pretest on attitudes allows the participants to examine their attitudes regarding cancer screening. The participants' responses on follow-up testing may differ from those of individuals who were given the education program and did not see the pretest. Therefore, when a study is conducted and a pretest is given, it may "prime" the participants and affect the ability to generalize to other situations.

> **TIP**
>
> When reviewing a study, be aware of the internal and external validity threats. These threats do not make a study useless—but actually more useful—to you. Recognition of the threats allows researchers to build on data and allows you to think through what part(s) of the study can be applied to practice. Specific threats to validity depend on the design type.
>
> There are other threats to external validity that depend on the type of design and methods of sampling used by the researcher, but these are beyond the scope of this text. Brincks and colleagues (2018) discuss challenges to internal and external validity using randomized trials as examples and offer techniques to minimize threats.

SYNTHESIS

Quantitative Research

Evaluating a study's design requires you to have knowledge of the overall implications that the choice of a design may have for the study as a whole. When investigators ask a research question, they (1) design a study, (2) decide how the data will be collected, (3) decide which instruments will be used, (4) identify the sample's inclusion and exclusion criteria, (5) determine how large the sample needs to be to diminish threats to the study's validity, and (6) choose the appropriate method of analyses. These choices are based on the nature of the research question or hypothesis. Minimizing threats to internal and external validity of a study enhances the strength of evidence. In this chapter, the meaning, purpose, and important factors of design choice, as well as the vocabulary that accompanies these factors, have been introduced.

Several criteria for evaluating the design related to maximizing control and minimizing threats to internal and external validity and, as a result, sources of bias can be drawn from this chapter. When evaluating the potential threats of internal and external validity of quantitative designs, it is important to refer back to the research question or hypothesis and aims of the study.

KEY POINTS

- How a researcher structures, implements, or designs a study affects the study's results, appraisal, and, ultimately, application of the results to practice.
- Evaluation occurs by synthesizing the overall strengths, quality, and consistency of the evidence provided by the studies retrieved.
- Control measures help manage threats to the study's internal and external validity and applicability of findings to practice.
- Internal validity is the degree to which one can infer that the intervention, rather than another condition or variable, resulted in the outcome or observed effects.
- External validity is the degree to which findings can be generalized to other populations or environments.
- Studies reviewed for an EBP project need to be evaluated for quality individually as well as a collective group.

REFERENCES

Brincks, A., Montag, S., Howe, G. W., Huang, S., Siddique, J., Ahn, S., et al. (2018). Addressing methodologic challenges and minimizing threats to validity in synthesizing findings from individual-level data across longitudinal randomized trials. *Prevention Science, 19*(Suppl. 1), 60–73. https://doi.org/10.1007/s11121-017-0769-1.

Donovan, N. J., Wu, Q., Rentz, D. M., Sperling, R. A., Marshall, G. A., & Glymour, M. M. (2017). Loneliness, depression and cognitive function in older U.S. adults. *International Journal of Geriatric Psychiatry, 32*(5), 564–573. https://doi.org/10.1002/gps.4495.

French, C. T., Diekemper, R. L., Irwin, R. S., Adams, T. M., Altman, K. W., Barker, A. F., & CHEST Expert Cough Panel., et al. (2015). Assessment of intervention fidelity and recommendations for researchers conducting studies on the diagnosis and treatment of chronic couch in the adult: CHEST guideline and expert panel report. *Chest, 148*(1), 32–54.

Gearing, R. E., El-Bassel, N., Ghesquiere, A., Baldwin, S., Gillies, J., & Ngeow, E. (2011). Major ingredients of fidelity: A review and scientific guide to improving quality of intervention research implementation. *Clinical Psychology Review, 31*, 79–88.

Knauert, M. P., Pisani, M., Redeker, N., Murphy, T., Araujo, K., Jeon, S., et al. (2019). Pilot study: An intensive care unit sleep promotion protocol. *BMJ Open Respiratory Research, 6*(1), e000411. https://doi.org/10.1136/bmjresp-2019-000411. PMID: 31258916; PMCID: PMC6561389.

Nelson, M. C., Corday, D. S., Hulleman, C. S., Darrow, C. L., & Somner, E. C. (2012). A procedure for assessing intervention fidelity in experiments testing educational and behavioral interventions. *The Journal of Behavioral Health Services & Research, 39*(4), 374–395.

Preyde, M., & Burnham, P. V. (2011). Intervention fidelity in psychosocial oncology. *Journal of Evidence-Based Social Work, 8*, 379–396.

Thiese, M. S. (2014). Observational and interventional study design types; an overview. *Biochemia Medica, 24*(2), 199–210. https://doi.org/10.11613/BM.2014.022.

Thomas, K. C., Stein, G. L., Williams, C. S., Perez-Jolles, M., Sleath, B. L., Martinez, M., et al. (2017). Fostering activation among Latino parents of children with mental health needs: An RCT. *Psychiatry Services in Advance, 68*(10), 1068–1075.

Yap, T. L., Horn, S. D., Sharkey, P. D., Zheng, T., Bergstrom, N., Colon-Emeric, C., et al. (2022). Effect of varying repositioning frequency on pressure injury prevention in nursing home residents: TEAM-UP trial results. *Advances in Skin and Wound Care, 35*(6), 315–325. https://doi.org/10.1097/01.ASW.0000817840.68588.04.

8

Intervention Studies

Lisa A. Wolf, Pamela B. DeGuzman, and Kathy Moore Baker

LEARNING OBJECTIVES

After reading this chapter, you should be able to do the following:
- Describe the purpose of an intervention study.
- Identify different intervention study designs.
- Identify potential threat to the internal and external validity of an intervention study.
- Identify the strengths and weaknesses of an intervention study.
- Synthesize evidence from intervention studies based on a PICOT question.
- Identify the contribution of intervention studies to an evidence-based practice review and its impact on healthcare.

KEY TERMS

Blinding
Control
Efficacy
Effectiveness
Exclusion criteria
Intervention fidelity
Pilot study
Power analysis
Quasi-experimental design
Randomized controlled trials
Randomization
Treatment fidelity

The purpose of an intervention study is to examine the causal relationship between an event or outcome (dependent variable) and an intervention (independent variable). An intervention study is the type of research design that is used when the research question is comparing the effect of a specific intervention on a designated study population. One methodological design often used for an intervention study is referred to as an **experimental design**. This type of design controls for human and environmental bias, producing results with the high degree of validity necessary to inform practice change (Tume et al., 2022). Also known as **randomized controlled trials** (RCTs), these intervention studies provide the highest level of evidence available to inform evidence-based practice (EBP) reviews. The level of evidence produced by an intervention study using an experimental design is generally designated at a Level II on most evidence hierarchy tables (Dang et al., 2022). Another type of research design used for an intervention study is termed **quasi-experimental**. Studies using this type of design generally do not have the same level of control measures as an experimental design but are still capable of producing highly valid results (Hariton & Locascio, 2018).

Based on the high level of validity the results of an intervention study can provide, nurses engaged in EBP work should include, when appropriate, intervention studies in their review. Conducting an intervention study for some clinical phenomena, however, can be more challenging than others. This is particularly true for many phenomena of interest to nursing scientists and other scientists studying the practice of nursing. Because of this, when including an intervention study in an evidence-based review, it is important to critically appraise (see Chapter 6) the intervention study based on the strength, quality, and consistency of the study findings as well as other characteristics of the study design that determine the validity of the study (Tume et al., 2022).

This chapter will provide you with an overview of various research designs that can be used when conducting intervention studies. The strengths and limitations of intervention studies and their specific design elements will be reviewed. Lastly, the skills and techniques needed to critically appraise the intervention studies for an EBP review will be described.

STUDY DESIGNS

Experimental Designs

An intervention study using an experimental design has three essential characteristics—randomization, control measures, and manipulation. Once the three elements are met, then, in general, data are gathered on all study participants both preintervention and postintervention to compare the responses. This represents the basic design of an experimental intervention study; however, more complex experimental designs can also be implemented using multiple types of randomization groups and interventions. For the EBP reviewer, it is important to understand each of the essential characteristics of intervention studies and have an appreciation of how they may be implemented in more complex study designs.

The first essential characteristic of an experimental intervention study is **randomization** of the sample population to either an intervention group or a control group. This allows the researcher to compare the effect of the intervention to a group of study participants who have been exposed to the intervention against a group of study participants who have not been exposed to the intervention (control group). There must be at least one control group and one intervention group, but more complex studies may have multiple intervention groups in the design. The purpose of the random assignment is to limit the effect of inherent differences in study populations that may influence their response to the intervention, and randomization helps ensure the comparison of the groups is conducted on study participants who share common characteristics. Second, there must be defined **control** measures to ensure the results of the study reflect the most direct relationship possible between the outcome being studied in the experiment and the intervention. Control measures minimize the possibility that factors other than the intervention in the study influence the presence or absence of the outcome being evaluated. There are many types of control measures that can be used in experimental designs. Two common control measures are the implementation of strict **inclusion and exclusion criteria** and **blinding (single, double, or triple blinding)** of the participants and/or personnel participating in the intervention. Implementing inclusion and exclusion criteria ensures that the sample populations are homogenous. For example, researchers frequently designate specific age ranges for study participants to limit age differences in study participants from influencing the results of the study. Blinding of the researcher to the randomization of study participants in both the control group and the intervention groups ensures that no one in the study environment can inadvertently influence the outcome of the study by behaving differently toward the study participants based on whether they were a part of the control or intervention group. In a double blind study, neither the research participant nor the researcher implementing the intervention are aware of whether the participant is part of the control or the experimental group. In a triple blind study, neither the research participant, the researcher implementing the intervention, nor the researcher conducting the data analysis are aware of whether the participant is part of the control or experimental group (Tume et al., 2022). Lastly, there must be **manipulation** of the control group. In other words, some type of intervention must be introduced to the study participants in the intervention group to measure their response. Once the three elements are met, randomization, controls, and manipulation, then, in general, data are gathered on all study participants both preintervention and postintervention to compare the responses.

There are other more complex ways that intervention studies may be conducted than just using the basic experimental design. The Solomon four-group uses two experimental groups and two control groups. All study participants are randomly assigned to one of the four groups. One control group and one intervention group receive a pretest and a posttest, and the second control group and intervention group receive a posttest only. This design is used when there is risk that the pretest may introduce a level of bias (pretest sensitization) and the posttest groups only offer a level of control for that concern. A repeated measures or cross-over experimental design uses random assignment to a control group and an intervention group, and there are initial pre- and postintervention measures for each group. Then the intervention is repeated with the initial control group receiving the intervention and the initial intervention group serving as the control group in the second arm of the study. A second posttest is then obtained. This design is effective for research questions with a limited number of available study participants resulting in low sample sizes (Tume et al., 2022).

Quasi-Experimental Designs

A quasi-experimental design is an intervention study that does not place people into groups using random assignment, and may lack a control group. In nursing a pre- and posttest design is often used. There is a measurement of the study population prior to the intervention and then a posttest intervention with the same population. There are several instances when randomization is not appropriate for the study population. There are times when it is logistically impossible to implement random assignment. This occurs when the intervention is a timed or naturally occurring event being introduced over a large population. An example of this is a study examining specific effects of an electronic health record (EHR) implementation in a single organization. This EHR is being implemented for an entire group of individuals and a researcher is unable to isolate a specific control group for the study. There are also times when it is unethical to limit an intervention to one group. This occurs when there are known positive outcomes of an intervention and the researcher is interested in another potential outcome of the intervention. An example of this is an intervention study involving an antidepressive medication. The medication may be known to decrease depression but the researcher is also interested in understanding the medication's effect on other variables. It would be unethical to withhold the medication in a control group in this situation (Siedlecki, 2020).

> **TIP**
>
> Randomized controlled trials (RCTs) provide a high level of evidence (Level II) secondary to the randomization and control measures used.

> **TIP**
>
> Quasi-experimental designs do not use randomization or the same level of control measures as an experimental design but are still capable of producing significant evidence (Level III).

INTENT TO IMPLEMENT

The purpose of an EBP review is to implement a change into practice that is proven to produce positive outcomes for patients. From an EBP perspective, intervention studies that are well designed and executed produce results that are highly valid and can demonstrate whether an intervention or practice change is efficacious. **Efficacy** refers to how well the intervention performs in well-controlled conditions. The intervention study must be well designed in order to produce results with a high degree of efficacy. The qualities of the research study that an EBP reviewer must consider and the methods they should use to appraise the intervention study will be reviewed in subsequent sections of this chapter, and the intervention study should not be considered for inclusion in the EBP recommendations unless efficacy is first established. Still, establishing that the results of the study are efficacious does not guarantee they will be effective and produce the desired outcomes in the real-world setting. Ironically, the tight controls that must be used to design an intervention study may limit the ability to translate the intervention into an effective strategy for the clinical setting. In the scientific nursing community, there are proponents of additional research strategies that can be used in conjunction with intervention studies to establish not the efficacy of the intervention but the **effectiveness** of the intervention.

Pilot Studies

To statisticians and methodologists, the term "**pilot study**" is strictly defined as a small-scale test of the methods and procedures to be used subsequently on a larger scale (Thabane et al., 2010), or an experimental, exploratory, test, preliminary, trial, or tryout investigation (Waite, 2002).

Pilot studies, therefore, aim to evaluate the viability and feasibility of critical research components and processes needed for larger studies to be successful. They play an important role in establishing realistic expectations, mitigating damage from unwanted surprises, and saving cost and time when later undertaking large trials. Pilot studies are useful in determining whether a larger project will succeed or fail by trialing logistic considerations, such as recruitment strategies.

Pragmatic Clinical Trials

In contrast to the controlled setting that is needed for an experimental or quasi-experimental intervention study, a pragmatic clinical design is conducted in the real-world setting with fewer controls on the study population. The research designs of experimental or quasi-experimental studies should not be considered an either/or approach with a pragmatic clinical trial; instead, the exploration of the intervention with a pragmatic clinical trial should be viewed on a continuum with experimental or quasi-experimental studies establishing efficacy and pragmatic clinical trials establishing effectiveness. The experimental and quasi-experimental intervention studies produce results that demonstrate the causal relationship between an intervention and an outcome, and the pragmatic clinical trials demonstrate that the intervention can be applied broadly in the clinical setting (Chen, 2014).

Factorial Designs

Another concern that has been raised by the scientific nursing community with translating evidence into practice using only experimental and quasi-experimental intervention studies is the result of nonsignificant findings when it is not due to poor study design. Rather, the nonsignificant findings are a result of interventions that have multiple components and it is impossible to discern, using traditional interventional study designs, the contributions of the individual or particular combinations of the intervention components. A factorial design called Multiphase Optimization Strategy (MOST) that was developed using engineering principles analyzes the components of a multicomponent intervention in isolation and in multiple combinations to determine which components have the most significant influence on the outcome (Collins, 2018). Another design called Sequential Multiple Assignment Randomized Trial (SMART) tailors interventions based on a study population's response and evaluates these tailored interventions over a sequence of interventions. Both designs represent innovative new models that nursing may use more and more in the future to allow rapid translation of evidence into practice (Collins et al., 2014).

THREATS TO VALIDITY

EBP is based on translating reliable evidence into practice. A process that does not include the critical appraisal of each study risks implementation of poorly designed or unsubstantiated interventions. In this section, we discuss how to evaluate threats to the validity of evidence, meaning elements of the design, sample selection, or implementation that may cause the evidence or data to be untrustworthy.

When evaluating intervention research for potential translation to implement in a patient care environment, it is important to evaluate the validity of each study. Critiquing validity allows the nurse to determine if the conclusion drawn by the researchers (i.e., that an intervention is effective at producing an outcome or not) is logical and not explained by other factors. Nurses should evaluate each intervention study for three types of validity: *internal validity*, *external validity*, and *validity of statistical conclusions*.

Threats to Internal Validity

Internal validity refers to the relationship between the independent variable and dependent variable of interest. When thinking about threats to internal validity, you want to have confidence that the intervention study you read actually suggested a strong relationship between the independent variable and clinical outcomes. Taylor (2013) describe several categories of internal validity that should be evaluated in intervention research, including: *person factors* related to study participants; *measurement or statistical factors* that occur during measurement or analysis of quantitative data; and *situational factors* that may be occurring when a trial is being conducted.

Person Factors

Bias in selection refers to changes in the dependent variable that may be attributed to differences in the groups themselves rather than the intervention. This can occur in quasi-experimental studies with more than one group when participants are not randomized to a study arm. Maturation can occur when there are changes in the dependent variable that are observed over time that may have occurred regardless of the intervention. This can occur in studies using a longitudinal or pre–posttest design with no control group. Attrition (also referred to as mortality or the dropout-rate) can occur when characteristics of participants fail to continue in a study over time. Characteristics of those who drop out can impact the dependent variable. Consider a study evaluating the impact of counseling sessions on the anxiety of patients with cancer. If participants choose to leave the study because they feel too overwhelmed to continue participation due to the added stress of living with cancer treatment, their withdrawal from the study could impact how much the dependent variable appears to improve as a result of the intervention.

Measurement or Statistical Factors

Threats to validity can occur during pre–posttest or longitudinal studies designed to evaluate changes in knowledge, because exposure to concepts during a pretest can impact participants' knowledge when they are retested. In this case, it is important for the researcher to address steps they took to minimize the knowledge of a pretest to influence later results. For example, a test in which participants need to write out nuanced answers will provide fewer threats to pretest validity than a true/false or multiple-choice test.

Intervention studies require precise measurement of independent variables (predictors) and dependent variables (outcomes), which is done with psychometric evaluation of instruments. There are multiple examples of how instrumentation can negatively impact validity because if researchers use surveys to measure phenomena that have not been demonstrated to be reliable and valid tools for measurement, the study's conclusions may be made in error. For example, when conducting research related to latent phenomena such as resilience, engagement, or anxiety, researchers should reference prior studies that evaluated the psychometrics of each survey tool being used to measure the concept of interest. The most common type of reliability evaluation is internal consistency. With this type of reliability, a report of an alpha of 0.70 is considered minimally acceptable (DeVellis & Thorpe, 2021). Content validity is the most common type of validity you will see presented in research articles. Construct validity is more often referred to in citations from original psychometric studies. Use of valid and reliable measures increases the likelihood that if a true difference exists between the intervention and the control condition, it is accurately captured. Similarly, if a study involves physiological measurements such as blood pressure or temperature, researchers should report how the measuring tools were assessed to ensure that the equipment measured accurately. For longitudinal studies, these physiological measuring instruments can lose their ability to measure accurately over the course of the study, and this should be addressed in the manuscript. Overall, when evaluating intervention studies, it is important to pay close attention to how the researchers report the measures they used to determine the outcomes.

A final statistical consideration is called statistical regression, or regression to the mean. This must be evaluated in pre–posttest or longitudinal designs because individuals who score extremely high or low on a measure compared to an average will typically score closer to the mean when measured again. Flannelly and colleagues (2018) describe an example in which interns who scored the lowest on an exam about end-of-life care are sent to an in-service as an exemplar of this phenomenon. The interns all scored much higher on the next exam, which makes sense because they were the lowest scoring interns on the initial exam and thus had the most room for improvement. When comparing posttests to pretests, the researchers would need to consider the potential factors that may have led to the original scores being very low, such as lack of motivation, fatigue, or distraction, and that scores will probably improve even without the intervention.

Situational Factors

History is a situational factor that a participant experiences during the intervention that can alter the impact of the intervention on the dependent variable. Consider if you are testing the impact of opening hospital room windows shades on intensive care unit patients' delirium. If the hospital's therapy dog typically comes by the unit to visit patients on the same days, this may alter the researcher's ability to draw conclusions about the impact of the intervention. Because hospital research is conducted in a complex environment, researchers are unlikely to be able to control all historical factors, but these should be acknowledged in the limitations section of the article.

Another situational factor to consider when critiquing research is the unreliability of the treatment intervention. **Intervention fidelity**, also called **treatment fidelity**, refers to processes used to make sure that the research intervention and all related activities were delivered exactly as planned to ensure that any treatment effect found or not found is a result of the intervention and not of alterations in execution of the study. Fidelity includes development of an intervention manual, training, monitoring, and supervision of research staff, measuring the consistency with which it is delivered, ensuring that there is consistent adherence to data collection protocols, and confirming that the intervention was delivered and received using a standardized protocol. Activities to maximize fidelity should be documented by a research team. For example, if there are multiple interventionists delivering the same intervention at different data collection sites, the researcher needs to describe how training was conducted and evaluated, and should provide evidence across interventionists. If researchers do not demonstrate that patients received interventions that were evaluated for fidelity to ensure consistent intervention delivery, the results can be called into question, and nurses may be unable to draw conclusions based on the findings.

> **TIP**
>
> When thinking about critically appraising intervention fidelity, assess whether:
> - An intervention manual was developed and used;
> - All research personnel were trained on the careful execution of the intervention;
> - The consistency with which the researchers executed the intervention was monitored; and
> - Adherence to the protocol (e.g., dose, timing) through supervision and booster sessions was measured.

Threats to External Validity

Understanding external validity is critical to the translation of evidence into nursing practice. External validity refers to the extent that results from the original intervention study may be generalizable, that is, that the same results can be expected if the intervention is tested under the same circumstances. Generalization should be evaluated not only to other groups, but also across times and situations (Taylor, 2013; Andrade, 2018). Given the continually changing nursing practice environment, it is important for nurses to understand how to evaluate external validity prior to adopting an intervention into practice.

It can be challenging for a nurse to find trials that are considered externally valid to their clinical setting given the limited number of rigorous nursing clinical trials (Baldi et al., 2014). This coupled with the continually evolving health care environment creates a challenge for nurses to find studies that are generalizable to their practice settings. As such, nurses evaluating studies for external validity may need to also consider the question of applicability, which refers to the question of whether results are valid for participants in a different treatment setting than where the study was originally conducted (Dekkers et al., 2010; Andrade, 2018).

Validity of Statistical Conclusions

The sample size in any intervention study must be evaluated carefully. Intervention studies typically use statistical power calculation procedures to make sure they enroll and retain an adequate number of research participants to address the study hypothesis. A **power analysis** provides the statistical projection based on the desired effect size. It is calculated to estimate the sample size needed to detect the treatment effect and calculated to reduce the probability of making a Type II error; that is, the likelihood of accepting that the intervention did not work when it really did. A power calculation should be evident in the article; it is used to determine the number of participants needed to detect a small, medium, or large treatment effect—that is, whether there is a difference between the intervention and control condition at a predetermined level of significance (typically $p < 0.05$ or $p < 0.01$). Studies that have high attrition rates because they are conducted over protracted time periods or with severely ill patient populations are more likely to have unavoidably high attrition and end up with a sample too small to accurately detect a significant treatment effect. In that case, researchers may factor dropout rates into the power analysis. In the case of a pilot study, researchers may be conducting an intervention solely to determine the effect size of an intervention with the purpose of calculating power for a future experimental study. In this case, a power analysis would not be expected when the study is published. Additional information regarding statistics can be found in Chapter 13.

> **TIP**
>
> As a clinical leader, you and your team need to assess whether the outcomes measured are clinically relevant for your clinical population, clinical setting, and available resources. You and your team need to use your clinical expertise and judgment—combined with the best available evidence, patient values, and preferences—to inform your decision about whether the outcomes of a study or group of studies are clinically important and applicable to improving patient care.

When critiquing intervention research, it is important to consider if the researcher violated any assumptions of statistical testing. Nurses may not always have access to trained statisticians, and can make statistical errors that invalidate seemingly statistically significant results. For example, several types of statistical tests are only intended to be used with normally distributed data (such as *t* tests and linear regression). If measured variables violate normality assumptions, researchers should either use nonparametric tests or normalize the data. When evaluating appropriateness of statistical testing, look to see if the researchers reported data about the normality of the distribution prior to using parametric tests. If not, the result may be invalid. It is also important to evaluate compatibility between the study design and the choice of test when evaluating the impact of an intervention. Imagine that you wanted to test a novel simulation with hospital nurses, and you wanted to measure the impact of the simulation on nurses' long-term knowledge retention. To provide anonymity, you do not ask individual nurses to provide their name or other identifying information. You give a knowledge test and then run the simulation, typically conducting multiple simulations to get people working on different shifts. One month after completing all intervention, you retest all the nurses on the unit to determine their knowledge retention. Typically, you would use a paired *t* test to analyze the impact of the simulation (assuming normally distributed data). However, because you did not identify the participants, assumptions of the paired *t* test are violated because the data cannot be paired. Furthermore, assumptions of the independent *t* test are violated because the conditions of the study violate the independence assumption. In this case, the researcher would need to use a nonparametric test such as a chi-square.

A Final Note About Validity

Nurses need rigorous intervention studies to guide practice. A strong understanding of research critique can help you ensure that the research driving your practice is of the highest quality. However, with limited rigorous nursing studies available (Baldi et al., 2014), nurses should critique the research to identify research gaps, and work to develop innovative studies to close those gaps. Furthermore, when evaluating literature for consideration of translation into the practice environment, you should be aware that the nature of the varied and continually changing practice environment can make it difficult to find studies that precisely match your practice environment. When reading research, determine if the researchers report these limitations and have attempted to address them in the research article. See Table 8.1 for a list of threats to validity to watch for.

SYNTHESIZING INTERVENTION STUDIES FOR AN EVIDENCE-BASED PRACTICE REVIEW

The systematic review, or the *research synthesis*, aims to provide a comprehensive, objective synthesis of multiple relevant studies (Aromataris & Pearson, 2014). A systematic review differs from a literature review in that it attempts to uncover all the evidence relevant to a question, focusing on research that reports data. Intervention studies provide the strongest level of evidence for designs of individual research studies. A systematic review of intervention studies is considered the gold standard for evidence, and a form of research itself. Some challenges to this process include heterogeneity of studies (i.e., different methodological approaches or outcomes measures around the same topic or problem) or just too few studies to synthesize (Cooper et al., 2019b). When attempting to synthesize studies, consider the scope of the question, and the various methods for synthesizing a limited number of studies to produce recommendations for practice. Additional information can be found in Chapter 10 regarding systematic reviews.

Scope of the Question

When reviewing the literature for synthesis, it is important to have a specific but not overly narrow question. An overly narrow question by its nature will limit the number of studies available for review. What may be more productive is to conduct a search based on the outcomes measure (e.g., "Reduction in A1c") rather than a specific intervention (e.g., "diet/nutrition counseling"). There will be many studies targeting the outcomes measure, and specific intervention components are likely to be similar across different interventions. That is, if there are 10 A1c reduction programs and each of these programs has five elements, it is safe to say that there will not be 50 unique components across the 10 programs. Carrying out separate reviews of each intervention can obscure the similarities across programs and will make it more difficult to assess the extent to which different

TABLE 8.1 Watch List for Threats to Validity

Type of Validity	Threat	What to Watch for
Internal	History: An event that occurs as the study is being conducted that could influence the outcome (the event could be global, national, local, or personal to individual research participants)	When was the study conducted? Were there any important events that could influence the study outcomes? Were new treatments made available during the study period? Did the researcher address this issue at all (try to collect data about it, control for it, or consider it in the analyses)?
Internal	Maturation: Changes that occur within individuals during the course of the study (i.e., changes in functioning, knowledge, cognition, developmental milestones, fragility, progression of disease state)	Did the study design take into account issues of maturation (especially in studies done with children and older adults)? Was the sample randomly assigned? Were there any differences in the characteristics of the groups that indicate maturation might be an issue (e.g., more adolescents in one group than in the other)?
Internal	Testing: Changes in response to measures that are caused by repeating the administration of the same measures multiple times	Are baseline and follow-up measures spaced far enough apart to prevent memory of prior responses? Are measures too brief so that easy recall is likely? Are number of data collection points supported by clear rationale? Note: Use of the Solomon four-group design reduces this threat.
Internal	Instrumentation: Changes to the instrument over time during the study (e.g., also can refer to changes in equipment such as changing scales to measure weight without calibration or changing to a new interviewer with minimal experience)	Is equipment being used in the study, and if so, is it calibrated each time it is used? Is there adequate training of all study personnel, including interviewers and observers? How often did the interviewers/observers change during the course of a study? Is there evidence that random checks were performed to make sure equipment and/or interviewers/observers were applying measures consistently?
Internal	Statistical regression to the mean: A tendency for those with extremely high and low scores on the baseline test to gradually move their scores toward the mean value	Did the researchers describe the distribution of scores at baseline and indicate any extremely high or low scores? Did the researchers discuss doing any statistical analyses to evaluate the effects for the total sample, as well as those with very high or low scores at baseline? Note: Randomization is used to reduce this threat and equalize groups.
Internal	Selection effect: When the research participants differ in some important ways from those who did not participate in the study, or between study groups, and this difference may potentially influence the study outcomes	Did the researchers describe a reliable means of randomizing research participants to groups? Did the researchers describe whether the intervention and control groups were the same or different on baseline characteristics? Did the researchers attempt to control for any differences in baseline characteristics by group in the main study analyses?

TABLE 8.1 Watch List for Threats to Validity—cont'd

Type of Validity	Threat	What to Watch for
Internal	Mortality, also known as attrition: When research participants drop out of the study	Did the researchers describe how many research participants in each group dropped out of the study? Was the dropout rate different between the two groups? Was the power calculation done to estimate the potential attrition rate? Was there a plan in place to reduce attrition? Did the researchers compare the characteristics of those who dropped out with those who completed the study? If there was a difference, did the researcher attempt to control for this in the final analyses? Did the researchers conduct an intent-to-treat analysis?
Internal	Contamination: When some or all of the components of the intervention are shared with or experienced by the control group	Did the researchers discuss how they controlled for any possible contamination between groups? Were separate individuals delivering the intervention and control conditions? Did research participants from both groups have the opportunity to interact with each other?
External	Interaction of selection and treatment effects: When research participants are different from the target population in important ways, and this difference has the potential to influence how they respond to the intervention being studied (i.e., more positively or more negatively)	Are the inclusion/exclusion criteria clearly outlined? Is the recruitment site located in a setting that may attract only a certain subgroup of study participants? How many research participants are approached, and how many decline to participate in the study? Did the researchers detail the study participant characteristics so you can judge how the results might be applied to the target population?
External	Interaction of setting and treatment effects: When the study setting is unique in some way or may attract only a certain type of subject	Is the setting unique in any important way that might influence how research participants evaluate the intervention? If there are multiple sites, did the researchers describe these settings and analyze the data by setting to evaluate any effect of the setting on study outcomes?
External	Interaction of history and treatment effect: When the period in history in which the study is conducted may be unique in some way that would reduce the likelihood that an attempt to replicate the findings would be successful	Did the researchers report the dates when data were collected? Is there anything historical about this time period related to the research study that might reduce the generalizability of the findings? Was there an extraneous variable occurring during the study period (e.g., television, radio, or social media ads)?
Statistical conclusion	Low or no statistical power	Was a power analysis done and reported? Was an adequate sample recruited and retained?

Continued

TABLE 8.1 Watch List for Threats to Validity—cont'd

Type of Validity	Threat	What to Watch for
Statistical conclusion	Assumptions underlying statistical tests are not met	Did the researchers use the correct statistical procedures for answering the research questions? Did the researchers provide enough data to know whether normal distributions were present when parametric analyses were performed? Did the researchers need to transform data, and did data meet statistical assumptions? Did the researchers use nonparametric analyses when data were not normally distributed?
Statistical conclusion	Fishing expedition: When researchers do multiple comparisons without accounting for the probability of committing a Type I error; exploring the data and doing analyses that are not originally planned	Did the researcher stick to the original analysis plan? Is the analysis plan consistent with the conceptual/theoretical framework? If multiple tests were performed, was the p value adjusted to account for the multiple comparisons (i.e., Bonferroni correction)?
Statistical conclusion	Unknown or poor reliability of scales used in the study: Random error associated with the reliability of a scale—the lower the reliability, the larger the amount of random error present; thus, it is essential to know the reliability of each scale for each study	Did the researchers report the reliability of all scales used in the study in their sample? Were any of the alphas for the scales less than 0.7?

intervention components are associated with program success (Cooper et al., 2019b). Generally, it is best to have all the available literature on an intervention or outcomes measure when synthesizing the evidence, understanding the effect of publication bias. Publication bias occurs because researchers are less likely to submit negative findings for publications (Wolf, 2017); however, understanding what does not work is just as important as understanding what does work. Publication bias may mean that the effectiveness of an intervention is overstated. A second consideration when searching literature is our own bias of intentionally selecting studies with particular characteristics or from particular sources for review. These actions limit the literature reviewed from the beginning, and certainly impact the availability of studies for review and synthesis.

> **TIP**
> When beginning a literature search for a systematic review, keep a very open mind. Search broadly and do not limit your search until later in the process. This mitigates selection bias.

Selecting Studies for Inclusion in a Synthesis

Because a systematic review seeks to synthesize and summarize existing literature, the first consideration is the available literature on the topic. Nurses with experience in EBP and database searching may use the PICOT mnemonic (Patient, Intervention, Comparison, Outcome, and Timing), which informs the concepts to be captured in the search. For a systematic review evaluating the effectiveness of an intervention, RCTs are considered the most reliable evidence. Because of the design of an RCT, it is assumed to be possible to determine causal relationships between the intervention and outcome more so than from other study designs that lack randomization and experimental control (Aromataris & Pearson, 2014). However, because interventions in health tend toward the more complex and contextual, results from RCTs should be critically appraised for real world usefulness (Minary et al., 2019). Other types of studies, such as nonrandomized intervention studies (NRISs) and mixed-methods studies may be included in a systematic review under certain conditions, which will be discussed later. Finally, it is important to also search the "gray literature," which generally consists of theses and dissertations that often do not get published in peer-reviewed journals but may provide additional literature and, more importantly, negative findings.

> **TIP**
>
> When searching the literature, pay attention to the methods (RCT vs. mixed methods or NRISs) to get a broad look at evidence. Check for implementation strategies, especially feasibility. Search the gray literature and note studies and EBP projects with negative findings.

Data extraction from the included studies usually comprises the following: review date, participant population, outcomes measures, intervention design, and patient outcome findings, to ensure that you are synthesizing the same *types of studies*, with the same *interventions*, and the same *outcomes measures*. Quality assessment is done with a standard tool, such as the AMSTAR-2 tool (A Measurement Tool to Assess Systematic Reviews [Shea et al., 2017]), which is a validated tool for assessing quality in systematic reviews. When you evaluate the strength of the evidence based on quality of studies included in the synthesis, you can be more confident that the intervention you are choosing for your own site is the most effective one for the outcomes you are hoping to affect.

Synthesizing the Studies

Once you've selected the studies that meet inclusion criteria and have done the data extraction, "synthesizing" the studies really means determining what the studies *collectively* tell us about the efficacy of an intervention. Because meta-analyses of RCTs allow researchers to (a) transparently reach a conclusion about the extent to which an intervention is effective and (b) statistically investigate sources of heterogeneity (Higgins & Green, 2011), when multiple studies that examine the same outcome are available, there is little debate among statisticians that the best way to integrate the results of the studies is by using some form of meta-analysis.

There is also a process for synthesizing NRISs, which can provide additional evidence for the review (Saldanha et al., 2022). Consider the following as you look at an NRIS for inclusion: *selection bias in the sample*, *confounding variables (known or unknown at the time the study was conducted)*, and *misclassification of outcomes*. In an exploration of the validity of NRISs in cardiovascular outcomes, it was reported that there was 80% agreement between RCTs and NRISs, suggesting that with data that are fit for purpose and proper design and analysis, causal treatment effects can be estimated through both randomized trials and nonrandomized real-world evidence studies (Franklin et al., 2021). In a systematic review, if conclusions in RCTs and well-done NRISs agree, the inclusion of NRISs may further support conclusions from RCTs and/or broaden the applicability of the conclusions. If they disagree, NRIS evidence contributes new evidence and/or can serve as a complement to the RCT data (Saldanha et al., 2022).

> **TIP**
>
> Consider a comparison of NRISs and RCTs to explore alignment of conclusions and recommendations.

A third approach especially important in nursing science is the process by which mixed-methods studies can be evaluated for evidence to strengthen practice recommendations (Calonge et al., 2023). While Calonge and colleagues (2023) used an adapted Grading of Recommendations Assessment, Development, and Evaluation (GRADE) tool for mixed-method studies specifically to grade evidence for public health emergency preparedness, the implications for nursing science are considerable.

In the real world, however, there are a variety of ways in which researchers can come to a conclusion or be able to make a statement about the effectiveness of a given intervention(s). These alternate methods include *narrative reviewing, vote counting, setting rules regarding the number of studies that have statistically significant results*, and a variety of forms of *meta-analysis* (Cooper et al., 2019b). We have given a brief description of these approaches and their limitations below.

Narrative reviewing: In short, this is a description of the available literature and the conclusions of the studies contained within that literature. The most obvious shortcoming of this method is that there is no real grading of the studies discussed, that is, little attention is paid to the strength of each study. In general, this method does not meet the standards of rigor and transparency and has fallen out of use with the advent of systematic review methods (Cooper et al., 2019a; Noble & Smith, 2018).

Vote counting: This method counts the numbers of studies about the intervention that accept or reject the null hypothesis, and those that show harm, so the group that has the most "votes" wins in terms of a conclusion as to effectiveness, benefit, or harm. The challenge with this method is that for it to be reasonably useful, each study being voted on needs to be appropriately powered, which is unlikely, and can result in a high error rate (Cooper et al., 2019b).

Rule setting: This is essentially a different type of vote counting, where generally two "good" studies are identified, informing the conclusions about effectiveness. The problem is the percentage of studies that meet this criterion. For example, if two out of two studies are "good," that translates into more confidence about effectiveness than if two of 30 studies are considered "good." This is not considered a good way to synthesize for evidence because of the high error rate.

Meta-analysis: Meta-analysis is the preferred method of synthesis when the review includes RCTs. The benefits of a meta-analysis include:
- Increased statistical power as a statistical test over simpler methods
- Greater precision (as reflected in overall effect size and smaller confidence intervals, indicating a more precise estimate)
- Information on the magnitude of the effect
- Ability to investigate reasons for variations between studies
- Ability to weight information from studies according to the amount and significance of information they contribute to the analysis
- Ability to investigate differences between studies and groups of studies and settle conflicting claims (Munn et al., 2014)

Factors in Implementation

Other things to consider as you evaluate and synthesize your evidence are such things as factors that influence dissemination and implementation of EBPs. Tierney and colleagues (2020) suggest considering the following as part of the synthesis review: *acceptability, adoption, appropriateness, feasibility, fidelity, implementation cost, intervention complexity, penetration, reach,* and *sustainability*. Including these elements as part of the review can inform evidence not just about clinical effectiveness, but also about implementation strategies. It helps translate RCTs and quasi-experimental designs into the real world. Specifically, the inclusion of multiple designs in a systematic review using the GRADE adaptation for mixed-methods studies (Calonge et al., 2023) can also help identify facilitators and barriers to the intervention, as well as the lived experience of people participating.

It is useful when your search of the literature finds intervention studies that can be used to answer your PICOT question. As a clinical leader, you and your team need to use your critical appraisal skills to determine the overall strengths and weaknesses of the study or studies and whether the findings of an intervention study or a group of studies can be applied to your patient population and clinical setting. A cost–benefit analysis may need to be completed and added to your team's overall appraisal before a final decision is made about implementing a change in practice (see Chapter 16). Because the goal of EBP is to achieve positive clinical outcomes and improve quality of life (Sidani et al., 2016), it is important for you as a clinical leader to participate in translating evidence about new interventions into practice.

SYNTHESIS

In this chapter, we have reviewed the purpose of an intervention study, different intervention study designs, and identified strengths and weaknesses of different design approaches, including potential threats to internal and external validity. We have also discussed the process of synthesizing evidence from intervention studies based on a particular PICOT question, how good intervention studies contribute to an EBP review, and the potential impact on health care practices. Importantly, we stress the use of considerations for implementation; the evidence derived from intervention studies must translate to real-world circumstances to be useful.

KEY POINTS

- Intervention studies, also called RCTs, provide the strongest Level II evidence for an individual study.
- Quasi-experimental designs are intervention studies that provide Level III evidence but lack randomization or a control group.
- Intervention studies are characterized by three features: control, randomization, and manipulation.
- Newer study designs are emerging that may help researchers identify the most important components of nursing interventions and show how well these

- new interventions work in the real world of clinical care.
- Critical appraisal of intervention studies is a multistep process that focuses on assessing how effectively the researchers minimized bias by controlling threats to internal and external validity.
- Results of intervention studies need to be critically appraised based on whether the data analysis is appropriate for answering the research question and significance of the evidence.
- Synthesizing the overall strengths and weaknesses of a group of intervention studies will inform clinical decision making about applicability of the findings to practice.

REFERENCES

Andrade, C. (2018). Internal, external, and ecological validity in research design, conduct, and evaluation. *Indian Journal of Psychological Medicine, 40*(5), 498–499. https://doi.org/10.4103/ijpsym.ijpsym_334_18.

Aromataris, E., & Pearson, A. (2014). The systematic review: An overview. *American Journal of Nursing, 114*(3), 53–58.

Baldi, I., Lago, E. D., Bardi, S. D., Sartor, G., Soriani, N., Zanotti, R., & Gregori, D. (2014). Trends in RCT nursing research over 20 years: Mind the gap. *British Journal of Nursing, 23*(16), 895–899.

Calonge, N., Shekelle, P. G., Owens, D. K., Teutsch, S., Downey, A., Brown, L., et al. (2023). A framework for synthesizing intervention evidence from multiple sources into a single certainty of evidence rating: Methodological developments from a US National Academies of Sciences, Engineering, and Medicine Committee. *Research Synthesis Methods, 14*(1), 36–51.

Chen, M.-L. (2014). Are trials with nursing interventions pragmatic? *The Journal of Nursing Research, 22*(3).

Collins, L. M. (2018). Conceptual introduction to the multiphase optimization strategy (MOST). In *Optimization of Behavioral, Biobehavioral, and Biomedical Interventions. Statistics for Social and Behavioral Sciences*. Cham: Springer. https://doi.org/10.1007/978-3-319-72206-1_1.

Collins, L. M., Trail, J. B., Kugler, K. C., Baker, T. B., Piper, M. E., & Mermelstein, R. J. (2014). Evaluating individual intervention components: Making decisions based on the results of a factorial screening experiment. *Translational Behavioral Medicine, 4*(3), 238–251.

Cooper, H., Hedges, L. V., & Valentine, J. C. (Eds.). (2019a). *The handbook of research synthesis and meta-analysis*. Russell Sage Foundation.

Cooper, H., Hedges, L. V., & Valentine, J. C. (2019b). Potentials and limitations of research synthesis. *The Handbook of Research Synthesis and Meta-analysis* (PP. 517–525). Russell Sage Foundation.

Dang, D., Dearholt, S., Bissett, K., Ascenzi, J., & Whalen, M. (2022). *Johns Hopkins evidence-based practice for nurses and healthcare professionals: Model and guidelines* (4th ed.). Sigma Theta Tau International.

Dekkers, O. M., von Elm, E., Algra, A., Romijn, J. A., & Vandenbroucke, J. P. (2010). How to assess the external validity of therapeutic trials: A conceptual approach. *International Journal of Epidemiology, 39*(1), 89–94. https://doi.org/10.1093/ije/dyp174.

DeVellis, R. F., & Thorpe, C. T. (2021). *Scale development: Theory and applications*. Sage Publications.

Flannelly, K. J., Flannelly, L. T., & Jankowski, K. R. B. (2018). Threats to the internal validity of experimental and quasi-experimental research in healthcare. *Journal of Health Care Chaplaincy, 24*(3), 107–130.

Franklin, J. M., Patorno, E., Desai, R. J., Glynn, R. J., Martin, D., Quinto, K., et al. (2021). Emulating randomized clinical trials with nonrandomized real-world evidence studies: First results from the RCT DUPLICATE initiative. *Circulation, 143*(10), 1002–1013.

Hariton, E., & Locascio, J. J. (2018). Randomised controlled trials—the gold standard for effectiveness research. *BJOG: An International Journal of Obstetrics & Gynaecology, 125*(13), 1716–1716. https://doi.org/10.1111/1471-0528.15199.

Higgins, J. P. T., & Green, S. (2011). *Cochrane handbook for systematic reviews of interventions version 5.0*. Internet.

Minary, L., Trompette, J., Kivits, J., Cambon, L., Tarquinio, C., & Alla, F. (2019). Which design to evaluate complex interventions? Toward a methodological framework through a systematic review. *BMC Medical Research Methodology, 19*(1), 1–9.

Munn, Z., Tufanaru, C., & Aromataris, E. (2014). JBI's systematic reviews: Data extraction and synthesis. *AJN The American Journal of Nursing, 114*(7), 49–54.

Noble, H., & Smith, J. (2018). Reviewing the literature: Choosing a review design. *Evidence-Based Nursing, 21*(2), 39–41.

Saldanha, I. J., Adam, G. P., Bañez, L. L., Bass, E. B., Berliner, E., Devine, B., et al. (2022). Inclusion of nonrandomized studies of interventions in systematic reviews of interventions: Updated guidance from the Agency for health care research and quality effective health care program. *Journal of Clinical Epidemiology, 152*, 300–306.

Shea, B. J., Reeves, B. C., Wells, G., Thuku, M., Hamel, C., Moran, J., et al. (2017). AMSTAR 2: A critical appraisal tool for systematic reviews that include randomised or non-randomised studies of healthcare interventions, or both. *BMJ, 358*.

Sidani, S., Fox, M., Epstein, D. R., & Miranda, J. (2016). Challenges in using the randomized trial design to examine the influence of treatment preferences. *The Canadian Journal of Nursing Research = Revue Canadienne de Recherche En Sciences Infirmieres, 48*(1), 7–13. https://doi.org/10.1177/0844562116665274.

Siedlecki, S. L. (2020). Quasi-experimental research designs. *Clinical Nurse Specialist, 34*(5), 198–202. https://doi.org/10.1097/NUR.0000000000000540.

Taylor, C. S. (2013). *Validity and validation*. Oxford University Press.

Thabane, L., Ma, J., Chu, R., Cheng, J., Ismaila, A., Rios, L. P., et al. (2010). A tutorial on pilot studies: The what, why and how. *BMC Medical Research Methodology, 10*(1).

Tierney, A. A., Haverfield, M. C., McGovern, M. P., & Zulman, D. M. (2020). Advancing evidence synthesis from effectiveness to implementation: Integration of implementation measures into evidence reviews. *Journal of General Internal Medicine, 35*, 1219–1226.

Tume, L. N., Mcevoy, N. L., & Vollam, S. (2022). Randomized controlled trials in critical care nursing: Essential to move practice forward. *Nursing in Critical Care, 27*(4), 477–479. https://doi.org/10.1111/nicc.12773.

Waite, M. (2002). *Concise Oxford thesaurus*. Oxford University Press.

Wolf, L. (2017). Giving the complete picture: Why publishing negative results is important. *Journal of Emergency Nursing, 43*(3), 289–290.

9

Observational Studies

Geri LoBiondo-Wood and Barbara Delmore

LEARNING OUTCOMES

After reading this chapter, you should be able to do the following:
- Apply critical appraisal criteria to observational studies.
- Differentiate between the types of observational studies.
- Synthesize evidence from observational studies based on a PICOT question.
- Summarize information from observational studies to formulate clinical decisions based on evidence.
- Apply findings from observational studies to formulate evidence-based clinical decisions.

KEY TERMS

Case series
Case-control study
Cohort study
Cross-sectional study
Exposure
Longitudinal study
Observational study
Outcome
Repeated measures study
Retrospective study

A critical focus for supporting your practice based on evidence is the ability to assess and implement interventions in a specific population that will lead to improvement of health care outcomes. A key benchmark for evidence-based practice (EBP) is intervention studies, but often, health care practice issues do not lend themselves to intervention studies. For example, assume that you are providing care for an adolescent population with cancer-related fatigue from undergoing chemotherapy. You may be interested in the amount of fatigue, variations in fatigue, and timing of patient fatigue in response to chemotherapy. You and your team would not be interested in therapy studies addressing interventions to relieve fatigue until you understand the patterns of fatigue over the course of treatment. Reviewing the evidence from intervention studies would not answer your clinical question. Instead, you and your team would need to examine the factors that contribute to the variability in adolescent cancer-related fatigue by reviewing observational studies. Observational studies are used when researchers intend to explore events, people, or situations as they naturally occur, or test relationships and differences among variables. Observational studies construct a picture of variables at one point or over a period of time, and the variables are not manipulated or randomized as in a randomized controlled trial (RCT). The purpose of this chapter is to provide an overview of observational designs with questions and issues to raise when critically appraising observational studies for EBP decision making.

OBSERVATIONAL STUDIES

The major types of observational studies are: cohort, case-control, cross-sectional, and survey. When you are reading studies classified as observational, it is key to remember that the researchers did not directly control or manipulate the variables, but measured the

105

variables as they naturally occurred. Observational studies are considered nonexperimental designs because the researcher does not actively manipulate the variables nor does the researcher randomly assign participants to groups. However, in retrospective studies such as a case-control study, researchers can randomly select (choose) cases and controls from a compiled database. Randomly selecting cases and controls may be desired by a researcher to add stringency to the selection process so that the study population is as representative or comparable as can be in a retrospective design (Talari & Goyal, 2020). Data for observational studies may be gathered on one or several occasions. The data can be gathered prospectively—that is, moving forward in time, or retrospectively looking back in time, or working in a **cross-section**, collecting data at one point in time (Talari & Goyal, 2020). As you review observational studies, the concepts of control and potential sources of bias (see Chapter 8) must be considered.

Observational studies are classified by the features of the study's design and data collection timing, and provide Level IV evidence (see Chapter 3). The information yielded by these types of studies is critical to developing a practice that is based on evidence and may also represent the best evidence available to answer either research or clinical questions.

The variables or conditions in observational studies are referred to as exposure and outcomes. An **exposure**, past, present, or future, can be either a harmful or beneficial condition that can affect the outcome of illness or health. An **outcome** is the consequence of the exposure.

Observational research is used when researchers wish to assess exposure to a condition and when manipulation is neither theoretically nor ethically possible, nor the aim of the study. Cigarette smoking and its relationship to lung cancer is a classic example of an observational study. For ethical reasons, individuals cannot be randomized to smoking or nonsmoking groups. Only the outcomes of long-term cigarette use versus nonuse in existing groups can be measured. As you evaluate observational studies, be aware of the sources of bias and internal and external validity issues that may affect study outcomes. Observational studies also are used to provide preliminary data for RCTs.

The conduct of observational studies in healthcare is appealing. Vast existing data sources, such as individual charts in electronic health records or large databases that contain health-related or all-payer data, can

TABLE 9.1	Types of PICOT Questions for Observational Studies
Design	PICOT Question Type
Cohort	Prognosis, Etiology, Diagnosis, Harm, Intervention
Case Series	Harm, Etiology, Prognosis, Diagnosis
Case-Control	Intervention, Prognosis, Case-Control

be used to study clinical issues. As described in Chapter 5, there are different types of PICOT questions. Answering a PICOT question requires a search of the best evidence. RCTs and quasi-experimental designs (see Chapter 8) are the gold standard for answering PICOT questions about the efficacy or effectiveness of an intervention, but not all PICOT questions are focused on the efficacy or effectiveness of an intervention. Questions related to diagnosis, prognosis, harm, and etiology may best be answered by reviewing observational studies (see Chapter 5). The types of PICOT questions related to observational designs are listed in Table 9.1. As you follow the steps of your chosen model (see Chapter 4) for your evidence-based project, you will most likely include several types of observational studies that must be evaluated within the parameters of their respective design elements as described in this chapter. Before discussing the observational design types that you will review and critically appraise for your EBP project, it is important to understand the principles underpinning observational study designs. When reviewing observational studies, you will find that the classifications of the designs are, at times, used interchangeably to categorize the components of a study. Fig. 9.1 provides a Decision-Making Algorithm for observational studies.

PURPOSE OF OBSERVATIONAL STUDIES

Several key overall concepts are operative in observational studies. One key concept is that the independent variable is not manipulated. It is observed and measured quantitatively, but not manipulated. Observational studies can use data from large data sets or collect data directly from participants. Data may be collected once or on several occasions.

Observational studies are valuable when relationships, differences, and comparisons need to be

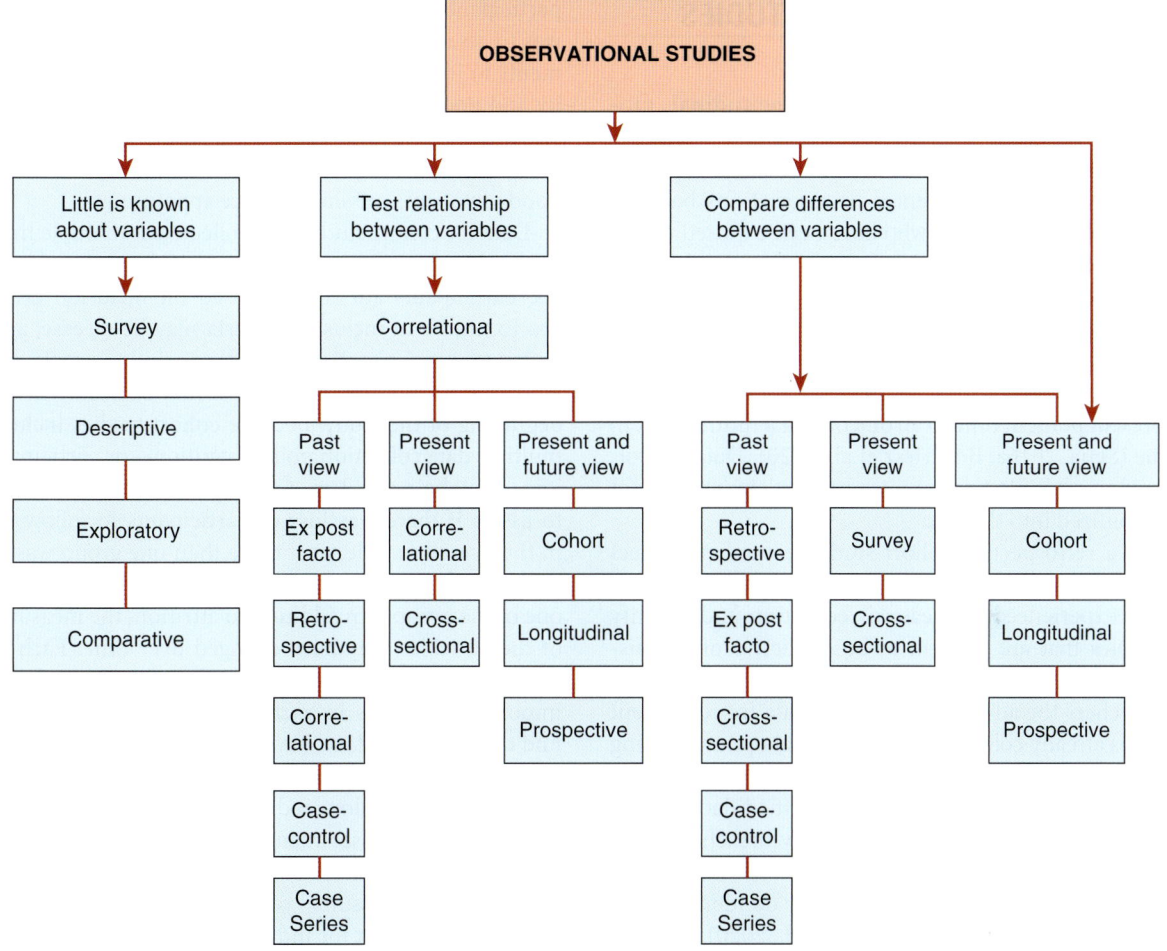

Fig. 9.1 Decision-Making Algorithm for Observational Studies.

assessed. Observational studies also are used to assess comparative effectiveness of interventions. Observational studies are useful when researchers wish to make comparisons among various treatments and randomization of participants is not possible, practical, or ethical. Large observational studies provide an avenue for researchers to obtain data from a diverse array of patients, providers, and treatment facilities (Delmore et al., 2019; Jagsi et al., 2014; Stellflug et al., 2022). Observational studies can test treatments retrospectively, cross-sectionally, or prospectively when studying cohorts in relation to an outcome of interest when a clinical trial and randomization are not possible. Because observational studies lack some of the elements of control, issues related to internal validity such as sampling, instrumentation, and testing must be closely assessed (see Chapter 8). As stated earlier, cohort studies are useful when your clinical question is focused on diagnosis, harm, causation, or prognosis.

> **TIP**
>
> Your question is what determines whether you should be conducting an EBP or research project. Therefore, it is important to consider ahead of time what your project's goal is and how it can best be accomplished. Your question is also what determines the design most appropriate to complete your project's goals. When conducting an EBP project, more than one design may be found and used to answer your PICOT question.

TYPES OF OBSERVATIONAL STUDIES
Cohort Studies

Cohort studies also are known as longitudinal, prospective, repeated measure, or retrospective studies. Cohort studies are those in which investigators compare or assess the differences or associations between and among participants who have been exposed or not exposed to an outcome. Cohort studies can be prospective or retrospective. In a prospective cohort study, researchers assess a group of participants experiencing an exposure—that is, either an intervention or a condition. The sample or study participants are followed from a present point in time to an outcome at a future point in time (Setia, 2016a; Bosdriesz et al., 2020). Data are collected at multiple time points and participants are not randomized into the study.

In a retrospective cohort study, researchers collect data from a sample of participants who have previously experienced a disease or condition and identify variables that are thought to be predictive of the disease or outcome identified. Retrospective studies offer researchers the advantage of having data from different groups already collected. The additional option of using de-identified versus identified participant data in retrospective research is possible. De-identified data may be preferred by a researcher to avoid any breaches in the participant's identity and preserve confidentiality. Generally, a sanctioned intermediary party de-identifies the data for the researcher (Yogarajan et al., 2020). The disadvantage of retrospective studies is that the data may be incomplete, inaccurate, or measured in a manner that is not ideal for answering a research or clinical question. These issues largely occur because the data used retrospectively was not initially collected for research purposes and therefore may not be fully aligned with the goals of a study (Talari & Goyal, 2020).

There are various reasons for conducting a retrospective cohort study. For example, assume that you are working in an outpatient setting and the focus of your clinical question is understanding the factors that influence missed outpatient appointments. Identifying the factors from the literature can potentially help improve patient appointment attendance. As part of the literature search in this area, you found an article that assessed potential demographic, disease, and practice factors extracted from chart data that predicted nonattendance in primary care settings in a sample of 550,083 participants (Ellis et al., 2017). The purpose of this study was to assess individuals who missed multiple appointments to identify potential risk markers for vulnerability and poor health outcomes. By including this article and other similar studies, you potentially could identify patient and practice factors that contribute to the likelihood of patients missing practice appointments.

Data for cohort studies are collected at multiple time points. Participants are not randomized in cohort studies. Participants are chosen based on inclusion criteria. Examples of inclusion criteria may be disease, age, or treatment. Cohort studies may include participants who have a condition or disease or may be healthy at the beginning of the study. Because cohort studies include multiple data collection points, attrition—or participant loss—may be a problem. Consequently, it is important to assess if there was loss of participants to follow up in the overall sample, or if more than one group was in the study, was there differential loss of participants in one of the groups? In addition to attrition, the measures of the variables may have changed over time. Each of the threats to internal validity outlined in Chapter 8 is important to assess in each study reviewed. You may find that a study did not have mortality issues, but selection issues were a problem. The participants in cohort studies are not randomized. The lack of randomization also requires an assessment of the threats to external validity (see Chapter 8).

For example, assume you are considering an EBP intervention project for individuals who have sustained an involuntary job loss, and you want to review interventions that have been tested. When conducting your literature review, you find the cohort study by Haynes and colleagues (2017). In this study, the researchers prospectively examined social rhythms, sleep, dietary intake, energy expenditure, waist circumference, and weight gain over 18 months in a group of individuals who had sustained involuntary job loss. Participants were evaluated on six occasions over the 18 months. The study overenrolled participants to account for attrition and missing data. When reviewing studies such as this, it is key to assess participant dropout, testing, and issues related to data collection at multiple time points. Although there are issues to consider if using such a study in an EBP project, data from this and similar studies can provide information for the development of evidence-based clinical programs aimed at implementing supportive interventions and prevention of negative outcomes. As you review this and other studies in this area, it is also important to assess how the variables were measured at multiple time points. Was there participant attrition or loss during the course of the study and if so, at what point(s) in the study? Synthesizing the findings—that is, the overall strengths and weaknesses of this and other similar studies—can help you decide what interventions to include in your support program.

A cohort study can provide both prospective and retrospective data. The Nurses' Health Study (NHS I) is a prospective, longitudinal study of nurses' health and health habits. This large study of 121,700 registered nurses began in 1976 and has expanded to two additional iterations, NHS II and NHS III (Bao et al., 2016). In these studies, nurses were sent questionnaires at specific time intervals and queried about their health status and health risk factors related to cancer, cardiovascular disease, and other disease processes. Initially, the study only included female nurses, but it was later expanded to male nurses. The data from this study enable researchers to prospectively gather information on several health issues, such as cardiovascular disease risk factors, cigarette smoking, and diet. Retrospectively, researchers have used this data to study the impact of cigarette smoking and diet on health over time. Data from these studies have assisted and will continue to assist care providers in developing new evidence-based avenues of health assessments and interventions in diabetes and cancer care and further aid development of evidence-based health care strategies for both women and men.

Another example of a retrospective cohort study was conducted by Kok and colleagues (2017). The study assessed the impact of obesity in cirrhotic patients with septic shock. In this study, the research team was able to assess the relationship of obesity using body mass index (BMI), septic shock, and mortality in a sample of 362 cirrhotic patients. The data obtained were from 1995 to 2015, taken from 28 medical centers across the United States and Canada. As you review the study, you find that it did not include data regarding presence or absence of ascites, potential variability in the sample in terms of treatment, or lack of a more accurate method of assessing obesity other than BMI (Kok et al., 2017). The authors acknowledged that the data do not imply causation but only that an association about the impact of obesity in cirrhotic patients with septic shock could be inferred. The researchers also acknowledged the lack of a more accurate method of assessing obesity other than BMI (Kok et al., 2017).

The studies reviewed point to several of the components of cohort studies, which often cannot be avoided. Because the exposure is not controlled in cohort studies and the samples are not randomized, it is difficult to conclude that the outcomes are truly caused by the intervention. When samples are not randomized, it is important to note that researchers can use various statistical procedures to assess for differences in the samples. Other previously identified issues to be aware of that may influence the results of cohort studies are:
- Missing data
- Participants' similarity
- Sample size
- Reliability of the data collection measures
- Time points of data collection

As you critically appraise cohort studies, remember that they provide useful information for practice. However, it is always important to assess how the variables were measured and identify each of the internal and external validity issues that can affect a study's outcome.

Case-Control Studies

Case-control studies are those designed to assess the association between an exposure (independent variable) and an outcome (dependent variable). Participants with the outcome of interest are compared with participants without the outcome. In this instance, a participant labeled as a "case" already has the outcome (e.g., disease, condition) whereas a "control" does not have the outcome. As a reminder, because the outcome already exists, there is no manipulation of the independent variable (exposure) as in an experimental design. (Talari & Goyal, 2020). Examples of exposure can be variables such as drug usage, symptoms, and diagnosis. Examples of outcomes may be a disease or a psychological or physiological condition. Case-control studies also may be labeled as *ex post facto*, *retrospective*, or *comparative*. Case-control studies can help identify risk factors related to disease or health conditions. Data from participants in these studies are typically retrospective—that is, data are abstracted from charts or other databases. Participants who have the intervention or condition are the cases, and those who do not have the intervention are the controls. Participants in case-control studies are *not* randomized to a group as in experimental studies but can be randomly selected to the case or control group to strengthen the selection process (Talari & Goyal, 2020). The case-control design is also strengthened by "matching." Matching is used to ensure that cases and controls are similar on specific characteristics, and may help to control certain types of confounders (Setia, 2016b). Although the data are retrospective, these designs can assist you in identifying risk factors related to health and illness outcomes.

Assume you are working on a complex medical unit in an acute care hospital that has a higher prevalence of heel pressure injuries as compared to other nursing units. The PICOT question leads you to a case-control study that was conducted by Delmore and colleagues (2019). The purpose of the study was to determine significant predictors as risk factors for heel pressure injury development in hospitalized adult patients (≥ 18 years old). This study was a continuation of these researchers' previous work that had found four significant predictors. The study's population was drawn from the New York state all-payer database governed by the New York State Department of Health. Cases were hospitalized patients admitted to a New York state hospital between January 2014 and June 2015, and had a documented hospital-acquired heel pressure injury. Controls were hospitalized patients who were admitted during the same time but did not have a documented hospital-acquired heel pressure injury. Data were de-identified and assigned a unique identifier by a sanctioned intermediary department so that the same patient was not selected twice. A 1:2 selection ratio was used to obtain cases and controls. In the main analysis, there were 1,697 patients (323 cases, 1,374 controls). The validation analysis, used to confirmed the predictive model in the main analysis, was 240 patients (80 cases, 160 controls). Findings revealed seven variables that were significant and independent predictors associated with heel pressure injuries. Using the seven variables, the researchers created an enabler in mnemonic form to help staff identify those hospitalized patients at risk for a heel pressure injury and apply the appropriate prevention strategies.

When considering the data for application to practice from case-control studies such as this, it is essential to assess how similar the sample was in each group, especially in the instance when the data were gathered over a long period; how and when the data were collected from the patients' records; and what policies and interventions were at the time of data collection, because practice changes over time.

Another example is a retrospective case-control study conducted by Dabroski and colleagues (2017). The aim of this multicenter study was to identify gender differences in risk factors for the development of cancer between men and women with type 2 diabetes. The study included 118 women and 98 men who developed cancer and the same number of participants who had type 2 diabetes but did not develop cancer. If considering these findings for practice, it would be important to note that the data for the 216 participants were gathered from charts at different centers over an extended period (January 1998 to September 2016). Additionally, when the participants were broken down in groups for analysis, there were small numbers of participants in each cancer diagnosis group related to gender. Also, smoking habits were categorized into never smokers, past smokers, and current smokers and reported in percentages. These categories do not provide an indication of the multiple aspects of cigarette smoking, such as number of cigarettes or packs per week, amount of nicotine in the cigarettes, and type of cigarette smoked. Also, all comorbidities were classified into three categories: hypertension, hyperlipidemia, and cardiovascular disease. The data from these and other retrospective studies are not useless, but must be understood within the context of current practice and knowledge.

In the study above, data were collected over a long period of time and, over time, policies change, as do interventions and practice. When assessing case-control studies, as these studies highlighted, it is critical to assess not just the design type but the methodology used in the studies.

> **TIP**
>
> When critically appraising observational studies, it is important to assess whether the sample is representative of the population, especially if more than one group is being studied.

Case Series

Case series designs are studies that collect data from a consecutive sample of patients treated in a similar manner without a control group or comparison group. As you read case studies, it is important to understand that these studies include one group only and have no control group, and the sample is one of convenience. Assume you and your clinical team are interested in interventions that would support compensatory memory after a traumatic brain injury (TBI) in your patients. In your search of the literature, you find a case series study conducted by Bos and colleagues (2017) that aimed to investigate the efficacy of a memory notebook and a smartphone as compensatory memory aids after TBI. Individuals with TBI commonly experience difficulties with prospective memory. The researchers postulated that an electronic memory notebook could potentially assist prospective memory. The study's methods included one group of seven participants. Each participant's memory was assessed to establish a no-intervention baseline, followed by intervention training and the intervention with either a smartphone alone or a memory notebook followed by a smartphone. Participants who used a smartphone demonstrated improvement in their ability to complete memory tasks within the assigned time frame. The study results also supported that smartphone use provided additional benefits over a memory notebook. In this study, the participants were not randomized to the study and the sample was one of convenience; the group comprised those willing to participate and the sample size was very small. Although the study identified the potential of smartphone use in the neurorehabilitation sample, it would be important to assess if other studies were completed in this area before a practice change could be instituted. Other studies in this area may have used different designs and larger samples, but similar methods.

When you are conducting an EBP project and you locate case series studies related to your clinical question, it is important to review and consider each of the threats to internal and external validity. Case series also may be labeled as *longitudinal* because the data may be collected from the same group over a period of time. Case series also may be referred to as *case reports*.

Survey Studies

Studies classified as **surveys** provide information in areas where little is known, often ask broad questions, and generally have large sample sizes. Survey studies can be classified as descriptive, exploratory, or comparative. These terms can be used alone, interchangeably, or together to describe a study. Surveys can be distributed anonymously electronically by email or texting, mail carrier delivery, or in person. Surveys focus on studying attitudes, preferences, and behaviors, and assist in establishing patterns and gaining information in an area where little is known. Surveys collect detailed descriptions of variables and use the data to justify and assess conditions and practices or make plans for improving health care practices. You will find that the terms *exploratory, descriptive, comparative,* and *survey* are used alone, interchangeably, or together to describe this type of study design. A survey is used to search for information about the characteristics of particular participants, groups, institutions, or situations or about the frequency of a variable's occurrence, particularly when little is known about it. Variables in surveys can be classified as opinions, attitudes, or facts. Surveys are useful because they can provide data for the development of intervention studies. Surveys can also be described as comparative when used to determine differences between variables. Survey data can be collected with a questionnaire or an interview and can have large or small samples of participants drawn from defined populations. Surveys can be either broad or narrow and can be composed of people or institutions. Surveys relate one variable to another or assess differences between variables, but do not determine causation.

The advantages of surveys are that a great deal of information can be obtained from a large population in a fairly economical manner, and that survey research information can be surprisingly accurate. If a sample is representative of the population, even a relatively small number of participants can provide an accurate picture of the population. Additionally, if an electronic platform is used to collect data and no names or identifiers from respondent are obtained, respondents are afforded anonymity. Anonymity means that the participant's responses cannot be linked to the data provided, increasing the integrity of the responses.

Survey studies do have disadvantages. The information obtained in a survey tends to be superficial. The breadth, rather than the depth, of the information is emphasized. A practice change would not be based on survey data alone.

An example of a survey is a study conducted by Huijten and colleagues (Huijten et al., 2023). The researchers conducted a cross-sectional, multicenter survey aimed to explore the perceived support needs of hospital nurses providing quality palliative care for persons with dementia in the Netherlands. Additionally, the researchers wanted to also identify differences between nurses in different ward types and at different educational levels. A convenience sample of a heterogeneous group of nurses were surveyed between January 2021 and April 2021 using a web-based questionnaire on the topics of palliative caregiving communication, collaboration, and hospital admissions. The 235 nurses that comprised the final sample had confirmed that they worked in hospice within the prior 10 years. The survey instrument was adapted from an instrument used in a former study performed in the nursing and home care setting, which was part of larger project called Desired Dementia Care Towards End of Life (DEDICATED). The researchers adapted the instrument for the hospital setting in consultation with the questionnaire developer, and researchers and nurses who were geriatric and palliative care specialists. Survey results showed that the hospital nurses perceived themselves as "competent" in caring for the patient with severe dementia at life's end regardless of education level, but differences were detected by nursing unit types. Findings identified three support needs indicated by the nurses: (a) support when caring for this population, (b) support when dealing with disagreement among family members concerning end-of-life care, and (c) support when trying to determine a consistent caregiver for the patient. This study demonstrates the adaptability of surveys and their instruments to query other facets of care aspects from for a patient population, especially when a population traverses the health care continuum.

Survey studies such as the Huijten and colleagues (2023) study can provide useful background information for a clinical project, but would require more specific data from other observational studies to answer a clinical question.

> **TIP**
>
> Evidence gained from a survey may be coupled with clinical expertise and applied to a similar population to develop an educational program and to enhance knowledge and skills in a clinical area (e.g., a survey designed to measure the nursing staff's knowledge and attitudes about EBP where the data are used to develop an EBP staff development course).

> **TIP**
>
> When you are establishing evidence for practice, each step of a study must be assessed. The design type is one element of assessment. Be aware that possible sources of bias can be introduced at any point in the study.

TYPES OF DATA AND DATA ANALYSES IN OBSERVATIONAL STUDIES

Data found in observational studies can be collected directly from individuals at one or more data points. In this instance, data and any subsequent analyses are from a primary source. Data can also be obtained from secondary sources. Secondary sources can be patient charts, all-payer databases, registries, claims, or databases such as Surveillance, Epidemiology, and End Results (SEER), which provides information on cancer incidence, prevalence, and survival statistics in the United States. Observational studies also use data from sources such as Medicare and Medicaid, and other large clinical databases such as the Healthcare Cost and Utilization Project (HCUP) from the Agency for Healthcare Research and Quality (AHRQ). When data is from a secondary source, subsequent analyses are termed secondary data analysis. Data also are obtained from self-report questionnaires. These may be continuous data, such as pulse rates or blood pressure readings. Data may also be from questionnaires that require a participant to respond to questions on a Likert scale from "strongly agree" to "strongly disagree." Survey data also can be categorical or dichotomous, such as a "yes" or "no" response.

Both primary and secondary data sources are valid and useful for asking clinical questions. It is important to note, however, that using a secondary data source has its caveats. While secondary sources are economical and offer the ability to explore and manage diverse data, the user must be mindful that: (a) the data was originally collected for another purpose and may be subject to multiple sources of biases, (b) the data may not be accurate or complete, or may be limited, and (c) permission is often required before obtaining and using a secondary data source (Martin-Sanchez et al., 2017).

Data for observational studies such as age, gender, medications, and disease characteristics are also abstracted from patient records. Information found in cohort studies includes actively collected questionnaire data that measure psychosocial variables from a sample or samples of individual participants who meet a study's inclusion criteria. As you review the data found in cohort studies, consider the data sources, time of data collection, how the data collection was standardized, its original purpose for being collected, and whether the measures were reliable and valid.

The sample and sample size in the studies reviewed within this chapter also must be evaluated. Chapter 7 discusses sample size in relationship to testing an intervention. Not all observational studies will have a sample size calculation. For example, surveys do not, but you will find a sample size calculation in cohort or case-control studies.

> **TIP**
>
> When you are reviewing cohort and case-control studies, remember that the lack of randomization and manipulation of the variables can affect the results and your interpretation of the results.

Data analyses found in observational studies include both descriptive and inferential data (see Chapter 13). The descriptive data will describe the participants and the study's variable characteristics, while the inferential statistics aid the researcher in drawing conclusions about the data that can be applied to the sample. When you are conducting an EBP project, the data analysis will differ from study to study, based on the variables' level of measurement, the instruments used, and the sample size (see Chapter 13). Because the data analyses vary from study to study, it is important to evaluate not just the statistic used but the issues previously identified, such as sample, instruments, and time period of data collection and if it is helping you answer your question.

When you are evaluating studies for an EBP, consider the clinical significance as well as the statistical significance (see Chapter 13). The results of the data analysis in each study set the stage for the interpretation, discussion, and limitations sections that follow the results. The "Results" section should reflect analysis of each research question and/or hypothesis tested. The information from each hypothesis or research question should be presented sequentially. The tests used to analyze the data should be identified. If the exact test that was used is not explicitly stated, the values obtained should be noted. The researcher does this by providing the numeric values of the statistics and stating the specific test value and probability level achieved.

CRITICALLY APPRAISING OBSERVATIONAL STUDIES

When moving through the steps of a model (see Chapter 4) and conducting an EBP project, it is key to assemble the relevant research and related literature to move to effective EBP changes. It is important to critique each study individually and collectively for strengths and weaknesses. You will find that working with a team to assemble and evaluate the literature will help you move through the steps of an EBP model (see Chapter 4) more efficiently. When you locate multiple studies related to your clinical question, it may be useful to pair a novice and expert to complete the critiques.

The variables or conditions in observational studies are not controlled using random assignment or manipulation as they are in RCTs. As such, these designs place the interpretation of findings at a higher risk for bias related to the threats of internal and external validity. It is important that you ask several key questions about each study that you review related to your clinical question (Table 9.2). Because observational studies lack the control associated with RCTs, it is important to assess for bias in each step of the study. The assessment of bias requires a review of each of the threats to internal validity (see Chapter 7). First, because the samples in these studies are generally convenience samples and participants are not randomized into groups, it is important to assess the specific inclusion and exclusion criteria, and assess whether the participants are similar or dissimilar in relation to the study objectives and demographics at baseline and in all the key elements of treatment or disease condition. Assessment of the measurement of variables is also key. Points to assess are:

- Were the data collected in real time?
- Did data collection depend on participants' recall (which can lead to recall bias)?
- Were the instruments reliable and valid?
- Were the instruments administered in the same manner to all participants?
- Were the conditions of data collection similar for all participants to maximize fidelity?
- If a study collected data on several occasions, was there participant loss?
- How many participants were approached to participate, and how many agreed?

Participants may be lost to follow-up if the data collection takes more time than a participant is willing to give. Understanding the questionnaires also can be an issue for participants. Participant dropout and incomplete questionnaire data may be issues, especially if there are multiple data collection periods. This situation is caused by respondent burden, which is the degree that

TABLE 9.2 Critical Appraisal and Sources of Bias—Observational Studies

Study Component	Potential Source of Bias
Design	Was the design consistent with the research problem or hypothesis studied?
Sample	Observational studies do not include randomization of participants to groups. Review the inclusion criteria and assess how the participants' characteristics were alike or dissimilar at baseline on key variables related to the study questions and relevant demographics. Was the sample representative of individuals experiencing the same condition or health issue? Were the overall characteristics of the participants alike? If more than one group, were their characteristics alike? Was the sample size adequate? Was the sample representative of the disease or condition being studied? Was a sample size calculation using power analysis reported? If a cohort study, was there participant attrition? If there was a comparison group, were the groups similar to each other regarding data collection points? How did the researchers control for bias in the sample?
Instruments	Were the instruments reliable, valid, and consistent with the variables measured?
Data Collection	What were the sources of data? Were the data collected consistent with the research question or hypothesis? If data were collected over time, was the follow-up adequate and were the time periods valid? Were the data sources the same for all participants? Were the data collection procedures consistent to maximize fidelity? If more than one group of participants, were the groups similar and the data collected at the same time? If the data were collected longitudinally as in a cohort, longitudinal, repeated measures study, was the follow-up adequate for the outcome to occur, and were the data collected at the same time for all groups?
Data Analysis	Was there missing data (especially important in cohort studies)? Was the analysis consistent with the question? Was the follow-up period adequate for the outcomes to occur? Was the analysis adjusted for confounding variables?
Findings	Were internal and external validity threats identified and discussed? Were the limitations of the study addressed?

the respondent perceives participating in a survey as problematic (Aiyegbusi et al., 2022). Respondent burden is caused by several reasons and if not addressed, the risk of increased missing and poor-quality data is greater. Care should be taken to address and avoid the issues of respondent burden expeditiously as poor-quality data can lead to poor health care decisions (Aiyegbusi et al., 2022). To avoid respondent burden, consider the following:
- Did the respondent detect a bias in the questions?
- Was the respondent able to comprehend the questions?
- Did the questions trigger an emotional response?
- How many questionnaires were they asked to complete, and what was the length of each?

Lengthy questionnaires can contribute to missing data and increase bias in study results. It is difficult to control confounding variables in observational studies. If confounding variables affected the study's outcome, it would be important for researchers to address this in the findings and conclusions sections of the article.

Because there are different types of observational studies with different strategies for sampling, data collection, and analysis, it is important to assess each study. Standardized critical appraisal tools such as those offered by the Center for Evidenced-Based Medicine (CEBM), Critical Appraisal Skills Programme (CASP), and Joanna Briggs Institute (JBI) are geared to assessing specific types of designs. For example, the CASP website offers checklists for diagnostic, case-control, and cohort studies. The checklist questions will help guide you through the process of evaluating the different types of designs you will encounter as you answer your PICOT question. As you review studies in this category, also consider the key concepts of critical appraisal identified within this chapter and in Box 9.1 and Table 9.2.

> **TIP**
>
> Collaboration is an essential feature of EBP projects. Critical appraisal of studies is most effectively accomplished by having at least two team members critically appraise each study using a CASP, CEBM, or JBI critical appraisal tool to establish interrater agreement by having them compare their respective critiques and arrive at a consensus about the strength and quality of the evidence.

> **TIP**
>
> Generalizability of studies from one sample to another depends on who participated in a study. When you are reviewing studies, the sample from each study must also be assessed. As you review studies, think about how well the participants represent the population of interest.

SYNTHESIS

Observational studies do not control interventions as do RCTs. As such, it is important to interpret the results of observational studies with caution. What strengthens the findings of observational studies is ensuring that all components of a study are clearly identified and consistent. Included in the assessment of individual observational studies is consideration not only of the design but also of the appropriateness of the measures, including the reliability and validity of the measures, sample size, sample characteristics, and analyses. Synthesis of the overall strengths and weaknesses of the findings of a group of observational studies advances your clinical team's ability to make recommendations about the applicability of findings to your clinical population and setting. This will be enhanced by a final assessment that includes the evaluation of similar studies conducted in the same or similar populations, using similar methods that concur with each other.

> **BOX 9.1 Critical Appraisal for Observational Studies**
>
> - Was the risk for the dependent variable or outcome the same for the exposed and control groups?
> - Were the inclusion and exclusion criteria clearly identified?
> - If there was a comparison group, how alike were the participants in each group in terms of participant characteristics and time of data collection?
> - If there was a comparison group, were the participants in both groups similar in terms of predictive factors related to the study's outcomes?
> - When were the data collected for the groups? Practice and interventions change rapidly, so data from studies that are several years old may not be relevant to current therapies.
> - Were the data from the groups collected simultaneously?
> - Where were the studies conducted, and were the settings similar to your setting?
> - Were there any intervening variables?
> - What were the threats to internal and external validity (see Chapter 7)?
> - Were the data sources from charts or directly from participants?
> - If data were collected from participants, was participant recall the basis of data collection?
> - Are the results relevant to my patients?
> - How strong is the relationship between independent variable/exposure and the dependent variable/outcome?

KEY POINTS

- Observational studies lack randomization.
- Observational studies can be prospective, retrospective, cross-sectional, or longitudinal.
- Observational studies also include case-control and survey studies.
- If an intervention is included, participants are not randomized to the intervention nor are the methods controlled as in an RCT.
- Bias or threats to internal and external validity need to be considered in each study reviewed.

REFERENCES

Aiyegbusi, O. L., Roydhouse, J., Rivera, S. C., Kamudoni, P., Schache, P., Wilson, R., et al. (2022). Key considerations to reduce or address respondent burden in patient-reported outcome (PRO) data collection. *Nature Communications, 13*(1). https://doi.org/10.1038/s41467-022-33826-4

Bao, Y., Bertola, M. L., Lenart, E. B., Stampfer, M. J., Willett, W. C., Speizer, F. E., et al. (2016). Origins, methods, and evolution of the three nurses' health studies. *American Journal of Public Health, 106*(9), 1573–1581.

Bos, H. R., Babbage, D. R., & Leathem, J. M. (2017). Efficacy of memory aids after traumatic brain injury: A single case series. *Neurorehabilitation, 41*(2), 463–481.

Bosdriesz, J. R., Stel, V. S., van Diepen, M., Meuleman, Y., Dekker, F. W., Zoccali, C., et al. (2020). Evidence-based medicine—when observational studies are better than randomized controlled trials. *Nephrology, 25*(10), 737–743. https://doi.org/10.1111/nep.13742

Dabroski, M., Szymanska-Garbacz, E., Miszczyszyn, Z., Derezinski, T., & Czupryniak, L. (2017). Differences in risk factors of malignancy between men and women with type 2 diabetes: A retrospective case control study. *Oncotarget, 8*(40), 66940–66950.

Delmore, B., Ayello, E. A., Smith, D., Rolnitzky, L., & Chu, A. S. (2019). Refining heel pressure injury risk factors in the hospitalized patient. *Advances in Skin and Wound Care, 32*(11). https://doi.org/10.1097/01.ASW.0000579704.28027.d2

Ellis, D. A., McQueenie, R., McConnachie, A., Wilson, P., & Williamson, A. E. (2017). Demographic and practice factors predicting repeated non-attendance in primary care: A national retrospective cohort analysis. *The Lancet, 2*, e551–e559.

Haynes, P. L., Silva, G. E., Howe, G. W., Thomson, C. A., Butler, E., Quan, S. F., et al. (2017). Longitudinal assessment of daily activity patterns on weight change after involuntary job loss: The ADAPT protocol. *BMC Public Health, 17*, 793.

Huijten, D. C. M., Bolt, S. R., Meesterberends, E., & Meijers, J. M. M. (2023). Nurses' support needs in providing high-quality palliative care to persons with dementia in the hospital setting: A cross-sectional survey study. *Journal of Nursing Scholarship, 55*(2), 405–412. https://doi.org/10.1111/jnu.12828. Epub 2022 Oct 11. PMID: 36218182.

Jagsi, R., Bekelman, J.E., Chen, A., Chen, R.C., Hoffman, K., Tina Shih, Y.C., Smith, B.D., & Yu, J.B. (2014). Considerations for observational research using large data sets in radiation oncology. *International Journal of Radiation Oncology Biology Physics, 90*(1), 11–24. https://doi.org/10.1016/j.ijrobp.2014.05.013.

Kok, B., Karvellas, C. J., Abraldes, J. G., Jalan, R., Sundaram, V., Gurka, D. P., et al. (2017). The impact of obesity in cirrhotic patients with septic shock: A retrospective study. *Liver International*.

Martin-Sanchez, F. J., Aguiar-Pulido, V., Lopez-Campos, G. H., Peek, N., & Sacchi, L. (2017). Secondary use and analysis of big data collected for patient care. *Yearbook of Medical Informatics, 26*(1), 28–37. https://doi.org/10.15265/IY-2017-008

Setia, M. (2016b). Methodology series module 2: Case-control studies. *Indian Journal of Dermatology, 61*(2), 146–151. https://doi.org/10.4103/0019-5154.177773

Setia, M. S. (2016a). Methodology series module 1: Cohort studies. *Indian Journal of Dermatology, 61*(1), 21–25. https://doi.org/10.4103/0019-5154.174011

Stellflug, S. M., Buerhaus, P., & Auerbach, D. (2022). Characteristics of family nurse practitioners and their preparation for practice in rural vs urban employment settings. *Nursing Outlook, 70*(3), 391–400. https://doi.org/10.1016/j.outlook.2021.12.007

Talari, K., & Goyal, M. (2020). Retrospective studies—utility and caveats. *Journal of the Royal College of Physicians of Edinburgh, 50*(4), 398–402. https://doi.org/10.4997/JRCPE.2020.409

Yogarajan, V., Pfahringer, B., & Mayo, M. (2020). A review of Automatic end-to-end de-identification: Is high accuracy the only metric? *Applied Artificial Intelligence, 34*(3), 251–269. https://doi.org/10.1080/08839514.2020.1718343

10

Systematic Reviews and Clinical Practice Guidelines

Amy Witkoski Stimpfel and Jin Jun

LEARNING OUTCOMES

After reading this chapter, you should be able to do the following:
- Differentiate among specific types of systematic reviews.
- Assess the quality of evidence from systematic reviews using standardized critical appraisal tools and criteria, including assessment of bias.
- Determine clinical relevance of a systematic review's conclusion and recommendation.
- Determine applicability of systematic review recommendations for clinical practice, policy, research, and/or education.
- Judge the quality of clinical practice guidelines using standardized critical appraisal tools and criteria.
- Differentiate among clinical practice guidelines developed by professional health care organizations and single health care institutions.

KEY TERMS

Clinical practice guidelines
Effect size
Fail safe number
Forest plot
Funnel plot
GRADE
Gray literature
Integrative review
Meta-analysis
Narrative review
Publication bias
Rapid review
Realist review
Review
Scoping review
Sensitivity analysis
Systematic review
Test for heterogeneity

Public and private agencies, payors, accreditation bodies, and patient advocacy groups (e.g., Centers for Medicare and Medicaid Services [CMS], Joint Commission, and American Nurses Credentialing Center [ANCC] Magnet Recognition Program) require that health care organizations demonstrate how they meet the Quadruple Aim of providing high-quality, cost-effective, satisfying care experiences, and improved workforce engagement. Clinical leaders are challenged to document how an evidence-based approach is used to meet those standards within their organizations. Given the growth in the breadth and depth of clinical research, it is a challenge for you as a clinical leader and your team to critically appraise studies that offer the strongest evidence to achieve the Quadruple Aim, and to remain current about clinical practice guidelines that inform adoption or revision of practices in your clinical setting.

Systematic reviews (SRs) and clinical practice guidelines (CPGs) offer clinicians a strategy for translating the best available evidence into clinical practice. Both focus on assessing multiple studies that answer a clinical question. A **review** is an evidence summary that synthesizes information from various sources to provide a comprehensive overview of the topic (Fink, 2014). You will note that there is no emphasis on a formal quality assessment of the included literature. Often, a review article aims to map out and categorize existing literature on a specific topic and identify gaps in the literature. Identifying gaps in the literature can serve as a basis for further reviews (e.g., SRs) or quality improvement projects or scholarship initiatives.

Common types of reviews include, but are not limited to, meta-analysis, integrative, and **scoping reviews**. A **systematic review** is a collection of research studies based on a clearly focused question that uses a defined search strategy to locate, assess, critically appraise, and synthesize relevant evidence to determine clinical practice recommendations. Other types of evidence reviews include **rapid**, **realist**, and **narrative reviews**. The different types of systematic reviews and review types are highlighted in Tables 10.1 and 10.2. Definitions and examples of these reviews and how they vary are described in Table 10.3.

Clinical practice guidelines are systematically developed statements or recommendations that link research and practice and provide an evidence-based best practice guide for clinicians. SRs of randomized controlled trials (RCTs) are considered to provide Level I evidence on the Evidence Hierarchy, found at the top of the evidence pyramid (see Chapter 3). CPGs are based on evidence ranging from Level I meta-analyses to those at Level VIII based on expert opinion.

In Chapters 8 and 9, you were introduced to quantitative designs focused on intervention and observational studies and how to critically appraise those studies for quality and applicability to practice. The purpose of this chapter is to expose you to SRs and CPGs that assess and/or provide evidence from multiple studies focused on answering a specific question. They provide a bridge between research and practice, offering clinicians a vital link for developing and implementing quality improvement initiatives.

> **TIP**
>
> Systematic reviews (SRs) and clinical practice guidelines (CPGs) are developed by interprofessional teams reflecting both diversity of professions and their expertise. The quality of the SRs and CPGs is, in part, evaluated by the quality of the team conducting the project. Screening of studies and evaluation of the strength and quality of those meeting inclusion criteria should be carried out by at least two members of the team with a third available to resolve differences.

TYPES OF REVIEWS

Based on a clearly formulated question, an SR represents an assessment and summation of a group of research studies found in the literature. An SR uses explicit, replicable criteria and methods to search for, identify, select, critically appraise, and analyze relevant data from the selected studies. The final step in an SR is summarizing the findings and making recommendations about applicability of the evidence to practice, policy, research, or education (Deeks et al., 2022). Other types of reviews also are guided by a focused question that may target a clinical, policy, research, or education topic or issue. The Decision-Making Algorithm in Fig. 10.1 provides a guide to assist you in deciding which type of SR is appropriate to answer a specific PICOT (Patient, population or problem, Intervention, Comparison or control, Outcome, and Time frame), or clinical question. A meta-synthesis is a review and analysis comprised of qualitative studies that is described further in Chapter 11.

A plethora of review article types has emerged in clinical and nonclinical disciplines that aim to demonstrate that the authors have searched the literature extensively using a clearly defined search strategy. Review articles cover a wide range of subject matter and study designs, including case study, qualitative, and quantitative research findings. Theoretical works and policy reports can also be used as the focus of a review to inform organizational or policy decision making. Tables 10.2 and 10.3 provide definitions and examples of different types of reviews.

SRs are guided by a PICOT question. They use search strategies to identify quantitative studies that focus on the same clinical question. The goal is to locate relevant studies that provide the strongest evidence with which to answer your clinical question and assess the strengths and weaknesses of the evidence in each study. In your search to find the best available evidence, you and your team will strive to locate RCTs. However, the reality of evidence-based practice is that cohort and case-control studies may provide the strongest level of evidence and design type to answer your clinical question.

SRs are often completed by clinical teams that may include a combination of clinicians, health science librarians, epidemiologists, and statisticians. Each study is critically appraised for validity and reliability—that is, quality, quantity, and consistency of the evidence, using

TABLE 10.1 Systematic Review and Meta-Analysis

Systematic review	Assessment of a group of quantitative studies with similar designs based on a focused clinical PICOT question that uses systematic and explicit methods and criteria to search for, identify, critically appraise, and analyze relevant data from the selected studies to summarize and communicate the findings and implications for applicability of evidence in a focused area (Page et al., 2021).
Meta-analysis	Statistical approach to analyzing the data from a group of studies included in a systematic review that allows statistical integration and combination of data across studies to quantify the effect using a larger sample size, thereby generating a more accurate estimate of the magnitude of the effect that informs an answer to a PICOT question (Hansen, Steinmetz, & Block, 2022).

TABLE 10.2 Types of Reviews

Integrative review	Critical appraisal of the literature in an area of interest that does not include a statistical analysis due to the limitations of the study designs or the heterogeneity of the designs and samples. A systematic approach using explicit criteria is often used (Whittemore & Knafl, 2005).
Narrative review	Review of the literature that includes a comprehensive, critical analysis of the current state of knowledge on a topic. They are often used to provide an overview of a topic, to identify gaps in the literature, or to develop a theoretical framework for future research. A systematic approach to searching for and appraising papers is not typically used (Onwuegbuzie & Frels, 2016).
Scoping review	A preliminary search and assessment of the potential size and scope of available research literature, including ongoing research. It aims to determine the value of undertaking a full systematic review. They use a variety of methods to synthesize the evidence, including thematic analysis, content analysis, and narrative synthesis. They focus on identifying the key concepts, research gaps, and methodological issues in a research area. (Munn et al., 2018).
Rapid review	A research methodology that uses shorter time frames than other evidence-based summaries. It provides a timely and valid view of evidence but sacrifices rigor. As such, rapid reviews are both review and assessment, and respond to urgent clinical and public health-related questions. They are used frequently in policy and practice settings to assist in decision making (Tricco et al., 2015).
Realist review	A realist review is a type of systematic review that focuses on understanding the context, mechanisms, and outcomes of interventions (CMO). It is a theory-driven approach to reviewing the literature, and its goal is to produce one or more theories to explain particular phenomena. Realist reviews are particularly useful for making sense of complex interventions, and are growing in popularity in the fields of health, education, and social policy. These interventions are often difficult to evaluate using traditional systematic review methods, because they are often implemented in different ways in different contexts, and their effects can be difficult to measure (Duddy & Wong, 2023).

standardized evaluation criteria and tools. The SR uses rigorous inclusion and exclusion criteria, an explicit and reproducible search methodology to identify all studies that meet the eligibility criteria, and assessment of the methods and findings from the included studies (Page et al., 2021; see Chapter 6). When completing the critical appraisal of an SR using one of the standardized critical appraisal tools identified in the IT Resources box, the following issues are addressed for each study:

- A focused clinical question
- Search strategy
- Sampling issues (e.g., inclusion and exclusion criteria, and sampling strategy)
- Methods and instrumentation
- Sources of bias (e.g., internal and external validity)
- Data analysis
- Findings
- Applicability of findings to practice

TABLE 10.3 Examples of Reviews

Type	Example
Integrative review	The purpose of "An integrative review of empirical literature on Indigenous cognitive impairment and dementia" (Racine, Johnson, & Fowler-Kerry, 2021) was to answer the research question: What are Indigenous perspectives on cognitive impairment and dementia? The authors conducted a literature search and used the integrative review methodology of Whittemore and Knafl (2005) and PRISMA (Moher et al., 2015). Synthesis and thematic analysis of 34 studies, which included 4 excellent quality systemic reviews, revealed 4 themes: frequency of cognitive impairment and dementia in Indigenous populations; culturally appropriate assessment techniques; tools for use in the clinical settings; and intersectoral collaboration. The findings highlight the need for community-led discussions and community engagement around Indigenous perspectives, needs, and understandings of aging, cognitive impairment, and dementia care.
Narrative review	The objective of "A Narrative Review of the Assessment of Depression in Chronic Pain" by Tenti, Raffaeli, & Gremigni (2022) was to explore the main critical issues in the assessment of depression in chronic pain and to identify self-report tools that can be reliably used for measuring it. Articles were obtained through a search of 3 databases and a hand search of the references of full-text papers for a total of 66 studies. Two authors independently scrutinized the selected articles to take note of the critical issues outlined by their authors, and they then identified relevant categories to group together articles that raised or discussed similar issues. Assessment of quality was not specified, and a statistical analysis of the data was not indicated for this narrative review.
Scoping review	A scoping review is a type of narrative review. Gifkins and colleagues (2020) explored "Fatigue and recovery in shiftworking nurses" using a scoping review to identify factors impeding or enhancing recovery from fatigue. Using the scoping review methodology based on Arksey and O'Malley's (2005) framework to identify existing research, they searched across 5 databases and identified and analyzed 31 studies. The evidence was assessed in narrative form without a quality assessment, and four themes were identified around factors impeding and enhancing recovery from fatigue both at work and home in shiftworking nurses. The findings had implications for individual nurses, mangers, and health care organizations while also noting the lack of intervention and longitudinal studies on the topic and an area for future research.
Rapid review	With the emergence of the novel coronavirus in 2020, assessment of the safety of vaccination during pregnancy was urgently needed. Ciapponi et al. (2021) completed a rapid review on the safety of COVID-19 vaccines for pregnant persons. The authors followed the Cochrane methods and the 2020 Preferred Reporting Items for Systematic Reviews and Meta-Analyses (PRISMA) statement for reporting results; they included 38 clinical and nonclinical studies, involving 2,398,855 pregnant persons and 56 pregnant animals from 39 reports. None of the adjusted relative effects comparing exposed vs. not exposed pregnant participants of the available exposure results were statistically associated with adverse outcomes. Thus, the authors concluded no evidence of safety concerns regarding the vaccines that the COVID-19 Vaccines Global Access Facility (COVAX MIWG) selected for review in August 2020, their components, or platforms used in other vaccines during pregnancy.
Realist review	van Dael and colleagues (2020) conducted a realist review "Learning from Complaints in Healthcare: A Realist Review of Academic Literature, Policy Evidence and Front-Line Insights" to address the translational gap between developments in complaints research and current complaint handling practice. Given the complexity of health care and policy interventions, they appropriately chose a realist review, which examines how and why interventions work, in what contexts, and for whom. After completing the stages of the review, including diverse evidence sources, the authors tested and refined their program theories assessing sources to develop the context, mechanism, and outcome (CMO) configurations. The authors followed the Realist and Meta-Narrative Evidence Syntheses: Evolving Standards (RAMESES) publication standards guided the reporting of the review (Wong et al., 2013).

CHAPTER 10 Systematic Reviews and Clinical Practice Guidelines

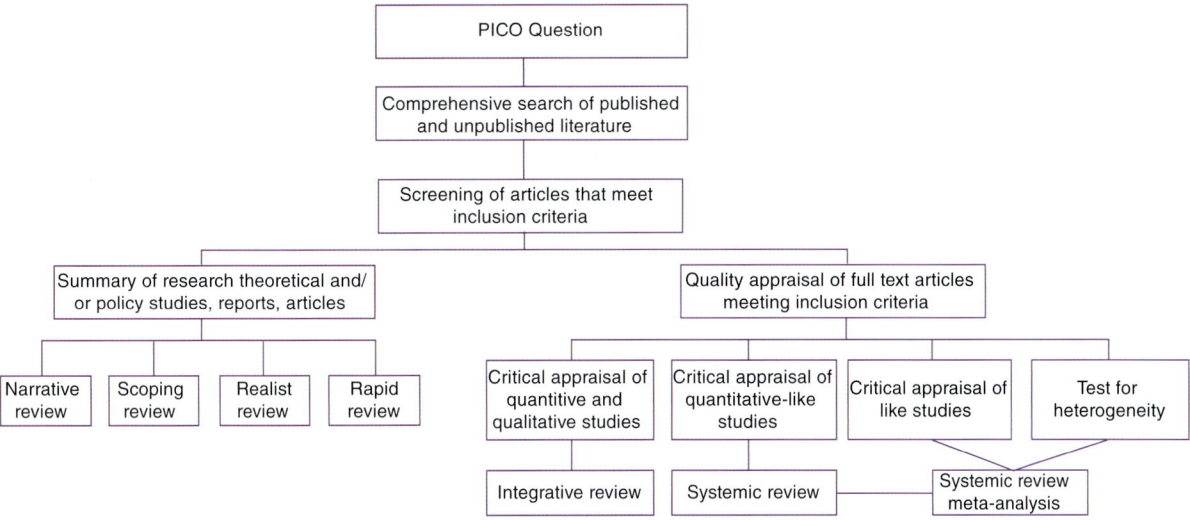

Fig. 10.1 The Decision-Making Algorithm.

More than one person on the SR team will evaluate the studies independently to be included or excluded from the review, a process sometimes called data extraction. A comprehensive search strategy will include both published and unpublished studies (often called gray literature; see Chapter 6). Similarly, you will note that at least two members of the SR team serve as independent judges to rate the quality of the studies using a standardized tool such as Consolidated Evidence for Reporting Trials (CONSORT) for RCT studies and Strengthening the Reporting of Observational Studies in Epidemiology (STROBE) for cohort studies. Once the studies in an SR are assessed for quality and synthesized according to a quality score or focus, practice recommendations are made and presented. The components of the SR are the same as a meta-analysis except there is no statistical analysis of the studies' data (Fig. 10.2 and Table 10.4).

> **TIP**
>
> An SR is an example of a secondary source because it uses previously conducted research studies. The individual studies that make up an SR, covered in Chapters 8, 9, and 11, are examples of primary sources.

An example of an SR was conducted by Bryant, Alonzo, and Schmillen (2017). The purpose of the SR was to review self-care interventions for adults with heart failure and describe direct provider involvement versus no direct provider involvement on patient self-care behaviors. The review was based on a PICOT question, had predetermined inclusion/exclusion criteria, described a detailed search strategy, and used the Preferred Reporting Items for Systematic Reviews and Meta-Analyses (PRISMA) and the PRISMA Checklist to ensure appropriate reporting of results to minimize bias. A strength of the SR was that assessment of studies for inclusion in the SR was completed independently by the two researchers. Based on grounding in the PICOT question and the inclusion/exclusion criteria, 29 studies were selected. Quality appraisal of the studies was completed using CONSORT for the RCT studies and STROBE for the observational studies. The majority of the studies in the SR were RCTs (n = 23). The remainder were quasi-experimental, cohort, mixed methods, or single-group designs. Studies included heart failure interventions, measurement of a self-care behavioral change as the outcome, and identification of provider involvement in the research. The majority of the studies' quality was moderate to low,

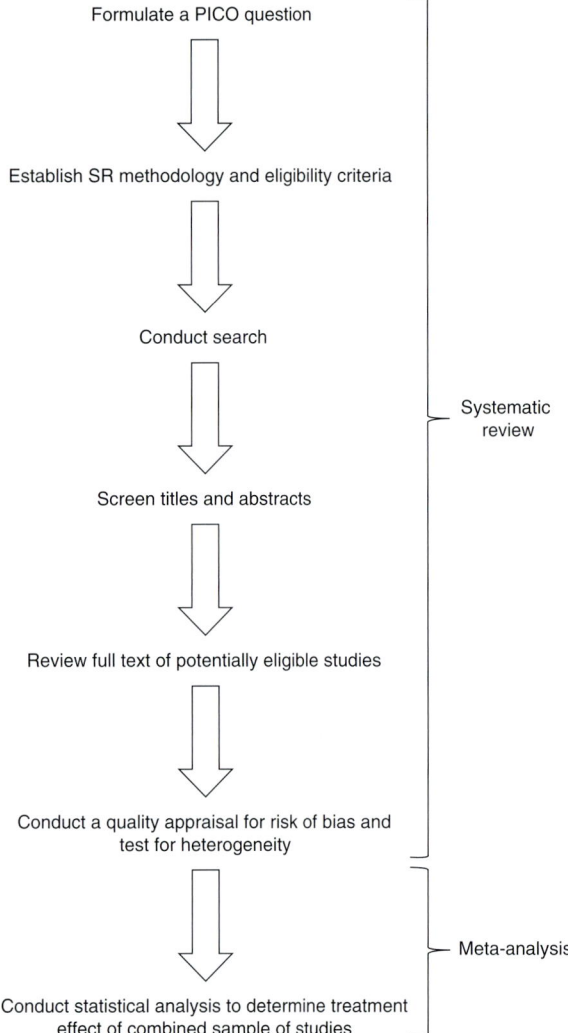

Fig. 10.2 Difference Between a Systematic Review and Meta-Analysis.

which can affect validity. Weaknesses of the studies reviewed included the heterogeneous nature of the study designs, interventions and their delivery (lack of consistent provider involvement), confounding strategies between studies, and limited generalizability that precluded statistical analysis of the studies as would be done with a meta-analysis. The authors appropriately concluded that there was a lack of data and quality of research studies to answer the PICOT question and demonstrated a significant gap in the literature. Additional rigorous explanatory research that focuses on the patient and provider interactions, including self-care communication strategies, is needed.

The individual studies in a systematic review are assessed and presented in a Table of Evidence (TOE) (see Chapter 3). The studies are synthesized as a group in a Synthesis TOE that highlights the overall strengths and weaknesses of the studies (see Chapter 6). Conclusions are based on your evaluation of the synthesized evidence:

- Does the SR answer my clinical (PICOT) question?
- Was the SR unbiased in its methodological quality?
- Are the SR results clinically important?
- Are the results useful and applicable to practice?

If you and your team have decided that the evidence is valid and important, you need to think about how it applies to your clinical question. For example, does your patient or population have characteristics similar to or different from those in the study? Is it feasible to apply the evidence in your practice setting in terms of resources or patient preferences? Recommendations can be made using standardized systems such as the Grading of Recommendations Assessment, Development, and Evaluation (GRADE) system (see Chapter 6). **GRADE** recommendations range from a strong recommendation based on high-quality evidence to a weak recommendation based on very low-quality evidence. You can download the GRADE Handbook (2013) that walks you through making recommendations about applicability to practice based on the extant evidence provided by the systematic review you and your team have critically appraised (https://gdt.gradepro.org/app/handbook/handbook.html).

Six recommended standards for SR teams are (Eden et al., 2011):
- Establish the review team with appropriate expertise of users and stakeholders
- Ensure user and stakeholder input
- Manage bias and conflict of interest of the reviewers and stakeholders
- Formulate the topic for the review
- Provide for peer review of the review protocol
- Make the review publicly available

TABLE 10.4	Systematic Review Components With or Without Meta-Analysis
Introduction	• Review of background, rationale for conducting the systematic review, and a clear clinical (PICOT) question
Methods	• Search strategy described, inclusion and exclusion criteria identified, databases used for obtaining published and unpublished studies (gray literature), how studies and data were selected and extracted, at least two independent judges specified • Description of methods to assess quality and risk of bias, obtaining a quality appraisal score for each individual study and an overall quality score • Description of summary methods used to assess the findings descriptively and/or quantitatively
Results	• Number of studies screened and characteristics (e.g., design types) • Risk of bias in each study • Narrative or quantitative reporting of results for all outcomes being investigated for strength, quality, quantity, and consistency of evidence • Table of Evidence (TOE)
Discussion	• Synthesis of findings including the strength, quality, and consistency of the evidence for each outcome, limitations of the studies, conclusions and recommendations for application of findings for practice • Synthesis TOE
Funding	• Sources of funding for the systematic review

> **TIP**
>
> Examples of SR standardized critical appraisal tools to make sense of evidence include but are not limited to:
> - Center for Evidence-Based Medicine (CEBM)—Systematic Review Critical Appraisal Worksheet (https://www.cebm.ox.ac.uk/)
> - Critical Appraisal Tools Programme (CASP)—Systematic Review Checklist (https://casp-uk.net)
> - Joanna Briggs Institute (JBI) Critical Appraisal Tools—JBI Evidence Implementation Manual; JBI Evidence Synthesis Manual (JBI's comprehensive guide to conducting systematic reviews); and Critical Appraisal Tools (includes checklists for randomized control trials, qualitative research, economic evaluations, and prevalence studies) (https://jbi.global/critical-appraisal-tools)
> - Preferred Reporting Items for Systematic reviews and Meta-Analyses (PRISMA), 2020 (https://www.prisma-statement.org/)
> - Strengthening the Reporting of Observational Studies in Epidemiology (STROBE) Checklists (https://www.strobe-statement.org)
>
> These are free to download and can be used by evidence-based practice teams or individual clinicians.

Regardless of the type of SR, for the SR to be valuable to the end user, the authors should be complete and transparent in their review process to ensure replicability and explain why and how they drew their conclusions (Page et al., 2021). Although SRs are highly useful, they must be reviewed and critiqued carefully for scientific rigor and applicability of the evidence to support continuing or discontinuing a practice, or making a minor or major change in practice.

Meta-analysis is a type of SR that involves the statistical combination of results from at least two or more separate studies (Deeks et al., 2022). Meta-analysis is used to statistically assess a group of systematically collected and completed studies that yield an overall statistic to derive conclusions about that body of research. Systematic methods including a quantitative component strive to minimize bias, thereby providing more reliable findings from which conclusions can be drawn and clinical decisions made. Outcomes of a meta-analysis may include a more precise quantitative estimate of the effect of treatment or risk factor for disease, or other outcomes, than any *single* study by contributing to the summarized results of *all* studies included in the pooled analysis. Using meta-analysis may also serve to resolve controversies arising from apparently conflicting studies by statistically synthesizing findings and formally assessing the degree of conflict and reasons for differences in results.

A meta-analysis is a complex and time-consuming undertaking. It is completed by an interprofessional team including, but not limited to, clinicians, statisticians, epidemiologists, public health experts, health science librarians, and informaticians. You will find that although the components of a meta-analysis sound complicated, your role as a clinician, educator, or administrator does not require an in-depth understanding of statistics. Your job is to read, understand, and, most importantly, interpret the findings of a meta-analysis; determine whether the results are of sufficient quality and consistency to consider applying them to practice; and think about their relevance for your patient, student, or staff resources, and setting.

The protocol for a meta-analysis, like all SRs, begins with and includes a research or clinical (PICOT) question and search strategy. For example, in the meta-analysis by te Velde et al. (2022) the objective of the review was to determine the efficacy of neurodevelopmental therapy (NDT) in children and infants with cerebral palsy (CP) or at high risk of CP. The clinical question asked, "What is the efficacy of NDT for any outcome in children and infants with cerebral palsy (CP) and infants with high risk of CP?" Components necessary to incorporate into a meta-analysis are:

1. Method for locating studies to be included in the analysis
2. Methods for evaluating the quality of the studies
3. Statistical testing of the combined sample for assessment of the effect

The clinical question will guide establishment of your search strategy. Identifying the inclusion/exclusion criteria is the first step. You will find that meta-analyses strive to include studies of similar design that provide the strongest evidence and, as such, predominantly include RCTs that provide Level II evidence (see Chapter 8). However, some clinical questions cannot be answered due to ethical or practical reasons through RCTs and thus use the next highest levels of evidence for inclusion in the meta-analysis. For example, in the Lake et al. (2019) meta-analysis, the search strategy inclusion criteria required the article to report odds ratios (ORs) or beta coefficients or adjusted ORs/beta coefficients with standard errors (SEs) or confidence intervals (CIs) from a regression model in their meta-analysis associating the nurse work environment with outcomes (Lake et al., 2019). Identifying electronic databases and search terms used by databases such as PUBMED, EMBASE, PsychINFO, CINAHL, Scopus, and the Cochrane Register of Controlled Trials (CENTRAL) with Boolean operators is extremely important in searching the published literature.

Depending on the amount of existing literature on your topic, you may observe that the search results are like an inverted pyramid; the search starts off by locating many more studies than are used in the meta-analysis. Limits that decrease the number of studies include design type, language restrictions, and funding source. Based on the inclusion/exclusion criteria, studies are screened for inclusion by at least two independent judges.

The inclusion of literature produced outside of traditional commercial or academic publishers, often called **gray literature**, in the search strategy is more common in meta-analyses than in other types of SRs. Inclusion of unpublished studies is thought to decrease bias associated with availability, cost, familiarity, and language used in traditionally published studies (Hansen et al., 2022). **Publication bias** is defined as the selective publishing of research based on the nature and direction of findings, where studies with significant or favorable results have greater likelihood of publication than those with nonsignificant or unfavorable findings (Marks-Anglin & Chen, 2020). Including *only* published literature can result in misleading conclusions since the set of published data may not be a representative sample of the overall body of evidence. To help reduce publication bias, Section 801 of the Food and Drug Administration Amendments Act (FDAAA 801) requires responsible parties to register clinical trials and submit summary results to ClinicalTrials.gov. The law applies to certain clinical trials of drug, biological, and device products, which has been in effect since September 27, 2007. Unpublished clinical trials can be found in the Clinical Trials Register (https://ClinicalTrials.gov; https://www.anzctr.org.au/) (see Chapter 6).

Publication bias can be assessed using a **funnel plot**. This is a graph based on ORs (see Chapter 13) that detects small study treatment effects. Lack of observed studies in certain regions of the plotted data that correspond to nonsignificant results may indicate that studies with nonpositive findings have not been published.

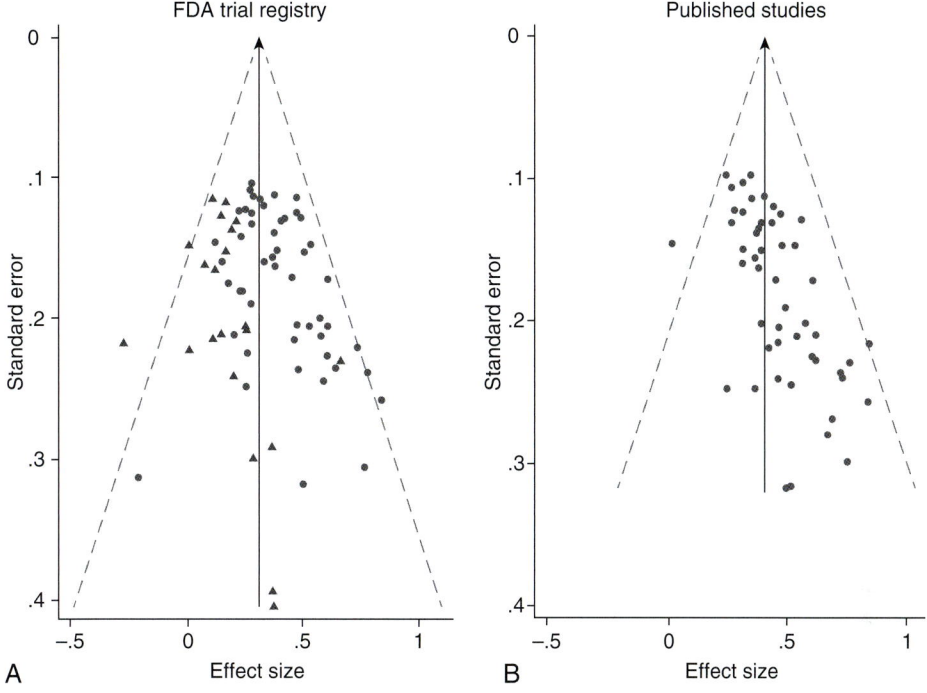

Fig. 10.3 (A) and (B) Funnel Plots Illustrating Publication Bias.

If you examine Fig. 10.3A and B, you will see an example of symmetrical and asymmetrical funnel plots. Fig. 10.3A illustrates a symmetrical funnel plot of a Food and Drug Administration (FDA) registry of 73 published and unpublished studies comparing 12 antidepressants to placebo (Turner et al., 2022). Fig. 10.3B illustrates an asymmetrical funnel plot of 50 studies published in scientific journals, skewed to the right side of the vertical axis, suggesting publication bias. Unpublished data, which can include studies, conference proceedings, preprints, and personal communications, usually have not been through a peer review process.

Another test, the **fail-safe number**, also known as the "file drawer" method, is used to quantify the impact of selective publishing (Marks-Anglin & Chen, 2020). Meta-analysis teams need to be concerned about studies that have been conducted but not published because of negative or neutral results. One way to assess for publication bias is to report the fail-safe N that uses an OR (see Chapter 13) to calculate the number of studies reporting no treatment effect that would need to be included in the analysis to reduce the pooled odds ratio to a nonsignificant value. When the fail-safe N is small, the results of the meta-analysis are uncertain and could easily change if a small number of unpublished studies with negative treatment effects were identified and included in the meta-analysis statistical testing. On the other hand, if the fail-safe N is large, many studies would be needed to overturn the treatment effect results and you would feel more confident about the reported findings.

It is also very important to examine whether and how the researchers assessed the quality of the studies selected for inclusion in the meta-analysis. Measuring the quality of the studies is essential since bias exists in all study designs, even though researchers attempt to minimize it. Even research from established teams published in high-impact journals can have methodological flaws, biases, and limited generalizability and applicability. Using a quality appraisal tool to evaluate sources of bias allows uniformity in the critical appraisal process of the findings and conclusions (Smith & Noble, 2014). You want to document that quality appraisal of studies was completed by at least two independent judges using a standardized quality assessment tool. For example, Lake and colleagues (2019) used the Johns Hopkins Nursing Evidence-Based Practice Rating Scale to evaluate the studies included in their meta-analysis, while te Velde et al. (2022) performed a risk of bias assessment using the Cochrane Risk of Bias Tool 2.0 for randomized clinical trials (The Cochrane Collaboration, n.d.). Risk of bias categories included:

- **Selection bias** by assessing the method of random assignment and process of allocation concealment
- **Performance and detection bias** or blinding of participants, providers, and outcomes assessors
- **Attrition bias** or assessing how incomplete data were managed
- **Reporting bias** or assessing whether all intended outcomes were reported

Each study was rated "high risk," "low risk," or "unclear risk" for each of those bias risk domains. Fig. 10.4 provides a methodological quality summary for the studies included in the te Velde meta-analysis. No studies were "high risk" across all categories while many studies were "low risk" across all categories.

> **TIP**
>
> When studies other than randomized controlled trials are included in an SR, quality appraisal tools specific to the design types should be used. For example, STROBE is used for quality appraisal of observational designs with high quality (7 to 8 criteria met), moderate quality (4 to 6 criteria met), and low quality (1 to 3 criteria met).

Quantitative synthesis by testing the effect of the intervention is what differentiates a meta-analysis from other types of systematic reviews. Examining the heterogeneity of studies is a key component of a meta-analysis. The **test of heterogeneity**, sometimes referred to as the test of homogeneity, is calculated to determine that the hypothesis that each study is measuring is similar across studies and for the same population. If the null hypothesis is supported, and the studies do not differ significantly from each other at the $p < 0.05$ level of significance, the studies would be considered similar and appropriate for a combined statistical analysis. If the null hypothesis was rejected, then the studies would be considered too diverse or heterogeneous to be pooled legitimately and analyzed statistically as a pooled sample in a meta-analysis, and might conclude as a nonquantitative systematic review (see Chapter 13). When results from the test of heterogeneity reject the null hypothesis, revealing that at least some of the studies are significantly different from the others in terms of design, results, or influence in the analysis, **sensitivity analysis** can be used to examine the effect of those studies that are "outliers." Traditionally, the Cochrane's Q test is used to assess for heterogeneity in meta-analyses; you will see the I^2 index in more recent meta-analyses. The I^2 gives an estimate of the percentage of variability in results across studies that is a result of real differences, not by chance (West, Gartlehner, & Mansfield, 2010).

Evaluating the treatment effect is an important component of a meta-analysis. The focus of combining studies in a meta-analysis is determining the treatment effect or effect size for each study. The **effect size** is a measure of the degree to which the null hypothesis is false; that is, the treatment (or intervention) makes a significant difference. Various statistics are used to calculate effect sizes, including t-tests, F-values, and correlation coefficients. One commonly used effect size measure that you will see reported in the literature and that you need to be able to interpret is Cohen's d, which derives the effect size for continuous data (e.g., HgbA1c levels) by subtracting the mean of the treatment group from the mean of the control group in each study and dividing by the pooled standard deviation. Cohen (1988) classifies effect sizes of 0.2 as small, 0.5 as moderate, and 0.8 as large. In the case of binary or dichotomous variables (e.g., quit smoking vs. did not quit smoking), the OR and 95% CIs are used to express the magnitude (size) of the treatment effect (see Chapter 13).

Once individual study effect sizes have been calculated, the effect sizes are pooled to obtain a pooled treatment effect or effect size that is reported in different ways, depending on the types of variables (continuous or dichotomous) involved and related statistical tests used. One of the most common graphics you will see is the **forest plot**, which features a visual reporting of the individual study ORs and the CIs as well as the pooled OR and CI for the combined studies, as illustrated in Fig. 10.5. An advantage of a meta-analysis is that combining the results of a group of studies results in a larger sample size, so you have more power to detect the magnitude of the effect of the intervention. The question you and your team need to answer is, "How large and precise is the treatment effect?"

The meta-analysis by te Velde (2022) provides continuous data for the PICOT question, "What is the efficacy of NDT for any outcome in children and infants with CP and infants with high risk of CP?" Results

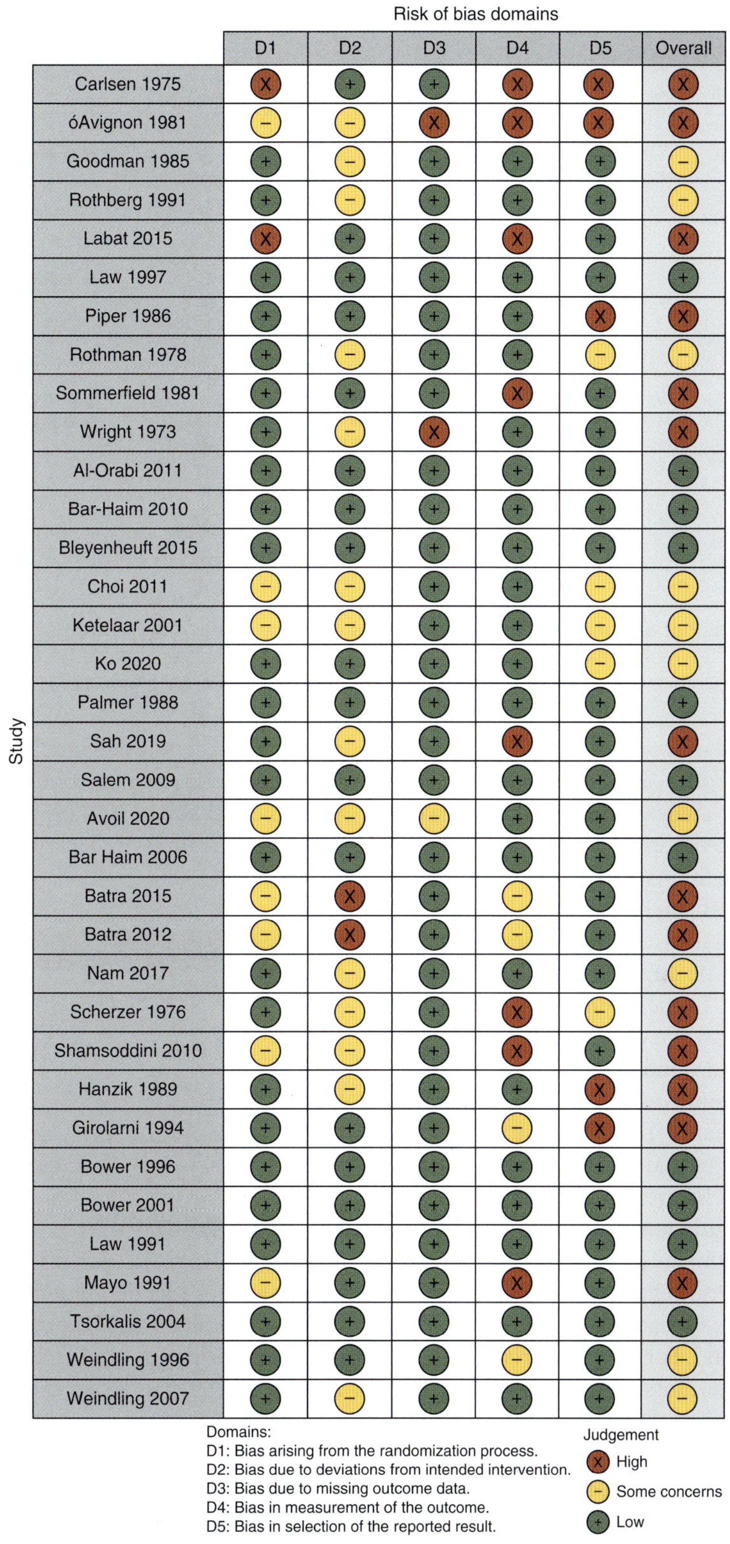

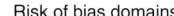

Fig. 10.4 Risk of Bias of Included Studies on Motor or Primary Outcome Measure by Domain Using Risk of Bias Tool 2.0. (From te Velde, A., Morgan, C., Finch-Edmondson, M., McNamara, L., McNamara, M., Paton, M. C. B., Stanton, E., Webb, A., Badawi, N., & Novak, I. (2022). Neurodevelopmental therapy for cerebral palsy: A meta-analysis. *Pediatrics*, *149*(6), e2021055061.)

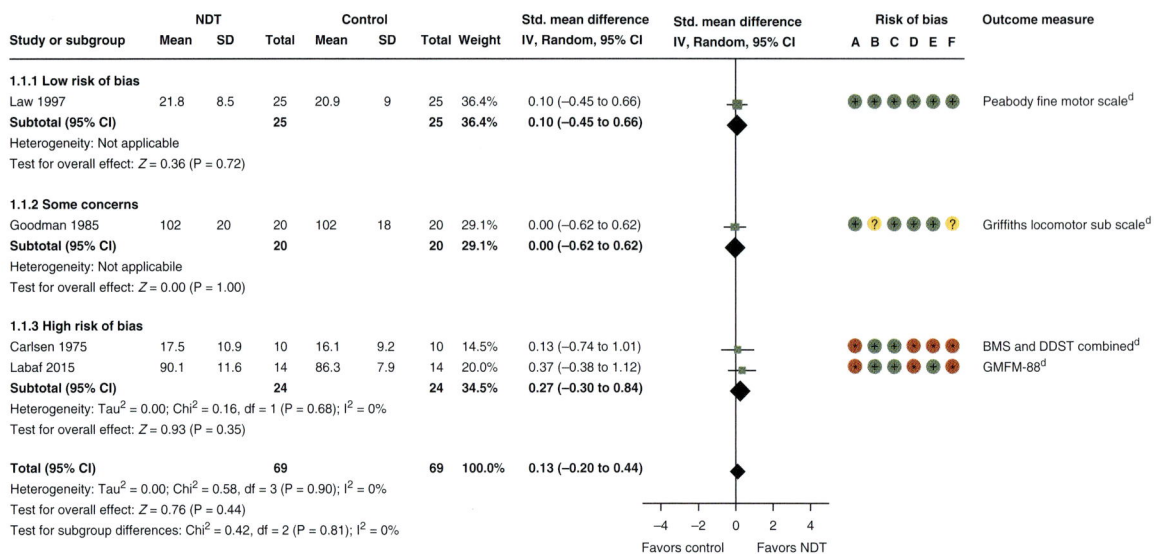

Fig. 10.5 Forest Plot Stratified by Study Risk of Bias. (From te Velde, A., Morgan, C., Finch-Edmondson, M., McNamara, L., McNamara, M., Paton, M. C. B., Stanton, E., Webb, A., Badawi, N., & Novak, I. (2022). Neurodevelopmental therapy for cerebral palsy: A meta-analysis. *Pediatrics*, *149*(6), e2021055061.)

were reported as standardized mean differences with 95% CIs. For dichotomous data, ORs and 95% CIs would be reported. For analysis, the types of interventions were categorized. For example, Fig. 10.5 reports the subgroup effects by the risk of bias: low, some risk, and high risk for NDT. If you inspect Fig. 10.5, you will see on the left side the subgroup of studies all testing the same outcome and the sample size in the NDT versus the control groups. In the middle of Fig. 10.5, you will see the vertical axis line of no effect that reports the individual effect and standardized mean difference (little squares), and the individual study CI (horizontal line with each little square). The larger the square, the larger the contribution of that study to the measure of effect. On the right of the vertical axis is the weight contributed by each study and the CI for each study. Studies with smaller samples generally contribute less to the estimates of overall effect. The summary combined treatment effect is located at the bottom of the vertical axis as a diamond. For the comparison of NDT against a control, the authors identified 9 studies (in 10 publications) comprising 418 participants. Controls consisted of no therapy (six studies in seven publications) or passive movement approaches with no child self-generated movements. In total, six publications did not meet inclusion for meta-analysis while four publications met inclusion criteria for meta-analysis for motor function outcome. No difference was found between NDT and control for motor function with a pooled effect size of 0.13 (95% CI, 0.20 to 0.46, I^2 0%). Chapter 13 addresses data analysis for SRs in greater depth.

> **TIP**
>
> As a clinical leader or graduate student beginning a project, you should include in your search strategy search terms and filters to locate meta-analyses that provide the highest level of evidence to answer your PICOT question.

Integrative Reviews

An *integrative review* is a critical appraisal of the literature in an area that does not include a statistical analysis due to the limitations of the study designs or the heterogeneity of the designs and samples; however, a systematic approach is used to locate and evaluate the studies (see Chapter 6). Integrative reviews are the broadest category of reviews and can include theoretical literature, research literature, or both. An integrative review can include quantitative or qualitative research, or both. When a review includes studies using qualitative and quantitative designs, it is called a mixed-methods review.

An example of an integrative review was conducted by Blakeman and Stapleton (2018), who explored the extant literature for key features of prodromal and acute myocardial infarction (MI) fatigue experienced by women. Based on Whittemore and Knafl's (2005) approach and the Theory of Unpleasant Symptoms, they conducted a comprehensive search, screening, and analysis of the evidence. The search revealed diverse types of evidence that included nonexperimental and qualitative studies (all of which were considered to provide Level II evidence) and doctoral dissertations. They used the Johns Hopkins Nursing Evidence-Based Practice Model (Dang et al., 2022) for their quality appraisal of the 21 studies that met the inclusion criteria. Results were summarized by fatigue characteristics such as frequency, quality, distress and intensity, and timing. They concluded that fatigue is the most common prodromal MI symptom experienced by women and is also a common acute symptom. The authors appropriately point out the limitations posed by inconsistent nomenclature or tools to differentiate reporting of fatigue when assessing women, and they highlight the need for additional research to fully explore fatigue and understand the multidimensional nature of MI-related fatigue. The high rate of morbidity and mortality that is exacted by MI makes the evidence reported by this team especially relevant to clinical practice and the assessment of women who often present with atypical prodromal symptoms of MI.

If you and your team have decided that the evidence is valid and important, you need to think about how it applies to your clinical question. For example, does your patient or population have characteristics similar to or different from those in the study? Is it feasible to apply the evidence in your practice setting in terms of resources or patient preferences? Recommendations can be made using standardized systems such as GRADE (see Chapter 6). GRADE recommendations range from a strong recommendation based on high-quality evidence to a weak recommendation based on very low-quality evidence. You can download the GRADE Handbook (2013) that walks you through making recommendations about applicability to practice, based on the extant evidence provided by the SR you and your team have critically appraised.

Critically Appraising Systematic Reviews

When you are critically appraising an integrative review, SR, or meta-analysis, remember the differences between the types of methods. Using a specific search strategy, reviews provide a broad overview of the literature related to a focused PICOT or clinical question. A weakness is that it often does not include quality appraisal of individual conceptual or policy literature or of quantitative and/or qualitative studies included in the review. SRs without a meta-analysis, as illustrated in Fig. 10.2, also begin with a focused PICOT or clinical question, should use an exhaustive search strategy that targets the published and gray literature, and should use independent judges to screen studies for inclusion and quality appraisal. The unique feature of an SR that is a meta-analysis is the statistical analysis to determine a single combined pooled estimate of effect, with a related CI for each relevant outcome.

Judging the credibility of integrative reviews, SRs, and meta-analyses is essential. We will focus on critical appraisal of SRs and meta-analyses in the following discussion. Use the Critical Appraisal Box as a guide for what we will discuss in this section of the chapter. The strengths and weaknesses of data for each critical appraisal component can be extracted and summarized in a TOE similar to the example in Chapter 3.

Critical appraisal begins by assessing whether the study poses a clearly stated question. For example, can you tell from reading the question what type of question is being asked, and what is the exposure, such as a therapy or diagnostic test, and are the outcome(s) of interest clearly stated?

The search strategy is the next SR critical appraisal component. A high-quality search is comprehensive and exhaustive. It identifies clearly stated inclusion and exclusion criteria, search terms, key words, MeSH (Medical Subject Headings) terms used by specific databases, Boolean operators, and filters to narrow the search and align with inclusion and exclusion criteria. A high-quality search includes published and unpublished literature using major bibliographic databases such as PubMed, Cochrane, CINAHL, Scopus, and EMBASE, as well as dates searched. The search should also include evidence that the researcher attempted to minimize publication bias by reviewing reference lists from relevant studies, contacting experts particularly to inquire about unpublished studies, reviewing conference proceedings, and searching the Clinical Trials Register (see Chapter 6). As discussed earlier in the chapter, funnel plots (see Fig. 10.3A and B) may be used to illustrate that publication bias has been evaluated. Make sure that at least two independent judges have screened the identified studies and arrived at a consensus about those to be included in the SR.

It is important for you and your team to determine whether a quality appraisal to evaluate the quality of the included studies was completed by at least two independent judges using a standardized quality appraisal tool appropriate to the type of clinical question and design. It is common for each study to have a quality rating, either numerical or high/medium/low, and for there to be an overall quality rating for the combined group of studies. When you are critically appraising a systematic review or meta-analysis, you will want to document the individual and collective quality appraisal data on your TOE. For example, in the SR by Bryant and colleagues (2017) assessing the impact of provider involvement on heart failure self-care, the quality assessment based on CONSORT and STROBE identified 10 studies as providing high-level quality of evidence, 10 moderate-level, and 9 low-level.

Do not assume that because an SR is comprised of RCTs or includes a meta-analysis that you will have confidence in the strength and quality of the evidence provided by the results. When you and your team critically appraise the SR, common reasons for low confidence include:

- An unfocused clinical/PICOT question that guided implementation of the SR
- Lack of description of a detailed search strategy that included published and unpublished literature
- Studies with high risk of bias
- Small sample size for individual and pooled studies
- Studies that differ in hypotheses or research questions tested
- Study participants who may differ in important ways from those in whom we are interested
- Inconsistent results across studies

You will find that the studies included in an SR will vary in design and results. This may result in a descriptive evaluation of the studies in a systematic review. In the Bryant et al. (2017) SR, combining studies for analysis was problematic because of the heterogeneous nature of the designs, type of educational delivery, and confounding strategies between studies. When studies are similar enough in design and hypothesis being tested or research question being answered, they potentially can be combined for quantitative analysis in a meta-analysis.

When you and your team are critically appraising an SR that includes a meta-analysis, it is important to assess whether the appropriate criteria were met to justify proceeding with the statistical testing of effect associated with meta-analysis. The main question is whether the results were similar from study to study. The results of the studies should be similar or homogeneous. As discussed earlier in the chapter, the test for heterogeneity estimates whether the differences are significant; the chi square test should report a $p > 0.05$ difference supporting that the results of the studies are similar. If the test for heterogeneity reveals that there is a significant difference, a sensitivity test can be used to systematically eliminate studies that account for the differences until the test for heterogeneity reveals the required homogeneity of the studies to be included in the effect analysis.

In the te Velde (2022) meta-analysis, random effects were used because of the varied nature of outcome measures with 95% CIs for certainty and I^2 for heterogeneity. If meta-analyses had considerable heterogeneity ($I^2 > 75\%$), subanalyses were conducted to determine the heterogeneity source. Sensitivity analysis using fixed effects was also conducted. Clinically relevant subgroup analyses were conducted. Forest plots, like the one in Fig. 10.5, provide for visual interpretation of the overall and/or subgroup results. Subgroup analyses are particularly common when no overall effect is found. Subgroups may be analyzed by type of design, intervention, setting, or quality.

When the results are reported, you want to think about whether the evidence provided by the findings aligns with the authors' conclusions. Consider whether the conclusions are justified by the strength, quality, and consistency of the evidence. Remember that the essence of evidence-based practice is integrating the best available evidence with patient preferences (values, choices, resources, and concerns) and clinical judgment. There are high- and low-quality systematic reviews just as there are for individual studies. Clinical leaders must evaluate whether the conclusions and recommendations are justified and appropriate for informing clinical practice decisions based on the strength and quality of the evidence presented in the SR. For example, the authors of the te Velde meta-analysis concluded that the studies overall were of low risk to bias; using the GRADE system, the evidence for outcomes was rated as moderate quality. This is shown in Fig. 10.6. They further concluded that NDT for children and infants with CP was, first, strongly recommended for the use of activity-based approaches in preference to NDT for improving motor function, and, second, they strongly recommended against using NDT at any dose for improving motor function. Thus, the authors appropriately concluded that the evidence supports the deimplementation of NDT in clinical practice.

Final critical appraisal considerations are pragmatic and focus on applicability:
- Is the study population similar to that of my patients?
- What are the risks and benefits of implementing the findings in my setting for my patient population?
- Is it feasible to implement the findings in my setting?
- Does my organization have the resources to implement the findings reported in this SR? What is the cost/benefit?
- What are the values and preferences of my patients and their families?

> **TIP**
> 1. Does the review explicitly address a focused clinical/PICOT question?
> 2. Does the PICOT question match the studies included in the review?
> 3. Are the inclusion and exclusion criteria clear and comprehensive?
> 4. Was the search for relevant studies exhaustive, including both published and gray literature?
> 5. Were there at least two independent judges assessing whether the studies met the criteria for inclusion in the review?
> 6. What is the level of evidence provided by the studies included in the review?
> 7. Was a quality appraisal conducted according to specific criteria to assess for risk of bias?
> 8. If the studies were critically appraised individually, were the strengths and weaknesses clearly reported?
> 9. Were the appropriate analyses completed to determine whether a meta-analysis could be conducted?
> 10. If a meta-analysis was conducted, how large was the effect, and did the review address confidence in effect estimates?
> 11. Was a synthesis reported for the overall strengths and weaknesses of the included studies?
> 12. Are the conclusions and recommendations relevant and supported by the review?

CLINICAL PRACTICE GUIDELINES

Clinical practice guidelines (CPGs) are systematically developed statements and recommendations intended to optimize care and link research and practice by providing a guide for practitioners (Informed, 2016). CPGs are one of the foundations of efforts to improve healthcare and health care delivery. They are developed through a rigorous systematic methodology synthesizing the ever-increasing amounts of published literature into a practical and digestible set of clinical recommendations to be used in a health care setting (Vandvik et al., 2013). Organizations such as the U.S. Preventive Services Taskforce (USPSTF), clinical specialty organizations, and providers develop CPGs globally and use to reduce health care service variability and improve resource utilization and clinical outcomes. CPGs are also used by clinicians at the point of care, or system-level administrators conducting cost/benefit analyses to improve clinical outcomes, reduce cost of care, and create satisfying patient and provider experiences.

Subject matter experts write evidence-based CPGs and regularly update them based on the need for practice changes, complemented by internal quality improvement (QI) data derived from problem-focused triggers. As a result, clinical teams and QI committees are encouraged to critically appraise and adopt new CPGs (see Chapter 3). For example, based on QI data for a sample of adult patients at high risk for diabetes, the QI team of a large primary care system was considering a policy change regarding allocation of fiscal resources for a routine diabetes screening and lifestyle modification program for adults at high risk for diabetes as part of cardiovascular risk assessment. Their search for a recent CPG found that in 2015, the USPSTF updated its 2008 recommendation statement that found insufficient evidence to assess the benefits and harms of diabetes screening for asymptomatic adults who did not have hypertension (Siu, 2015). Siu (2015) reports that since the 2008 recommendation, six new lifestyle intervention studies that incorporate long-term follow-up consistently have shown the benefit of lifestyle modifications to prevent or delay diabetes progression and improve clinical outcomes. As such, the newer evidence led the USPSTF to conclude that there is a moderate net benefit to measuring blood glucose in adults who are at increased risk for diabetes, and it recommends screening (B recommendation) as

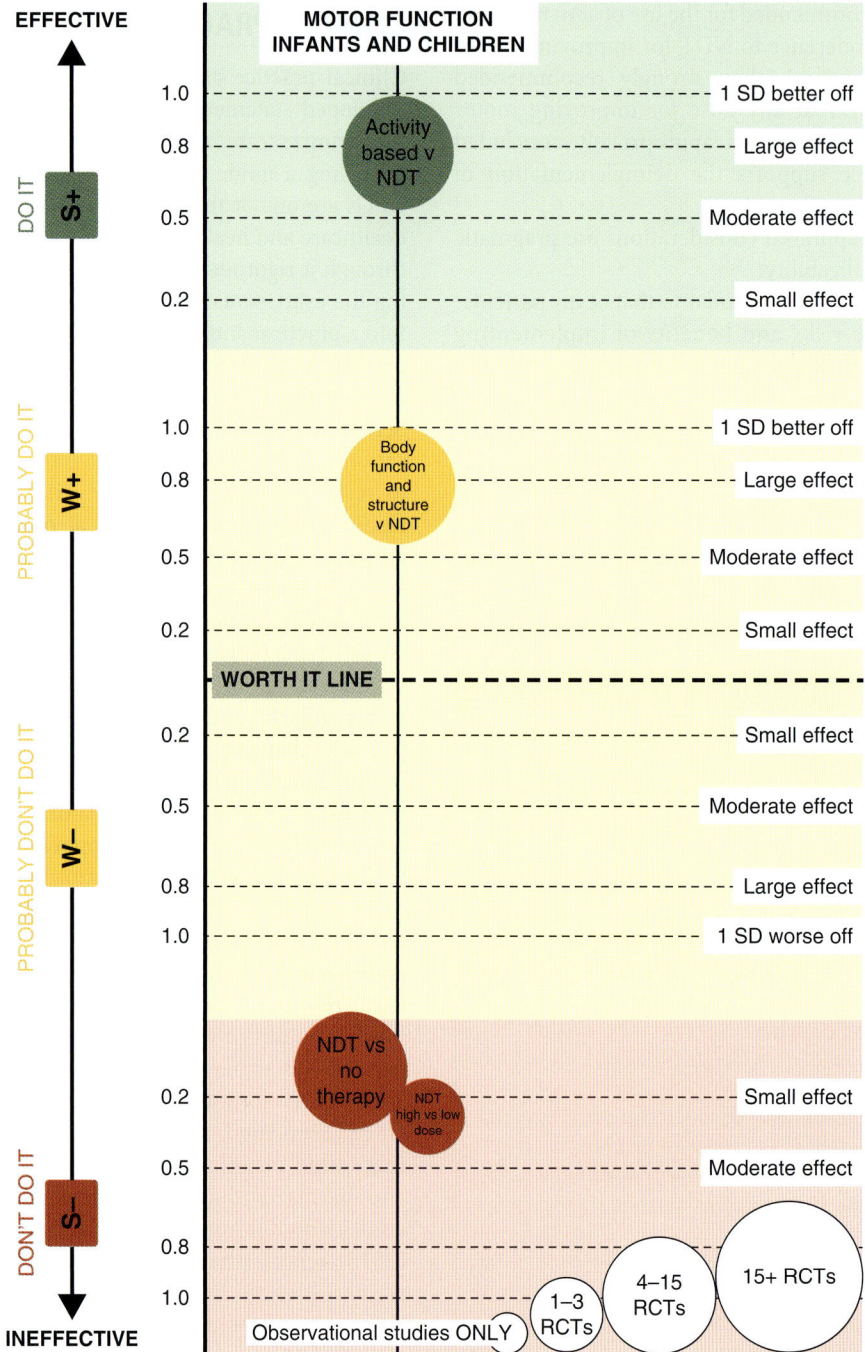

Fig. 10.6 GRADE Assessment. Note: Recommendations from the GRADE evidence alert indicate green as strong recommendation for, yellow as a conditional recommendation, and red as strong recommendation against use of an intervention. (From te Velde, A., Morgan, C., Finch-Edmondson, M., McNamara, L., McNamara, M., Paton, M. C. B., Stanton, E., Webb, A., Badawi, N., & Novak, I. (2022). Neurodevelopmental therapy for cerebral palsy: A meta-analysis. *Pediatrics*, *149*(6), e2021055061.)

part of cardiovascular risk assessment in adults aged 40 to 70 years who are overweight or obese. It also is recommended (B recommendation) that clinicians offer or refer patients with abnormal blood glucose levels to intensive behavioral counseling to promote a healthy diet and physical activity (Siu, 2015). Based on the USPSTF Grade B recommendation, the clinical team was confident about the benefit and decision to recommend allocation of resources to offer screening and lifestyle modification. A cost/benefit analysis would be the next step in the decision-making process.

It is important to understand the issues surrounding emergence of CPGs and the factors contributing to their use or lack of use by nurses, nurse practitioners, physicians, and other health care professionals (Jun et al., 2016). The rapid growth in CPG development has resulted in a wide variation in the rigor and reporting of how a CPG was formulated and how the recommendations are graded. Keep in mind that CPGs can range from scientifically rigorous based on Level Ia meta-analysis evidence to Level IV expert opinion. Pragmatically, CPGs sometimes are developed and written in complicated formats that clinicians and organizations find challenging to implement, which limits effectiveness in influencing clinical practice and improving patient outcomes (Jun et al., 2016). The Institute of Medicine (2011) has identified eight standards for developing trustworthy CPGs:

1. Establishing transparency
2. Management of conflict of interest
3. Guideline development group composition
4. Clinical practice guideline (systematic review intersection)
5. Establishing evidence foundations for and rating strength of recommendations
6. Articulation of recommendations
7. External review
8. Updating

> **TIP**
>
> Many CPGs are very long and address multiple clinical issues. You and your team may find that only specific sections of a CPG apply to your specific clinical issue, type of practice, and setting.

CPGs should be informed by the best available evidence and provide clinicians with an algorithm for clinical management or decision making for specific diseases (e.g., diabetes), conditions (e.g., obesity, hypertension), or treatments (e.g., pain management). Evidence-based practice guidelines are those developed using the scientific process. This includes convening an interprofessional team of experts in the field who are charged with developing guidelines and making recommendations using a scientific protocol similar to the steps of a systematic review (see Table 10.4). Ideally, evidence-based CPGs should comprise Level I SRs that are meta-analyses providing high-quality supporting evidence. When SRs are not extant, teams developing an evidence-based CPG search the literature for the best available evidence provided by individual studies using Level II, III, and IV RCTs and quasi-experimental, cohort, and case-control designs.

For a variety of reasons, not all areas of clinical practice have a sufficient research base. You will observe that expert-based practice guidelines that provide Level VII evidence are developed by consensus panels and expert opinion groups. When this approach is used, nationally known experts in a field are convened to develop a CPG guideline based on their opinions along with research evidence available to date. If only limited research is available for inclusion, a rationale should be presented for the practice recommendations made. The Institute of Medicine (2011) also identified eight attributes of guideline development:

1. Validity
2. Reliability and reproducibility
3. Clinical applicability
4. Clinical flexibility
5. Clarity
6. Documentation
7. Development by a multidisciplinary team
8. Plans for periodic review and update

Guidelines that are formulated using rigorous methods provide a useful starting point for understanding the evidence base of practice. Although information in well-developed national guidelines is a starting point, it is usually necessary to localize the guideline using institution-specific, evidence-based policies, procedures, or standards before applying a guideline in a specific setting. However, because guideline vary in quality, it is essential that health care teams and organizations appraise the quality of a CPG to determine whether it should be implemented in a primary care practice, home care setting, or acute care institution.

The National Comprehensive Cancer Network (NCCN), a consortium of 33 leading cancer centers worldwide, is an organization that develops guidelines. The NCCN guidelines are accessible at https://www.nccn.org/guidelines/nccn-guidelines. For example, the NCCN-sponsored guideline for Supportive Care has multiple CPGs within that broad category, including cancer-related fatigue, antiemesis, and survivorship. CPGs are frequently located on organizations' websites and are either open-access or available only to members. More accessible guidelines are available through several different guideline repositories provided by different organizations including the World Health Organization (https://www.who.int/publications/who-guidelines) or the Guidelines International Network (https://g-i-n.net/international-guidelines-library). Box 10.1 provides a summary of the key features and criteria for development of a guideline. The next two IT Resource Boxes provide a selected list of digital databases and organization websites where you can locate guideline. These lists provide only a small sample of the abundantly available guideline dissemination and development resources.

> **TIP**
>
> **Selected Specialty Clinical Practice Guidelines Databases**
>
> - American College of Physicians: https://www.acponline.org/clinical-information/clinical-guidelines-recommendations
> - American Academy of Pediatrics: https://www.aap.org/en/patient-care/
> - American Psychiatric Association: https://www.psychiatry.org/psychiatrists/practice/clinical-practice-guidelines
> - Oncology Nursing Society: https://voice.ons.org/topic/clinical-practice-guidelines
> - American College of Obstetricians and Gynecologists: https://www.acog.org/clinical/clinical-guidance/practice-advisory
> - American College of Nurse-Midwives: http://www.midwife.org/
> - American College of Cardiology: https://www.acc.org/Guidelines
> - Veterans Administration: https://www.healthquality.va.gov/
> - American Geriatrics Society: https://www.americangeriatrics.org/publications-tools

> **TIP**
>
> **Selected Databases for Locating Clinical Practice Guidelines**
>
> - TRIP (Turning Research Into Practice) database: https://www.tripdatabase.com/ https://www.tripdatabase.com/
> - United States Preventive Taskforce (USPSTF): https://www.uspreventiveservicestaskforce.org/uspstf/
> - Cochrane Library: https://www.cochranelibrary.com/
> - National Center for Complimentary and Integrative Health, Clinical Practice Guidelines: https://www.nccih.nih.gov/health/providers/clinicalpractice
> - International Guideline Network: https://g-i-n.net/international-guidelines-library
> - Search Databases (access through your health care setting's library or direct links below, apply additional filters for "Practice Guideline," which will narrow down the search)
>   - Cumulated Index to Nursing and Allied Health Literature (CINAHL) with full text: https://www.ebsco.com/products/research-databases/cinahl-full-text
>   - DynaMed: https://www.dynamed.com/
>   - MedlinePlus: https://medlineplus.gov/
>   - PubMed: https://pubmed.ncbi.nlm.nih.gov/

IMPLEMENTING CLINICAL PRACTICE GUIDELINES IN CLINICAL PRACTICE

Locating and reviewing a guideline in a clinical area can be overwhelming. Even after a guideline has been located, it can be a challenge to wade through the lengthy document and determine the critical clinical information. Usually the background information including the sponsoring organization, funding source, guideline development panel, and dates covered by the literature review is evident. Evidence-based CPGs also include the system used for quality appraisal and recommendations (e.g., USPSTF rating system).

However, the challenges with reviewing CPGs is locating the relevant sections and assessing whether there is transparency about the rigor of the evidence review and critical appraisal. This step also involves reviewing whether the evidence supporting the recommendations is explicit and identifying the benefits and harms associated with the intervention or management protocol. CPGs based on low-quality evidence, such as expert opinion, have the potential to

> **BOX 10.1 Criteria for Developing a Clinical Practice Guideline**
>
> - Developed by a knowledgeable, multidisciplinary panel of experts and representatives from key affected groups
> - Considers important patient subgroups and patient preferences, as appropriate
> - Includes a structured abstract about the guideline and its development
> - Includes systematically developed statements that include recommendations and strategies that assist clinicians and patients in making decisions about appropriate care for specific clinical conditions
> - Produced under the sponsorship of government agencies at the local, state, or federal level
> - Produced under the sponsorship of professional organizations (e.g., medical, nursing, pharmacy), public or private foundations, or health plans
> - Guided by a systematic literature search and review of the existing scientific evidence published in peer review journals
> - Includes critical appraisal of scientific evidence using standardized critical appraisal tools
> - Includes graded recommendations based on the strength and consistency of evidence
> - Developed, reviewed, or revised within the past 5 years

be of no benefit or even harmful to patients, so they need to be appraised carefully before implementation (Boltin et al., 2020).

The 2017 Guidelines for the Prevention, Detection, Evaluation, and Management of High Blood Pressure in Adults (Whelton et al., 2017) is an update of the classic Seventh Report of the Joint National Committee on Prevention, Detection, Evaluation and Treatment of High Blood Pressure (JNC7), published in 2003. Developed jointly by the American College of Cardiology and the American Heart Association, it provides a good example of an interprofessional CPG representing experts from a broad array of backgrounds that demonstrates strong transparency about the rigor of its method, critical appraisal of the evidence, and recommendations. This CPG is comprehensive and incorporates new information regarding blood pressure (BP)-related risk of cardiovascular disease (CVD), ambulatory BP monitoring, home BP monitoring, BP thresholds to initiate antihypertensive drug treatment, BP goals of treatment, and strategies to improve hypertension treatment. The format for grading the quality of evidence and strength of recommendations appropriately appears at the beginning of the guideline. Presented in "modular knowledge chunk format," the CPG sections are accompanied by the strength of the evidence and recommendation. For example, the recommendation that reads "Out-of-office BP measurements are recommended to confirm the diagnosis of hypertension and for titration of BP-lowering medications in conjunction with telehealth counseling or clinical interventions" is supported by Level A evidence (e.g., > 1 RCT, meta-analysis of RCTs) and a Level I recommendation (strong). In comparison, a recommendation about BP treatment threshold and use of CVD risk states, "Use of BP-lowering medications is recommended for primary prevention of CVD in adults with no history of CVD and with an estimated 10-year risk of ASCVD < 10% and a systolic blood pressure (SBP) of 140 mmHg or higher or a diastolic (DBP) blood pressure of 90 mmHg or higher." This was based on a Level A strong recommendation, but only C-LD level of evidence (e.g., nonrandomized observational or registry studies, meta-analyses of such studies), which was the best available evidence.

Despite the proliferation of RCTs conducted over the past four decades, there remains a paucity of high-quality RCTs and meta-analyses that provide strong and consistent evidence to inform CPG development and recommendations. The recommendations are based on the strength of the evidence for each of the questions identified at the beginning of the CPG. As you read CPGs, even those from prestigious groups like the USPSTF, you may be surprised that few recommendations are based on Level A evidence. Remember that evidence-based CPG recommendations are based on the best available evidence per the quality appraisal model used for a specific CPG (Box 10.2). Some CPG panels choose to make recommendations based on expert opinion when the evidence is poor or lacking. When expert opinion is used, it should be identified as such and aggregated using a systematic protocol.

CPGs also do not necessarily provide a "cookie-cutter" approach with a "one size fits all" formula (Alonso-Coello et al., 2010; Kung et al., 2012; Mickan et al., 2011). Use of a CPG must be for the right person, at the right time, and in the right way (Rosenfeld & Shiffman, 2009). Thinking about how useful the recommendations are to your patient population, you may

> **BOX 10.2 Examples of Clinical Practice Guidelines Appraisal Tools**
>
> - AGREE II Tool (Brouwers et al., 2010): https://www.agreetrust.org/
> - AGREE GRAS (shortened version of AGREE II; (Brouwers, Kho, & Browman, 2012): https://www.agreetrust.org/resource-centre/agree-ii-grs-instrument/
> - Johns Hopkins Nursing Evidence-Based Practice Non-Research Evidence Appraisal Tool to assess non-evidence-based guideline: https://www.hopkinsmedicine.org/evidence-based-practice/model-tools
> - Johns Hopkins Nursing Evidence-Based Practice Research Evidence Appraisal Tool (2012) to assess evidenced-based guideline: https://www.hopkinsmedicine.org/evidence-based-practice/model-tools

use the section(s) of a CPG that apply to your patient population while considering patient preferences and available resources. Keep in mind that it is nearly impossible for clinicians to keep up with the proliferation of individual research studies; that is why evidence-based CPGs are so important to clinicians who seek to provide high-quality, cost-effective, satisfying care to their patients.

Implementation of CPGs in clinical settings involves both an individual and system-level commitment. Despite the increasing availability of high-quality CPGs, their use remains low. The top three barriers that inhibit nurses from using guidelines are (Correa et al., 2020; Jun et al., 2016):

- Lack of orientation and education
- Amount of time it takes to implement them
- Workload issues such as lack of staffing

Assessing your organization's readiness to implement a best practice guideline is a critical step and must involve all relevant levels of administrative and clinical leadership (Iowa Model Collaborative et al., 2017). Studies report effective CPG implementation and improvements in clinical outcomes when a multilevel plan is developed and implemented (Iowa Model Collaborative et al., 2017; Jun et al., 2016). Essential ingredients for success in transferring evidence into practice include:

- Organizational support
- Unit-based champions
- A positive clinical milieu
- Resources to facilitate day-to-day implementation
- Interactive professional development sessions that focus on education and skill building
- Integration of CPGs into the electronic health record with required prompts, reminders, and point-of-care clinical decision tools
- Changing organizational policies to reflect CPGs as a required standard of care
- Incentives to disseminate new CPGs as a best practice internally and externally

In your role as a clinical leader, you can be an evidence-based practice mentor who supports interprofessional teamwork, collaboration, and unit-based champions. You can play a pivotal role as a liaison between the team charged with CPG implementation and administrative leadership. Evaluating the impact of the CPG on clinical and financial outcomes is an important factor in promoting organizational adoption and sustainability. Evidence-based practice models provide a framework for you and your team to monitor and evaluate the CPG structure, process, and outcome data (see Chapter 18). Quality improvement data and feedback provide evidence of whether the CPG is being used in practice and how it is affecting patient care. Disseminating the results of a CPG implementation project internally and externally is another area for staff development (see Chapter 19). For example, coaching your staff, especially the unit-based champions, to develop short but compelling CPG presentations to educate about and market to internal and external stakeholders is an excellent leadership skill to cultivate. Strategically planned presentations are excellent vehicles for obtaining organizational leaders' buy-in, which is vital to ensuring sustainability. Ongoing administrative support and staff engagement are critical elements in supporting long-lasting practice changes associated with improved clinical outcomes and evidence of organizational effectiveness.

> **TIP**
>
> Use of the Interprofessional Education Collaborative (IPEC) Competencies provides a useful framework for your team in developing the trust, respect, and effective communication skills a CPG team needs to undertake implementation of a CPG in a practice setting.

CRITICAL APPRAISAL OF CLINICAL PRACTICE GUIDELINES

Appraising Clinical Practice Guidelines

As evidence-based CPGs proliferate, it becomes increasingly important to critically appraise them regarding the methods used for guideline formulation and their potential applicability. Like research studies, guidelines must be critically appraised by clinical teams like yours before adoption and implementation. The findings of a systematic review by Alonso-Coello and colleagues (2010) concluded that although the quality of guideline was improving, quality scores as measured by the Appraisal of Guidelines Research and Evaluation (AGREE) Instrument have remained moderate to low over the last two decades. Thus, critically appraising the scientific rigor of a guideline is a part of locating an appropriate guideline to use. The general areas of appraisal include the following:

- Date of publication or release and authors
- Endorsement of the guideline
- Clear purpose of the guideline
- Patient population and subpopulation
- Types of evidence (research, theoretical) used in guideline development
- Inclusion criteria for types of studies used in formulating the guideline
- Description of the method or model for grading the evidence
- Search terms and retrieval methods used to acquire evidence in the guideline
- Practice statements supported by citations
- Practice recommendations supported by graded recommendations
- Comprehensive reference list
- Review of the guideline by external experts
- Evidence of whether the guideline has been used or tested in practice. If yes, in what types of settings, and with which patient groups and subgroups?

Completing a guideline appraisal will also enhance your team's position in making a convincing argument to your health care colleagues and/or administrators about why or why not to adopt or revise a guideline as a policy or practice standard. For example, Westwell Hospital had been prescribing antiemetic medications for their pediatric oncology patients utilizing an algorithm based on a 2013 guideline published in a relevant oncology journal. However, the clinicians learned of a more current guideline from Pediatric Oncology Group of Ontario published in 2018 that no longer recommended a previously used medication for antiemetic purposes and allowed another antiemetic to be used in younger patients. The clinical team evaluated the guideline systematically and reached the consensus to change their practice to be better aligned with the current guideline (Beauchemin et al., 2019).

Appraising guideline is a systematic process. Thus, locating an appropriate and reliable instrument is the first step. A team of researchers (Siering et al., 2013) conducted a systematic review of 40 appraisal tools for evaluating guidelines and concluded that the most comprehensively validated appraisal tool is the Appraisal of Guidelines Research and Evaluation II (AGREE II) instrument (https://www.agreetrust.org/agree-ii/). However, Siering and colleagues (2013) also noted that the research or clinical question should dictate the choice of appraisal tool. The AGREE II instrument is one of the most widely used appraisal tools to evaluate the applicability of a guideline to practice (Brouwers et al., 2010). AGREE II was developed to help assess guideline quality, provide a methodological strategy for guideline development, and inform practitioners about information that should be reported in guidelines and how it should be reported. As you can see from the list in Box 10.2, AGREE II is available online and is user friendly. It focuses on 6 domains with a total of 23 questions rated on a 7-point scale and 2 final assessment items that require appraisers to make overall judgments about the guideline based on how they rated the 23 questions. Along with the instrument itself, the AGREE Enterprise website offers excellent guidance on tool usage and development that you will find very helpful, especially when you begin your guideline critical appraisal journey. Table 10.5 highlights the structure and content of the six domains of the AGREE II tool.

A recent update indicates that the AGREE II tool has been reformatted and renamed the AGREE Global Rating Scale (AGREE GRS) to facilitate clinician use (n.a. & Canadian Institutes of Health Research, 2017). You can download it as a PDF at https://www.agreetrust.org/resource-centre/agree-ii-grs-instrument/. The AGREE GRS tool is shorter, has been tested since 2012, and has acceptable validity, but its sensitivity to detecting differences is low. Therefore, the AGREE Trust still recommends the use of the valid and reliable AGREE II tool (Brouwers et al., 2010, 2012).

TABLE 10.5 Structure and Content of AGREE II's Six Domains

Structure of Domain	Content of Items
Domain 1: Scope & Purpose	Is the overall aim of the CPG clear, including specific health-related questions and its specific population (items 1–3)?
Domain 2: Stakeholder Involvement	Were the appropriate health professionals involved in its development, and does it represent the intended users (items 4–6)?
Domain 3: Rigor of Development	Was an appropriate and clear method used to search and synthesize evidence, including recommendations and methods for updating them (items 7–14)?
Domain 4: Clarity of Presentation	Is the language of the CPG clear, organized, and appropriately formatted, including recommendations (items 15–17)?
Domain 5: Applicability	Are facilitators and barriers to implementing the CPG and necessary resources identified (items 18–21)?
Domain 6: Editorial Independence	Are the recommendations unbiased in relation to the funding source or member's organizational affiliation (items 22–23)?

> **TIP**
>
> The quality of a CPG is only as good as the quality of the evidence used to support it. It is essential to critically appraise a CPG using the Appraisal of Guidelines Research and Evaluation II (AGREE II) tool before implementation to determine its quality and fit for your patient population.

Another important point to consider is the grading of the recommendations. Guidelines are inconsistent in how they rate the quality of evidence and strength of recommendations. As a result, guideline users like you are challenged to understand the information that grading systems are trying to communicate (Guyatt et al., 2008). Although there is a variety of rating frameworks, the Grading of Recommendations Assessment, Development, and Evaluation (GRADE) system is increasingly becoming the gold standard for rating guideline recommendations (https://www.gradeworkinggroup.org/). For a detailed discussion of the GRADE rating system, consult the online GRADE Handbook (https://gdt.gradepro.org/app/handbook/handbook.html). The MAGIC (Making Grading the Irresistible Choice) Evidence Ecosystem Foundation is an international nonprofit organization providing software service for evidence synthesis and guidelines (https://magicevidence.org/about/). Additionally, the USPSTF is another esteemed recommendation rating system (https://www.uspreventiveservicestaskforce.org/uspstf/about-uspstf/methods-and-processes/grade-definitions), as is the one developed by the Agency for Health Research and Quality (AHRQ). Clinicians make health care decisions by weighing the potential benefit and/or harm of alternative treatment options based on the best available evidence. Guideline recommendations and quality ratings provide an estimate of the confidence clinicians can have in expected advantages or disadvantages of the intervention effect. Clinical leaders need to carefully assess the quality of evidence that provides the rationale for recommendations. A classic example is that for a decade, guidelines recommended that clinicians encourage postmenopausal women to use hormone replacement therapy (HRT) to decrease cardiovascular risk. Had a rigorous system for rating the quality of recommendations been used, it would have revealed that the evidence came from observational studies with inconsistent evidence of low quality. Ultimately, RCTs showed that HRT does not reduce cardiovascular risk and may even increase it in some cases (Rossouw et al., 2002). In contrast to the earlier recommendation, the 2017 Final Recommendation Statement by the USPSTF cites a "D" recommendation against the use of combined estrogen and progestin for the primary prevention of chronic cardiovascular conditions in postmenopausal women. A "D" recommendation indicates a high degree of certainty that the service has no net benefit and that the harm outweighs the benefit. Critical appraisal of guideline is implemented using a standardized critical appraisal tool like the AGREE II instrument and applying the criteria to the attributes of the guideline. The answers to the questions and the accompanying score reveal data about the strength and quality of the evidence provided in the guidelines.

> **TIP**
> *Clinical Practice Guidelines*
>
> 1. Is the date of publication, release, or update cycle current?
> 2. Are the authors of the CPG clearly identified and appropriate to the guideline?
> 3. Were the authors representative of key interprofessional stakeholders in this specialty?
> 4. Who sponsored and/or funded development of the CPG?
> 5. Are the CPG problem, purpose, and population clearly addressed?
> 6. Was there a clearly identified CPG development methodology?
> 7. Was a clearly identified method used to grade the evidence and make recommendations?
> 8. Was there an explicit search strategy?
> 9. Did the CPG team conduct a comprehensive review and critical appraisal of the literature?
> 10. Were all the relevant outcomes specified?
> 11. Was each recommendation stated explicitly and accompanied by strength of evidence and a graded recommendation?
> 12. Are the recommendations clinically relevant?
> 13. Was the CPG subjected to peer review and testing?
> 14. Will the recommendations be helpful in caring for my patient population?
> 15. Does my health care organization or practice have the resources to implement the recommendations of this CPG?
> 16. Does implementation support current practice or require a minor or major change in practice?
> 17. Can the outcomes be measured in my clinical setting?

Critical appraisal is not just about evaluating the quality of the evidence and strength of the recommendations. As you can see in critical appraisal criteria 14 to 17, you and your team must assess whether the CPG will be helpful in providing care for your patient population (e.g., age, gender, comorbidities). Beyond considering whether the guideline applies to your patient population, is it feasible to implement it in your practice setting? For example, a CPG on fall prevention in the hospital setting is not the same as fall prevention in a home or long-term care setting. A guideline for adult asthma management is not the same as asthma management in children. As a clinical leader, you also must be aware of the financial resources needed to implement a practice change; you need to determine whether they are available in your practice setting. Finally, you want to make sure that the outcomes of implementing a CPG are measurable in your clinical setting so it can be integrated into your quality improvement program.

SYNTHESIS

SRs and CPGs are powerful sources of evidence and recommendations with which to guide clinical, educational, or administrative practices. Evidence-based practice requires that you determine whether you and your team would consider proposing a change in practice based on the strength and quality of evidence provided by an SR and coupled with your clinical expertise and patient preferences. SRs, especially meta-analyses comprising multiple RCTs, offer stronger evidence in estimating the magnitude of the effect of an intervention. The strength of evidence is a key component of building a practice based on evidence. CPGs vary widely in the rigor with which they are developed and the strength of evidence to support recommendations. However, well-developed guidelines and their recommendations do inform practice and provide an important approach to making evidence-informed changes that enable clinicians to provide high-quality, cost-effective, and satisfying care to their populations.

KEY POINTS

- A systematic review is guided by a focused clinical/PICOT question and uses electronic searches to identify quantitative studies that use similar designs to answer a clinical question.
- A review is a type of systematic analysis guided by a focused clinical question. It includes an extensive search of the literature and can include a theoretical review of the literature or a review of both qualitative and quantitative research literature.
- Meta-analysis is a quantitative epidemiological study design, a subset of systematic reviews that quantitatively summarizes the findings of a group of studies using the same design to obtain an estimate of the impact of an intervention.
- Standardized tools for critically appraising a systematic review and meta-analysis are available from the Center for Evidence-Based Medicine (CEBM), the Critical Appraisal Skills Programme (CASP), and the Cochrane Collaboration.
- Clinical practice guidelines (CPGs) are systematically developed statements or recommendations that link research and practice.
- There are two types of guidelines, evidence-based and expert-based.
- Evidence-based CPGs search the research literature, assess the strength and quality of the evidence provided by the studies that meet the inclusion criteria, and make graded recommendations to guide practice.
- Expert-based CPGs are developed when the research literature is sparse. A panel of experts in an area of interest develops the CPG based on their expert opinions and critical appraisal of existing research.
- The AGREE II tool is the gold standard instrument for critical appraisal of CPGs.
- Clinicians need to determine whether the findings of systematic reviews and CPGs are relevant for their patient populations, applicable in their clinical settings, and financially feasible to implement.
- Systematic review and CPG teams should be interprofessional and represent diverse stakeholders including patients.

REFERENCES

Alonso-Coello, P., Irfan, A., Soia, I., Gich, I., Delgado-Noguera, M., Rigau, D., et al. (2010). The quality of clinical practice guidelines over the last two decades: A systematic review of guideline appraisal. *Quality and Safety in Health Care*, 19(e58), 1–7.

Arksey, H., & O'Malley, L. (2005). Scoping studies: Towards a methodological framework. *International Journal of Social Research Methodology*, 8, 19–32. https://doi.org/10.1080/1364557032000119616.

Beauchemin, M., Cohn, E., & Shelton, R. C. (2019). Implementation of clinical practice guidelines in the healthcare setting: A concept analysis. *ANS. Advances in Nursing Science*, 42(4), 307–324. https://doi.org/10.1097/ANS.0000000000000263.

Blakeman, J. R., & Stapleton, S. J. (2018). An integrative review of fatigue experienced by women before and during myocardial infarction. *Journal of Clinical Nursing*, 00, 1–11.

Boltin, D., Lambregts, D. M., Jones, F., Siterman, M., Bonovas, S., Cornberg, M., & Quality of Care Taskforce, UEG., et al. (2020). UEG framework for the development of high-quality clinical guidelines. *United European Gastroenterology Journal*, 8(8), 851–864. https://doi.org/10.1177/2050640620950854.

Brouwers, M. C., Kho, M. E., & Browman, G. P. (2012). The global rating scale complements the AGREE II in advancing the quality of practice guidelines. *Journal of Clinical Epidemiology*, 65(5), 526–534.

Brouwers, M. C., Kho, M. E., Browman, G. P., Burgers, J. S., Cluzeau, F., Feder, G., Fervers, B., Graham, I. D., Grimshaw, J., Hanna, S. E., Littlejohns, P., Makarski, J., Zitzelsberger, L., & AGREE Next Steps Consortium. (2010). AGREE II: Advancing guideline development, reporting and evaluation in health care. *CMAJ: Canadian Medical Association Journal [Journal de l'Association medicale canadienne]*, 182(18), E839–E842. https://doi.org/10.1503/cmaj.090449.

Bryant, R., Alonzo, A., & Schmillen, H. (2017). Systematic review of provider involvement in heart failure self-care. *Journal of the American Association of Nurse Practitioners*, 29(11), 682–694.

Center for Evidence-Based Medicine. (2016). *Critical Appraisal Tools*. https://www.cebm.net/critical-appraisal.

Ciapponi, A., Bardach, A., Mazzoni, A., et al. (2021). Safety of components and platforms of COVID-19 vaccines considered for use in pregnancy: A rapid review.

Vaccine, 39(40), 5891–5908. https://doi.org/10.1016/j.vaccine.2021.08.034.

The Cochrane Collaboration. (n.d.) Cochrane Risk of Bias Tool 2.0. https://methods.cochrane.org/bias/resources/rob-2-revised-cochrane-risk-bias-tool-randomized-trials.

Cohen, J. (1988). *Statistical power analysis for the behavioral sciences* (2nd ed.). Academic Press.

Correa, V. C., Lugo-Agudelo, L. H., Aguirre-Acevedo, D. C., Contreras, J. A. P., Borrero, A. M. P., Patiño-Lugo, D. F., et al. (2020). Individual, health system, and contextual barriers and facilitators for the implementation of clinical practice guidelines: A systematic metareview. *Health Research Policy and Systems, 18*(1), 74. https://doi.org/10.1186/s12961-020-00588-8.

Critical Appraisal Skills Programme. (2017). *CASP Systematic Review Checklist*. http://www.casp-uk.net/.

Dang, D., Dearholt, S., Bissett, K., Ascenzi, J., Whalen, M., & Sigma Theta Tau International, & Johns Hopkins University School of Nursing. (2022). *Johns Hopkins evidence-based practice for nurses and healthcare professionals: Model and guidelines* (4th ed.). Sigma Theta Tau International.

Dearholt, S., & Dang, D. (2012). *Johns Hopkins nursing evidence-based practice model and guidelines* (2nd ed.). INL Sigma Theta Tau International.

Deeks, J. J., Higgins, J. P. T., & Altman, D. G. (2022). Chapter 10: Analysing data and undertaking meta-analyses. In J. P. T. Higgins, J. Thomas, J. Chandler, M. Cumpston, T. Li, M. J. Page, & V. A. Welch (Eds.), *Cochrane Handbook for Systematic Reviews of Interventions*. Cochrane. Version 6.3. https://www.training.cochrane.org/handbook.

Duddy, C., & Wong, G. (2023). Grand rounds in methodology: when are realist reviews useful, and what does a "good" realist review look like? *BMJ Quality & Safety, 32*(3), 173–180. https://doi.org/10.1136/bmjqs-2022-015236.

Eden, J., Levit, L., Berg, A., & Morton, S. (Eds.), Institute of Medicine (US) Committee on Standards for Systematic Reviews of Comparative Effectiveness Research. (2011). *Finding what works in health care: Standards for systematic reviews*. National Academies Press (US). https://doi.org/10.17226/13059.

Fink, A. (2014). *Reviewing the literature. Conducting research literature reviews: From the Internet to paper*. Sage, 2–45.

Fink, L., & Lewis, D. (2017). Exercise as a treatment for fibromyalgia: A scoping review. *The Journal for Nurse Practitioners, 13*(8), 546–551.

Gifkins, J., Johnston, A., Loudoun, R., & Troth, A. (2020). Fatigue and recovery in shiftworking nurses: A scoping literature review. *International Journal of Nursing Studies, 112*. https://doi.org/10.1016/j.ijnurstu.2020.103710.

Grant, M. J., & Booth, A. (2009). A typology of reviews: An analysis of 14 review types and associated methodologies. *Health Information and Libraries Journal, 26*, 91–108.

Guyatt, G. H., Oxman, A. D., Vist, G. E., et al. (2008). GRADE: An emerging consensus on rating quality of evidence and strength of recommendations. *British Medical Journal, 336*, 924–926.

Hansen, C., Steinmetz, H., & Block, J. (2022). How to conduct a meta-analysis in eight steps: A practical guide. *Management Review Quarterly, 72*, 1–19. https://doi.org/10.1007/s11301-021-00247-4.

Haynes, R. B. (1993). Where's the meat in clinical journals. *ACP Journal Club, 119*, A22–A23.

Informed. (2016). What are clinical practice guidelines? In *InformedHealth.org [Internet]*. Institute for Quality and Efficiency in Health Care (IQWiG). https://www.ncbi.nlm.nih.gov/books/NBK390308/.

Institute of Medicine. (2011). Consensus report: Clinical practice guidelines we can trust. http://data.care-statement.org/wp-content/uploads/2016/12/IOMGuidelines-2013-1.pdf.

Iowa Model Collaborative, Buckwalter, K. C., Cullen, L., Hanrahan, K., Kleiber, C., McCarthy, A. M., & on behalf of the Iowa Model Collaborative., et al. (2017). Iowa Model of Evidence-Based Practice: Revisions and Validation. *Worldviews on Evidence-Based Nursing, 14*(3), 175–182. https://doi.org/10.1111/wvn.12223.

Jun, J., Kovner, C. T., & Stimpfel, A. W. (2016). Barriers and facilitators of nurses' use of clinical practice guidelines: An integrative review. *International Journal of Nursing Studies, 60*, 54–68. https://doi.org/10.1016/j.ijnurstu.2016.03.006.

Kung, J., Miller, R. R., & Mackowiak, P. A. (2012). Failure of clinical practice guidelines to meet institute of medicine standards. *Archives of Internal Medicine, 172*(21), 1628–1633.

Lake, E. T., Sanders, J., Duan, R., Riman, K. A., Schoenauer, K. M., & Chen, Y. (2019). A meta-analysis of the associations between the nurse work environment in hospitals and 4 sets of outcomes. *Medical Care, 57*(5), 353–361. https://doi.org/10.1097/MLR.0000000000001109.

Liberati, A., Altman, D. G., Tetzlaff, J., et al. (2009). The PRISMA statement for reporting items for systematic reviews and meta-analyses of studies that evaluate health care interventions: Explanation and elaboration. *Annals of Internal Medicine, 15*(4), w65–w94.

Marks-Anglin, A., & Chen, Y. (2020). A historical review of publication bias. *Research Synthesis Methods, 11*(6), 725–742. https://doi.org/10.1002/jrsm.1452. PMID: 32893970.

Mickan, S., Burls, A., & Glasziou, P. (2011). Patterns of "leakage" in the utilisation of clinical guidelines: A systematic review. *Postgraduate Medical Journal, 87*, 670–679.

Moher, D., Shamseer, L., Clarke, M., et al. (2015). Preferred reporting items for systematic review and meta-analysis protocols (PRISMA-P) 2015 statement. *Systematic Reviews*, 4(1), 1.

Munn, Z., Peters, M. D. J., Stern, C., Tufanaru, C., McArthur, A., & Aromataris, E. (2018). Systematic review or scoping review? Guidance for authors when choosing between a systematic or scoping review approach. *BMC Medical Research Methodology*, 18(1), 143. https://doi.org/10.1186/s12874-018-0611-x.

n.a., & Canadian Institutes of Health Research. (2017). AGREE GRS instrument. https://www.agreetrust.org/resource-centre/agree-ii-grs-instrument. [Accessed 26 July 2024].

Onwuegbuzie, A. J., & Frels, J. K. (2016). A typology of literature reviews: Evolution and future directions. *Review of Educational Research*, 86(2), 436–477.

Page, M. J., McKenzie, J. E., Bossuyt, P. M., et al. (2021). The PRISMA 2020 statement: An updated guideline for reporting systematic reviews. *BMJ (Clinical research ed.)*, 372, n71. https://doi.org/10.1136/bmj.n71.

Racine, L., Johnson, L., & Fowler-Kerry, S. (2021). An integrative review of empirical literature on indigenous cognitive impairment and dementia. *Journal of Advanced Nursing*, 77(33), 1155–1171.

Rosenfeld, R. M., & Shiffman, R. N. (2009). Clinical practice guideline development manual: A quality-driven approach for translating evidence into action. *Otolaryngology—Head and Neck Surgery: Official Journal of American Academy of Otolaryngology—Head and Neck Surgery*, 140(6 Suppl. 1), S1–43. https://doi.org/10.1016/j.otohns.2009.04.015.

Rossouw, J. E., Anderson, G. L., Prentice, R. L., et al. (2002). Risks and benefits of estrogen plus progetin for secondary prevention of coronary heart disease in postmenopausal women: Principal results from the Women's Health Initiative randomized controlled trial. *Journal of the American Medical Association*, 288, 321–333.

Siering, U., Eikermann, M., Hausner, E., Hoffmann, E., & Neugebauer, E. A. (2013). Appraisal tools for clinical practice guidelines: A systematic review. *PLOS ONE*, 8(12), e82915. http://journals.plos.org/plosone/article?id=10.1371/journal.pone.0082915.

Siu, A. (2015). Screening for abnormal glucose and Type 2 diabetes mellitus: U.S. preventive services task force recommendations statement. *Annals of Internal Medicine*, 163(11), 861–871.

Smith, J., & Noble, H. (2014). Bias in research. *Evidence-Based Nursing*, 17(4), 100–101.

Tenti, M., Raffaeli, W., & Gremigni, P. (2022). A narrative review of the assessment of depression in chronic pain. *Pain Management Nursing: Official Journal of the American Society of Pain Management Nurses*, 23(2), 158–167. https://doi.org/10.1016/j.pmn.2021.03.

te Velde, A., Morgan, C., Finch-Edmondson, M., McNamara, L., McNamara, M., Paton, M. C. B., et al. (2022). Neurodevelopmental therapy for cerebral palsy: A meta-analysis. *Pediatrics*, 149(6), e2021055061. https://doi.org/10.1542/peds.2021-.

Tricco, A., Lillie, E., Zarin, W., & for the PRISMA-Rapid Review Group., et al. (2015). A scoping review of rapid review methods. *BMC Medicine*, 13(1), 142.

Turner, E. H., Cipriani, A., Furukawa, T. A., Salanti, G., & de Vries, Y. A. (2022). Selective publication of antidepressant trials and its influence on apparent efficacy: Updated comparisons and meta-analyses of newer versus older trials. *PLoS Medicine*, 19(1), e1003886. https://doi.org/10.1371/journal.pmed.1003886.

van Dael, J., Reader, T. W., Gillespie, A., Neves, A. L., Darzi, A., & Mayer, E. K. (2020). Learning from complaints in healthcare: A realist review of academic literature, policy evidence and front-line insights. *BMJ Quality & Safety*, 29(8), 684–695. https://doi.org/10.1136/bmjqs-2019-009704.

Vandvik, P. O., Brandt, L., Alonso-Coello, P., Treweek, S., Akl, E. A., Kristiansen, A., et al. (2013). Creating clinical practice guidelines we can trust, use, and share: A new era is imminent. *Chest*, 144(2), 381–389. https://doi.org/10.1378/chest.13-0746.

West, S., Gartlehner, G., Mansfield, A., et al. (2010). *Comparative effectiveness review methods: Clinical heterogeneity [Internet]*. Agency for Healthcare Research and Quality. https://www.ncbi.nlm.nih.gov/books/NBK53310/.

Whelton, P. K., Carey, R. M., Aronow, W. S., et al. (2017). 2017 ACC/AHA/AAPA/ABC/ACPM/AGS/APhA/ASH/ASPC/NMA/PCNA guideline for the prevention, detection, evaluation, and management of high blood pressure in adults. *Journal of the American College of Cardiology*. https://doi.org/10.1016/j.jacc.2017.11.006.

Whittemore, R., & Knafl, K. (2005). The integrative review: Updated methodology. *Journal of Advanced Nursing*, 52(5), 546–553.

Wong, G., Greenhalgh, T., Westhorp, G., Buckingham, J., & Pawson, R. (2013). RAMESES publication standards: Meta-narrative reviews. *BMC Medicine*, 11, 20. https://doi.org/10.1186/1741-7015-11-20.

11

Qualitative Studies

Kathleen Evanovich Zavotsky and Marie Foley

LEARNING OUTCOMES

After reading this chapter, you should be able to do the following:
- Describe the role of qualitative research in evidence-based practice, nursing, and healthcare.
- Synthesize the value and rigor of qualitative research as it relates to healthcare.
- Incorporate the role of critical appraisal of qualitative studies as it relates to evidence-based practice, nursing, and healthcare.
- Apply qualitative measures of rigor when critiquing qualitative research findings and applying it to practice.
- Apply critical appraisal criteria to evaluate a qualitative study.
- Synthesize evidence provided by a group of qualitative studies.
- Evaluate meta-syntheses of qualitative findings and how this approach can strengthen internal and external validity.
- Integrate qualitative evidence and clinical judgment in the planning and implementation of evidence-based practice, nursing, and healthcare.

KEY TERMS

Auditability
Bracketing
Case study
Confirmability
Credibility
Data saturation
Dependability
Emic
Ethnography
Etic
Grounded theory
Meta-synthesis
Phenomenology
Purposive sampling
Qualitative research
Transferability
Trustworthiness

Evidence-based practice (EBP) is acknowledged as important in professional nursing practice and has made significant contributions to health care outcomes over the past two decades. EBP integrates the best available research evidence, patient preferences, and clinical expertise to provide patient care that achieves the best outcomes for patients in any given clinical situation. Fundamental to reliable patient care is the development of your skill set to include critical thinking, critical reasoning, process and outcome evaluation, and synthesis of all evidence available in an effort to make sound clinical decisions in your nursing practice (Ravindran, 2019). **Qualitative research** is explanatory, descriptive, and inductive in nature and comprises methods that help us formulate an understanding of phenomena and their context answered by discovery-oriented research questions. As noted in Chapter 3, the current state of knowledge related to EBP provides you and your colleagues with well-defined criteria with which to appraise quantitative research. Criteria to evaluate qualitative findings have been evolving but may not be as transparent as quantitative critiquing guidelines. This is intrinsically related to the subjective nature of the findings and the ongoing dialogue concerning rigor in qualitative research. It is important for you to note that the evidence hierarchy presented in Chapter 3, Fig. 3.1 does include qualitative studies; however, they are ranked as providing weaker, Level VI evidence. As long as hierarchical evidence pyramids are used to rank the level of evidence provided by specific types of designs, the strength of evidence provided by qualitative studies will continue to be misrepresented because the linear approach used to evaluate quantitative studies such as randomized controlled trials does not align with the nonlinear nature of qualitative research. This supports the need for a different paradigm for critically appraising the strength and quality of the evidence provided by the findings of qualitative studies so the evidence provided by the findings are valued as important data that inform clinical practice about the patient experience.

The purpose of this chapter is to describe the significance of qualitative research as it relates to EBP in nursing and healthcare. Qualitative research methods are defined, strategies to determine scientific rigor are addressed, and guidelines for critical appraisal and synthesis of qualitative research findings are described.

Qualitative research findings have a place in EBP and are an important component of quality improvement (QI). Findings from qualitative research can be linked to the Institute for Healthcare Improvement (Nundy et al., 2022) Quadruple Aim Initiative. These include reducing cost and improving population health, patient experience, and health care team well-being (Arnetz et al, 2020). The National Academies of Sciences, Engineering, and Medicine (2021), formerly called the Institute of Medicine (IOM), defines well-being as an inherently complex concept, encompassing an individual's appraisal of physical, social, and psychological resources needed to meet a psychological, physical, or social challenge (Dodge et al., 2012). There is existing evidence that supports the fact that health care team well-being can impact the quality of healthcare related to compassion fatigue, medical errors, and impaired decision making (National Academies of Sciences, Engineering, and Medicine, 2021).

Qualitative research methodologies provide a relationship between what patients and health care teams aspire to in terms of improving the quality of health care services. One component of QI is the focus on the patient experience. An important measure of quality is the extent to which patients' needs and expectations are met. This directly connects to qualitative methodologies in which researchers are working to operationalize theoretical explanations of life experiences derived from actual described patient experiences. One example might be found in transgender patient care, where the nursing literature is sparse, contributing to confusion, discomfort, and misunderstandings regarding how to provide the best evidence-based care for this population. In a study by Rossman and colleagues (2017), young adult patients described feeling uncomfortable, judged, and exposed to harsh consequences of being transgender. The findings also revealed nurses' discomfort with and lack of knowledge about people who identify as transgender and their health care needs. Some studies (Kattari et al., 2021; Kcomt, 2019) noted that transgender patients frequently report encountering verbal abuse and condescending and humiliating treatment from health care providers. If we are to provide effective evidence-based care for this population, qualitative research will be critical to developing the thematic elements about the lived health care experiences of this patient population that will contribute evidence to develop best practices that inform high-quality, cost-effective, and satisfying care tailored to this patient population. Since there is limited amount of research related to LGBTQIA and transgender care, this is a perfect opportunity to utilize qualitative methodologies to future advance the science thereby improving health care quality for this vulnerable population.

The Institute for Healthcare Improvement (Nundy et al., 2022) Quadruple Aim Initiative includes patient experience, population health, health care cost, and health care team well-being. Qualitative research can contribute to the attainment of the Quadruple Aim by better describing health care needs and understanding those needs from the perspective of the lived experience of both the patients and providers. Describing the patient's and provider's lived experience can improve healthcare overall and ensure that providers feel healthy, well, and supported.

> **TIP**
>
> Seek out researchers experienced in qualitative research, educational opportunities, and conferences to improve your understanding of qualitative research and its relevance to your role as a nurse and a nurse leader.

QUALITATIVE METHODOLOGIES AND WORLDVIEW

Researchers using qualitative methodologies approach their work with a worldview that is holistic, values subjectivity, and believes that each individual attributes meaning to their experience based on past, present, and possibly future experiences. For example, Ranjbar and colleagues (2017) studied the development of moral competency in Iranian nursing students. Using a constructivist grounded theory method, they found that during the students' education experience three levels of moral development occurred that helped the formation of a professional identity. The levels included moral transition, moral reconstruction, and professional morality. This model provides insight into the development of professionalism in nursing, something that concerns every faculty member as it is noted as an area for nursing competency development in the *Essentials* set forth by the American Association of Colleges of Nursing for nursing education (AACN, 2021). Their study emphasizes how the worldview of students, in terms of professionalism, changes based on past, present, and possibly future experiences.

Qualitative research methods are selected to describe phenomena about which little is known. These methods capture meaning as it is lived and pay close attention to the experience as lived by the participants. An example of capturing meaning as it is lived can be understood in the work of Wolf and colleagues (2018) and their work on exploring the experience of emergency department (ED) nurses conducting the triage process and the influences on their decisions. The participants described processes that were unit- and/or nurse-dependent and were manipulations of the triage system to "fix" problems in ED flow, rather than a standard application of a triage system. The participants reported that, in practice, the use of triage scales to determine acuity and route patients to appropriate resources varies in accuracy and application among ED nurses and in their respective EDs. These qualitative findings led the authors to the conclusion that future research should focus on intervention and comparison studies examining the effect of staffing, nurse experience, hospital policies, and length of shift on the accuracy of triage decision making. In the preceding example, qualitative research explores and describes more fully the complexities of caring for the patients in an ED. The approach seeks to understand what is occurring in the triage nurses' decision making in the ED as it is lived. Thousands of reports of well-conducted qualitative studies exist on topics germane to nursing practice. Findings from qualitative research provide valuable insights into understanding and improving patient care from both nurse and patient perspectives.

The intended goal of qualitative research is to describe phenomena relevant to nursing that is lacking in theoretical information or requires a better understanding of a particular phenomenon. You cannot study an issue using quantitative research methods if you do not have a theoretical basis to develop your study (van Manen, 2017; Doyle et al., 2020). Qualitative research methods are often used when few studies are available on one particular topic or when the researcher wants to obtain an alternate view of an issue (Meadows-Oliver, 2014). The sample size in qualitative studies is relatively small. The sampling method is often described as **purposive**; that is, the sample is homogeneous and reflects the population being studied. Subjects are often identified as participants or key informants. The common data collection method is interview with verbatim transcription of exactly what the participants have said. When no new data emerge, often referred to as *saturation*, data collection ends. **Data saturation** is determined by the researcher when no new information emerges from the informants. All data collection procedures result in large amounts of narrative data with the descriptive phrases, words, and quotes of the participants. Findings of the study have the potential to improve patient care, prevent comorbidities, or lead patients to recovery that is free of complications.

Raw data are a narrative compilation of exactly what both researcher and participant said during the interview that is then transcribed verbatim, as well as the participant's observed behaviors. Data analysis processes are systematic and rigorous to ensure that findings can be confirmed with qualitative analytic methods (Turale, 2020).

Qualitative research is most valuable when expressing patients', families', students', and health care providers' stories and should be applied in areas where there is a need to build knowledge that may then lead to theory development, quantitative studies, and instrument development. For example, Arbour and Wiegand (2023) used a phenomenological method to explore the lived experiences of critical care nurses while providing end-of-life care. They found that many critical care nurses were unprepared for their emotions and reactions when caring for dying patients. The study findings demonstrated the need for education, support, and debriefing for the nursing staff after a patient death. The intended purpose of qualitative research and the types of data analysis used in these projects are significantly different from those of quantitative studies.

Qualitative approaches:
- Must be appropriate for the phenomenon being studied;
- Must be relevant to the PICOT question; and
- Focus on the values and opinions most important to patients, families, and staff to deepen the understanding of the impact of care on health care outcomes (Doyle et al., 2020).

The qualitative paradigm is used to explore the meaning of experience that can be missed by quantitative studies. Qualitative studies build conceptual frameworks and theoretical understanding of the phenomenon being studied. By examining issues crucial to patients and families, it provides more complete information regarding the best evidence on which to build professional nursing practice and support care and health care outcomes. Caring for the transgender patient is a contemporary example of a topic that needs a theoretical foundation that can be built from qualitative methods. How can we possibly know what various populations need in terms of quality healthcare if we do not listen to the stories of their experiences as patients?

There are a variety of approaches to qualitative research (Fig. 11.1). The most commonly used, described in this chapter, are phenomenology, grounded theory, ethnography, case study, and mixed methods. Metasynthesis of qualitative research is also addressed. It is important for you to remember that when qualitative researchers develop their expertise and select a methodology, they immerse themselves in the seminal work related to each method.

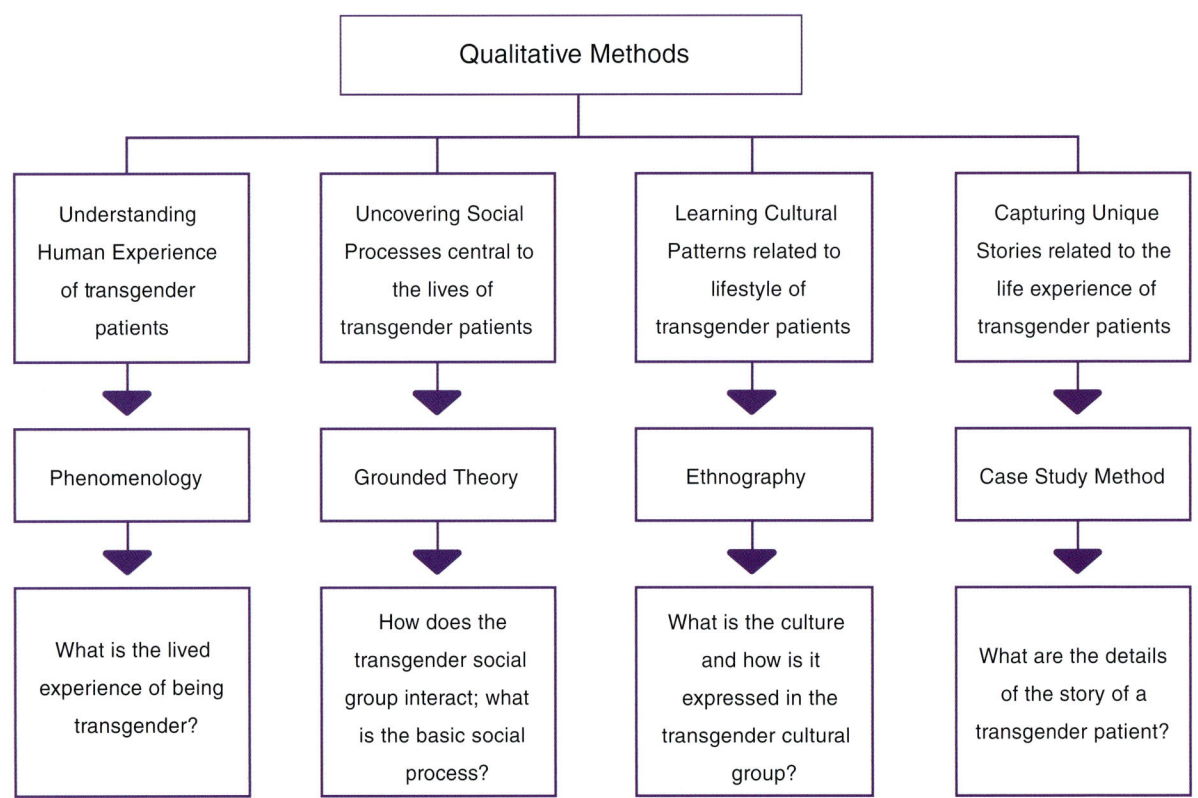

Fig. 11.1 Decision-Making Algorithm: Qualitative Research Methods to Study Transgender Patient Needs.

> **TIP**
>
> Incorporate evidence from qualitative research into clinical practice by developing your critical appraisal skills for evaluating qualitative research. There are multiple critical appraisal tools that can guide you such as Joanna Briggs Institute Critical Appraisal Tools (https://jbi.global/critical-appraisal-tools), Critical Appraisal Skills Programme (CASP) International Network Checklists (https://casp-uk.net/casp-tools-checklists/), and Grading of Recommendations, Assessment, Development, and Evaluations (GRADE; see Chapter 4) (https://bestpractice.bmj.com/info/us/toolkit/learn-ebm/what-is-grade/).

PHENOMENOLOGY

Phenomenology is a qualitative research method derived from philosophy with the purpose of describing particular phenomena, or the appearance of things, as lived experience. The phenomenological term "lived experience" is critical for the understanding of phenomenological reflection, meaning, analysis, and insights. Data are collected via interviews guided by open-ended questions and prompts, then transcribed verbatim. Lived experiences are the data of phenomenological research; interviews with informants continue until data saturation occurs. The researcher then "dwells" with the data, reading and rereading the raw data until common thematic elements emerge. Developing a rich, thick description of the phenomenon under investigation is important for health care providers and helps identify health care needs. The primary goal of phenomenology is to peel back the layers of current beliefs to eventually get to the true raw description of the phenomenon (van Manen, 2017; Zahavi & Martini, 2019). Keller and Evanovich Zavotsky (2023) conducted a phenomenological study to explore the perception of the future role of the nurse manager working in an academic health system peri-pandemic and identify the variability in levels of experience. The study clearly showed that regardless of the level of experience, opportunity and resources are needed for leadership development, innovative communication strategies, contemporary business acumen, and workforce wellness techniques to support the role of nurse manager (NM) in healthcare. This study concluded that preparing NMs is critical for the success of any health care organization and to ensure quality outcomes for patients, families, and providers.

GROUNDED THEORY

Grounded theory research is used to generate theories about clinical practice and understanding about multiple aspects of healthcare. Grounded theory as a method is rooted in sociology—specifically, symbolic interactionism, which describes the relationship between people and society. The approach is inductive and has clearly developed systematic procedures designed to develop a theory or basic social process. The emergent theory is based on observations and perceptions of the social processes and evolves during data collection and analysis (Corbin & Strauss, 2015). The constant comparative method of data analysis, an iterative approach, is used to examine data from interviews, identify gaps in understanding from the data, and conduct additional interviews until data saturation occurs. For example, Berthelsen (2020) studied nurse researchers employed in clinical hospital research positions. Using a constructivist grounded theory method, they found that the theory of Positioning showed how nurse researchers tried to establish their positions in acute care settings. The nurse researchers' choice of path was found to be guided by personal and professional beliefs. Overall, the nurse researchers' behavior was discovered as seven interconnected behavioral actions of building an identity and transforming themselves. This theory of Positioning provides a framework of nurse researchers' work and shows that there is diversity in their actions, tasks, and ambitions. Therefore, nursing leaders can use this theory to match the needs of their acute care departments.

ETHNOGRAPHY

Ethnography is associated with anthropology, the work of describing culture and the people of a particular culture. The purpose of ethnographic research is to discover and understand the social and psychological culture within a group of people. Within ethnography, culture is defined as the collective understanding and influences of shared behaviors and understandings and the deeper influences being placed on the group being studied.

Derived from the Greek term *ethnos*, meaning people, race, or cultural group, the ethnographic method focuses on the scientific description and interpretation of cultural or social groups and systems (Malik et al., 2017). The goal of the ethnographer is to understand the participants' views of their world, or the emic view.

The emic view, the insiders' view, is contrasted with the etic view, the outsiders' view. The ethnographer's approach requires that the researcher enter the world of the study participants to observe what happens, listen to what is said, ask questions, and collect whatever data are available. Data can include artifacts of the culture such as clothing, jewelry, cooking implements, and ceremonial objects. Researchers use the method to study cultural variations in health and patient groups as subcultures within the larger culture of healthcare. Black and colleagues (2021) suggest through their scoping review that ethnographic research has benefit for health care improvement and is considered an acceptable methodology. For example, Martin-Ferres and colleagues (2019) examined the study of human dignity in nursing practice utilizing an ethnographic approach. Two themes emerged from their analysis of semi-structured interviews. They found factors of, and the delivering of, dignified care were guided by respect, confidentiality, privacy, and communication. These were often times in conflict, and it was through both the observation and interviews that discrepancies were noted. The results of this study suggest that professional forums should be provided and need to be developed to help nurses be more aware of their practice.

CASE STUDY

Case study research is rooted in sociology and focuses on describing elements of an individual case, both the commonalities and the peculiarities. A single case may be an individual, a family, a community, or an organization (Sibbald et al., 2021). Case studies emphasize a holistic approach to the research that may lead to identification of patterns consistent across a set of cases that contribute to a more global understanding of a particular problem. The selection of cases can range from those that are most common to those that are most unusual. It is recommended that you choose cases that provide the best opportunity for learning. Case study data are gathered using interviews, field observations, and review of documents, diaries, and transcripts for evidence to describe and explain the complexity of a case (Sibbald et al., 2021). Although researchers pose questions to begin a case study data collection, the initial questions are never all inclusive. Instead, the researcher uses an iterative process of "growing questions" in the field. As data are collected, other questions emerge and serve to guide the researcher's quest to untangle the complexities of the case. Eppel-Meichlinger and colleagues (2022) conducted a research study utilizing case study design in order to gain insight into the experiences of family caregivers who accompanied a loved one during voluntary stopping of eating and drinking during end of life. They identified similarities and differences between cases of voluntary stopping of eating and drinking, which helped them develop a conceptual model to use in future practice.

MIXED METHODS

According to Younas and colleagues (2019) **mixed-methods research**, which combines both qualitative and quantitative methods, is still in its infancy in nursing, and researchers encounter challenges during its conduct, analysis, and reporting. Inadequate justification for utilizing mixed methods and inadequate data integration compromise the rigor of mixed-methods studies, and data integration remains a challenge for nurse researchers. There is a need to determine researchers' attitudes and challenges toward using mixed methods and to educate them about advanced mixed methods. Emphasis should be placed on use of advanced data integration methods so that the rigor and quality of mixed-methods research can be enhanced in nursing research.

An example of a study that utilized mixed methods was conducted by Witkoski Stimpfel and colleagues (2022). They studied the complex phenomena of individual and work factors associated with the health and well-being of registered nurses during the COVID-19 pandemic. The data were collected through survey as well as one-on-one interviews to help capture the qualitative comments. Through their analysis they found that nurses reported high levels of depressive symptoms, anxiety, and insomnia, which can contribute to overall nurse wellness.

> **TIP**
>
> Qualitative research teams are comprised of stakeholders, the research team members, and the key informants who are partners in dialogue and discovery. Through observation and dialogue, the meaning of the lived experience, culture, social process, or historical period are revealed and represent a cohesive mutual representation of reality that can impact health care outcomes.

META-SYNTHESIS

Meta-synthesis, sometimes call a meta-summary, is a rigorous synthesis of a critical mass of qualitative research evidence that relates to answering a specific research question. Meta-synthesis is a method for synthesizing knowledge, for example, relating to service users' healthcare-related experiences and the factors that facilitate their involvement in their own care and commitment to a healthy lifestyle (Thorne, 2022). Meta-synthesis reviews attempt to overcome possible biases at all stages by following a rigorous methodology. Meta-syntheses involve further extraction and further abstraction of qualitative findings and include calculation of the manifest frequency effect sizes (Butler et al., 2016). The methods include constant comparison, taxonomic analysis, the reciprocal interpretation of in vivo concepts, and the use of imported concepts to frame data (Butler et al., 2016). Inferences about the findings are derived from taking all of the reports in a sample of studies as a whole to offer a cohesive description or explanation of the phenomenon while retaining the essence and unique contribution of each study (Butler et al., 2016).

Researchers must make several decisions when preparing a meta-synthesis, including:
- Formulating a qualitative research question;
- Identifying, selecting, and critically appraising relevant studies;
- Abstracting, synthesizing, and lending further interpretation to the body of study findings; and
- Drawing overall conclusions.

This type of knowledge is needed in EBP. Meta-synthesis is a concept that includes several methodologies in synthesizing qualitative research findings. It focuses on combining data from original studies and follows the principles of scientific rigor seen in systematic reviews that synthesize the best available and critically appraised knowledge. Systematic review of qualitative studies is significant for implementation of EBP as it helps ensure that when making both clinical and administrative decisions, it is done by including a depth and breadth of the latest science related to the specific topic (Thorne, 2022).

Equally important is the need to examine the validity of the results and decide how you and your team can apply the meta-synthesis findings to patient care and QI. Similar to systematic reviews, meta-synthesis of qualitative findings may be the best way to integrate evidence across a wider range of scientific methodologies. In particular, this approach may help clinical leaders and their teams work within the qualitative evidence-based movement with greater assurance that scientifically sound reference points have not compromised the complexity, richness, and diversity inherent in clinical practice. Newer approaches to research synthesis and integration hold promise for increasing confidence about what might constitute a qualitatively derived evidentiary knowledge claim (Thorne, 2022). Qualitative synthesis has the ability to create a systematic logic within which findings from distinct studies in a field can be rigorously integrated into stronger and more generalizable knowledge claims (Butler et al., 2016; Thorne, 2022). Qualitative data from a meta-synthesis provides stronger qualitative evidence that you and your team can use to validate and support the Quadruple Aim and patient experience and use in evidence-based QI initiatives aimed at improving the clinical experience of individuals, families, and communities.

> **TIP**
>
> Participating in the development of a meta-synthesis related to a clinical question of interest to you or your clinical team will enable you to ensure that you are integrating and evaluating the most up-to-date evidence.

KEY DIFFERENCES IN QUALITATIVE METHODOLOGIES

Sampling strategies in qualitative research have as their primary goal the collection of raw data, from individuals experiencing the phenomena being studied, with the goal of describing the phenomena from the perspective of the individuals actually living it (Duggleby & Williams, 2016; Vasileiou et al., 2018). The specific sampling strategy, usually purposive, is driven by the phenomenon under investigation. Box 11.1 highlights common types of sampling strategies used in qualitative studies. For example, if a researcher was interested in the lived experience of having an implantable cardiac defibrillator, the researcher would need to sample individuals with defibrillators. Sampling is purposeful in that participants are selected because they can best inform the research question and have experience with the phenomenon under investigation. However, you will

> **BOX 11.1 Common Types of Sampling Strategies Used in Qualitative Research**
>
> **Purposive sampling**—the intentional selection of participants or events consistent with the focus of the study
> **Snowball sampling**—recruitment of participants from social networks of informants already enrolled in the study
> **Convenience sampling**—recruitment of participants who meet the study inclusion criteria and volunteer to enroll in the study

notice that sample size in qualitative studies is expected to be small; a predetermined sample size is not the norm, although it is recommended that you start with an estimate (Vasileiou et al., 2018).

> **TIP**
>
> Often the standard of saturation is used to determine sample size. When you can say to yourself, "I am no longer hearing anything new," then the assumption is made that saturation has been reached. Choose participants carefully, ensuring that those selected can best inform the question.

Data gathered via qualitative research methods include thoughts, feelings, behaviors, and actual lived experiences as told by the individuals experiencing the phenomenon under investigation. By listening to patients' voices through analysis of their words and behaviors, scientific evidence can be enriched through narrative data that may not be heard or fully understood by filling out questionnaires or computing statistics (Renjith, et al., 2021). Whereas quantitative research methods strive to eliminate or control for contextual elements, qualitative research methods encompass these elements and construct studies that examine relevant issues related to individual life experiences (Danford, 2023, van Manen, 2017). Appraising the best evidence to inform practice should include qualitative findings as a source of critical evidence. However, thorough evaluation of qualitative findings is essential if they are to be incorporated into patient care and EBP (Chicca, 2020). Data collection ends when the researcher is no longer hearing anything new or different and is referred to as saturation, as noted earlier.

> **TIP**
>
> Practice interviewing and focus group facilitation skills and have them evaluated by an expert before beginning data collection.

DATA ANALYSIS

Qualitative data are words rather than numbers. As such, they are analyzed by interpretation rather than mathematical manipulation. Meaning is extracted from the repetitive patterns of words emerging from the raw data that coalesce into thematic patterns that provide a rich description that explains the behavior or experience. This is where it becomes critically important that the researcher use a systematic process to describe thoroughly to the reader the process of how the researcher arrived at their conclusions (Ravindran, 2019). By doing so, the researcher establishes the authenticity and trustworthiness of the data.

> **TIP**
>
> Consider how you can apply qualitative findings to your clinical decision making and EBP or QI projects.

SCIENTIFIC RIGOR IN QUALITATIVE RESEARCH

Criteria for determining the trustworthiness of qualitative research were introduced by Lincoln and Guba (1985) in the 1980s when they replaced terminology for achieving rigor, reliability, validity, and generalizability with **dependability**, **credibility**, and **transferability**. Strategies for achieving **trustworthiness** were also introduced. The literature reflects ongoing discussion of these original criteria (Ravindran, 2019); however, this sentinel work remains in use today.

To conduct research that reflects precision and rigor, regardless of the paradigm, the researcher must first select the methodology most appropriate to study the research problem at hand (see Fig. 11.1). Qualitative approaches are used to describe the "why," whereas quantitative approaches address what has occurred, how many times something occurred, relationships among variables, or the effect of an intervention on an outcome (see Chapters 8 to 10). Qualitative approaches describe experiences about which little is known in the form of individuals' thoughts, feelings, and behaviors instead of numbers. Data are gathered in settings where what is being studied is actually occurring. Process is of primary concern rather than outcomes (Ravindran, 2019). Table 11.1 lists methodological differences between qualitative and quantitative research studies.

> **TIP**
>
> As a nurse and nursing leader, think about a bias you may have about a clinical situation or patient population. Talk through your bias with a neutral party or write your assumptions, bias experiences, and beliefs in a journal. Qualitative researchers suspend or bracket their biases to maximize their objectivity before launching a qualitative research study.

The criteria to critique the quality and rigor of quantitative and qualitative research are extremely different and grounded in each paradigm's specific end goals. In quantitative research, rigor is judged in terms of a study's validity, reliability, generalizability, and objectivity (see Chapter 7). Quantitative results are intended to be free from bias, to be replicable across contexts, and to generalize from the sample under study to the full target population. Qualitative research has its own, separate measures of quality: credibility, transferability, dependability, and confirmability as defined in Table 11.2 (Lincoln & Guba, 1985; Baillie, 2015).

Ensuring credibility refers to the conscious effort to establish confidence in an accurate interpretation of the meaning of the data (Cypress, 2017). Do the results of the research reflect the experience of participants or

TABLE 11.1 Process-Related Differences in Qualitative Research

Qualitative Research Methods Naturalistic Paradigm	Quantitative Research Methods Positivist Paradigm
Grounded in qualitative methods, research conducted within this paradigm reflects a research process that lends focus to the complexities of phenomena as they exist in the world.	Grounded in quantitative methods, research conducted within this paradigm allows researchers to conduct studies that are more fundable and seek the facts of social phenomena.
Methods are generated from the disciplines of anthropology, psychology, history, and philosophy.	Methods are derived from logical positivism and empiricism.
The focus is on understanding and describing phenomena as they are experienced.	The focus is on controlling and predicting: Can we control the outcome?
Qualitative data collection methods include participant observation, interview, and retrospective description.	Quantitative data collection methods include experiments, quasi-experiments, and physiological, psychological, and sociological measures.
Knower and known are interactive and inseparable. The researcher is the instrument.	Knower and known are independent.
Approaches are subjective, holistic, and process oriented.	Approaches are objective and outcome oriented.
Data are thick and rich, providing for detailed analysis. Hundreds of pages of verbatim transcripts comprise the data.	The purpose is to predict relationships achieved by testing and validating hypotheses with a given statistical probability.
Data collection and analysis occurs over an extended period of time. Interviews may need to be repeated two or three times to clarify information and ensure accuracy of analysis.	Data are analyzed through statistical inference.
Sample sizes in qualitative research are small due to rich, thick data gathered and the depth of analysis required. The researcher determines when to end collection of data. This is generally referred to as "saturation," or the point at which no new information is being noted during the data collection phase.	Quantitative designs use power analysis to ensure that enough subjects are recruited so that statistically meaningful results can be detected.
The purpose is to develop theory.	The purpose is to test theory.

TABLE 11.2 Comparison Criteria: Critical Evaluation of Authenticity and Trustworthiness of Data

Quantitative Language	Qualitative Language	Definition	Example Techniques
Internal Validity: the degree to which it can be inferred that the experimental treatment, rather than an uncontrolled condition, resulted in the observed effects	Credibility, dependability/auditability	When the exhaustive description is returned to the participants to review, they recognize it as their reality. The findings make sense to the participants.	Prolonged time in the field: evidence is supplied that indicates the researcher spent prolonged engagement in the field collecting data. Triangulation: two or more theories, groups of participants, methods instruments, or investigators were included. Peer debriefing: the researcher and the research are peer reviewed by another researcher who can challenge the method and offer guidance. The research can be audited in such a way that the reader can follow the line of thinking used by the researcher in the development of thematic elements and exhaustive description. Here, the researcher should offer raw data and demonstrate how that data were translated in the researcher. Audit trail of decision making occurs throughout the research process.
External Validity/Generalizability: the degree to which the findings of a study can be generalized to other populations or environments.	Transferability	The purpose of qualitative research is theory development. The important question to be asked is whether the findings may be transferred to another similar setting.	Thick, rich descriptions of the setting and participants: findings are recognized by participants and possibly those not included in the study, but with similar experiences.
Objectivity	Confirmability	Provides confirmation of the researcher's influence.	Bracketing. Journal writing, reflecting the researcher's thoughts and interpretations during data collection; also referred to as reflexivity.
Reliability	Authenticity and trustworthiness of the data/credibility	Do the participants recognize the experience as their own? Has adequate time been allowed to fully understand the phenomenon?	Exhaustive description and synthesis of raw data with development of thematic elements is returned to the participants for them to validate accuracy of interpretation.
Generalizability	Transferability/fittingness	Are the findings applicable outside the study situation?	Comprehensive descriptions of the setting and participants are produced.

Adapted from Lincoln & Guba, 1985.

the context in a believable way? Does the explanation fit the description? Thorne (2019) identified the need to ensure that interpretations are trustworthy and reveal some truth external to the investigators' experience. Authenticity is closely linked to validity and involves the portrayal of research that reflects the meanings and experiences that are lived and perceived by the participants (Doyle et al., 2020).

Because qualitative research is based on entirely different epistemological and ontological assumptions compared with quantitative research, quantitative validity criteria are inappropriate for evaluation purposes (Cypress, 2017). For example, the important distinction between internal and external validity in quantitative research holds less meaning and applicability within a framework where generalizability to populations is not a significant research goal (see Chapter 7).

The expansion, proliferation, and evolution of qualitative research approaches have created a tension that has influenced validity criteria. Phenomenology, ethnography, grounded theory, case study, and mixed-methods methodologies set the stage for the development of numerous other qualitative methods applicable to nursing science. Much discussion has ensued regarding the alignment of philosophy, epistemology, and methodology. The divergence of the interpretive perspective from the positivistic perspective required in-depth analysis. Selecting research methods was viewed not simply as a technological choice; rather, methods were proposed to be based on philosophical, ideological, ethical, and political assumptions (Doyle et al., 2020).

> **TIP**
>
> Work diligently and consistently to incorporate qualitative research into your clinical practice.

Creativity must be preserved within qualitative research, but not at the expense of the quality of science. Therefore, in order to use qualitative research findings to implement evidence-based care, rigorous appraisal of qualitative research to evaluate trustworthiness is paramount, as in any other type of research (Williams et al., 2020). Table 11.3 provides a detailed summary of critiquing guidelines for qualitative research.

Promoting and evaluating scientific rigor in qualitative research is critical if these methodologies are to be used by clinicians in EBP. Criteria for assessing quality in qualitative research must differ from that of quantitative research. There is a range of techniques that can be used to promote, evaluate, and critique qualitative research and, when consistently applied, provide practitioners with solid evidence to inform their practice. Remember that qualitative critiquing criteria are no less rigorous than those used to assess quantitative data; they are simply different and require different steps and measures to ensure quality data. You will note that the primary methods used to control internal validity in qualitative studies are those aimed at controlling bias relative to the researcher and the subjects. Qualitative researchers use bracketing as a method of recognizing and setting aside their knowledge or opinions about the study. **Bracketing** involves being self-aware or freeing oneself of assumptions and making the researcher's own perspective explicit and putting this knowledge aside (Johnston et al., 2017).

Additional steps may include, but are not limited to:
- Prolonged engagements in the field,
- Persistent observation,
- Peer debriefing,
- Member checks,
- Audit trails,
- Mixed methods, and
- Establishing interrater reliability as data are analyzed and thematic elements emerge.

These steps are key for increasing both the dependability and credibility of the researcher's findings. The strongest qualitative evidence will emerge from studies that incorporate most of these common methods to enhance internal validity. See Table 11.3 for qualitative critique guidelines.

SYNTHESIS

From a philosophical viewpoint, the study of humans is deeply rooted in descriptive modes of science. With regard to safe patient care and accountability, remember that EBP has clear roots in quantitative and qualitative research. This has enlivened the debate about what constitutes evidence and reinvigorates the conversation about the merits of qualitative research and its contribution to EBP and healthcare (Ravindran, 2019). As a clinical leader, you want to think about the contribution to the quadruple aim (Institute for Healthcare Improvement, 2017) that is made by evidence from qualitative research studies; the four aims provide rich data about the patient

TABLE 11.3 Critical Appraisal of Qualitative Research

Stylistic Considerations	1. Was the report well written, grammatically correct, and well organized? 2. Was there sufficient detail to enable critical appraisal? 3. Is there evidence that the researcher has the qualifications, knowledge, and expertise to conduct the research? 4. Does the abstract give a clear summary of the study, including the main findings and recommendations?
Statement of the Phenomenon of Interest	1. Was the title clear, accurate, and related to the research question? 2. What is the phenomenon of interest, and is it clearly stated for the reader? 3. What is the justification for using a qualitative method? 4. Is there a clearly defined qualitative research method?
Purpose	1. Is the purpose of the study appropriate for the research question? 2. Does the researcher describe the projected significance of the work to nursing?
Ethical Considerations	1. Is protection of human participants addressed? 2. Did the author address institutional review board approval? 3. Were the participants fully informed about the nature of the research? 4. Did the researcher address participant autonomy and confidentiality? 5. Were participants protected from harm?
Method	1. Is the method used to collect data compatible with the qualitative research question? 2. Is the qualitative method adequate to address the phenomenon of interest? 3. If a particular approach is used to guide the inquiry, has the researcher completed the study according to the processes described?
Sampling	1. What type of sampling is used? Is it appropriate given the particular method? 2. Are the informants who were chosen appropriate to inform the research? 3. Were the participants and setting adequately described and appropriate for informing the research? 4. Was saturation achieved?
Data Collection	1. Is data collection focused on human experience? 2. Does the researcher describe data collection strategies (i.e., interview, observation, field notes)? 3. Were the data gathered of sufficient depth and richness? 4. Were the questions asked and observations made and recorded in an appropriate way? 5. Is saturation of the data described? 6. What are the procedures for collecting data?
Data Analysis	1. Are the data analysis strategies consistent with the qualitative method? 2. Has the researcher remained true to the data? 3. Does the reader follow the steps described for data analysis?
Authenticity and Trustworthiness of Data	1. Does the researcher address the credibility, auditability, and fittingness of the data? Credibility • Do the participants recognize the experience as their own? Auditability • Can the reader follow the researcher's thinking? • Does the researcher document the research process? Fittingness • Are the findings applicable outside the study situation? • Are the results meaningful to individuals not involved in the research? • Is the strategy used for analysis compatible with the purpose of the study?
Findings	1. Are the findings presented within a context? 2. Is the reader able to comprehend the essence of the experience from the report of the findings? 3. Are the researcher's conceptualizations true to the data? 4. Does the researcher place the report in the context of what is already known about the phenomenon? Was the existing literature on the topic related to the findings?

Continued

TABLE 11.3	Critical Appraisal of Qualitative Research—cont'd
Conclusions, Implications, and Recommendations	1. Do the conclusions, implications, and recommendations give the reader a context in which to use the findings? 2. How do the conclusions reflect the study findings? 3. What are the recommendations for future study? Do they reflect the findings? 4. How has the researcher made the significance of the study explicit to nursing theory, research, or practice?
References	Were the books, journals, and other materials referred to in the study accurately referenced?

and health care provider experience and the context of care, and also help build theories about those lived experiences in healthcare. The purpose of qualitative research is about understanding phenomena and finding meaning through examining the pieces that make up the whole.

Evidence from the most commonly used qualitative nursing research methods—grounded theory, case study, mixed methods, ethnography, and phenomenology—provide valuable insights into why an intervention may or may not work, and help us consider patient preferences when designing best practice guidelines, develop healthy work environments, and influence our QI strategies about how to provide a satisfying experience for patients, families, and providers.

KEY POINTS

- Qualitative research findings are important components of EBP and QI.
- The purpose of qualitative research is to understand phenomena and find meaning by examining pieces that make up the whole.
- Qualitative research findings are linked to the component of the Quadruple Aim related to improving the patient and health care provider experience, including quality and satisfaction.
- Researchers using qualitative methods have a holistic worldview, value subjectivity, and believe that individuals attribute meaning to their experiences.
- Five types of qualitative methods include phenomenology, grounded theory, ethnography, case study, and mixed methods.
- The qualitative equivalent of a systematic review is a meta-synthesis, sometimes called a meta-summary.
- Qualitative research methods do not include a predetermined sample size; data collection continues until data saturation occurs.
- Qualitative data collection includes thoughts, feelings, observations, behaviors, and actual lived experiences as told by the informants experiencing the phenomenon under consideration.
- Qualitative data are words or artifacts, not numbers, that are analyzed by interpretation; narrative presentation of data is the norm.
- Scientific rigor is determined by critical appraisal criteria focused on dependability, credibility, transferability, and trustworthiness

REFERENCES

American Association of Colleges of Nursing (AACN. (2021). *The essentials: Core competencies for professional nursing education.* https://www.aacnnursing.org/Portals/0/PDFs/Publications/Essentials-2021.pdf.

Arbour, R. B., & Wiegand, D. L. (2023). Self-described nursing responses experienced during care of dying patients and their families: A phenomenological study. *Journal of Hospice & Palliative Nursing, 25*(2), E49–E56. https://doi.org/10.1097/NJH.0000000000000936.

Arnetz, B. B., Goetz, C. M., Arnetz, J. E., Sudan, S., vanSchagen, J., Piersma, K., & Reyelts, F. (2020). Enhancing healthcare efficiency to achieve the Quadruple Aim: An exploratory study. *Biomedical Research Notes, 13*(1), 362. https://doi.org/10.1186/s13104-020-05199-8.

Baillie, L. (2015). Promoting and evaluating scientific rigor in qualitative research. *Nursing Standard, 29*(46), 36–42.

Berthelsen, C. (2020). Positioning: A classic grounded theory on nurse researchers employed in clinical practice research positions. *Grounded Theory Review, 19*(1).

Black, G. B., van Os, S., Machen, S., & Fulop, N. J. (2021). Ethnographic research as an evolving method for supporting healthcare improvement skills: A scoping review. *Biomedical Research Methodologies*, *21*(1), 274. https://doi.org/10.1186/s12874-021-01466-9.

Butler, A., Hall, H., & Copnell, B. (2016). A guide to writing a qualitative systematic review protocol to enhance evidence-based practice in nursing and health care. *Worldviews on Evidence-Based Nursing*, *13*(3), 241–249.

Chicca, J. (2020). Introduction to qualitative nursing research. *American Nurse*, *15*, 28–32.

Corbin, J. M., & Strauss, A. L. (2015). *Basics of qualitative research techniques and procedures for developing grounded theory* (4th ed.). Sage.

Cypress, B. S. (2017). Rigor or reliability and validity in qualitative research: Perspectives, strategies, reconceptualization, and recommendations. *Dimensions of Critical Care Nursing*, *36*(4), 253–263. https://doi.org/10.1097/DCC.0000000000000253.

Danford, C. A. (2023). Understanding the evidence: Qualitative research designs. *Urologic Nursing*, *43*(1), 41–45.

Dodge, R. ,A., Daly, J., Huyton, L., & Sanders, L. (2012). The challenge of defining wellbeing. *International Journal of Wellbeing*, *2*(3), 222–235. https://doi.org/10.5502/ijw.v2i3.4.

Doyle, L., McCabe, C., Keogh, B., Brady, A., & McCann, M. (2020). An overview of the qualitative descriptive design within nursing research. *Journal of Research in Nursing*, *25*(5), 443–455.

Duggleby, W., & Williams, A. (2016). Methodological and epistemological considerations in utilizing qualitative inquiry to develop interventions. *Qualitative Health Research*, *26*(2), 147–153.

Eppel-Meichlinger, J., Stängle, S., Mayer, H., & Fringer, A. (2022). Family caregivers' advocacy in voluntary stopping of eating and drinking: A holistic multiple case study. *Nursing Open*, *9*(1), 624–636. https://doi.org/10.1002/nop2.1109.

Johnston, C. M., Wallis, M., Oprescu, F. I., & Gray, M. (2017). Methodological considerations related to nurse researchers using their own experience of a phenomenon within phenomenology. *Journal of Advanced Nursing*, *73*(3), 574–584.

Kattari, S. K., Bakko, M., Langenderfer-Magruder, L., & Holloway, B. T. (2021). Transgender and nonbinary experiences of victimization in health care. *Journal of Interpersonal Violence*, *36*(23–24), NP13054–NP13076. https://doi.org/10.1177/0886260520905091.

Kcomt, L. (2019). Profound health-care discrimination experienced by transgender people: Rapid systematic review. *Social Work in Health Care*, *58*(2), 201–219. https://doi.org/10.1080/00981389.2018.1532941.

Keller, R., & Evanovich Zavotsky, K. (2023). The nurse manager role of yesterday, today, and tomorrow: A qualitative study in an academic health system. *Nurse Leader*, *21*, e28–e34. https://doi.org/10.1016/j.mnl.2022.10.006.

Lincoln, Y. S., & Guba, E. G. (1985). *Naturalistic inquiry*. Sage.

Malik, G., McKenna, L., & Griffiths, D. (2017). Using pedagogical approaches to influence evidence–based practice integration–processes and recommendations: Findings from a grounded theory study. *Journal of Advanced Nursing*, *73*(4), 883–893.

Martin-Ferreres, M. L., de Juan Pardo, M. A., & Medina Moya, J. L. (2019). An ethnographic study of human dignity in nursing practice. *Nursing Outlook*, *67*(4), 393–403. https://doi.org/10.1016/j.outlook.2019.02.010.

Meadows-Oliver, M. (2014). Meta-ethnography. *Nursing Research Using Ethnography: Qualitative Designs and Methods in Nursing*, *171*.

National Academies of Sciences, Engineering, and Medicine. (2021). *The future of nursing 2020–2030: Charting a path to achieve health equity*. The National Academies Press. https://doi.org/10.17226/25982.

Nundy, S., Cooper, L. A., & Mate, K. S. (2022). The quintuple aim for health care improvement: A new imperative to advance health equity. *JAMA*, *327*(6), 521–522. https://doi.org/10.1001/jama.2021.25181.

Ranjbar, H., Joolaee, S., Vehadhir, A., & Bernstein, C. (2017). Becoming a nurse as a moral journey: A constructivist grounded theory. *Nursing Ethics*, *24*(5), 583–597.

Ravindran, V. (2019). Data analysis in qualitative research. *Indian Journal of Continuing Education*, *20*(1), 40–45. https://doi.org/10.4103/IJCN.IJCN_1_19.

Renjith, V., Yesodharan, R., Noronha, J. A., Ladd, E., & George, A. (2021). Qualitative methods in healthcare research. *International Journal of Preventive Medicine*, *12*(20). https://doi.org/10.4103/ijpvm.IJPVM_321_19.

Rossman, K., Salamanca, P., & Macapagal, K. (2017). A qualitative study examining young adults' experiences of disclosure ad non-disclosure of LGBTQ identity to healthcare providers. *Journal of Homosexuality*, *64*. https://doi.org/10.1080/00918369.2017.1321379.

Sibbald, S. L., Paciocco, S., Fournie, M., Van Asseldonk, R., & Scurr, T. (2021). Continuing to enhance the quality of case study methodology in health services research. *Healthcare Management Forum*, *34*(5), 291–296. https://doi.org/10.1177/08404704211028857.

Thorne, S. (2019). On the evolving world of what constitutes qualitative synthesis. *Qualitative Health Research*, *29*(1), 3–6. https://doi.org/10.1177/1049732318813903.

Thorne, S. (2022). Quantitative meta-synthesis. *Nurse Author Editor*, *32*(1), 15–18. https://doi.org/10.1111/nae2.12036.

Turale, S. (2020). A brief introduction to qualitative description: A research design worth using. *Pacific Rim International Journal of Nursing Research*, *24*(3), 289–291. https://he02.tci-thaijo.org/index.php/PRIJNR/article/view/243180.

van Manen, M. (2017). Phenomenology in its original sense. *Qualitative Health Research*, *27*(6), 810–825.

Vasileiou, K., Barnett, J., Thorpe, S., & Young, T. (2018). Characterizing and justifying sample size sufficiency in interview-based studies: Systematic analysis of qualitative health research over a 15-year period. *BMC Medical Research Methodology*, *18*, 1–18.

Williams, V., Boylan, A. M., & Nunan, D. (2020). Critical appraisal of qualitative research: Necessity, partialities, and the issue of bias. *BMJ Evidence-Based Medicine*, *25*(1), 9–11.

Witkoski Stimpfel, A., Ghazal, L., Goldsamt, L., & Vaughan Dickson, V. (2022). Individual and work factors associated with psychosocial health of registered nurses during the Covid-19 pandemic: A mixed methods study. *Journal of Occupational and Environmental Medicine*, *64*(6), 515–524. https://doi.org/10.1097/JOM.0000000000002495.

Wolf, L. A., Delao, A. M., Perhats, C., Moon, M. D., & Zavotsky, K. E. (2018). Triaging the emergency department, not the patient: United States emergency nurses' experience of the triage process. *Journal of Emergency Nursing*, *44*(3), 258–266.

Younas, A., Pedersen, M., & Tayaben, J. L. (2019). Review of mixed-methods research in nursing. *Nursing Research*, *68*(6), 464–472. https://doi.org/10.1097/NNR.0000000000000372.

Zahavi, D., & Martiny, K. M. M. (2019). Phenomenology in nursing studies: New perspectives. *International Journal of Nursing Studies*, *93*, 155–162. https://doi.org/10.1016/j.ijnurstu.2019.01.014. 30795899.

12

Sources of Data to Drive Evidence-Based Practice and Quality Improvement

Patricia Maria Lavin and Mary Jo Vetter

LEARNING OUTCOMES

After reading this chapter, you should be able to do the following:
- Recognize internal and external sources of evidence and information to describe the current and future state of organizational performance.
- Describe the value of an organizational strategic plan in identifying high-priority areas for evidence-based quality improvement (QI) initiatives.
- Differentiate structure, process, and outcome measures.
- Describe the value of conceptual and operational definitions in measuring outcomes.
- Identify sources of internal and external benchmarking data.
- Describe the value of nursing-sensitive indicators in the delivery of high-quality care.

KEY TERMS

Conceptual and operational definitions
Culture of inquiry
Internal and external benchmarks
Internal evidence
Nursing-sensitive indicators
Outcome measure
Performance improvement
Process measure
Public reporting
Strategic plan
Structure measure

In addition to external evidence obtained from research studies, you can access other sources of evidence that will inform the design, implementation, and evaluation of an evidence-based practice/quality improvement project. Organizations collect data internally from various sources to assess performance on clinical, financial, operational, quality, and safety outcomes. Internal data can be shared with leaders and staff in various ways, such as scorecards, analytic dashboards, and unit-based report cards on organizational outcomes including performance metrics associated with quality and safety and historical trends. Established performance benchmarks inform expectations and goals for organizational performance. Examples of benchmark categories that are used to determine aspirational outcomes of improvement efforts include government and private insurance payer expectations, performance levels achieved by similar practice settings that can be found in external analytics platforms such as the National Database of Nursing Quality Indicators (NDNQI) or the Vizient Clinical Database, health care analytics platforms that are used for performance improvement as well as regulatory guidance on minimum requirements for quality and safety.

> **TIP**
>
> Examine performance data at the organizational or unit level to identify areas in need of improvement based on evidence.

One example of an agency responsible for public reporting that sets benchmarks for performance is the Centers for Medicare and Medicaid Services (CMS) value-based program. The CMS program rewards providers through a reimbursement structure that focuses on the quality, not the quantity, of care provided to Medicare and Medicaid patients. This information is translated to consumers through the CMS Star Rating System (see https://www.cms.gov/medicare/quality-initiatives-patient-assessment-instruments/hospitalqualityinits/hospitalcompare). The Star Rating methodology is calculated as a determination of the overall hospital-level quality based on a star rating system. The overall rating ranges from one to five stars, with more stars indicating higher quality. The Star Rating empowers consumers by providing a rating methodology to decide where to seek care by comparing quality, benefits, and costs across providers. The quality rating for hospitals is based on five areas: mortality, safety of care, readmission, patient experience, and timely and effective care that is aggregated into one single star rating for each hospital (https://www.medicare.gov/care-compare/resources/hospital/overall-star-rating). CMS recently shifted more weight to the patient experience, thus joining payers and providers to improve patient experience, increasing the attainment of a five-star rating.

The CMS Star Rating and other external regulatory bodies, such as the Joint Commission (https://www.jointcommission.org/measurement/), have developed many standardized core performance measures that impact health care organizations' strategic planning and internal performance measures. Health care organizations use **strategic planning** to prioritize efforts and allocate resources to improve targeted performance areas. Strategic plans are socialized across an organization by leaders who seek to galvanize improvement initiatives to align with strategic goals based on current evidence-based practices (EBPs) and internal and external performance measures. Priorities can be set to meet or exceed external benchmarks, establish and maintain a reputation of excellence in care delivery, or provide health care consumers with information about services that differentiate the organization from others. Quality measurements are aligned with strategic priorities and provide the nurse with a blueprint for those areas of practice improvement deemed mission-critical to the practice setting or organization.

As nurses, we must be able to "read the room" to understand how to move the evidence into practice changes within an organizational setting. Nurses are in a pivotal position to know the areas of opportunity for improvement. However, even the best efforts will only succeed when a culture of inquiry and support for the practical nature of integrating evidence into practice exists. We need to understand the organizational culture to implement effective and impactful change projects that address the organization's and patients' needs or contribute to the body of nursing knowledge. Creating a culture of clinical inquiry involves fostering an environment that values and supports the continuous pursuit of knowledge, EBP, and patient care and outcomes improvement. Essential ingredients of a **culture of inquiry** include:

- Leadership demonstrating a commitment to EBP and quality improvement (QI)
- Providing ongoing education and training to equip staff with the necessary skills to engage in clinical inquiry
- Establishing clear expectations through job descriptions, performance appraisals, and development plans that engaging in clinical inquiry activities is a professional responsibility
- Encouraging critical thinking, curiosity, questioning, and challenging the status quo in practice to drive improvement
- Providing access to resources to engage in clinical inquiry, such as library services, literature search support, database access, and analytic support
- Promoting collaboration and networking to facilitate a positive professional practice environment that supports data transparency, sharing ideas, experiences, and research findings in forums such as journal clubs, shared governance committees, QI, and EBP rounds
- Celebrating clinical inquiry efforts by recognizing achievements, sharing success stories, providing incentives and awards, and promoting dissemination
- Promoting a continuous learning culture where lessons learned are shared and used as an opportunity for growth
- Developing infrastructure for research, EBP, and QI

As fixers, nurses sometimes act hastily to solve a problem by putting band-aids on the obstacles we see in practice. Often, these quick and usually ineffective solutions to a problem only address the symptom and not the root cause of the problem. Einstein is quoted as having said, "If I had an hour to solve a problem, I would spend 55 minutes thinking about the problem and five minutes thinking about solutions." A critical step in problem solving is preparation. Sufficiently rigorous data and information gathering from various sources is essential in defining multiple contributors to the problem before implementing change strategies to solve it. In Lean Management, this is the Gemba Walk (Lot et al., 2018), which involves mapping the journey of the patient or the staff to understand how a process is operationalized. Understanding the practice environment and the impact of the critical strategies for change is a precursor for success. When seeking to understand a clinical problem or issues, you should seek to illuminate the steps in a process that may need modification to facilitate practice change. Valuable information can be obtained by gathering preintervention data that reflects the current state of the practice prior to implementing interventions. You can then conduct a pre- and post-implementation comparative analysis by:

- Interviewing staff individually or in groups
- Administering surveys by asking relevant questions about the problem
- Conducting medical record audits
- Observing work patterns and documenting process flow
- Reviewing current policies and procedures related to the practice issue
- Understanding interprofessional roles and responsibilities
- Examining communication patterns between and among staff and the health system

> **TIP**
>
> Before attempts are made to solve or improve a clinical practice problem, it is essential to fully understand the current state of the problem from the perspective of all stakeholders. Use a variety of methods to gain a deep appreciation of the factors contributing to an issue.

QI, according to the Institute for Healthcare Improvement (IHI), must be: (1) guided by alignment with organizational strategy, (2) evidence based, (3) strongly supported by leadership, and (4) aimed at promoting excellence at all levels of an organization. Translating quality goals and objectives into actionable plans requires strategic alignment, which involves translating the organization's priorities and goals for quality into actionable plans (Scoville & Little, 2014). QI efforts are the most effective when they cascade down from the senior organizational leaders to frontline staff who then keep leaders informed of progress with practice change initiatives.

Health system **strategic plans** have goals driven by value-added strategic priorities impacted by internal and external factors that drive the focus on quality and safety, finance, patient experience, and the management of resources, especially people. By linking the aims of an evidence-based/QI project to organizational strategic goals, you will optimize stakeholder buy-in, access to resources, and the sustainability of attained outcomes.

Once a problem is defined, organizational alignment with the strategic plan is established, and leadership support is secured, determining how outcome improvement is measured is essential. Measurement plans are the foundation for demonstrating the success/value of EBP or QI projects. They provide the structure to monitor performance and to measure the impact of interventions in reaching the aim(s) of the project. Understanding what type of measure is needed for a change project is the key to a successful change project. The Donabedian model of Structure-Process-Outcomes measures is familiar to nursing as it is the core framework for the American Nurses Credentialing Center (ANCC) Magnet Designation (Lal, 2021). It can guide the identification of the measurement that best fits your aim. Gupta & Kaplan (2020) offer a healthcare-specific definition of the components of the Donabedian model:

Structure measures describe the health care setting and environment. They can include assessments of the physical environment, human resources, and organizational configuration.

Process measures examine the delivery of care and describe activities of the health care system. Process measures capture what we do as health care providers, are more precise reflections of care delivery, and are more amenable to change. Therefore, they are often the primary targets of improvement efforts.

Outcome measures focus on the impact of care on patients or populations. They can include health status, disease outcomes, patient satisfaction, and knowledge. Outcome measures are often the most rigorous to achieve.

A link between the process of care measures and the targeted outcomes measures is essential to facilitate evidence-based improvement. **Process measures** focus on the activities, tasks, or steps involved in a process and help evaluate the process's quality, consistency, and efficiency. **Outcome measures** focus on the results or consequences of the process in order to determine its success in meeting performance goals. It is expected that improvement in processes will lead to improved outcomes. A good example of this is the process of handwashing and educating communities about handwashing, which impacts the health of communities. According to the Centers for Disease Control and Prevention (CDC, see https://www.cdc.gov/cleanhands/data-research/facts-stats/), handwashing education in a community can impact the following:

- 23% to 40% reduction in the number of people who get sick with diarrhea
- 16% to 21% reduction in respiratory illnesses, like colds, in the general population
- 29% to 57% reduction in absenteeism due to gastrointestinal illness in schoolchildren

Once measures are identified, the next essential step is to clearly define the details of what is being measured before initiating a change in practice. Often, evidence-based definitions accompanied by consensus among those involved in the improvement effort are needed to know definitively when an improvement has occurred. Both conceptual and operational definitions of the phenomena being examined are necessary and serve complementary purposes. A **conceptual definition** provides an abstract and theoretical understanding of a concept and helps stakeholders understand the clinical phenomenon within a particular context. **Operational definitions** further define the concept in terms of specific observable and measurable actions, operations, or procedures. It translates an abstract definition into practical terms that can be observed, quantified, or tested. For example, the conceptual definition of pain can be stated as an unpleasant sensory and emotional experience associated with actual or potential tissue damage that involves both physiological and psychological components. The operational definition could be the self-reported pain intensity rating on a numeric rating scale ranging from 0 to 10, where 0 represents no pain and 10 represents the worst imaginable pain. Pain can be measured at different times using this scale to facilitate pain management. In different contexts, the operational definition of pain may include additional measurement factors such as pain duration, location, or other descriptors depending on the factors relevant to the improvement effort. Operational definitions must be clear and unambiguous to bring a measure from a general concept to a precise tool to evaluate the aims of the change project (Gupta & Kaplan, 2020).

BENCHMARKING

How can the impact of the evidence-based change or QI intervention on preestablished goals and aims be determined? One approach is setting realistic improvement goals informed by the results of similar change projects in comparable practice settings. Published reports of QI efforts can provide you with information about achievements in similar circumstances. An **external benchmark** compares performance to other organizations while an **internal benchmark** compares performance within an organization. Both can also be used to set targets for performance improvement. A benchmark refers to a standard, reference point, or comparison to another organization, system, or quality performance indicator. Using benchmarks enables the identification and quantification of performance gaps in order to focus organizational efforts and resources where they are needed most and predicted to have the most significant impact (Donaldson et al., 2005). Benchmarking provides a means of tracking progress toward a goal, assessing organizational performance in relation to competitors, and ensuring compliance with best practices and recognized standards. Organizations often compare their performance to others but can also compare current performance against established improvement targets or historical trends (see Chapter 14).

> **TIP**
>
> When trying to determine the measures you will use to determine when improvement has occurred, consult with organizational departments who are knowledgeable about the data being collected to support the strategic plan. Consider these data as readily available sources of outcome measurements.

Multiple sources may be available when seeking internal or external evidence to describe the current state of a problem or establish improvement targets and measures. These data, information, and insights are generated and collected within an organization to drive improvement in quality and outcomes. Some measures are reported to external agencies such as

CHAPTER 12 Sources of Data to Drive Evidence-Based Practice and Quality Improvement

the NDNQI, the Joint Commission Resource Portal, Vizient, and the CDC's National Healthcare Safety Network. Internal data sources and analyses express the state of current practice, identify areas of concern, and monitor progress toward improvement goals. Common areas of data collection captured through internal and external data reporting are discussed in the following sections.

THE VOICE OF THE PATIENT AND FAMILY

Patients and families voice their concerns, challenges, and ideas for change through many vehicles. The patient's voice is heard in organization-based patient and family advisory councils, and patient comments are collected in surveys and garnered through nurse leader rounding, patient complaints, and formal grievances. Another source of the patient's voice is patient experience surveys, a foundational tool to improve patients' perception of care delivery. The patient experience focuses on whether and how often a patient experiences critical aspects of healthcare, including communication with clinicians, understanding medication instructions, and coordinating health care needs (see https://www.ahrq.gov/). CMS produces a variety of setting-specific Consumer Assessment of Healthcare Providers and Systems (CAHPS) surveys (see https://www.cms.gov/data-research/research/consumer-assessment-healthcare-providers-systems, n.d.) that are officially designated and offer organizations the ability to benchmark their performance by comparing their rating to those achieved by other health systems.

The voice of the patient is also captured in patient-reported outcomes (PROs) in the delivery and coordination of care. PROs are standardized assessments for data collection from patients about their health status or experience with a health condition. PROs support patient–provider communication, detection, and management of health conditions and improve patient experience (Austin et al., 2020). See Table 12.1 for more.

TABLE 12.1	The Voice of the Patient	
Data Sources	**Description**	**Location**
Hospital-based patient complaints and grievances	Patient complaints range from minor, easily resolved at the point of care, to major, also known by CMS as grievances (CMS, 2016).	Some examples of departments that may handle patient complaints and grievances are the departments of: patient relations, patient experience, patient advocacy, corporate compliance, nursing quality, patient safety officer
U.S. Department of Health and Human Services	If a concern, problem, or complaint related to any aspect of care during a patient's hospital stay from a Medicare provider then submit your concerns to your state's Beneficiary and Family Centered Care Quality Improvement Organization (BFCC-QIO).	(https://www.medicare.gov/claims-appeals/file-a-complaint-grievance/filing-a-complaint-about-your-quality-of-care; https://health.data.ny.gov/Health/Hospital-Profile/7a62-tptu)
Patient and family advisory boards/committees	The patient and family advisory council (PFAC) is an organizational council of current and former patients, family members, and caregivers working together to improve and implement best practices at a hospital or health care organization.	Examples of contacts for PFAC would be a hospital department of patient experience or patient relations

Continued

TABLE 12.1 The Voice of the Patient—cont'd

Data Sources	Description	Location
Patient experience surveys: CAHPS	CAHPS surveys ask patients to report on their experiences with a range of health care services at multiple levels of the delivery system. CMS CAHPS surveys - Hospital CAHPS (https://www.cms.gov/research-statistics-data-and-systems/research/cahps/hcahps1) - Home Health CAHPS (https://www.cms.gov/research-statistics-data-and-systems/research/cahps/hhcahps) - HCBS CAHPS Survey (https://www.medicaid.gov/medicaid/quality-of-care/performance-measurement/cahps-hcbs-survey/index.html) - Fee-for-Service CAHPS (https://www.cms.gov/node/178911) - Medicare Advantage and Prescription Drug Plan CAHPS (https://www.cms.gov/research-statistics-data-and-systems/research/cahps/mcahps) - In-Center Hemodialysis CAHPS (https://www.cms.gov/research-statistics-data-and-systems/research/cahps/ichcahps) - Nationwide Adult Medicaid CAHPS (https://www.cms.gov/research-statistics-data-and-systems/files-for-order/limiteddatasets/cahps) - CAHPS Hospice (https://www.cms.gov/research-statistics-data-and-systems/research/cahps/cahps-hospice-survey) - Outpatient and Ambulatory Surgery CAHPS (https://www.cms.gov/research-statistics-data-and-systems/research/cahps/oas-cahps) - CAHPS for MIPS (https://www.cms.gov/research-statistics-data-and-systems/research/cahps/mips) - Emergency Department CAHPS (https://www.cms.gov/research-statistics-data-and-systems/research/cahps/ed)	Contact the department of patient experience, hospital quality department, or nursing quality department for access to survey results

TABLE 12.1 The Voice of the Patient—cont'd

Data Sources	Description	Location
Patient experience surveys: • NRC Health • Press Ganey • Picker	• NRC Health is a patient experience company that surveys between 35 and 50 million patients annually globally (https://nrchealth.com/) • Press Ganey is a health care performance improvement company that specializes in patient experience surveys and is global (https://www.pressganey.com/consulting/industry-initiatives/) • Picker is a health care performance company that measures patient experience and is global (https://picker.org/)	Contact the department of patient experience or quality for access to survey results
Q Reviews	The Q Reviews platform is a digital patient engagement solutions across the care continuum (https://q-reviews.com/about-quality-reviews/)	Contact the department of patient experience or quality for access to survey results
Care Compare Website/ Centers for Medicare and Medicaid Services (CMS) Star Ratings	CMS and the nation's hospitals work collaboratively to publicly report hospital quality performance information on Care Compare website (https://www.medicare.gov/care-compare/) and the Provider Data Catalog (https://data.cms.gov). This tool can be used to find and compare different types of Medicare providers (like physicians, hospitals, nursing homes, and others) and the quality of the care that they render based on the CMS Star Rating.	Find Healthcare Providers: https://www.medicare.gov/care-compare/ (an official website of the U.S. government)

EMPLOYEE ENGAGEMENT AND SATISFACTION SURVEYS

Ensuring the safety and resiliency of the workforce is a necessary precondition to advancing patient safety. It is a unified, total systems-based perspective and approach to eliminating harm to both patients and the workforce, according to the National Steering Committee for Patient Safety's *Safer Together: A National Action Plan to Advance Patient Safety*. Engaging employees within organizational decision making, collaboration, and providing opportunities for professional development is essential to employee engagement. Broader clinician participation in multidisciplinary and cross-departmental activities promotes alignment with institutional priorities and policies regarding patient care requirements by actively engaging those with the most contact with patients and families, according to *Safer Together: A National Action Plan to Advance Patient Safety*. High levels of nurse engagement have been linked to better workforce outcomes, including lower staff turnover, lower burnout, and higher reports of job satisfaction (Niskala et al., 2020). See Table 12.2 for more.

INTERDISCIPLINARY RELATIONSHIPS

The impact of interdisciplinary approaches to care is a critical focus of improvement on patient-reported

TABLE 12.2 Employee Engagement and Satisfaction Surveys

Data Sources	Description	Location
Employee engagement survey tools	Examples of surveys that measure employee engagement: • Utrecht Work Engagement Scale • Gallup Q • The Safety, Communication, Operational Reliability, and Engagement (SCORE) survey	• UWES (https://wilmarschaufeli.nl) • Connect employee engagement with performance – Gallup (https://www.gallup.com/workplace/229424/employee-engagement.aspx?utm_source=google&utm_medium=cpc&utm_campaign=gallup_access_branded&utm_term=gallup%20employee%20engagement&gclid=EAIaIQobChMIh-eguf2OgAMVk43ICh3qNgOhEAAYAyAAEgIO2PD_BwE) • The Psychological Safety Scale of the Safety, Communication, Operational, Reliability, and Engagement (SCORE) survey (a brief, diagnostic, and actionable metric for the ability to speak up in health care settings) (https://psnet.ahrq.gov/issue/psychological-safety-scale-safety-communication-operational-reliability-and-engagement-score)
The NDNQI RN Survey with Practice Environment Scale	The NDNQI RN Survey with Practice Environment Scale contains the Practice Environment Scale of the Nursing Work Index (PES-NWI) (Lake et al., 2024), in addition to Nurse-Nurse Interaction (from NDNQI Job Satisfaction Scales-R survey)	Index of Work Satisfaction (https://info.pressganey.com/press-ganey-blog-healthcare-experience-insights/your-comprehensive-guide-to-the-press-ganey-national-database-of-nursing-quality-indicators-ndnqi)

outcomes, essential to treatment evaluation, quality, and shared decision making. Interdisciplinary relationships have many synonyms, such as interdisciplinary, interprofessional, multidisciplinary or comprehensive, enhanced intensive, complex, and integrating care (Kaiser et al., 2022). Data sources describing interprofessional relationships include previously listed employee engagement surveys, CAHPS surveys, and the NDNQI RN Survey with Practice Environment Scale. See Table 12.3 for more.

PATIENT SAFETY

The World Health Organization states that Patient Safety is a health care discipline that emerged with the evolving complexity of health care systems and the resulting rise of patient harm in health care facilities. It aims to prevent and reduce risks, errors, and patient harm while providing healthcare. A cornerstone of the discipline is a continuous improvement based on learning from errors and adverse events (see Patient Safety, https://www.who.int/news-room/fact-sheets/detail/patient-safety). Patient safety, as Thomas Lee, chief medical officer of Press Ganey, proposed, goes beyond achieving zero harm in hospitals. It must apply to the health care continuum, including ambulatory care and telemedicine (Lee, 2023). There are many roadblocks in building a culture of safety, from resistance to change and adherence to the status quo, silos of care, a lack of cohesive communication structures, and a lack of transparency of data and knowledge. Pursuing patient safety is an iterative process that requires the work of interprofessional team members. Given the fragmented nature of healthcare, the challenges are complex (Henriksen et al., 2005). It requires continuous improvement due to the learnings from opportunities from adverse events (see Patient Safety, https://www.who.int/news-room/fact-sheets/detail/patient-safety), and it is fundamental to delivering quality essential health services. See Table 12.4 for more.

NURSING-SENSITIVE INDICATORS

Nursing-sensitive indicators (NSIs) are measures sensitive to the input of nursing care. NSIs have a high degree of specificity to nursing, can be trended, and

TABLE 12.3 Interdisciplinary Relationships

Data Sources	Description	Location
Employee engagement surveys and patient experience surveys	The assessment of interdisciplinary relationships are included in employee engagement surveys and patient experience surveys such as: • Gallup's Engagement Survey • NDNQI RN Satisfaction • Picker Survey • HCAHPS (Hospital Consumer Assessment of Healthcare Providers and Systems)	• Connect employee engagement with performance – Gallup (https://www.gallup.com/workplace/229424/employee-engagement.aspx?utm_source=google&utm_medium=cpc&utm_campaign=gallup_access_branded&utm_term=gallup%20employee%20engagement&gclid=EAIaIQobChMIh-eguf2OgAMVk43ICh3qNgOhEAAYAyAAEgIO2PD_BwE) • Index of Work Satisfaction (https://www.ache.org/learning-center/publications/books/1003) • Picker (https://picker.org/) • HCAHPS: Patients' Perspectives of Care Survey (https://www.cms.gov/medicare/quality-initiatives-patient-assessment-instruments/hospitalqualityinits/hospitalhcahps)
Examples of instruments frequently used in practice to evaluate teamwork among health care professionals	• Collaborative Practice Assessment instrument (CPAT): General tool applicable to a variety of clinical settings • Mayo High Performance Teamwork Scale (MHPTS): Explores explicit goals and accountability, heedful interrelating, communication, adaptability, conflict resolution, and leadership • Modified Index for Interdisciplinary Collaboration (MIIC): Founded on four perspectives: a multidisciplinary theory of collaboration, services integration, role theory, and ecological systems theory • ICU Nurse Physician Collaboration: Catered toward working relationships between nurses and physicians • Observational Teamwork Assessment for Surgery (OTAS): Catered toward teamwork in a surgical environment • Team Climate Inventory (TCI): Grounded in the four-factor theory of climate for innovate: participative safety, support for innovation, vision, and task orientation • Team Emergency Assessment Measure (TEAM): Covers three core categories: leadership, teamwork, and task management	Kang et al., 2022

TABLE 12.4 Patient Safety Databases

Data Sources	Description	Location
• Agency for Healthcare Research and Quality's (AHRQ) Hospital Survey on Patient Safety Culture • Agency for Healthcare Research and Quality (AHRQ): Network of Patient Safety Databases (NPSD) • Joint Commission: National Patient Safety Goal	• The AHRQ released the Surveys on Patient Safety Culture (SOPS) Hospital Survey for providers and other staff to assess patient safety culture in their hospitals. • The AHRQ presents the dashboards of patient safety data received for analysis and publication. NPSD contains nonidentifiable data from patient safety work products (PSWP) submitted by Patient Safety Organizations (PSOs) nationwide. • Joint Commission: National Patient Safety Goals: The National Patient Safety Goals aim to improve patient safety.	• Hospital Survey on Patient Safety Culture | Agency for Healthcare Research and Quality (https://www.ahrq.gov/sops/surveys/hospital/index.html) • NPSD Dashboards | Agency for Healthcare Research and Quality (https://www.ahrq.gov/npsd/data/dashboard/index.html) • National Patient Safety Goals | The Joint Commission (https://www.jointcommission.org/standards/national-patient-safety-goals/)
Hospital Care Compare	Hospital Care Compare displays hospital performance data in a consistent, unified manner to ensure the availability of credible information about the care delivered in the nation's hospitals. The hospitals displayed on Care Compare are generally limited to acute care hospitals, acute care veteran's hospitals, Department of Defense hospitals, critical access hospitals, and children's hospitals.	https://www.cms.gov/medicare/quality-initiatives-patient-assessment-instruments/hospitalqualityinits/hospitalcompare
CDC's National Healthcare Safety Network	The nation's most widely used healthcare-associated infection tracking system.	https://www.cdc.gov/nhsn/index.html
Joint Commission: Sentinel Event Database	This data also supports the importance of establishing National Patient Safety Goals.	https://www.jointcommission.org/-/media/tjc/documents/resources/patient-safety-topics/sentinel-event/sentinel-event-general_information-june-2022.pdf
AHRQ NPSD: Data Reporting Tools—Falls Supplement	This dashboard includes information organized by fall at a glance (by age), commonly reported patient activities prior to fall.	Falls Supplement | Agency for Healthcare Research and Quality (https://www.ahrq.gov/npsd/data/dashboard/falls-supplement.html)

have a solid link to nursing quality (Gallagher & Rowell, 2003). NSIs should be *essential* to improving the quality of care delivered, *sensitive to nursing care*, measured by a *scientifically reliable and valid* method, feasible to collect, and *valuable* to end users (Start, 2018). NSIs are factors in a person's health status that nursing care can directly affect. They form the foundation for monitoring the quality of nursing care, which assists in establishing a common ground for benchmarking and providing evidence of the cost-effectiveness of nursing care, planning quality improvements, launching local improvement projects, and evaluating and comparing the performance of nursing staff (Siaki et al., 2022).

The American Nurses Association, the U.S. National Quality Forum, and the U.S. Agency for Healthcare Research and Quality have attempted to standardize the development of NSIs. However, there has yet to be a universal consensus on what constitutes an NSI. Different measures to quantify the quality of nursing care have been developed in different countries. NSIs are included in the U.S. NDNQI. The Canadian Health Outcomes for Better Information and Care have also developed standardized patient outcomes that reflect the quality of nursing care. Similar initiatives have been taken in European countries such as the United Kingdom, Ireland, and the Netherlands (Siaki et al., 2022). NSIs that can be used to measure patient safety and the efficiency of nursing care include central line bloodstream infections, catheter-associated urinary tract infections, hospital-acquired pressure injuries, and falls with injuries.

The American Academy of Ambulatory Care Nursing published an AAACN report on Ambualtory Care Nursing-Sensitive Indicator Industry Report (Start et al., 2016) on evidence-based recommendations for ambulatory care NSIs in order to conduct "constant surveillance so that departure from standards can be detected early and corrected" in the ambulatory setting (Start, 2018). A benchmarking structure was also developed, where clinical sites could compare across specialty, volume size, organizational service line, and system (Start, 2018). These measures and adjoining benchmarking databases are now a part of the Press Ganey database, which also offers inpatient nurse-sensitive measures through the NDNQI (Start, 2018). Examples of ambulatory NSIs are the perioperative clinical measure set, which includes patient burns, surgical errors, unplanned postoperative transfers/admissions, and fall with injury. See Table 12.5 for more.

WORKFORCE SAFETY

Ensuring the safety and resiliency of the organization and the workforce is a necessary precondition to advancing patient safety, according to the Institute for Healthcare Safety (Sampath et al., 2021). The work on eliminating harm cannot only be focused on patients but includes the health care workforce in order for an organization to take a unified, whole-system quality approach to eliminate harm (Sampath et al., 2021, see also *Safer Together: A National Action Plan to Advance Patient Safety*, https://www.ahrq.gov/patient-safety/reports/safer-together.html). See Table 12.6 for more.

HEALTH EQUITY

The Future of Nursing 2020–2030: Charting a Path to Achieve Health Equity calls for nurses to ensure equitable health care services within and across the care continuum and patient populations through identifying and disseminating EBPs. Nurses are challenged to improve and sustain a supportive culture of care for both staff and patients.

Advocating for policy changes that address population health and social determinants of health at the organizational and public policy levels is imperative in achieving health equity. Advancing health equity through creating a vision and a culture of health equity is a call for nursing leaders. *In the Future of Nursing 2020–2030* nurses are called to build the needed structures and processes and work within and across boundaries to achieve the vision of health for all (National Academies of Sciences, Engineering, and Medicine et al., 2021). See Table 12.7 for more.

SYNTHESIS

Today's nurses are called on to lead in the development of effective strategies for improving the nation's health

TABLE 12.5 Nursing-Sensitive Indicators

Data Sources	Description	Location
National Database of Nursing Quality Indicators (NDNQI)	NDNQI is the leading nursing quality indicators database that contains unit-level information about 600+ measures relevant to nursing performance, patient and workforce experience, and health outcomes. The data is derived from a combination of administrative documentation and medical records. Across ambulatory and inpatient care settings, nursing sensitive indicators are measured with the NDNQI.	NDNQI Nursing Quality Indicators Database | Press Ganey (https://www.pressganey.com/platform/ndnqi/) In hospitals settings inquiries can be made to the NDNQI Nursing Coordinator.

TABLE 12.6 Worker Safety Databases

Data Sources	Description	Location
Occupational Safety and Health Administration (OHSA) OHSA-Ergonomics OSHA: Preventing Workplace Violence: A Road Map for Healthcare Facilities	OSHA ensures safe and healthful working conditions for workers by setting and enforcing standards and by providing training, outreach, education and assistance. Prevention of Musculoskeletal Disorders in the Workplace Workers in hospitals, nursing homes, and other healthcare settings face significant risks of workplace violence. This road map describes the five core components of a workplace violence prevention program.	Data | Occupational Safety and Health Administration (https://www.osha.gov/data) Preventing Workplace Violence: A Road Map for Healthcare Facilities Preventing Workplace Violence: A Road Map for Healthcare Facilities (osha.gov) www.osha.gov/sites/default/files/OSHA3827.pdf

TABLE 12.7 Health Equity Databases

Data Sources	Description	Location
National Healthcare Quality and Disparities Reports (NHQDR)	The NHQDR provides a unique set of AHRQ data tools to assist in focusing efforts on identifying areas for improvement in the delivery of healthcare in the United States. These tools can be used to inspect states as geographic areas for quality disparities in vulnerable populations to pursue improvement activities.	National Healthcare Quality and Disparities Reports | Agency for Healthcare Research and Quality (https://www.ahrq.gov/research/findings/nhqrdr/index.html)
American Association for Cancer Research (AACR) Cancer Disparities Progress Report	The AACR Disparities Progress Report outlines the cancer health disparities are adverse differences in cancer burden experienced by racial and ethnic minorities and other medically underserved populations that include those living in rural areas; individuals from sexual and gender minorities; and those living in persistent poverty.	The State of Cancer Health Disparities in 2022 | AACR (https://cancerprogressreport.aacr.org/disparities/cdpr22-contents/cdpr22-the-state-of-cancer-health-disparities-in-2022/)
Health Equity Research Guide	Selected scholarly literature databases and journals available to help you find research about health equity.	CDC Library | Health Equity Research Guide (https://www.cdc.gov/library/researchguides/healthequity.html)

(Ogbolu et al., 2018). Nurses must lead across the continuum of care from the bedside to the boardroom, and beyond. To sit at the table to enhance organizational culture and clinical processes and to be agents of change, we must embed our practice in the best available evidence, and lead interprofessional QI and evidenced-based initiatives from the unit level and to the C-Suite, in our communities, and nationally. We must be well versed in QI methodologies and read, interpret, and use data to support and drive change.

It is imperative that we can know where to find the source data within and outside of our organizations to implement the needed changes to improve clinical, financial, operational, quality, and safety outcomes for our patients, for our workforce, and for the health of the communities that we serve.

CHAPTER 12 Sources of Data to Drive Evidence-Based Practice and Quality Improvement

KEY POINTS

- Source information from organizations is used to assess performance on clinical, financial, operational, quality, and safety outcomes. Organizational source information can be found in organizational strategic plans, scorecards, analytic dashboards, and unit-based report cards, and they can be utilized to establish targets for future states.
- Health system strategic plans can be used to identify high-priority areas for a change project. By linking the aims of a change project to organizational strategic goals, stakeholder buy-in, access to resources, and the sustainability of attained outcomes can be optimized.
- Sources of internal organizational evidence that are drivers of organizational performance can range from data for the "Voice of the Patient," employee engagement and satisfaction surveys, patient safety outcomes, nursing-sensitive indicators, and workforce safety.
- The Donabedian model of structure, process, and outcomes measures can guide the identification of the best measurement that meets the aim of a change project. Structure measures describe the health care setting and environment. Process measures examine the delivery of care and describe activities of the health care system. Outcome measures focus on the impact of care on patients or populations.
- Conceptual and operational definitions are valuable in measuring a change project's outcomes. Conceptual definitions provide an abstract understanding of a concept and clinical phenomenon. In contrast, operational definitions define specific observable and measurable actions, operations, or procedures within a concept and bring a measure from a general concept to a precise tool to evaluate the aims of the change project.
- Benchmarking enables the illumination of performance gaps in patient and staff safety, patient experience, or staff satisfaction in order to focus organizational efforts and resources to make the most significant difference in organizational outcomes.

REFERENCES

Agency for Healthcare Research and Quality. (n.d.). Hospital survey on patient safety culture. https://www.ahrq.gov/sops/surveys/hospital/index.html

Austin, E., LeRouge, C., Hartzler, A. L., Segal, C., & Lavallee, D. C. (2020). Capturing the patient voice: Implementing patient-reported outcomes across the health system. *Quality-of-Life Research: An International Journal of Quality-of-Life Aspects of Treatment, Care, and Rehabilitation*, 29(2), 347–355. https://doi.org/10.1007/s11136-019-02320-8.

Centers for Medicare and Medicaid Services (CMS). (2016). Public reporting. https://qualitynet.cms.gov/inpatient/public-reporting/public-reporting.

Centers for Medicare and Medicaid Services (CMS). (n.d.). Consumer assessment of healthcare providers and systems. https://www.cms.gov/research-statistics-data-and-systems/research/cahps

Donaldson, N., Brown, D. S., Aydin, C. E., Bolton, M. L., & Rutledge, D. N. (2005). Leveraging nurse-related dashboard benchmarks to expedite performance improvement and document excellence. *Journal of Nursing Administration*, 35(4), 163–172.

Gallagher, R. M., & Rowell, P. A. (2003). Claiming the future of nursing through nursing-sensitive quality indicators. *Nursing administration Quarterly*, 27(4), 273–284. https://doi.org/10.1097/00006216-200310000-00004.

Gupta, M., & Kaplan, H. C. (2020). Measurement for quality improvement: using data to drive change. *Journal of Perinatology*, 40(6), 962–971. https://doi.org/10.1038/s41372-019-0572-x.

Henriksen, K., Battles, J. B., Marks, E. S., & Lewin, D. I. (Eds.). (2005). *Advances in patient safety: From research to implementation (Volume 3: Implementation Issues)*. Agency for Healthcare Research and Quality. https://www.ncbi.nlm.nih.gov/books/NBK20545/.

Kaiser, L., Conrad, S., Neugebauer, E. A. M., Pietsch, B., & Pieper, D. (2022). Interprofessional collaboration and patient-reported outcomes in inpatient care: A systematic review. *Systematic Reviews*, 11(1), 169. https://doi.org/10.1186/s13643-022-02027-x.

Kang, H. (Joel), Flores-Sandoval, C., Law, B., & Sibbald, S. (2022). Interdisciplinary health care evaluation instruments: A review of psychometric evidence. *Evaluation & the Health Professions*, 45(3), 223–234. https://doi.org/10.1177/01632787211040859.

Lake, E. T., Gil, J., Moronski, L., McHugh, M. D., Aiken, L. H., & Lasater, K. B. (2024). Validation of a short form of the practice environment scale of the nursing work index: The PES–5. *Research in Nursing & Health, 47*(4), 450–459. https://doi.org/10.1002/nur.22388.

Lal, M. M. (2021). Introducing the 2023 Magnet Application Manual. *Journal of Nursing Administration, 51*(12), 593–594. https://doi.org/10.1097/NNA.0000000000001090.

Lee, Thomas H. (2023). *Healthcare's path forward: How ongoing crises are creating new standards for excellence.* McGraw Hill.

Lot, L. T., Sarantopoulos, A., Min, L. L., Perales, S. R., Boin, I. F. S. F., & Ataide, E. C. (2018). Using Lean tools to reduce patient waiting time. *Leadership in Health Services, 31*(3), 343–351. https://doi.org/10.1108/LHS-03-2018-0016.

National Academies of Sciences. (2021). Engineering, and Medicine; National Academy of Medicine; Committee on the Future of Nursing 2020–2030. In J. L. Flaubert, S. Le Menestrel, D. R. Williams, & M. K. Wakefield (Eds.), *The future of nursing 2020–2030: Charting a path to achieve health equity.* National Academies Press. https://www.ncbi.nlm.nih.gov/books/NBK573918/.

Niskala, J., Kanste, O., Tomietto, M., Miettunen, J., Tuomikoski, A. M., Kyngäs, H., & Mikkonen, K. (2020). Interventions to improve nurses' job satisfaction: A systematic review and meta-analysis. *Journal of Advanced Nursing, 76*(7), 1498–1508. https://doi.org/10.1111/jan.14342.

Ogbolu, Y., Scrandis, D. A., & Fitzpatrick, G. (2018). Barriers and facilitators of care for diverse patients: Nurse leader perspectives and nurse manager implications. *Journal of Nursing Management, 26*(1), 3–10.

Sampath, B., Rakover, J., Baldoza, K., Mate, K., Lenoci-Edwards, J., & Barker, P. (2021). *Whole system quality: A unified approach to building responsive, resilient health care systems.* IHI White Paper. Institute for Healthcare Improvement.

Siaki, L. A., Patrician, P. A., Loan, L. A., Matlock, A. M., Start, R. E., Gardner, C. L., & McCarthy, M. S. (2023). Ambulatory care nurse-sensitive indicators: A scoping review of literature 2006–2021. *Journal of Nursing Care Quality, 38*(1), 76–81. https://doi.org/10.1097/NCQ.0000000000000660. Epub 2022 Sep 21. PMID: 36166653.

Scoville, R., & Little, K. (2014). *Comparing lean and quality improvement.* IHI White Paper. Institute for Healthcare Improvement.

Start, R. (2018). Perspectives in ambulatory care. Realizing momentum and synergy: Benchmarking meaningful ambulatory care nurse-sensitive indicators. *Nursing Economics, 36*(5), 246–251.

Start, R., Matlock, A. M., & Mastal, P. (2016). Ambulatory care nurse-sensitive indicator industry report: Meaningful measurement of nursing in the ambulatory patient care environment. Ambulatory Care Nurse-Sensitive Indicator Industry Report – © 2016 AAACN.

World Health Organization & Patients Safety. (September 11, 2023). https://www.who.int/news-room/fact-sheets/detail/patient-safety.

13

Understanding Statistics for Evidence-Based Practice

Carl A. Kirton, Alexa Colgrove Curtis, and Courtney Keeler

LEARNING OBJECTIVES

After reading this chapter, you should be able to do the following:
- Identify the levels of measurement for research variables and implications for data analysis.
- Differentiate between descriptive and inferential statistics.
- Explain the concept of probability as it applies to hypothesis testing and interpretation of study findings.
- Distinguish between Type I and Type II error and their effects on study outcomes.
- Interpret common quantitative statistical analyses used to report data findings in published research studies.
- Critically appraise the strength and quality of the evidence provided by the statistical findings of a research study.
- Evaluate the applicability of research findings to evidence-based clinical practice and health care quality improvement.

KEY TERMS

a priori
Clinical meaningfulness
Confidence interval
Continuous variable
Descriptive statistics
Dichotomous variable
Inferential statistics
Interval data
Likelihood ratio
Mean
Median
Mode
Negative predictive value

Nominal data
Nonparametric statistics
Null hypothesis
Null value
Odds ratio
Ordinal data
Parameter value
Parametric statistics
Positive predictive value
Power analysis
Prevalence
p value
Qualitative analysis

Quantitative analysis
Range
Ratio data
Receiver Operating
 Characteristics (ROC) curve
Relative risk
Sensitivity
Specificity
Standard deviation
Type I error
Type II error
Variable

Statistics is the science of analyzing and interpreting quantitative data. Statistical techniques are powerful tools that enable us to make meaningful interpretations of quantitative data to guide evidence-based clinical practice and health care quality improvement. Statistical analysis can be used to describe a phenomenon of interest, explain differences and relationships between variables, and even predict clinical outcomes based on these relationships. When considering the strength and quality of evidence to make a practice change, it is essential

173

to understand the logic and information provided by the data in each of the studies you review. Appropriateness of the statistical techniques utilized within a study research design is also essential to consider. A high-quality research study will have a research design, methods, and statistical analyses that align with the research question(s) or hypotheses. This chapter provides an introduction to statistical concepts applicable to evidence-based clinical practice and health care quality improvement.

BASIC CONCEPTS APPLIED TO AN EVIDENCE-BASED PROJECT: DATA AND DESIGN

The analysis and interpretation of available research data to answer a PICOT question (see Chapter 5) is foundational to the completion of an evidence-based (EB) or quality improvement (QI) project. Effective interpretation requires an understanding of the type of data being utilized as the data drive the analytic strategies and outcome interpretation. Research design is broadly categorized as quantitative or qualitative analysis. **Quantitative analysis** applies statistical techniques to numeric data. **Qualitative analysis** utilizes interpretive methodologies to analyze nonnumeric data including narrative, textual, and visual data sources. This chapter is focused on statistical analysis within quantitative research design. The reader is referred to Chapter 11 for a consideration of the utilization of qualitative research in evidence-based practice (EBP).

Levels of Measurement

Quantitative research is shaped by theoretical concepts that are operationalized (or translated) into research variables. **Variables** are identified as either *dependent* or *independent*. A **dependent variable** (or outcome variable) represents the phenomenon of interest to the study, such as a target blood sugar. The **independent variable** (or explanatory variable) reflects the exposure or factor influencing the dependent variable, such as the consumption of a blood sugar-lowering medication. Put another way, variation in the independent variable theoretically influences variation in the dependent variable. In a research study, variables are measured using a variety of tools such as biometric measurements (e.g., finger stick blood sugar) and survey instruments (e.g., questionnaires). These measurement tools provide data on the variable that is categorized as either *nominal*, *ordinal*, *interval*, or *ratio*-level data.

Nominal data, also referred to as categorical data, are nonnumeric and have no established hierarchy between variable values. For example, consider state of residence. North Dakota does not have an intrinsic quantitative value; moreover, there is no hierarchy between states like Michigan and Iowa. Michigan is not of greater value than Iowa (or vice versa). Table 13.1 provides additional examples of nominal data. **Dichotomous variables** (also referred to as **binary variables**) are variables that can take on only two possible values, such as yes/no, present/not present, or history of/no history of. For instance, consider a dichotomous variable measuring whether an individual identifies as a current smoker (yes or no).

The next level is **ordinal data**, which is a set of data that has a hierarchical designation. Put another way, ordinal variables have an intrinsic order. The intervals between the hierarchical values are not assumed to be objectively and incrementally equal. Likert-style scale variables offer a great example of ordinal level variables—for instance, a variable measuring satisfaction level where the available choices are "satisfied," "neutral," and "not satisfied." While the data can certainly be ranked (e.g., those who report being "satisfied" are more content than those who respond "neutral"), the difference between categories, such as "satisfied" and "neutral," is not quantitatively defined. That said, ordinal-level measurement is often translated into numeric data, such as 0 for "not satisfied," 1 for "neutral," and 2 for "satisfied" so that the data can be analyzed using the statistical techniques for interval-level data. Again, Table 13.1 offers additional examples of ordinal variables.

Interval data are similar to ordinal data in that values can be placed in rank order; however, interval data categories take on numeric values and the spacing (or "intervals") between categories are incrementally consistent. Of importance, interval-level data do not include an "absolute zero." This means that a measurement of zero in interval-level data does not represent the absence of the characteristic being measured. For example, in the measurement of temperature on a Fahrenheit scale, the degrees have a set quantitative value such that the difference between 20 and 30 degrees is the same value as the difference between 40 and 50 degrees. However, a temperature reading of 0 degrees is a point on a measurement continuum that does not represent the actual absence of temperature.

TABLE 13.1 Levels of Measurement

Variable Type	Definition	Examples
Nominal	Data are grouped into distinct and exclusive categories that cannot be rank ordered.	• Blood type (A, B, AB, or O) • HIV-AIDS diagnosis (yes or no) • Smoking status (current smoker, never smoker, or former smoker) • Sex (male or female) • Marital status (married, never married, widowed, or divorced) • Geographic region of residence (West, Midwest, Northeast, or South)
Ordinal	Data are categorized into distinct and exclusive groups that can be placed in rank order.	• CES-D 10 scale, in which respondents are asked whether they have felt "bothered by things that usually don't bother me" in the last 7 days (possible answers: rarely or none of the time [less than 1 day], some or a little of the time [1–2 days], occasionally or a moderate amount of the time [3–4 days], or all of the time [5–7 days]) • Education (less than a high school degree, high school degree or equivalent, some college/associate degree, college degree or more) • Weight by category (low [BMI < 18.5], middle [BMI 18.5 < 25], or high [BMI > 25]) • Yearly household income by category (< $25,000, $25,000–$50,000, > $50,000)
Interval	Data reflect a chronological sequence with equal distances between data points across a continuum but do not contain a true zero value (a zero value does not make sense).	• Ambient temperature (measured in Celsius or Fahrenheit) • pH scale 0–14 (pH of 0 is the presence of high concentrations of hydrogen ions) • SAT scores (standardized range of 400–1,600)
Ratio	Data are measured continuously with equal spacing between intervals and include a true zero value.	• Weight (as a continuous scale measurement) • Yearly household income (a continuous measure reflecting the dollar value of household income, which could be zero) • Number of months in remission from Crohn's disease (a continuous measure reflecting the amount of time an individual has been in remission; a zero value indicates that an individual is not in remission)

BMI, Body mass index; *CES-D,* Center for Epidemiological Studies Depression.
Note: A variable can be operationalized in several ways. For instance, in this table, "weight" and "yearly household income" are defined in different ways. Researchers should consider their study objectives, desired statistical analysis strategies, and data limitations in defining their variables.
From Curtis & Keeler, 2021.

What about data that do include an absolute zero value? **Ratio data** have the same characteristics as interval data but also include an absolute zero. This means that when a variable has a value of zero, there is a complete absence of that variable. Consider a variable measuring the number of cigarettes smoked per day (or CPD): if the CPD variable has a value of 0, the respondent smokes 0 cigarettes. Both interval and ratio-level data provide measurement for **continuous variables**, variables that include the possibility of an infinite number of fractional values (i.e., decimals) within a range. Table 13.1 provides descriptions of data types with examples for each of the levels of measurement.

Why is this discussion so important? In the critical appraisal process to address a PICOT question, the researcher's EB or QI project can be investigated through statistical analysis strategies. For such an analysis to be meaningful, the research must be able to identify the appropriate statistical tools for their evaluation. Likewise, during the planning phase of an EB or QI implementation project, the project team (sometimes with the support of a data analyst or statistician) selects an appropriate method of analysis for the project given the levels of measurement of the variables.

Nominal and ordinal data are analyzed using what are called **nonparametric statistics** or distribution-free statistical methods. These statistical methods do not assume a probability-based normal sample distribution (i.e., a bell-shaped curve distribution of data values). On the other hand, interval and ratio scales are typically analyzed using **parametric statistics**, which do assume normal sample population probability distributions. The concept of probability distributions is discussed further later in this chapter. Overall, parametric statistics utilizing probability distributions are generally considered to be a more robust type of statistical analysis.

DESCRIPTIVE AND INFERENTIAL STATISTICS

Quantitative statistical analyses can be grouped into two major types: *descriptive* and *inferential*. **Descriptive statistics** are used to summarize, organize, and display a set of data. **Inferential statistics** are used to draw conclusions about a target population based on information obtained from a sample. The target population for a study reflects the underlying population of interest to the researcher, such as intensive care unit nurses. Typically, a researcher cannot feasibly collect data on the entire target population because of temporal, financial, or logistical constraints. As a result, the researcher will often collect and analyze data from a sample of the population. The use of descriptive statistics is limited to describing the study sample, while inferential statistics can be used to *infer* findings from the sample onto a target population. Using inferential statistics, a researcher can estimate the **parameter value** (i.e., the average variable score) for a variable within the target population from the study sample. The following sections describe some descriptive and inferential statistical tests common to EB projects.

Descriptive Statistics

There are three primary data analytic concepts examined and reported using descriptive statistical analyses: *frequencies, measures of central tendency,* and *data variability*. Frequency is another name for count. Frequencies are simply data counts within a data set (e.g., number of sample participants who identify as male). It is common to calculate these frequencies as a percentage to provide a perspective on the proportion of the sample represented by this characteristic.

Measures of central tendency are the most commonly reported descriptive measure. Measures of central tendency include the **mean**, **median**, and **mode** (Table 13.2). All three measures describe the central or middle values associated with the specified variable within a data set. The mean is the average of values, the median is the middle value when values are organized chronologically, and the mode is the most frequently reported value in a data set. Descriptive frequencies and

TABLE 13.2	Sample Data of Measure of Central Tendency
Data set: average BMI among adults in the sample	18.2, 20.1, 22.4, 22.4, 23.6, 23.8, 24.4, 25.2, 26.7, 27.9, 28.6, 30.1, 32.4
Mean	The average of all the data in a set. To determine the mean, add all of the numbers in the data set and divide by the number of data points. (18.2 + 20.1 + 22.4 + 22.4 + 23.6 + 23.8 + 24.4 + 25.2 + 26.7 + 27.9 + 28.6 + 30.1 + 32.4)/13 = 325.4/13 = 25.0
Median	The value in a set that is closest to the middle of a range. To find the median, order the numbers in the data set. The median is the number that appears in the middle of the data set. 18.2, 20.1, 22.4, 22.4, 23.6, **23.8**, 24.4, 25.2, 26.7, 27.9, 28.6, 30.1, 32.4
Mode	The value that occurs most frequently in a data set. 18.2, 20.1, **22.4, 22.4**, 23.6, 23.8, 24.4, 25.2, 26.7, 27.9, 28.6, 30.1, 32.4 22.4 (appears 2 times in the data set, more than any other value)

measures of central tendency (e.g., means) may be the only data reported in a nonresearch EB or QI project. If the primary purpose of the analysis is to determine the effectiveness of a practice change after project implementation, these descriptive values alone may be sufficient to evaluate the impact of implementation. Pre- and postintervention descriptive data may be displayed in a table or graph format to provide clarity through visual representation.

To adequately interpret measures of central tendency it is important to recognize the amount of variability that exists in a data set. The **range** reflects the distance between the lowest and highest values for a given variable in interval or ratio-level data. The range can be reported as two numbers (i.e., minimum value, maximum value) or as a single number (i.e., range = maximum value − minimum value). It is important to evaluate the range because a mean can be skewed by the presence of extreme scores. For example, a mean of 50 in a data set with a range of 5, for example, may be interpreted differently than a mean of 50 in a data set with a range of 30.

Means and ranges are commonly accompanied by a **standard deviation** (SD) calculation. An SD is the most frequently reported measure of variability in a data set. The SD reflects how far the variable values are spread from the mean. The higher the SD, the greater the variability in the data set. The SD formula for a sample is relatively simple: it is the square root of the variance, with variance being a calculation of the differences between each value in a data set and the mean.

Sample standard deviation
$$S = \sqrt{\frac{\Sigma(X_i - \bar{x})^2}{(n-1)}}$$
$\bar{x}$ = Sample average
x = Individual values in sample
n = Count of values in sample

SD can be easily computed using a spreadsheet program (e.g., Excel) or statistical software (e.g., SPSS). Through examination of four values (sample size, lowest value, highest value, and SD), the researcher can begin to appreciate the extent of the variability in the data set.

INFERENTIAL STATISTICS

The findings of descriptive statistics are limited to the sample data set and cannot be generalized to similar groups or the entire target population. This is where inferential statistics are utilized. Inferential statistics provide an analysis that allows the researcher to generalize, or infer, the results obtained from a sample to a target population. In doing so, researchers make assumptions about the distribution (or shape) of data to conduct statistical tests. The results of the statistical tests provide the basis for statistical inference. We discuss these topics and provide an example of a distribution in detail below.

THE NORMAL DISTRIBUTION

Normal distribution is a concept where the mean, median, and mode all align, with the distribution of the data points following the classic bell-shaped curve. In a perfectly normal distribution, not only are the mean, mode, and median exactly equal but there are the same number of data points above and below the mean. With normally distributed data, a majority of data are concentrated around the mean and become more spread out the further one gets from the mean.

The distances from the mean are described in terms of standard deviations from the mean, often represented with the Greek letter *sigma* (σ). When the data are *normally distributed*, approximately 68% of the values will fall within 1 standard deviation from the mean, 95% of values will fall within 2 standard deviations, and 99.7% of values will fall within 3 standard deviations. This is often referred to as the 68-95-99.7 Rule. As the one end of the distribution mirrors the other, these percentages reflect deviation above and below the mean. For instance, with a normal distribution, approximately 68% of the data fall between mean $-1*\sigma$ and mean $+1*\sigma$ while approximately 99.7% of the data fall between mean $-3*\sigma$ and mean $+3*\sigma$.

When the data are normally distributed, they are considered *parametric*. See Fig. 13.1; the classic bell-shaped curve is a graphic representation of data that are normally distributed. An important consideration in determining whether data are normally distributed is the number of observations included in the study sample. As a rule of thumb, distributions become more normal as sample size increases. The **central limit theorem** highlights the positive association between sample size and normality (review the concept of the central limit theorem in Box 13.1).

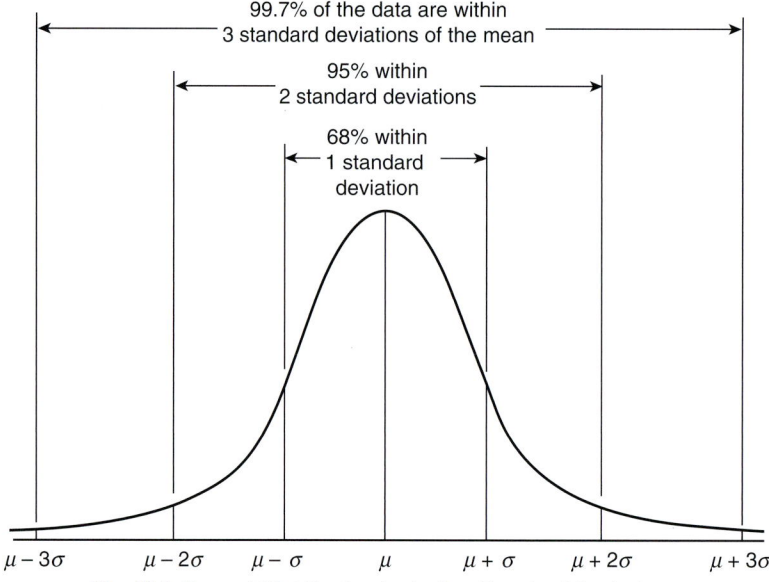

Fig. 13.1 Normal Distribution Including Standard Deviations.

BOX 13.1 The Central Limit Theorem

The central limit theorem can seem quite technical but can be understood if we think through the following steps. We begin with a simple random sample with n individuals from a population of interest. From this sample, we easily can form a sample mean that corresponds to the mean of the measurement we are curious about in our population.

A sampling distribution for the sample mean is produced by repeatedly selecting simple random samples from the same population and of the same size, and then computing the sample mean for each of these samples. The samples are to be thought of as independent of one another. The central limit theorem concerns the sampling distribution of the sample means.

We may ask about the overall shape of the sampling distribution. The central limit theorem says that this sampling distribution is approximately normal, commonly known as a bell curve (see Fig. 13.1). This approximation improves as we increase the size of the simple random samples that are used to produce the sampling distribution. There is a very surprising feature concerning the central limit theorem. The astonishing fact is that this theorem says a normal distribution arises regardless of the initial distribution. Even if our population has a skewed distribution, which occurs when we examine things such as incomes or people's weights, a sampling distribution for a sample with a sufficiently large sample size will be normal.

CENTRAL LIMIT THEOREM IN PRACTICE

Many inferential statistical techniques, such as those involving hypothesis testing, assume that a variable, such as systolic blood pressure or body mass index (BMI), is normally distributed. While normally distributed data simplifies matters, such an outcome is often unrealistic. Real-world data is typically characterized by outliers, skewness, multiple peaks, and asymmetry. Skewedness reflects a situation where data are concentrated above or below the mean. In this case, the mean, median, and mode do not align (Fig. 13.2).

What do we do if the data are not normally distributed? Even though we might not know the shape of the underlying distribution of our study sample, the central limit theorem states we can treat the sampling distribution as if it were normal given an adequate sample size. According to the central limit theorem, distributions become more normal as the sample size increases.

With this in mind, a mathematical procedure called a **power analysis** is used to calculate the participant number or sample size needed to effectively utilize inferential statistics. If the study sample is too small, researchers cannot assume that the data are normally distributed—that is, following the bell-shaped curve. Further, a study with a small sample size might be

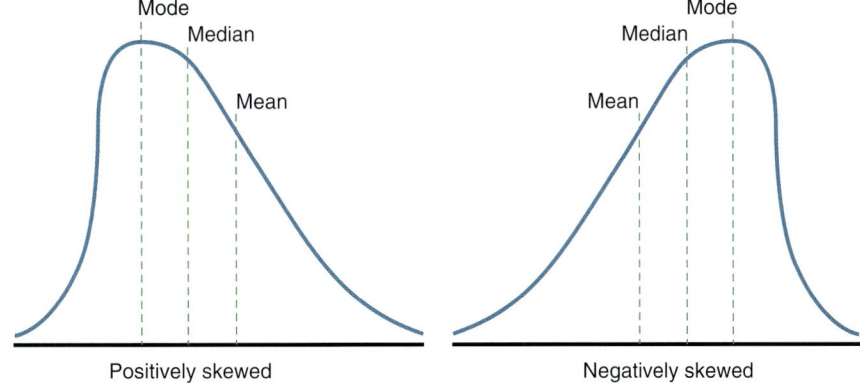

Fig. 13.2 Skewness. Set of Two Bell-Shaped Curves Depict Two Types of Skewness. The Curve on the Left, Skewed to the Right Representing a Positively Skewed Curve, Shows Mode, Median, and Mean Marked from Left to Right. The Curve on the Right, Skewed to the Left Representing a Negatively Skewed Curve, Shows Mean, Median, and Mode Marked from Left to Right. (From Cipher, D.J. (2021). Introduction to statistical analysis. In: Grove, S.K., Gray, J.R. (Eds.), *Burns & Grove's the practice of nursing research: appraisal, synthesis, and generation of evidence* (pp. 635-651). Elsevier Inc.)

considered "underpowered," meaning it will be difficult to establish whether statistically significant associations exist.

When the data are not distributed normally, the data are analyzed using *nonparametric* statistics (Box 13.2). When the data are distributed normally, the data are analyzed using parametric statistics (Box 13.3). There are statistical tests that can be conducted using data analysis software to determine whether the data are distributed normally (e.g., Kolmogorov-Smirnov and Shapiro-Wilk tests). You should consult a statistical text for a discussion of these tests.

NORMALITY EXAMPLE

Ebrahimi et al. (2022) conducted a randomized control trial to answer the clinical question, "Will the use of aromatherapy affect a patient's pain after coronary artery bypass surgery?" The investigator compared two groups after cardiac surgery: Group A, the intervention group, inhaled 5 drops of 20% lavandula essential oil. Group B, the placebo group, received 5 drops of distilled water. The sample size was 98. Both groups received each preparation every 24 hours for 3 days. Pain was measured using a visual analog scale measuring 0 for no pain to 10 for severe pain. The study found that the mean pain score achieved a significant decrease in the intervention group compared to the placebo group at day one and day two but not at day three.

BOX 13.2 Nonparametric Statistics

When the Author Is	Examples of Nonparametric Statistics Found in Studies
Comparing means between two distinct/independent groups	Wilcoxon rank sum test
Comparing two quantitative measurements taken from the same individual	Wilcoxon signed rank test
Comparing means among three or more distinct/independent groups	Kruskal-Wallis test
Estimating the degree of association between two quantitative variables	Spearman's rank correlation
Testing for relationships between two categorical data sets	Chi-squared test

If you were performing critical appraisal, at this point, you would identify that the variable pain is recorded as a numeric score measured as ratio-level data. This means that the appropriate statistical test would be a parametric test given an adequate study sample size. If you examine the data in Table 13.3 from this study, you will note that the authors compare the mean differences in pain scores between the two groups using a nonparametric statistical test (Mann-Whitney U). Why did the authors use a nonparametric test when a parametric test could have been used? The authors reported in the methods section that the variables in the study were determined, through statistical analysis, not to be normally distributed, which is a requirement for parametric testing. As a result, the appropriate statistical approach is the use of nonparametric testing.

HYPOTHESIS TESTING AND PROBABILITY VALUES

With statistical inference, often a researcher is trying to assess whether an effect or difference between the study groups exists. While these tests come in many forms (see Boxes 13.2 and 13.3), they all have the same purpose: *to tell us the probability that the study findings can be attributed to chance.*

In hypothesis testing, the researcher makes a prediction as to how changes in the experimental variable (independent variable) cause or explain changes in the outcome variable (dependent variable). In a research study, the investigators state a **null hypothesis** asserting that there is no relationship (i.e., no effect) between the two study variables. The null hypothesis is compared to the **research** or **alternative hypothesis**, which assumes that some effect or difference between study variables exists. The researcher conducts statistical hypothesis testing to seek evidence against the null hypothesis—namely evidence that a relationship or association exists. Through statistical testing (see Boxes 13.2 and 13.3), researchers gauge the probability of whether the null hypothesis is true, ultimately deciding whether to accept or reject the null hypothesis. The **p value** provides a metric for making this decision.

p values reflect the probability of an event or outcome occurring in repeated trials under similar conditions, and thus the study results are not simply a function of chance. Statistical significance is assessed by comparing p values to a designated α level. The α level reflects the probability of rejecting the null hypothesis when the null hypothesis is true. In other words, the α level reflects a researcher's risk preference (namely, the risk that the researcher identifies an association between

BOX 13.3 Parametric Statistics

When the Author Is	Examples of Parametric Statistics Found in Studies
Comparing means between two distinct/independent groups	Two-sample *t* test
Comparing two quantitative measurements taken from the same individual	Paired *t* test
Comparing means among three or more distinct/independent groups	Analysis of variance (ANOVA)
Estimating the degree of association between two quantitative variables	Pearson's coefficient of correlation

TABLE 13.3 Comparison of the Mean Pain Score Between the Placebo and Intervention Group Receiving Lavandula Aromatherapy

Pain	Groups	N	Mean	SD*	*p* Value**
The difference between the mean pain score preintervention and postintervention in the first day	Placebo	51	0.02	1.61	0.0001
	Intervention	61	1.98	1.95	
The difference between the mean pain score preintervention and postintervention in the second day	Placebo	51	−0.18	1.52	0.0001
	Intervention	54	0.98	1.61	
The difference between the mean pain score preintervention and postintervention in the third day	Placebo	49	0.18	0.73	0.183
	Intervention	49	0.41	0.91	

*Standard deviation.
**Mann-Whitney test.
Note: The change in state score (post/pre) was compared in the three groups using the Mann-Whitney U test.
From Ebrahimi et al., 2022.

variables when one does not actually exist). The higher the α level, the higher the risk.

Typically, α is set at 0.05, with p values less than or equal to this threshold qualifying as significant (p value ≤ 0.05). When the p value ≤ 0.05, the researcher can reject the null hypothesis (no effect or difference) in favor of the alternative hypothesis (an association or effect exists). In hypothesis testing the researcher decides in the design of the statistical analysis to conduct a **one-tailed** or **two-tailed** test. In a one-tailed test (focused on only the extreme end of one tail of the bell curve) the alternative hypothesis projects a unidirectional outcome of the dependent variable (e.g., the researcher hypothesizes that the intervention group will have a lower serum blood sugar than the control group). In a two-tailed test the research hypothesis is nondirectional, stating only that there is a difference between comparisons (i.e., lower or higher).

Because research is not an exact science, there is always a probability that an error can occur in the researcher's conclusion. These types of error are grouped into two categories: **Type I error** (the rejection of a true null hypothesis) and **Type II error** (failure to reject a false null hypothesis).

Type I error occurs when the researcher rejects a true null hypothesis, namely incorrectly concludes that there is an effect or an association when, in reality, such a relationship does not exist. The α level reflects the probability of committing a Type I error. As discussed, alpha is typically set at 0.05. This means that there is a 5% risk that the null hypothesis will be rejected when it is true. A researcher can have a higher degree of certainty by decreasing the α level to 0.01. However, lowering the α level increases the possibility of not identifying a clinically significant association between study variables. That said, the researcher should decide regarding the alpha level before the start of the study (i.e., **a priori**). A Type I error can lead to a wrong conclusion about an association between variables (i.e., you believe there are important differences when there really are not) and provoke an ineffective practice change.

A Type II error can occur when the researcher fails to reject the null hypothesis. Plainly speaking, Type II error occurs when the researcher fails to identify a significant effect or association when indeed such an impact or relationship does in fact exist. When a Type II error occurs, the researcher may fail to make an important change in practice because they believe there is no need to do so. The risk of making a Type II error is often denoted as β. Calculating β is complex and is best calculated using statistical software.

The risk of a Type II error is directly related to statistical power. Statistical power reflects the probability of correctly rejecting a null hypothesis when the null hypothesis is false. It is influenced by sample size, effect size (i.e., strength of the impact), significance level, and a variety of other factors including the research design. Increasing sample size is one of the easiest ways to boost power. The smaller the sample size, the more difficult it is to detect a difference between study variables. As power increases, the probability of avoiding a Type II error decreases. To reduce the probability of a Type II error, researchers often conduct a prospective power analysis to determine the necessary sample size for a sufficiently powered analysis.

Effect size is the magnitude of the strength of the relationship between the independent and dependent variables. This is quantified as the expected percentage of change in the dependent variable as influenced by the independent variable. During the planning stage of a study, researchers select a significance level for the study and then estimate the effect size. To do this, they may ask themselves, "How large of an effect do I want to observe in the dependent variable—10%, 20%, 50%?" This question is important because at the conclusion of the study, a 10% effect size might be statistically significant but clinically insignificant, whereas a 50% effect size might be both statistically and clinically significant. Effect size can be calculated using a Cohen's d statical procedure or a Pearson's r (discussed later in this chapter). Effect size may also be determined through a previous pilot investigation or gleaned from the available literature. It is important to remain mindful that effect size and sample size are linked. Detecting small effects requires larger samples, and conversely larger effect sizes reduces the sample size requirements.

Understanding effect size helps us move beyond the simplistic question of "Does this intervention work or not?" (i.e., is the association statistically significant) and challenges researchers to consider far more sophisticated questions like, "How well does this intervention work?" and "What is the **clinical meaningfulness**?" For these reasons, effect size is an important tool in reporting and interpreting effectiveness and should be reported with intervention studies.

Confidence intervals (CIs) are reported in the research literature to provide a range of values within which a given population parameter may be expected to fall based on an analysis of the study sample results. The confidence level (commonly identified as 95%) describes the chance that the lower and upper bounds of the CI capture the true parameter (or target population) value. For instance, a researcher might be interested in average BMI of a U.S. pediatric population aged 8 to 10. While the researcher will never know the underlying mean BMI value for all children in this age range (population parameter), the researcher can sample from within this population, estimate the mean, and construct a CI. Typically, investigators record their CI results as a 95% degree of certainty. At times, you also may see the degree of certainty recorded as 99%. Returning to the above example, suppose a researcher constructs a 95% CI. The researcher could than say, with 95% confidence, that the true BMI parameter value falls within a given range of BMIs.

CIs can be calculated for a variety of descriptive and inferential statistics. More and more professional journals require investigators to include CIs as one of the statistical methods used to interpret study findings. Even when CIs are not reported, they can be calculated easily from the available study data as long as a mean and standard error values are provided. The method for performing these calculations is widely available in statistical texts.

Kratovil et al. (2023) conducted a study of nurses working in a hospital setting regarding their attitudes on caring for patients with substance use disorders (SUDs). Examine Table 13.4 from the study, which compares the mean difference score of nurse's knowledge about substance use by unit, with lower scores indicating better knowledge. If you examine the data, you will see that the nurses on a mental health unit had much lower scores suggesting they have better knowledge about substance use than nurses in all other hospital units. You will also notice that the study investigators provide CIs to accompany the mean differences (these are in parenthesis). The CIs provide the reader with a range for the mean differences for the variable that might be found in the population. Said another way, if you were to repeat the study repeatedly, you would be 95% certain to obtain a mean difference within this range of scores.

CIs also provide an indication of statistical significance. When a CI contains a **null value** (that may be 0 or 1 depending on the test statistic used), the researcher cannot definitively rule out that the true population (or parameter) value is 0 or 1. This, in turn suggests, that the researcher finds no evidence of a significant effect or relationship. On the other hand, if the CI does not include a null value, the researcher can report evidence of a significant association or effect. For numeric values determined by a mean difference between the scores in the intervention group and the control group, the null value is "0." If the CI does not include the null value of "0," the result is statistically significant as illustrated in Fig. 13.3. For numeric values determined by proportion or ratio (e.g., relative risk, odds ratio, discussed later in this chapter), the null value is "1."

TABLE 13.4 Comparison of Mean Differences on Drug and Drug Problems Questionnaire on Knowledge by Hospital Unit

Hospital Unit Pairs		Mean Difference (95% CI)	P Value
ED	ICU	025 (–0.041 to 0.54)	0.13
	Medical-surgical	031 (0.04 to 053)	0.023
	Mental health	–0.45 (–0.87 to –0.04}	0.023
	Mother-baby	0.33 (–0.01 to 0.67)	0.07
ICU	Medical-surgical	0.06 (–0.20 to 0.32)	0.98
	Mental health	–0.71 (–1.12 to 0.30)	< 0.0011
	Mother-baby	0.08 (–0.26 to 0.41)	0.97
Medical-surgical	Mental health	–0.77 (–1.16 to –0.37)	< 0.0011
	Mother-baby	0.02 (–0.30 to 0.33)	> 0.99
Mental health	Mother-baby	0.78 (0.34 to 123)	< 0.0011

From Kratovil et al., 2023.

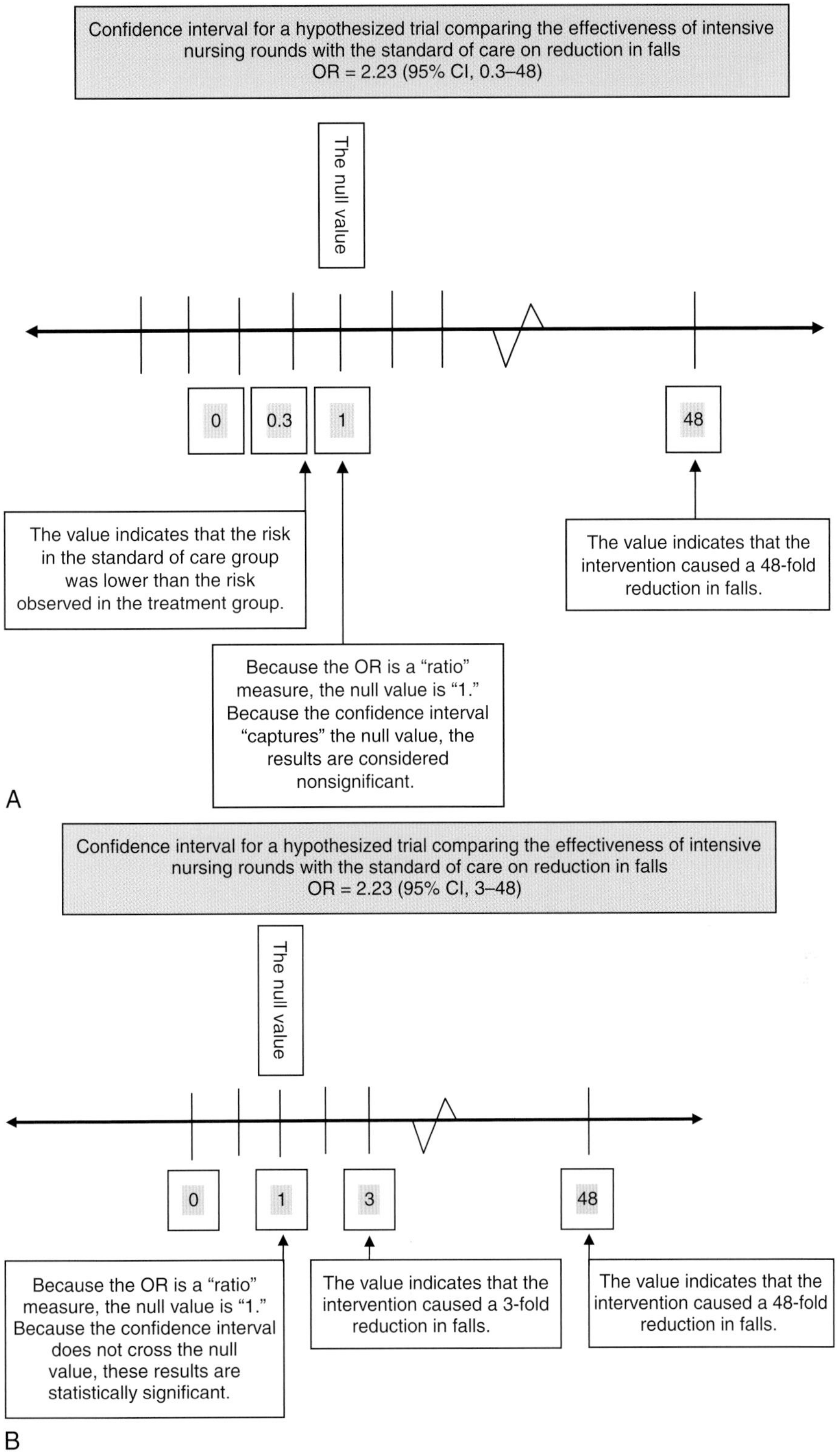

Fig. 13.3 (A) Confidence Interval (Nonsignificant) for a Hypothesized Trial Comparing the Ratio of Events in the Experimental Group and Control Group. (B) Confidence Interval (Significant) for a Hypothesized Trial Comparing the Ratio of Events in the Experimental Group and Control Group.

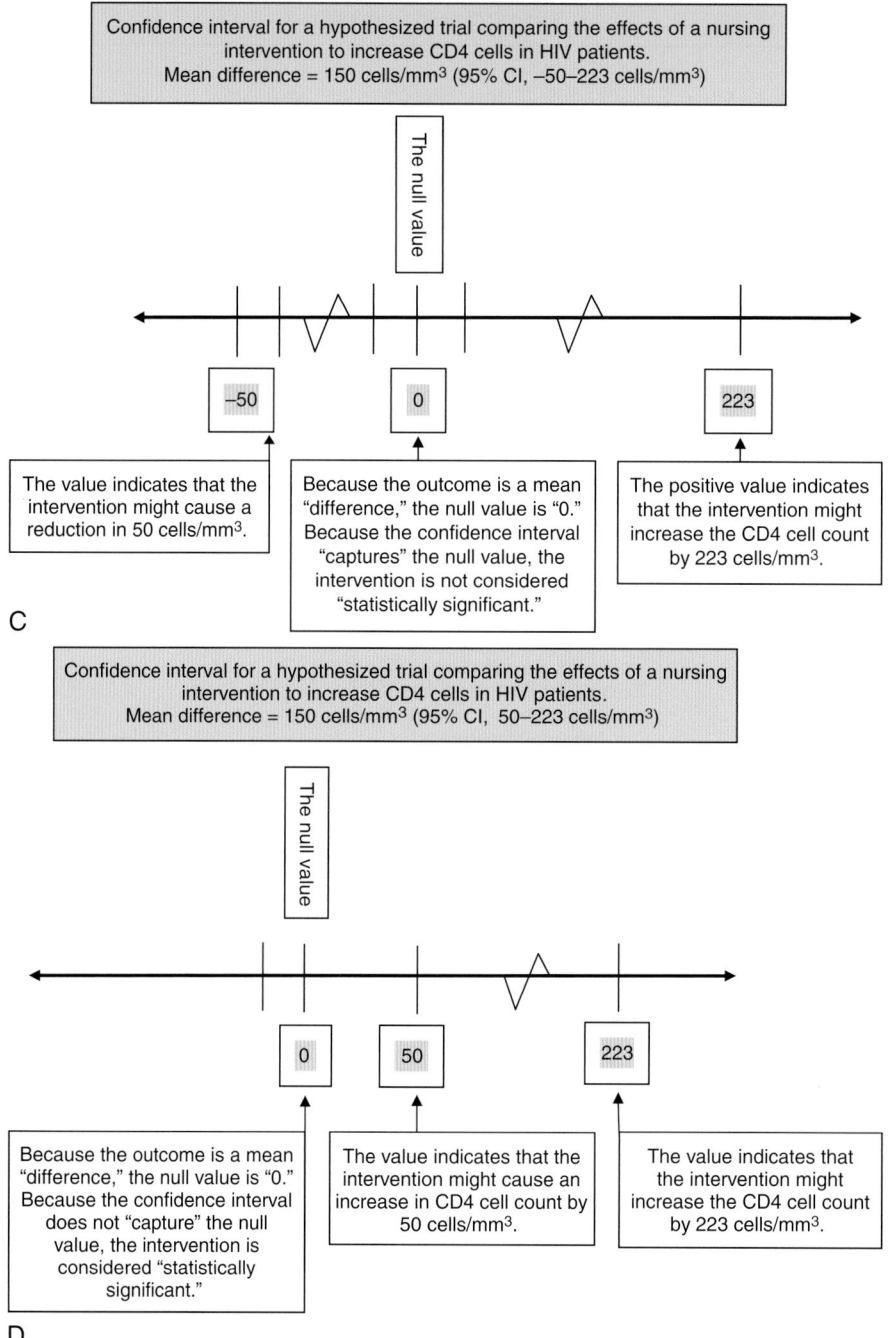

Fig. 13.3, cont'd (C) Confidence Interval (Nonsignificant) for a Hypothesized Control Trial Comparing the Difference Between Two Treatments. (D) Confidence Interval (Significant) for a Hypothesized Control Trial Comparing the Difference Between Two Treatments. *OR,* Odds ratio.

CRITICAL APPRAISAL OF EVIDENCE-BASED LITERATURE STATISTICS

During the critical appraisal process, you will likely encounter a wide range of research study designs that utilize a considerable variety of statistical techniques. Research design is broadly categorized as either descriptive (limited to describing the outcomes of the study sample) or analytical (using inferential statistics to generalize from the sample to the population). Analytical research designs are categorized as observational (studies that identify associations between conditions that are present within a population without researcher intervention) or experimental (studies that examine relationships between variables by intentionally exposing comparison groups to different conditions).

Generally, all quantitative studies will report some descriptive statistics, including frequencies, measures of central tendency, and measures of variability as discussed previously in this chapter. Most articles will describe their study samples using descriptive and analytical methods. If the study uses a descriptive study design, the research results will be reported using only descriptive statistics. If the study is an analytical research design the results with be reported using both descriptive *and* inferential statistics.

COMPARING DIFFERENCES BETWEEN GROUPS

Analytical research studies often contrast data from two or more different groups of subjects using parametric or nonparametric inferential statistics. The statistics used depend on the level of measurement of the variable (nominal, ordinal, interval, or ratio), how many groups are being compared, and whether the data are normally distributed, recalling that data that are not normally distributed are analyzed using nonparametric statistics.

One of the most commonly used parametric statistical tests is the **Student's *t* test**, more commonly referred to as simply a *t* test. The *t* test examines whether statistically significant differences exist between the mean score of a continuous, interval, or ratio-level outcome (dependent) variable. An *independent* samples *t* test is used to compare groups that are not related to one another, such as in examining the difference in outcomes between study participants from two different hospital facilities. A *dependent* or paired samples *t* test is used to compared groups that are related, such as in the examination of pre- and postintervention outcomes on the same participant sample. The *t* test provides a t statistic value. The researcher can interpret this test statistic to infer how closely aligned the study scores are with the expected normal distribution if the null hypothesis were true (i.e., there is no relationship between variables). A t value of 0 indicates that there is no difference between the sample mean and the hypothesized mean for the null hypothesis. The *t* test also provides a p value, which indicates how likely the study findings can be explained by chance. A statistically significant *t* test (generally p value ≤ 0.05) indicates that there is a 5% risk that the null hypothesis will be rejected when it is true (a Type I error).

Like the *t* test, the **one-way ANOVA** (analysis of variance) test that can be used to compare the means from three or more independent groups. The **repeated measures ANOVA** is used to analyze three or more dependent groups. Like the *t* test, ANOVA analyses produce a test statistic, in this case an F statistic value, as well as a p value. As with any statistical test, the researcher can use the test statistic and p value to interpret relative statistical significance. Analogous statistical tests of difference between groups (*t* test and ANOVA) are available for nonparametric analysis of nominal or ordinal level variables. These tests are listed in Box 13.2.

MEASURING RELATIONSHIPS BETWEEN VARIABLES

Some research studies are designed to assess an association or relationship between the independent and dependent variables. For interval and ratio-level data this is generally accomplished using the **Pearson's correlation coefficient (r),** commonly called the Pearson's r. The Pearson's r tests the statistical significance of a linear relationship between two interval/ratio-level variables and provides information on the direction and strength of that relationship. For example, is there a relationship between body temperature and heart rate? As body temperature rises, does heart rate rise or fall? The direction of the relationship in a Pearson's r is identified as a positive or negative association. If the heart rate rises when the body temperature rises, that is identified as a positive association. Conversely, if heart rate falls while body temperature rises, that would be considered a negative association. The strength of the association is indicated by the absolute value of the correlation coefficient. If the correlation coefficient is 0, there is no relationship between variables. A perfect negative correlation is identified as −1 and a perfect positive correlation is +1. In hypothesis testing, the outcome of the Pearson's r calculation, strength and direction, is additionally considered for statistical probability using the p value determinations as described previously.

The researcher can also use the Pearson's r to determine the percentage of variance (i.e., change) in one variable that is explained by the influence of the second variable (and vice versa). This variation is calculated by multiplying r^2 (referred to as the **coefficient of determination**) by 100, which provides the percentage of variance. The percentage of variance can be used to determine the study effect size for the consideration of clinical significance, as well as used in sample size calculations. Using the Pearson's r, a value of 0.1 to 0.3 is considered a small effect, 0.3 to 0.5 a medium effect, and 0.5 and above a large effect. As previously discussed, a larger sample size will be needed to identify a relationship with a small effect.

A researcher can also assess linear association through linear regression analysis. A simple linear regression analysis creates a linear model of the relationship between a single, independent variable and a single, continuous dependent (outcome) variable such that the slope of the line predicts the change of the dependent variable for every one-unit change of the independent variable. As with the other analytical research strategies, the regression model is tested for statistical significance using a p value calculation. Like the Pearson's r, the regression model provides an R^2, which identifies the amount of variance in the outcome variable that is explained by the independent variable. An advantage of the regression model is the ability to predict an outcome variable measurement based on an independent variable. Multiple regression can be used to assess the relationship between an outcome variable and more than one independent variables. Logistic regression is used when the outcome variable is a nominal binary variable (e.g., disease or no disease)—importantly, in this circumstance, the relationship is not assumed to be linear. Depending on your research question and what you hope to explore, some study designs (and associated statistical) techniques may better suit your underlying objective. The specific statistics you will see in your review of the EB literature depends on the type of clinical question you are asking.

RISK REDUCTION ANALYSIS

Risk reduction estimates enable clinicians to assess potential changes in health outcomes associated with exposure and are frequently used in research on disease prevention and treatment. If an exposure and a given health outcome are associated, risk reduction calculations allow a clinician to estimate potential reductions in adverse health outcomes if a specific exposure were avoided. Within this context, one might consider absolute and relative measures of association. Before diving to this conversation, readers might consider reviewing definitions of incidence and prevalence, which are introduced in Chapter 25.

Absolute Measures of Association

Absolute measures of risk compare differences in prevalence, cumulative incidence, or incidence rate across exposed (E) and unexposed groups (U). Clinicians often rely on one of the **risk differences (RD) calculations** below to assess absolute measures of association (Aschengrau & Seage, 2020). Data used to consider the differences between exposed and unexposed groups can be organized using a 2 x 2 table, such as the hypothetical example provided here. In this table the exposure is a BMI > 30 and the outcome of interest is type 2 diabetes.

	Type 2 Diabetes (Yes)	Type 2 Diabetes (No)	Total
BMI ≥ 30	26	53	79
BMI < 30	5	68	73
Total	31	121	152

Prevalence Difference. **Prevalence** is the measure of a characteristic within a population. Prevalence difference (PD) is the difference in prevalence between the exposed and unexposed groups.

$$PD = PE - PU \text{ (no units)}$$

Using our hypothetical example:
Prevalence of type 2 Diabetes among persons with a BMI > 30 = 26/79 = 0.33
Prevalence of type 2 Diabetes among persons with a BMI < 30 = 5/73 = 0.07
PD type 2 Diabetes = 0.33 − 0.07 = 0.26 = 26 per 100

Thus, the interpretation of these data would be, among persons with a BMI > 30 there were 26 more cases of type 2 diabetes per 100 as compared to persons with a BMI of < 30.

Cumulative Incidence Risk Difference. Cumulative incidence risk difference (CIRD) is the proportion of candidates in a population that develop a condition over a designated specific period of time, interpreted as the average risk of a condition. It is calculated by dividing the number of new cases by the number in the candidate population, considered over a specified time period. The CI risk difference is the difference between the cumulative incidence in the exposed and unexposed groups.

$$CI\ RD = CI_E - CI_U \text{ (no units)}$$

Incidence Rate Difference. Incidence rate is the number of new cases of a condition that arise within the context of a "person-time" observation in the candidate population. Person-time calculations are different from calculation of the candidate population in cumulative incidence in that inclusion of "person-time" candidates continue only as long as the candidate is actively engaged in the study. This technique is particularly useful in dynamic populations where the population is fluid due to birth, death, and loss to follow up. The calculation of incidence rate is the number of new cases divided by the person-time observation in the candidate population. The incidence rate difference is the difference in incidence rate between the exposed and unexposed groups.

$$IR\ RD = IR_E - IR_U \text{ (person-time units)}$$

Risk reduction measures quantify "excess risk." Namely, by how much does prevalence or incidence of disease in the exposed population exceed that in the general population? This information provides clinicians and researchers with a numeric estimate of potential reductions in incidence and prevalence that might occur if the exposure were avoided. Using absolute measures of risk, a researcher can answer the following questions: "How much impact would prevention have?" and "How many people would benefit?"

Relative Measures of Association

Relative measures of association compare the ratio of disease in the exposed population to that in the unexposed population. Common measures of **relative risk** include prevalence ratio, risk ratio, and rate ratio (Aschengrau & Seage, 2020).

Prevalence ratio is the ratio of prevalence between exposed and unexposed groups.

$$PR = P_E / P_U \text{ (no units)}$$

Using our hypothetical example above, the PR for type 2 diabetes = 0.33/0.07 = 4.7. Thus, persons with a BMI > 30 have over 4 times the prevalence of type 2 diabetes as compared to persons with a BMI of < 30.

Risk ratio is the ratio of cumulative incidence between exposed and unexposed groups.

$$RR = CI_E / CI_U \text{ (no units)}$$

Rate ratio is the ratio of incidence rate between exposed and unexposed groups.

$$IRR = IR_E / IR_U \text{ (no units)}$$

Ratios equal to 1 imply that prevalence and/or incidence are approximately equal between the two groups, thus the exposure has minimal impact on rates of disease. Ratios greater than 1 imply that exposure is associated with increased risk of disease. Conversely, ratios less than 1 imply that exposure is protective, associated with decreased rates of disease. Relative measures of association enable clinicians to assess the strength of associations, by quantifying how much more likely are exposed persons to develop the outcome than the unexposed.

ODDS RATIO ANALYSIS

The **odds ratio** helps clinicians assess whether a given health outcome is associated with a specific exposure, particularly in the context of case-control research study designs. Recall from Chapter 9, case-control studies reflect an observational study framework, where the researcher observes (rather than assigns) whether: (1) exposure occurred and (2) a given health outcome manifests. In this context, the research begins by identifying "cases," namely individuals with a given (often rare) health outcome. These cases are than "matched" to "controls," namely patients without disease who are drawn from the at-risk population (Keeler & Curtis, 2022; Aschengrau & Seage, 2020). The researcher can then compare rates of exposure across the cases (those with disease) and controls (those without disease) by calculating a disease odds ratio (defined as the odds of being a case among the exposed divided the odds of being a case among the unexposed) or the exposure odds ratio (defined as the odds of being exposed among the cases divided by defined the odds of being exposed among the controls) (Keeler & Curtis, 2022; Aschengrau & Seage, 2020).

$$\text{Odd ratio (OR)} = \frac{\text{number of exposed cases} \times \text{number of unexposed controls}}{\text{number of unexposed cases} \times \text{number of exposed controls}}$$

The odds ratio can be interpreted as follows:
OR = 1 → no association between health outcome and exposure
OR > 1 → positive association between health outcome and exposure
OR < 1 → negative association between health outcome and exposure

For example, White et al. (2019) conducted a study to examine the relationship between registered nurse (RN) burnout, job dissatisfaction, and missed care in nursing homes. Missed nursing care, sometimes referred to as "unfinished nursing care," is an important metric of the quality of nursing care to patients. The researchers surveyed 687 registered nurses employed in U.S. nursing homes. Findings from this study indicate that nursing home RNs are often unable to complete needed nursing care due to inadequate time or resources, and that missed care is more common among RNs with high burnout or job dissatisfaction. Table 13.5 shows data from this study. RNs with burnout were 5.53 times more likely to leave necessary care undone (odds ratio [OR] = 5.53; 95% confidence interval [CI] = 2.79–10.06) than RNs without burnout. RNs who were dissatisfied were 2.3 times more likely to leave necessary care undone (OR = 2.33; 95% CI = 1.55–3.49) than RNs who were satisfied. Odds ratios are often accompanied by a confidence interval (CI) as noted in this study. See Fig. 13.3A-D to understand the correct interpretation of the confidence intervals.

STUDY DESIGN AND STATISTICAL TEST SELECTION

The statistical tests discussed in this chapter can be utilized across a variety of study designs. For instance, correlations and risk ratios can be calculated from both experimental and observational data. That said, in some study designs, some statistical tests are more common than others. With this in mind, it is worth reviewing interventional and observational study designs.

Interventional Study Designs

Interventional studies help researchers answer a question about the effectiveness of a particular treatment or intervention. Intervention studies are discussed in detail in Chapter 8. Intervention studies usually contrast data from two or more different groups of subjects. The EB statistics used in an intervention study depend on whether the numeric values of the study variables are **continuous** (a variable that measures a degree of change or a difference on a range, such as blood pressure) or **discrete**, also known as dichotomous (measuring whether an event did or did not occur, such as the number of people diagnosed or not diagnosed with type 2 diabetes).

Continuous outcomes (e.g., mean scores) often are analyzed by a basic statistical test called the *t* test, a method that assumes the data in the different groups come from populations where the observations have a normal distribution and the same variances (or standard deviations). Similar to a *t* test, the one-way ANOVA test can be used to compare the means from three or more groups. There also is the two-way ANOVA that allows you to compare the means of two or more groups in response to two different independent variables. The statistics used depend on the level of measurement, whether your data are normally distributed (parametric vs. nonparametric), and the category of data (see Boxes 13.2 and 13.3).

The goal of most intervention studies is to measure the effect of an intervention on an outcome. The effect on dichotomous outcomes (measuring whether an event did or did not occur) have common measures

TABLE 13.5 Bivariate Analysis Demonstrating Two Variables Associated With Missed Care by Registered Nurses

Variable	Bivariate	
	OR (95% CI)	p value
Burnout	5.53 (2.79–10.96)	< 0.001
Job dissatisfaction	2.33 (1.55–3.49)	< 0.001

From White et al., 2019.

that are important to EB practitioners. In such trials, we want to know whether the treatment or intervention results in positive or negative outcomes and by how much. Investigators use risk calculations to assist EB practitioners in considering whether to accept or reject a treatment. They are also used to help communicate risk-benefit information to patients and/or key stakeholders.

Observational Study Designs

In observational studies, a phenomenon of interest is observed from within a preexisting context rather than constructed by the researcher. Suppose that a researcher was interested in exploring the relationship between smoking status and heart disease. In an observational study, the researcher would "observe" smoking status within the sample, not assign participants into "smoking" and "nonsmoking" groups. This example highlights the necessity of an observational study design in some contexts, namely a researcher cannot ethically assign participants into dangerous exposure groups like smoking. With all observational study designs, causality is difficult to establish because of the absence of tightly controlled treatment groups (Capili & Anastasi, 2023). Observational studies include cross-sectional, cohort, and case-control study designs. Statistics common to observational study designs can be those associated with risk reduction analysis and odds ratio analysis. See Chapter 9 for a discussion of observational studies.

Studies Involving Diagnostic Tests

Fundamentally, clinicians need to understand the relative accuracy of the tests they use to diagnosis disease. While not all tests have binary outcomes, one can consider instances where, based on certain thresholds, a test yields a binary positive or negative result. That said, clinicians often want to know if the test result is indeed accurate? A test's validity reflects the ability of the test to accurately distinguish between those who have and do not have the disease (Curtis & Keeler, 2022). Four measures help gauge the validity: sensitivity, specificity, positive predictive value, and negative predictive value.

Sensitivity measures the ability of the test to correctly identify those who **have** the disease (Curtis & Keeler, 2022). A highly sensitive test generates few false negative results, meaning few actual positive cases are missed. Specificity measures the ability of the test to correctly identify those who **do not have** the disease (Curtis & Keeler, 2022). A highly specific test generates few false positive results; however, individuals with the disease may go undiagnosed. Tests with low specificity have the disadvantage that, among other things, many subjects without the disease will screen positive and potentially receive unnecessary and possibly invasive, risky, or expensive follow-up diagnostic or therapeutic procedures.

Sensitivity and specificity, although widely used, are just part of the story—although sensitivity and specificity describe the specific characteristics of diagnostic tests, we must also consider how well the test performs within a specific population. To measure performance of a test we use predictive values that account for the effect of the prevalence of a disease. Predictive values are highly influenced by the prevalence of the disease in the population, as prevalence increases so does the positive predictive value (PPV). Predictive values provide information about test performance that answer the questions: "What are the chances that the subject has the disease if they test positive?" and conversely "What are the chances that the subject does not have the disease if they test negative?" The PPV identifies the proportion of those with positive test results who truly have the disease. Similarly, negative predictive value (NPV) identifies the proportion of those with negative test results who truly do not have the disease. To calculate the PPV and NPV you need the sensitivity and specificity. If you refer to Box 13.4, you can see how easy it is to calculate

BOX 13.4 Positive Predictive Value and Negative Predictive Value

Positive predictive value (PPV)	The proportion of people with a positive test who have the target disorder	Formula for positive predictive value: PPV = True Positive/(True Positive + False Positive)
Negative predictive value (NPV)	The proportion of people with a negative test who do not have the target disorder	Formula for negative predictive value: NPV = True Negative/(True Negative + False Negative)

TABLE 13.6 Calculating Sensitivity and Specificity

	Disease Present	Disease Absent
Test positive	a (TP)	b (FP)
Test negative	c (FN)	d (TN)
	Sensitivity: a/(a + c)	Specificity: d/(b + d)

FN, False negative; FP, false positive; TN, true negative; TP, true positive.

TABLE 13.7 Serological Status by Self-Reported History of CT Infection

	Positive Serology (n = 146)	Negative Serology (n = 263)
Positive self-report (n = 108)	76	32
Negative self-report (n = 301)	70	231

Sensitivity is 52.1% (95% CI, 43.6%–60.4%). Specificity is 87.8% (95% CI, 83.3%–91.5%). Positive predictive value is 70.4% (95% CI, 60.8%–78.8%). Negative predictive value is 76.7% (95% CI, 71.6%–81.4%). CI, Confidence interval; CT, Chlamydia trachomatis.
From Frisse et al., 2017.

the PPV and NPV; most investigators also provide this information.

How do researchers and clinicians know if someone has disease? Well, in calculating sensitivity and specificity, test results can be compared to a gold standard test. The gold standard is the best single test or combination of tests that is considered the current preferred method of diagnosing a particular disease. For example, the gold standard test for diagnosing cancer is the surgical biopsy. If you were to introduce a new test to diagnosis cancer you would want to compare the performance of the new test to gold standard.

Table 13.6 walks readers through four possible outcomes.

- In cell "a," we enter those in whom the test in question correctly diagnosed the disease as determined by the gold standard. In other words, the test is positive, as is the gold standard. These are the true positives (TPs).
- In cell "b," we enter those who have positive results for the test in question but do not have disease according to the gold standard test. The newer test has wrongly diagnosed the disease. These are false positives (FPs).
- In cell "c," we enter those who have the disease according to the gold standard test but have negative results with the test in question. The test has wrongly labeled a diseased person as "normal." These are false negatives (FNs).
- In cell "d," we enter those who have no disease as determined by the gold standard test and are also negative according to the newer test. These are true negatives (TNs).

There are many examples of diagnostic tests in the literature. For instance, Frisse et al. (2017) conducted a study to evaluate the validity of women's self-reported history of Chlamydia trachomatis (CT) infection compared with CT serology, a marker for previous infection (Frisse et al., 2017). They compared participants' survey responses with the question, "Have you ever been told by a health care provider that you had chlamydia?" to serological test results indicating the presence or absence of antibodies to CT as assessed by a microimmunofluorescence assay. Prevalence of past infection, sensitivity, and specificity were calculated and are presented in Table 13.7.

Sensitivity of self-report (the new diagnostic test) was 52.1% and the specificity of self-report was 87.8%. The authors concluded, "When evaluating the validity of self-report in women enrolled in the FACT study, we found self-report to not be a valid marker of past CT infection status. Only 52% of women with positive serology reported a history of CT infection. This low sensitivity indicates a high false-negative rate. Specificity was higher at 88%, indicating a false-positive rate of 12%" (Frisse et al., 2017).

Additionally, if you look at Table 13.7 from the Frisse et al. study, you will see that the investigator provides that PPV is 70.4% and NPV is 76.7%. The PPV tells the clinician what percentage of those with a positive finding have the disease. The NPV reveals what percentage of those with a negative result do not have the disease. The interpretation for PPV and NPV for the Frisse et al. study is: "Our positive and negative predictive values of self-reported CT infection were 70% and 77%, respectively. Thus 30% of participants who reported a history of CT infection did not have a history of infection according to serology, and almost 25% of participants who reported not having a history of CT infection actually had serological evidence of infection" (Frisse et al., 2017).

Another statistic used in studies involving diagnostic tests is the **likelihood ratio (LR)**. The LR provides a measure of how likely a person is to have a disease or condition given a diagnostic test result. The LR calculation uses pretest odds of a condition (often determined using prevalence data) and an LR calculation for the diagnostic test to identify the degree to which the current diagnostic test result increases or decreases the odds of disease. The LR calculation for a positive diagnostic test (LR+) is sensitivity/1 − specificity, otherwise stated as the true positive rate divided by the false positive rate. The LR calculation for a negative diagnostic test (LR−) is 1 − sensitivity/specificity; or the false negative rate divided by true negative rate (Box 13.5). The practical advantage of the LR is the ability to interpret a diagnostic test result in the context of the individual patient and derive a posttest probability for disease. More and more journal articles require authors to provide test LRs; they also may be available in secondary sources.

Since LR calculations can be slightly complex, most EB practitioners use a likelihood ratio nomogram rather than perform mathematical calculations to avoid the necessary conversions between odds and probabilities. The Fagan Nomogram (Fig. 13.4) is a visual instrument sometimes used in clinical practice. It is made up of three parallel lines. On the left line, the clinician finds the pretest probability and connects a line from this number to the center line, which reflects the likelihood ratio (usually from the published data). The clinician continues a straight line through to the posttest probability. With this the clinician can evaluate the probability of disease (+LR) or no disease (−LR) after application of the test. Today, most clinician simply use widely available apps and enter the information to obtain this information.

As an example, suppose we take a sexual history on a sexually active woman of childbearing age whose male sexual partner was recently treated for a chlamydia infection. From epidemiological data, we know that the prevalence of asymptomatic chlamydia infection in the population is approximately 47% (HEDIS, n.d.). This could be used as our pretest probability; other sources of pretest probability can be based on patient-specific data (e.g., physical examination). We then apply the

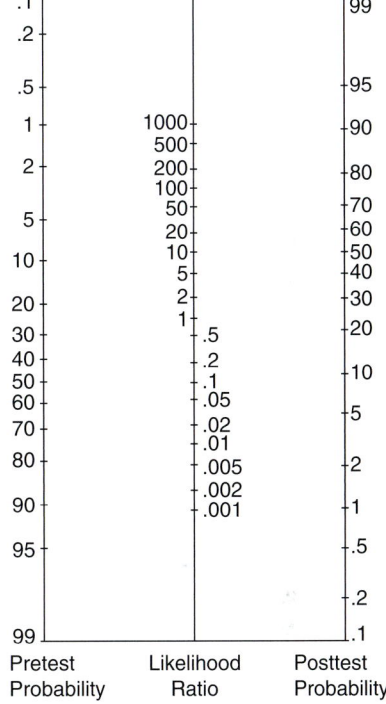

Fig. 13.4 The Likelihood Ratio Nomogram.

BOX 13.5	Positive Likelihood Ratio and Negative Likelihood Ratio		
Positive likelihood ratio (LR)	The LR of a positive test tells us how well a positive test result does by comparing its performance when the disease is present to when it is absent. The best test to use for ruling in a disease is the one with the largest likelihood ratio of a positive test.	Formula for positive likelihood ratio: Sensitivity/(1 − Specificity)
Negative likelihood ratio	The LR of a negative test tells us how well a negative test result does by comparing its performance when the disease is absent to when it is present. The better test to use to rule out disease is the one with the smaller likelihood ratio of a negative test.	Formula for negative likelihood ratio: (1 − Sensitivity)/Specificity

likelihood ratio of the diagnostic test, calculated using the known sensitivity and specificity. Using the nomogram, if we note our pretest probability (47%) and the test is positive with a known likelihood ratio (5), the probability that the patient has chlamydia is 70% (Fig. 13.5). With that level of probability, you are likely to treat the patient for chlamydia.

As displayed in Table 13.8, a test with a positive likelihood ratio of greater than 10 provides the clinician with a high degree of certainty that the patient has the suspected disorder. Conversely, tests with a low positive likelihood ratio (e.g., less than 2) provide you with little certainty that the patient has the suspected disorder. When a test has a likelihood ratio of "1" (the null value), it will not contribute to decision making in any meaningful way and should not be used. A test with a large negative likelihood ratio provides the clinician with a high degree of certainty that the patient does not have the disease. The farther away from "1" the negative LR is, the better the test will be for its use in ruling out disease (i.e., there will be few false negatives).

Although the authors of the Frisse et al. study did not provide a negative likelihood ratio (NLR), it is calculated easily from sensitivity and specificity (see Table 13.6); the NLR = 0.5. With a pretest probability of 45% and an NLR of 0.5 (and the test is negative), using our nomogram, our posttest probability of infection is 23%. Without any other compelling evidence to treat this patient, you are less likely to do so given this lowered probability of infection.

Likelihood ratios are useful when a test has only a single threshold or cut-point value (for instance, positive or negative for disease, such as a biopsy). Tests that yield results on a continuous scale (e.g., Braden score for pressure ulcer risk) require specification of a test threshold to define positive and negative results. Changing the threshold alters the proportion of false positive and false negative diagnoses.

This change in threshold for a given instrument or diagnostic test can be displayed in a specific type of graph known as the **Receiver Operating Characteristics (ROC) curve**. This graph can be extremely helpful in establishing an acceptable threshold or cutoff point for the instrument or diagnostic test. This graph plots the sensitivity and false positive rate at a given value for the instrument or diagnostic test (Fig. 13.6). The best cutoff has the highest true positive rate together with

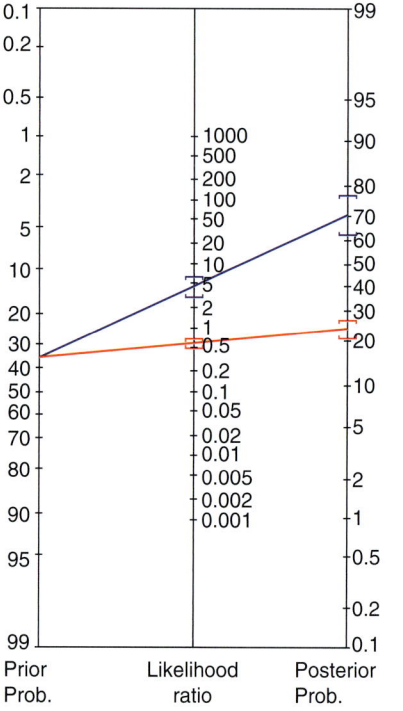

Fig. 13.5 Use of the Likelihood Ratio for Chlamydia Study Data.

TABLE 13.8 How Much Do Likelihood Ratio Changes Affect Probability of Disease?

Likelihood Ratio Positive	Likelihood Ratio Negative	Probability that Patient Has (LR) or Does Not Have (LR)
LR > 10	LR < 0.1	Large
LR 5–10	LR 0.1–0.2	Moderate
LR 2–5	LR 0.2–0.5	Small
LR < 2	LR > 0.5	Tiny
LR = 1.0		Test provides no useful information

LR, Likelihood ratio.

the lowest false positive rate. Examine Fig. 13.6; the false positive rate is on the X axis and the true positive rate is on the Y axis. All of the cutoff values are determined and plotted on the graph, creating a curve (the blue line in the figure). Thus, every point on the ROC curve represents a chosen cutoff, although you cannot see it. What you can see is the curve of the true positive fraction and the false positive fraction that you will get when you choose this cutoff. The important part of the ROC curve is the area under the curve. The area under the ROC curve (AUROC) of a test can be used as a criterion to measure the test's discriminative ability (i.e., how well the test can discriminate in a given clinical situation) (Fig. 13.7).

A perfect test can discriminate between healthy and sick persons with 100% sensitivity and 100% specificity (no such test), and would look like the curve in Fig. 13.8. When we have a test with no ability to discriminate between those with and without disease, we have a worthless test. A worthless test has a discriminating ability equal to flipping a coin. The ROC curve of the worthless test falls on the diagonal line. It includes the point with 50% sensitivity and 50% specificity (Fig. 13.9). The area under the ROC curve of the worthless test is 0.5.

By examining the graph, the researcher or clinician can better understand the tradeoffs that sometimes have to be made to increase sensitivity or specificity. The closer an ROC curve is to the upper left corner, the more efficient is the test. Computing the area is beyond the scope of this introductory material. Various computer

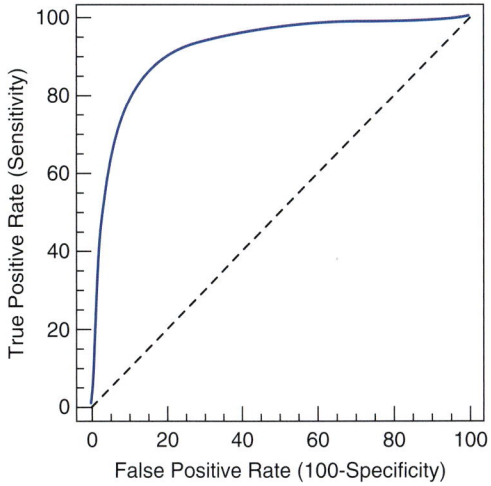

Fig. 13.6 Example of a Receiver Operating Curve.

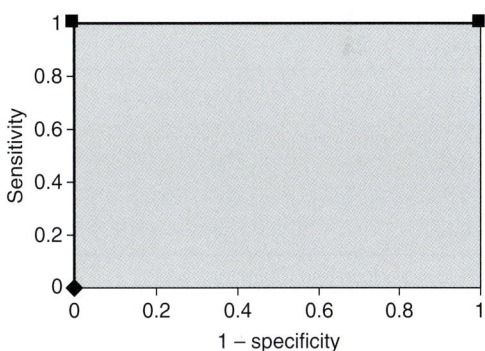

Fig. 13.8 AUROC of Test with 100% Sensitivity and Specificity.

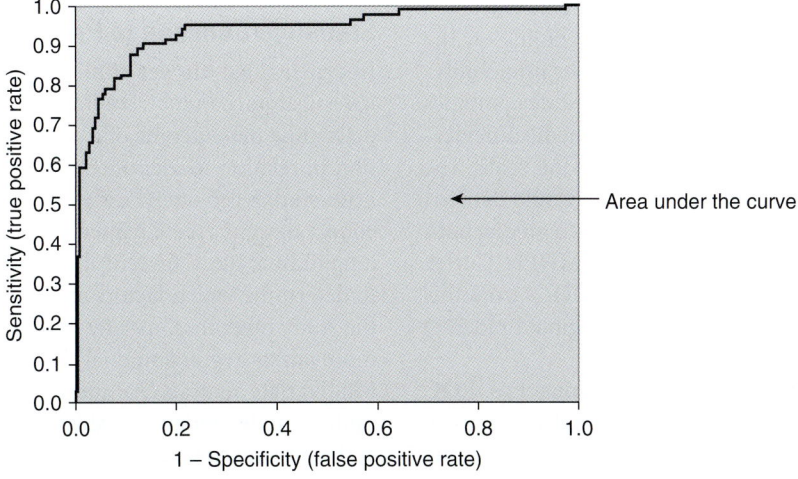

Fig. 13.7 The Area Under the ROC Curve (AUROC).

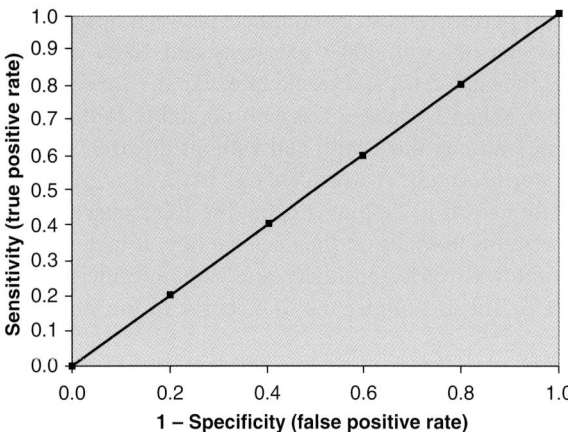

Fig. 13.9 The Area Under the ROC Curve (AUROC) for a Worthless Test.

TABLE 13.9 Guide for Interpreting the Area Under the ROC Curve (AUROC)

AUROC	Category
0.69–1.0	Very good
0.8–0.9	Good
0.7–0.8	Fair
0.6–0.7	Poor
0.5–0.6	Fail

ROC, Receiver Operating Characteristics.

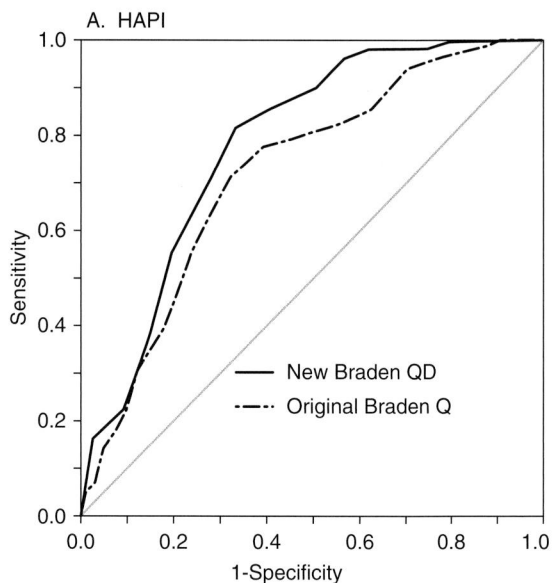

Fig. 13.10 AUROC Comparing Original Braden Q with Braden QD. *HAPI*, Hospital-Acquired Pressure Injuries. (From Curley et al. 2018.)

programs can calculate automatically the area under the ROC curve. Use the following guide in Table 13.9 when evaluating an ROC curve.

In a pediatric study designed to evaluate hospital-acquired pressure injury, investigators constructed a new tool, the Braden QD Scale, which builds on the Braden Q Scale that only measures risk for immobility-related pressure ulcers. The Braden QD Scale combines immobility-related pressure ulcer and medical device-related pressure injury (MDPI) risk in one scale. The authors' hypothesis was that a new scale would demonstrate sufficient sensitivity and specificity to predict both immobility-related pressure injuries and MDPIs (Curley et al., 2018). Fig. 13.10 is one of several ROCs from this study comparing the AUROC for the original Braden Q with the AUROC for the Braden QD.

You will note that the figure contains *two* ROC curves. In a diagnosis article, it is typical to compare the gold standard test with the new test. In this case, the original Braden Q is compared with the new Braden QD to predict hospital-acquired pressure injuries (HAPI). By examining the area under the curve (AUC), you can tell the scale with the greatest AUC (new Braden QD) has the greatest discrimination to predict pressure injuries. Table 13.10 provides the actual AUC data for this graph, along with many other variables. Here the study authors include confidence intervals for the data. When examining this data, be sure to check that the confidence intervals do not include the null value. If the null value is not included, the results are statistically significant.

Statistics Common to Prognosis Articles

In articles that answer clinical questions of prognosis, investigators conduct studies in which they want to determine the outcome of a particular disease or condition in relation to identified variables of interest. Prognosis studies can often be identified by their longitudinal cohort designs (see Chapter 9). At the conclusion of a longitudinal study, investigators statistically analyze data to determine which factors are strongly associated with the study outcomes, usually through a technique called multivariate regression analysis or multiple regression. Multivariate analysis examines the relationship between multiple independent variables on a dependent variable at the interval or ratio level of measurement. We will not examine the complex formulas and calculations used

TABLE 13.10 Comparing the AUC for Braden Q vs. Braden QD in the Overall Sample and Stratified by Enrollment Subgroups

Cohort	No. Subjects/Total	Braden Q AUC (95% CI)	Braden QD AUC (95% CI)
Overall—any HAPI	49/625	0.72 (0.65–0.79)	0.78 (0.73–0.84)
Any immobility-related pressure injury	14/625	0.78 (0.66–0.90)	0.86 (0.78–0.93)
Any MDPI[a]	42/625	—	0.78 (0.72–0.84)
Age category			
Preterm to < 1 month	7/109	0.61 (0.36–0.85)	0.65 (0.45–0.86)
1 month to 8 years	24/325	0.75 (0.65–0.84)	0.77 (0.69–0.86)
9 to 21 years	18/191	0.72 (0.61–0.83)	0.83 (0.77–0.90)
Diagnosis at admission			
Medical/surgical diagnosis	22/346	0.81 (0.74–0.87)	0.84 (0.76–0.91)
Cardiovascular diagnosis	27/279	0.67 (0.56–0.77)	0.73 (0.65–0.81)
Endotracheal intubation at enrollment[b]			
Intubated	33/193	0.64 (0.55–0.73)	0.64 (0.54–0.73)
Not intubated	16/432	0.66 (0.53–0.80)	0.77 (0.67–0.87)

[a]The Braden Q Scale was not designed to predict MDPIs; therefore, the AUC was not computed.
[b]AUC for each enrollment subgroup is reported for any HAPI development.
AUC, Area under the curve; *CI,* confidence interval; *HAPI,* hospital-acquired pressure injury; *MDPI,* medical device-related pressure injury.
From Curley et al., 2018.

to perform multivariate analysis; there are textbooks written on this subject alone and it is better left to an advanced statistics course or consultation.

Statistics Common to Meta-Analysis

A meta-analysis is a statistical analysis of pooled results from previous research studies. A meta-analysis is used to improve precision of previous research studies by providing more information through pooled results from multiple samples, to investigate the consistency of effect across studies using different populations, and to assess conflicts between studies with discrepant results. A methodologically sound meta-analysis is more likely than a single intervention study to be successful in identifying the true effect of an intervention because it limits bias. Most meta-analysis methods provide a weighted average of effect estimates of the included studies. Risk ratios or odds ratios are commonly reported statistics. Heterogeneity among the studies in the sample is explored often using a chi-squared statistical test.

The usual manner of displaying data in a meta-analysis is by a pictorial representation known as a forest plot (or *blobbogram*). Forest plots always list information about each study accompanied by a summary measure of effect size in relative risk, odds ratio, or mean difference. Let us see how a forest plot and effect size difference are used to summarize the studies in a meta-analysis on the use of aromatherapy on the sleep quality of registered nurses (Kang et al., 2020). See Fig. 13.11, which reports the mean difference in effect sizes of sleep quality scores in nurses that used aromatherapy as an intervention (experimental group) and those that did not use aromatherapy to sleep (control group). The most important information is contained in the figure at the right of the study. You see a vertical line that represents the null value; you now know that when the statistic is the odds ratio, the null value is "1." When the statistic is the mean difference, the null value is "0." The findings from each individual study are represented as a blob or square (the measured effect) on the vertical line, as a mean difference. Sometimes you also will note that each blob or square is a bit different in size. The size reflects the weight the study has on the overall analysis. This is determined by the sample size and the quality of the study. For this meta-analysis, all of the studies approximately have the same weight (observe column 8 in Fig. 13.11) so the squares appear to have the same size. The width of the horizontal line represents the 95%

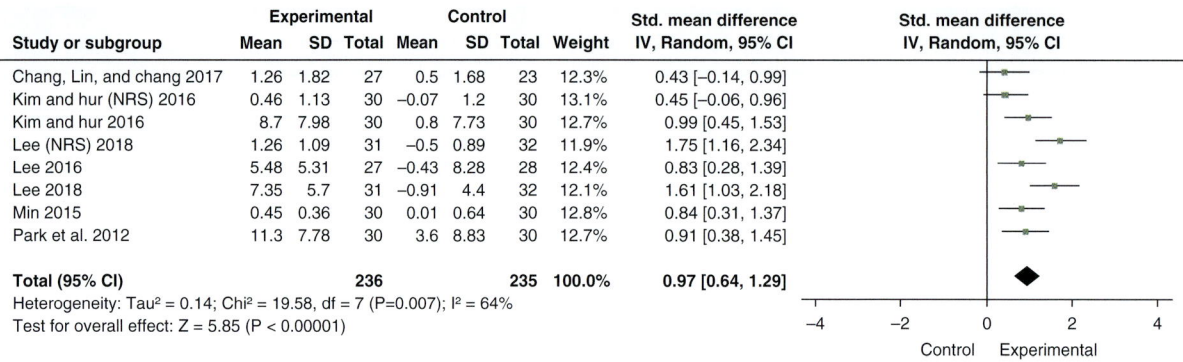

Fig 13.11 Forest Plot. (From Kang et al., 2020.)

confidence interval in the individual study. The vertical line is the line of no effect (i.e., the null value). When the confidence interval of the result (horizontal line) touches or crosses the line of no effect (vertical line), we can say that the study findings did not reach statistical significance. If the confidence interval does not cross the vertical line, we can say that the study results reached statistical significance. In the Kang et al. study, only two studies cross the line of no effect; all of the other studies are on one side of the null value favoring the experimental group.

You also will notice other important information and additional statistical analyses that may accompany the forest plot table, such as a test to determine whether the results of each of the individual trials are mathematically compatible (heterogeneity) and a test for overall effect. The reader is referred to a book of advanced research methods for discussion of these topics. There is a subtotal diamond for the study outcome statistically pooling the results of each of the controlled trials. Because the total diamond does not touch the line of no effect, the overall interpretation is that aromatherapy as an intervention improves the sleep quality in registered nurses.

IMPLICATIONS FOR PRACTICE SETTINGS

Nurses implementing EBP projects, QI initiatives, or a research project must understand the basics of descriptive and inferential statistical analysis to inform their work. Having fundamental knowledge of statistics commonly used in EBP projects helps the nurse synthesize and analyze evidence from practice. Although a nurse researcher is likely to collaborate with a biostatistician on the statistical analysis plan for a study, it is essential for the nurse to understand the analytical possibilities and limitations of the data in the design of the research project.

SYNTHESIS

Statistical analyses allow us to answer important questions about characteristics of populations, relationships between variables, and causative factors of conditions using scientifically rigorous methods. Statistical analysis is an integral element of any research study and other rigorous QI and EB evaluation processes. Whether you are critically appraising a research study or evaluating a QI or EBP project, the statistical analysis must align with the purpose of the study, research or clinical questions, research design, and data collection methods to achieve meaningful results. When you are designing or planning EB or QI projects, choosing the appropriate statistics is essential to project rigor and requires a deep appreciation of both descriptive and inferential methods. The specific statistic(s) you will encounter in your work will depend on the EB question you are trying to answer. The depth of detail you must know about EBP statistics depends on your role in evaluating a practice change or generating new knowledge. There are a variety of options for continued study of data analytical techniques including formal courses, online resources, and biostatistician consultation. Every nurse is encouraged to engage in the data of health and health care delivery to be fully prepared to improve the health outcomes of the populations we serve.

KEY POINTS

- A high-quality research study must have alignment among the research question(s), study design, study methods, and statistical analyses.
- Descriptive statistics are used to summarize, organize, and display a set of data. Inferential statistics are used to draw conclusions about a target population based on information obtained from a sample.
- It is appropriate to use less complex statistical analyses like descriptive statistics for quality improvement and EBP projects.
- The statistical analysis used will be driven by the research or project purpose, type and amount of data, and distribution of data.
- Data that normally is distributed utilizes parametric statistical tests, and data that is not normally distributed utilizes nonparametric statistical tests.
- Statistical analysis is an integral element of any research study and other rigorous QI and EB evaluation processes.

REFERENCES

Aschengrau, A., & Seage, G. R. (2020). *Essentials of epidemiology in public health*. Jones & Bartlett Learning, 237–266.

Capili, B., & Anastasi, J. K. (2023). Improving the validity of causal inferences in observational studies. *American Journal of Nursing*, *123*(1), 45–49. https://doi.org/10.1097/01.NAJ.0000911536.51764.47.

Curley, M. A. Q., Hasbani, N. R., Quigley, S. M., Stellar, J. J., Pasek, T. A., Shelley, S. S., et al. (2018). Predicting pressure injury risk in pediatric patients: The Braden QD scale. *Journal of Pediatrics*, *192*, 189–195.

Curtis, A. C., & Keeler, C. (2022). Diagnostic studies: Measures of accuracy in nursing research. *American Journal of Nursing*, *122*(6), 44–49. https://doi.org/10.1097/01.NAJ.0000833928.06431.8e.

Curtis, A. C., & Keeler, C. (2021). Measurement in nursing research. *American Journal of Nursing*, *121*(6), 56–60. https://doi.org/10.1097/01.NAJ.0000753668.78872.0f.

Ebrahimi, S., Paryad, E., Ghanbari Khanghah, A., Pasdaran, A., Kazemnezhad Leili, E., & Sadeghi Meibodi, A. M. (2022). The effects of lavandula aromatherapy on pain relief after coronary artery bypass graft surgery: A randomized clinical trial. *Applied Nursing Research*, *68*, 151638. https://doi.org/10.1016/j.apnr.2022.151638.

Frisse, A. C., Marrazzo, J. M., Tutlam, N. T., et al. (2017). Validity of self-reported history of *Chlamydia trachomatis* infection. *American Journal of Obstetrics and Gynecology*, *216*(4), 393.e1–393.e7. https://doi.org/10.1016/j.ajog.2016.12.005.

HEDIS. (n.d.). www.ncqa.or/hedis/measures/chlamydia-screening-in-women/.

Kang, J., Noh, W., & Lee, Y. (2020). Sleep quality among shift-work nurses: A systematic review and meta-analysis. *Applied Nursing Research*, *52*, 151227. https://doi.org/10.1016/j.apnr.2019.151227.

Keeler, C., & Colgrove, A. (2022). Case–control studies. *American Journal of Nursing*, *122*(2), 51–56. https://doi.org/10.1097/01.NAJ.0000820584.29051.80.

Kratovil, A., Schuler, M. S., Vottero, B. A., & Aryal, G. (2023). Original research: Nurses' self-assessed knowledge, attitudes, and educational needs regarding patients with substance use disorder. *American Journal of Nursing*, *123*(4), 26–33. https://doi.org/10.1097/01.NAJ.0000925496.18847.c6.

White, E. M., Aiken, L. H., & McHugh, M. D. (2019). Registered nurse burnout, job dissatisfaction, and missed care in nursing homes. *Journal of the American Geriatrics Society*, *67*(10), 2065–2071. https://doi.org/10.1111/jgs.16051.

PART III Implementation

14

Evidence-Based Approaches for Improving Health Care Quality

Maja Djukic, Mattia J. Gilmartin, and Marilyn Lopez

LEARNING OUTCOMES

After reading this chapter, you should be able to do the following:

- Discuss the clinical leader's role in health care quality improvement.
- Use national quality and safety resources, aims, priorities, and initiatives to lead team-based change initiatives.
- Evaluate the impact of context such as accreditation, payment, and public reporting systems on improvement efforts.
- Incorporate data-driven benchmarks to monitor and improve system performance and meet Quality Payment Program requirements.
- Differentiate the characteristics of the major quality improvement (QI) models used in healthcare.
- Analyze the steps of the improvement process and determine appropriate QI tools to use in each phase of the process.
- Analyze root causes of quality and safety problems to inform design of evidence-based improvement interventions.
- Implement evidence-based improvement strategies to optimize success and sustainability of QI interventions.
- Critically appraise a journal article reporting the results of a QI project using the SQUIRE guidelines.

KEY TERMS

Benchmarking
Cause and effect diagram
Clinical Microsystems
Common cause variation
Control chart
DMAIC improvement model
Fishbone diagram
Flowchart

High-reliability organizing/
  organization
Improvement cycle
Lean
Model for Improvement
Plan-Do-Study-Act
Public reporting
Quality healthcare
Quality improvement

Root cause analysis
Run chart
Six Sigma
Social determinants of health
Special cause variation
SQUIRE 2.0 guidelines
Total Quality Management/
  Continuous Quality
  Improvement

QUALITY IMPROVEMENT IN HEALTHCARE

The Institute of Medicine (IOM, 2001), now called the National Academy of Medicine, defines **quality healthcare** as care that is safe, effective, patient-centered, timely, efficient, and equitable (Box 14.1). The quality of the health care system was brought to the forefront of national attention in several important

> **BOX 14.1 Six Dimensions and Definitions of Health Care Quality**
>
> 1. **Safe:** avoiding injuries to patients from care that is intended to help them
> 2. **Effective:** providing services based on scientific knowledge to all who could benefit and refraining from providing services to those not likely to benefit
> 3. **Patient-centered:** providing care that is respectful of and responsive to individual patient preferences, needs, and values, and ensuring that patient values guide all clinical decisions
> 4. **Timely:** reducing waits and sometimes harmful delays for both those who receive and those who give care
> 5. **Efficient:** avoiding waste, including waste of equipment, supplies, ideas, and energy
> 6. **Equitable:** providing care that does not vary in quality because of personal characteristics such as gender, ethnicity, geographical location, and socioeconomic status
>
> From Institute of Medicine (2001).

reports (IOM, 1999, 2001), including *Crossing the Quality Chasm*, which concluded that "between the health care we have and the care we could have lies not just a gap, but a chasm" (IOM, 2001, p. 1). The report notes that "the performance of the health care system varies considerably. It may be exemplary, but often is not, and millions of Americans fail to receive effective care" (IOM, 2001, p. 3).

Since the IOM (2001) report was published, quality of care has improved for some conditions, but not for others (Dzau & Shine, 2020). For example, between 2000 and 2022, breast cancer deaths decreased by 28.7%, colorectal cancer deaths decreased by 37.5%, and deaths from HIV/AIDS decreased by 57.7% (Agency for Healthcare Research and Quality [AHRQ], 2022). On the other hand, maternal health, child and adolescent mental health, substance use disorders, and oral health quality have all worsened (AHRQ, 2022). For example, overall maternal mortality rate increased from 17.4 deaths per 100,000 live births in 2018 to 23.8 deaths per 100,000 live births in 2019; the rate of death from suicide among adolescents ages 12 to 17 increased by 70.3% between 2008 and 2020, rising from 3.7 to 6.3 deaths per 100,000 population; and overall rates of overdose deaths involving any opioid increased by 36.8% between 2019 and 2020, rising from 15.2 to 20.8 deaths per 100,000 population in 1 year (AHRQ, 2022). Furthermore, disparities in quality based on earnings, race/ethnicity, and geography continue to persist. For example, "in 2020, the percentage of individuals with a live birth in the last 12 months who received early and adequate prenatal care was lower for Hispanic (69.5%), non-Hispanic (American Indian/Alaska Native) (59.1%), non-Hispanic Asian (76.5%), non-Hispanic Black (67.3%), and non-Hispanic Native Hawaiian/Pacific Islander (47.1%) individuals than for non-Hispanic White individuals (79.6%)"; the care was also "lower for individuals in large central metro areas (71.9%) compared with individuals in large fringe metro areas (75.9%)" (AHRQ, 2022, p. 58). Despite these quality issues, the United States spends much more on healthcare (16.8% of gross domestic product) compared with other developed nations, but ranks last in health care quality in comparison with 10 other countries (Schneider et al., 2021).

The purpose of this chapter is to introduce you to the principles of **quality improvement** (QI) and provide examples of how to apply these principles in your practice so you can effectively contribute to needed health care improvements. QI "uses data to monitor the outcomes of care processes and improvement methods to design and test changes to continuously improve the quality and safety of health care systems" (Cronenwett et al., 2007, p. 127).

THE CLINICAL LEADER'S ROLE IN HEALTH CARE QUALITY IMPROVEMENT

Florence Nightingale championed QI by systematically documenting high rates of morbidity and mortality resulting from poor sanitary conditions among soldiers serving in the Crimean War of 1854 (McDonald, 2017). She used statistics to document changes in soldiers' health, including reductions in mortality resulting from a number of nursing interventions such as hand hygiene, instrument sterilization, changing bed linens, ward sanitation, ventilation, and proper nutrition (McDonald, 2017). Today, clinical leaders are vital to health system improvement efforts. One main initiative developed to bolster graduate nurses' education in health system improvements is the Quality and Safety Education for Nurses (QSEN) project (Pohl et al., 2009; Altmiller & Hopkins-Pepe, 2019). The overall goal of this project is to support the development of advanced practice nurses' competence in the areas of QI, patient-centered care, teamwork and collaboration, patient safety, informatics, and evidence-based practice (EBP). Other initiatives such as the Care Innovation and Transformation

BOX 14.2 National Quality Aims and Priorities

National Quality Aims	National Quality Priorities for Achieving the Aims
• **Better Care:** Improve the overall quality of care by making healthcare more patient-centered, reliable, accessible, and safe. • **Healthy People/Healthy Communities:** Improve the health of the U.S. population by supporting proven interventions to address behavioral, social, and environmental determinants of health in addition to delivering higher-quality care. • **Affordable Care:** Reduce the cost of quality healthcare for individuals, families, employers, and government.	• Make care safer by reducing harm caused in the delivery of care. • Ensure each person and family is engaged as a partner in their care. • Promote effective communication and care coordination. • Promote the most effective prevention and treatment practices for the leading causes of mortality, starting with cardiovascular disease. • Work with communities to promote wide use of best practices to enable healthy living. • Make quality care more affordable for individuals, families, employers, and governments by developing and sharing new health care delivery models.

From Agency for Healthcare Research and Quality (2017b).

Program (American Organization of Nurse Executives, n.d., https://www.aonl.org/education/cit) have been developed to increase engagement in QI. To influence improvements in the work setting effectively and ensure that all patients consistently receive excellent care, it is important to do the following:

- Align national, organizational, and unit level goals for QI
- Recognize external drivers of quality such as accreditation, payment, and performance measurement
- Develop skills to apply QI models and tools

NATIONAL GOALS AND STRATEGIES FOR HEALTH CARE QUALITY IMPROVEMENT

The National Quality Strategy was established by the Affordable Care Act and published in 2011 to pursue the triple health care improvement aims of better care, affordable care, and healthy people/healthy communities (AHRQ, 2017b). National goals focusing on improving quality and safety have evolved over time. For example, the Institute for Healthcare Improvement set forth the quadruple aim that includes population health, the experience of care, reducing the overall costs of care, and reducing clinician burnout (IHI, 2017). In 2022, the Centers for Medicare and Medicaid Services (CMS) announced a new national quality strategy to guide improvement across the health care system (Box 14.2). Achieving these national quality targets requires a major redesign of the health care system. One way you, as a clinical leader, can contribute to this redesign is to familiarize yourself with national priorities, corresponding improvement goals, and national initiatives (Table 14.1), and use them to guide improvements in your work setting.

QUALITY STRATEGY LEVERS

QI relies on aligning institutional priorities with several strategy levers that drive it. The National Quality Strategy encourages all members of the health care community, including individuals, family members, payers, providers, and employers, to collaborate in using one or more of the nine strategy levers (AHRQ, 2017b). We describe briefly how each lever is used for QI:

- **Measurement and feedback:** Provide performance feedback to plans and providers to improve care. National health care performance standards are developed using a consensus process in which stakeholder groups representing the interests of the public, health professionals, payers, employers, and government identify priorities, measures, and reporting requirements to document and manage the quality of care (National Quality Forum [NQF], 2004). See Box 14.3 for examples of groups responsible for developing measurement standards.
- **Public reporting:** Compare treatment results, costs, and patient experiences. Several major public reporting systems are described in Box 14.4.
- **Learning and technical assistance:** Foster learning environments that offer training, resources, tools,

TABLE 14.1 The Centers for Medicare and Medicaid Services (CMS) National Quality Strategy

Launched in 2022, the CMS National Quality Strategy is an ambitious long-term initiative that aims to promote the highest quality outcomes and safest care for all individuals. The CMS National Quality Strategy focuses on a person-centric approach from birth to end of life across setting of care and payors including Traditional Medicare, Medicare Advantage, Medicaid and Children's Health Insurance Program (CHIP), and Marketplace coverage. The Eight Goals of the CMS National Quality Strategy are Organized into Four Priority Areas:

Priority Area	Description
1. Outcomes and Alignment	Outcomes: Improve quality and health outcomes across the care journey Alignment: Align and coordinate across programs and care settings
2. Equity and Engagement	Equity: Advance health equity and whole person care Engagement: Engage individuals and communities to become partners in their care
3. Safety and Resiliency	Safety: Achieve zero preventable harm Resiliency: Enable a responsive and resilient health care system to improve quality
4. Interoperability and Scientific Advancement	Interoperability: Accelerate and support the transition to a digital and data-driven health care system Scientific Advancement: Transform healthcare using science, analytics, and technology

Data from https://www.cms.gov/Medicare/Quality-Initiatives-Patient-Assessment-Instruments/Value-Based-Programs/CMS-Quality-Strategy

---

BOX 14.3 Performance Measurement Standard Setting Groups

Introduction to Performance Measurement Standards

The National Quality Forum (NQF) is a nonprofit organization that seeks to measure and improve the quality of healthcare in the United States by establishing national health care quality and safety goals and priorities. The NQF's evidence-based measure endorsement process is the gold standard for health care quality measurement. The NQF endorsement process is a transparent, consensus-based model that brings together stakeholders from the private and public sectors to foster quality improvement. Approximately 300 NQF-endorsed measures are used by federal public and private pay-for-performance programs and in private-sector and state health care quality programs (National Quality Forum, 2023).

The Agency for Healthcare Research and Quality (AHRQ) Quality Indicators are standardized, evidence-based measures of the quality of hospital care that are readily available using hospital administrative data. There are 101 Quality Indicators organized into four main categories: inpatient quality for adult and pediatric patients; preventive quality indicators for ambulatory care; and avoidable complications. Approximately half of the AHRQ Quality Indicators are endorsed by the National Quality Forum and are used to support hospital quality improvement, health system planning, and pay for performance initiatives (Agency for Healthcare Research and Quality, n.d.).

---

and guidance to help organizations achieve QI goals.
- **Certification, accreditation, and regulation:** Adopt or adhere to approaches to meet safety and quality standards. Several accrediting bodies are listed in Box 14.5.
- **Consumer incentives and benefit designs:** Help consumers adopt healthy behaviors and make informed decisions.
- **Payment:** Incentivize and reward providers who deliver high-quality care that is designed to meet the specific health care needs of individuals and

BOX 14.4 Public Reporting Systems

- **Hospital Compare** allows consumers to compare information on hospitals. The database includes performance measures on timely and efficient care; readmissions and deaths; complications; use of medical imaging; survey of patients' experiences; and payment and value of care. For more information, visit https://www.medicare.gov/care-compare/?redirect=true&providerType=Hospital
- **Nursing Home Compare** allows consumers to compare information about nursing homes. It contains quality of care information on every Medicare and Medicaid-certified nursing homes in the nation. The database includes performance measures on health inspections, staffing, and clinical quality. For more information, visit https://www.medicare.gov/care-compare/?redirect=true&providerType=NursingHome
- **Home Health Compare** has information about the quality of care provided by Medicare-certified home health agencies that meet federal health and safety requirements throughout the nation. For more information, visit https://www.medicare.gov/care-compare/?guidedSearch=HomeHealth&providerType=HomeHealth
- **Hospital Consumer Assessment of Healthcare Providers and Systems (HCAHPS)** is developed by the Agency for Healthcare Research and Quality, and is a standardized survey and data collection method for measuring patients' perspectives on hospital care. The HCAHPS survey contains 32 questions about patient perspectives on care for eight key topics: communication with doctors, communication with nurses, responsiveness of hospital staff, pain management, communication about medicines, discharge information, cleanliness of the hospital environment and quietness of the hospital environment, post-hospital transitions, admissions through the emergency room, and mental and emotional health. HCAHPS performance is used to calculate incentive payments in the Hospital Value-Based Purchasing program for hospital discharges beginning in October 2012. For more information, visit https://www.cms.gov/Medicare/Quality-Initiatives-Patient-Assessment-Instruments/HospitalQualityInits/HospitalHCAHPS
- **Physician Quality Reporting Initiative** is a program administered by CMS that collects performance data at the physician/provider clinical level in the ambulatory and primary care sectors. For more information, visit https://www.cms.gov/medicare/quality-initiatives-patient-assessment-instruments/pqrs/downloads/pqrs_overviewfactsheet_2013_08_06.pdf
- **The Leapfrog Group** is an initiative of organizations that buy healthcare and are working to improve the safety, quality, and affordability of healthcare for Americans. The Leapfrog Group conducts a survey to compare hospitals' performance on the national standards of safety, quality, and efficiency that are most relevant to consumers and purchasers of care. For more information, visit https://www.leapfroggroup.org/
- *U.S. News & World Report.* Annual honor role of America's best hospitals helps guide patients, in consultation with their doctors, to the right hospital when they need care. Because each patient's needs are different, *U.S. News* offers rankings and ratings in three dozen different health care services. In each state and region, hospitals with a wide breadth of excellence are recognized as Best Regional Hospitals, and the best of them are also named to the national Honor Roll. For more information visit https://health.usnews.com/health-care/best-hospitals/articles/best-hospitals-honor-roll-and-overview

populations. Box 14.6 shows examples of payment incentives.
- **Health information technology:** Improve communications, transparency, and efficiency for better coordinated health and healthcare.
- **Innovation and diffusion:** Foster innovation in health care QI and facilitate rapid adoption within and across organizations and communities.
- **Workforce development:** Invest in people to prepare the next generation of health care professionals to bring about changes in health care quality and support lifelong learning for providers.

In addition to the listed quality strategy levers, CMS (2023), in their National Quality Strategy, highlighted the importance of advancing health equity to improve health care quality by focusing on **social determinants of health** (SDOH). SDOH include: education access and quality, health care access and quality, economic stability, neighborhood and built environment, and social and community context, for which health care delivery systems and providers need to account for in care delivery to mitigate health disparities and improve health care quality (Dzau et al., 2022; Office of Disease Prevention and Promotion, n.d.).

> **BOX 14.5 QI Accrediting Organizations**
>
> - **Joint Commission:** Responsible for ensuring a minimum standard of structures, processes, and outcomes for patient care. Accreditation by the Joint Commission is voluntary, but it is required to receive reimbursement for patient care services. For more information, see: www.jointcommission.org/
> - **National Committee for Quality Assurance Accreditation for Health Plans (NCQA):** A private not-for-profit organization dedicated to improving health care quality. The NCQA is responsible for accrediting health insurance programs. Accredited health insurance programs are exempt from many or all elements associated with annual state audits. The NCQA developed and maintains the Healthcare Effectiveness Data and Information Set (HEDIS). For more information, see: https://www.ncqa.org
> - **Healthcare Effectiveness Data and Information Set (HEDIS):** A tool used by the majority of America's health plans to measure performance on important dimensions of care and service. HEDIS allows for comparison of performance across health plans. For more information, see: http://www.ncqa.org/Programs/Accreditation/HealthPlanHP.aspx and http://www.ncqa.org/HEDISQualityMeasurement.aspx
> - **American Nurses' Credentialing Center Magnet Recognition and Pathway to Excellence Recognition Programs**: A voluntary program that recognizes health care organizations that provide the very best in nursing care and uphold the tradition of professional nursing practice. For more information, see: https://www.nursingworld.org/organizational-programs/

Measuring Health Care Quality

In alignment with the National Quality Aims for better care, better health, and lower costs, the Medicare program has initiated several value-based programs (e.g., Alternative Payment Models, Merit-Based Incentive Payment System, Hospital Value-Based Purchasing Program) to reward providers for the quality of care rather than the quantity of care they give to patients (CMS, 2022). As part of the value-based payment model, Medicare provides incentive payments to clinicians, hospitals, nursing homes, and home health agencies based on how well they perform on each measure or how much they improve their scores on quality measures compared with baseline performance. Therefore, as an advanced practice nurse or clinical leader, you are responsible for knowing which quality measures apply to your practice setting so you can ensure that the care you provide meets appropriate quality standards.

For example, if you are a clinician participating in Medicare Part B, you will be paid for your services through Medicare's Quality Payment Program (CMS, n.d.), the result of the Medicare Access and CHIP Reauthorization Act (MACRA) of 2015. For examples of measures that are part of Medicare's Quality Payment Program see Table 14.2.

> **TIP**
>
> To identify measures that best apply to your practice and that you can report to the Quality Payment Program, visit https://qpp.cms.gov/mips/quality-requirements. Select your specialty practice area and identify the level of reporting priority for the measures to prioritize your improvement efforts.

Benchmarking

Measurement of quality indicators must be done methodically using standardized tools. Standardized measurement allows for **benchmarking**. Benchmarking is the process of comparing the performance of one organization's performance with an external standard. Benchmarking is an important tool for managers and clinical leaders to motivate others to engage in improvement work and to help members of an organization understand where their performance falls in comparison to others (AHRQ, 2018).

Benchmarking is critical for QI because it helps identify when performance is below an agreed-upon standard, and it signals the need for improvement. For example, when you track a patient population's performance on standard measures defined by Healthcare Effectiveness Data and Information Set (HEDIS), such as pneumococcal vaccine coverage for older adults or breast cancer screening, it allows for comparison of your performance to those of providers in other organizations who care for similar patient populations and use the same measures to document provided care. Tracking changes in overall performance on quality measures over time allows you to intervene if the score falls below a set standard. Equally, after you implement

> **BOX 14.6 Financial Incentives to Promote Quality in the Health Care Sector**
>
> **Capitation:** A payment arrangement for health care services. Pays a provider (physician or nurse practitioner) or provider group a set amount for each enrolled person assigned to them, per period of time, whether or not that person seeks care. These providers generally are contracted with a type of health maintenance organization (HMO). Payment levels are based on average expected health care use of a particular patient, with greater payment for patients with significant medical histories (American Medical Association, 2022).
>
> **Bundled Payments Initiative:** Links payments for multiple services that patients receive during an episode of care. Payments seek to align incentives for hospitals, post-acute care providers, doctors, and other practitioners to improve the patient's care experience during a hospital stay in an acute care hospital through post-discharge recovery.
>
> **Pay for Performance:** An emerging movement in health insurance where providers are rewarded for meeting pre-established targets for health care delivery services. This model rewards physicians, hospitals, medical groups, and other health care providers for meeting certain performance measures for quality and efficiency.
>
> **Value-Based Health Care Purchasing:** A project of participating health plans, including the Centers for Medicare and Medicaid Services (CMS), where buyers hold providers of healthcare accountable for both cost and quality of care. Value-based purchasing brings together information on health care quality, patient outcomes, and health status, with data on dollar outlays going toward health. The focus is on managing health care system use to reduce inappropriate care and to identify and reward the best-performing providers.
>
> **Accountable Care Organization (ACO):** A payment and care delivery model that seeks to tie provider reimbursements to quality metrics and reductions in the total cost of care for an assigned population of Medicare beneficiaries enrolled in the traditional fee-for-service program. A group of coordinated health care providers forms an ACO, which then provides care to a group of patients. The ACO may use a range of payment models (e.g., capitation, fee-for-service). The ACO is accountable to patients and the third-party payer for the quality, appropriateness, and efficiency of the healthcare provided (Shartzer et al., 2021).

needed interventions focused on improving vaccination or cancer screening coverage in your patient population, you can track changes in those measures to determine whether the interventions were effective or not. Therefore, standardized measurement can tell you when changes in care are needed and whether the interventions that have been implemented resulted in actual improvement of patient outcomes.

When organizations document care in a uniform manner, it is possible to compare patient outcomes across units. These performance data are useful for benchmarking efforts where clinical teams learn from each other how to apply best practices from high-performing practices to the care processes of lower-performing practices. To support the validity of benchmarking, it is essential to ensure that the numerator and denominator for a specific quality measure are defined and measured in the same manner across time and among different clinical units. (AHRQ, 2018). For example, when you are trying to understand what percentage of the patients in your practice with a diabetes diagnosis have hemoglobin A1C (HgA1C) values above 8, the numerator should include all patients who have HgA1C values greater than 8 and a diabetes diagnosis, and the denominator should include all patients diagnosed with diabetes with available HgA1C levels. If you include patients with diabetes who do not have HgA1C values available in your denominator, your measure of the percentage of patients with elevated HgA1C levels will be falsely deflated. To see how your organization's performance compares to others on important quality measures, visit one of the **public reporting** system sites outlined in Box 14.4.

COMMON QUALITY IMPROVEMENT PERSPECTIVES AND MODELS

QI as a management model is both a philosophy of organizational functioning and a set of statistical analysis tools and change techniques to reduce variations in the quality of goods or services that an organization produces (Nelson et al., 2007). The QI model emphasizes customer satisfaction, teams and teamwork, and the continuous improvement of work processes (Box 14.7). Other defining features of QI include a proactive leadership style at all levels to set performance goals and expectations, use

TABLE 14.2 The Quality Payment Program 2023 Cross-Cutting Quality Measures

Measure Title and Description	Measure Type	Measure Steward
Advance Care Plan: Percentage of patients aged 65 years and older who have an advance care plan or surrogate decision maker documented in the medical record or documentation in the medical record that an advance care plan was discussed but the patient did not wish or was not able to name a surrogate decision maker or provide an advance care plan.	Process	National Committee for Quality Assurance
Preventive Care and Screening: Body Mass Index (BMI) Screening and Follow-Up Plan: Percentage of patients aged 18 years and older with a BMI documented during the current encounter or during the performance period AND who had a follow-up plan documented if most recent BMI was outside of normal parameters.	Process	Centers for Medicare & Medicaid Services
Documentation of Current Medications in the Medical Record: Percentage of visits for patients aged 18 years and older for which the eligible clinician attests to documenting a list of current medications using all immediate resources available on the date of the encounter.	Process	Centers for Medicare & Medicaid Services
Preventive Care and Screening: Tobacco Use: Screening and Cessation Intervention: Percentage of patients aged 18 years and older who were screened for tobacco use one or more times within the measurement period AND who received tobacco cessation intervention on the date of the encounter or within the previous 12 months if identified as a tobacco user.	Process	National Committee for Quality Assurance
Controlling High Blood Pressure: Percentage of patients 18–85 years of age who had a diagnosis of essential hypertension starting before and continuing into, or starting during the first 6 months of the measurement period, and whose most recent blood pressure was adequately controlled (< 140/90 mmHg) during the measurement period.	Intermediate Outcome	National Committee for Quality Assurance
Preventive Care and Screening: Screening for High Blood Pressure and Follow-Up Documented: Percentage of patient visits for patients aged 18 years and older seen during the measurement period who were screened for high blood pressure AND a recommended follow-up plan is documented, as indicated, if blood pressure is elevated or hypertensive.	Process	Centers for Medicare & Medicaid Services
Screening for Social Drivers of Health: Percentage of patients aged 18 years and older screened for food insecurity, housing instability, transportation needs, utility difficulties, and interpersonal safety.	Process	Centers for Medicare & Medicaid Services

From the Quality Payment Program website: https://qpp.cms.gov/mips/explore-measures?tab=qualityMeasures&py=2023

of data to make decisions, and standardization of work processes to reduce variation across providers and service encounters (Nelson et al., 2007). The key principles associated with QI are shown in Table 14.3.

Although QI has its roots in the manufacturing sector, many of the ideas, tools, and techniques used to measure and manage quality have been applied in health care organizations to improve clinical outcomes and reduce waste (McConnell et al., 2016). The major QI models used in healthcare include the following:

- **Total Quality Management/Continuous Quality Improvement** (TQM/CQI)
- **Six Sigma**
- **Lean**
- **Clinical Microsystems Model**
- **High Reliability Organizing/Organizations** (HRO)

The key characteristics of each of these models are described in Table 14.4. Because QI uses a holistic approach, leaders often select one quality model that is used to guide the organization's overarching improvement agenda.

It is important to note that health care organizations have adopted principles and practices associated with the industrial QI approach relatively recently. Historically,

BOX 14.7 DNP Practice Improvement Example

Medication Fall Safety in the Older Hospitalized Adult: A Case Study in Excellence

Background

Falls are the leading causes of injury and death in older adults and associated with a health care cost of approximately $31 billion each year in the United States (Moreland et. al., 2020; Burns et al., 2016). High reliability organization (HRO) principles used with interdisciplinary unit-based huddles help identify issues and examine processes to detect root causes and develop solutions to minimize risk of hospital acquired conditions (Cantu et al., 2021; The Joint Commission, 2019; IHI, 2017). Registered nurses (RNs) play a key role in reducing patients' fall risk by identifying common medications associated with increased fall risk (Haddad et al., 2018). Based on analyses of an academic medical center's internal data, National Database of Nursing Quality Indicators fall data, fall case reviews, and consensus from key stakeholders, it was decided to launch a quality improvement (QI) initiative to reduce medication-related fall risks and prevention strategies.

Step 1: Assessment

The QI project was launched to help decrease falls and improve patient satisfaction with communication about medication fall safety in hospitalized adults 65 years and older. The Plan-Do-Study-Act (PDSA) method assessed the impact of nurses' confidence with teach-back utilizing the patient and family medication fall safety measures guide (Reed and Card, 2016; Knudsen et al., 2019). Short PDSA cycles allowed for revisions to project and intervention modifications as needed (Coury et al., 2017). The PICOT question for this team QI project:

PICOT Question:

P-In hospitalized older adults 65 years and older,
I-how effective is receiving care from nurses that have received training on medication fall safety,
C-as compared to current standard fall education,
O-to improve communication about medication satisfaction on a medicine inpatient care unit,
T- from admission to discharge.

Improvement Step 2: Analysis

An extensive literature search was conducted to identify recent studies that explored the effects of nursing medication safety interventions in older adults. A root-cause analysis with medication-related fall case reviews provides high reliability teams an understanding of current state processes and opportunities to targeted solutions and standardize practice (Hibbert et. al., 2018). Nurses had opportunities to collaborate with team experts to detect, prevent, and improve safety. Therefore, creating the right environment and identifying gaps help nurses develop grit to learn and how to improve and integrate new knowledge.

Improvement Step 3: Develop a Plan for Improvement

This QI project incorporated evidence-based practice (EBP) guidelines and an eLearning module to address educational gaps that include current state, desired state, and learning outcomes in recognizing and mitigating medication fall risks and prevention strategies (Lopez et al., 2023). The plan for improvement also included developing and implementing materials around medication fall prevention strategies for older patients and their families to be used on HRO rounds and during medication fall safety teach-back.

The eLearning content was created with evidence-based guidelines, geriatric resource nurse champions, advanced practice nurses, pharmacy, and patient and family education team (Lopez, 2019). Patient education health literacy specialists were instrumental to assure educational materials and resources to incorporate plain language principles into oral and text-based for patients and families (Coleman, 2020). Moreover, clear communication skills on HRO rounds to improve nurses' confidence in caring for patients. Lastly, they evaluated strategies for medication fall safety prevention in a patient's plan of care (Yen & Leasure, 2019).

A patient medication fall safety prevention measures guide was adapted from national guidelines with the teach-back method (Montero-Odasso et al., 2022; 2019 Beers Criteria, 2019). A plain language guide created easy-to-understand concepts for all patients. It is important to minimize the risk that an individual patient will not understand the information provided to them (AHRQ, 2021). Additionally, a nurse medication fall risk resource guide was developed with common medication-related fall categories and side effects in keeping with a health literate friendly approach utilized on HRO team rounds to facilitate team medication fall safety communication.

Improvement Step 4: PDSA Method to Test and Implement the Improvement Plan

Data collection involved PDSA cycles process improvement techniques in real time. This also allowed us to act

Continued

BOX 14.7 DNP Practice Improvement Example—cont'd

on nurse feedback and tweak the educational materials in continuous small tests of change. The PDSA method was used to assess the impact of nurses' confidence with teach-back utilizing the patient and family medication fall safety measures guide.

HRO Concepts Applied at the Bedside by RNs[1]
1. Culture of safety
   - Reports a fall without fear.
   - Assess risk fall factors with EBP tools.
   - Reconciliation of current medications and adjustment with team experts.
   - Communicates and determines interventions for post fall on team rounds and handoffs.
2. Patient safety interventions
   - Incorporates preventive interventions into daily existing workflow.
   - Identifies EBP with fall early prevention & management.
   - Ensures patient and family teach-back on medication fall safety measures.
3. Training and learning opportunities
   - Implements specific EBP tools into plan of care to address early prevention & new change management (e.g., UB-CAM, Beer Criteria Guidelines, Morse Fall Risk Scale & Braden Scale for Predicting Pressure Ulcer Risk [Husser et al., 2021; AGS, 2020 & 2019; Fick et al, 2022 & 2015; Morse, l997; Braden & Bergstrom, 1994]).
   - Conducts safety rounds with other staff nurses and team experts to provide new understanding of EBP tools use in complex inpatient case.
4. Developing leadership
   - Geriatric resource nurse to other staff nurses.
   - Participants in unit team HRO and safety huddles post falls.
   - Member of root cause analysis and fall prevention committees.
5. Data systems/fall event report
   - Collects daily fall data and enter in Patient Safety Indicator organizational software reporting system to provide information on potentially avoidable safety events that represent opportunities for improvement in delivery of care.
   - Reviews falls and injurious falls unit rate trends with team experts.

Results
Ninety-one percent of RNs completed the module and improvement was noted with nurses' knowledge on medication fall risks and reported confidence using new teach-back guide from a low of 50% to 83%. Medication patient satisfaction increased to 63.8% (Unit #1) and 65.0% (Unit #2). Case reviews showed an 8% reduction in fall counts with patients at a higher risk. Also, an increase overall (2.2%) in patient satisfaction scores.

Implications for Clinical Practice and Sustainability
As frontline advance practice nurse (APN) responders to recent COVID surge challenges, the momentum of integrating complex pharmacotherapeutics into new care practices continues to have a stronger sense of priorities and purpose with medication fall safety and prevention. The APN leader role in nurse educational training initiatives is essential to meet the unique needs of our vulnerable older adults. Furthermore, aligning organizational priorities with numerous departments is important in the success of leading QI HRO teams.

To this end, utilizing HRO principles and PDSA cycles is an effective way to generate change and increase nurses' confidence with teach-back overtime to improve patient satisfaction scores. This QI project provided a team and family-centered approach to medication falls risks and needed prevention strategies. Furthermore, it is necessary to create partnerships with team experts and families to promote clinically effective evidence-based quality care utilizing a patient-centric approach to medication fall risk safety, satisfaction, and cost.

[1] Adapted from Quigley & White (2013).
Box, generally, adapted from Lopez et al. (2023).

the quality of healthcare was assessed retrospectively using the quality assurance (QA) model. The QA model uses chart audits to compare care against a predetermined standard. Corrective actions associated with QA focus on assigning individual blame and correcting deficiencies in operations. Another model commonly associated with health care QI is the Structure-Process-Outcome Framework (Donabedian, 1966/2005). This framework is used to examine the resources that make up health care delivery services, clinicians' work

TABLE 14.3 Principles of Quality Improvement

Improvement Principle	Key Benefits
• Principle 1—Customer focus/patient focus 　• Health care organizations rely on patients and therefore should understand current and future patient needs, meet patient requirements, and strive to exceed patient expectations.	• Increased customer value • Increased revenue and market share obtained through flexible and fast responses to market opportunities • Increased effectiveness in the organization's resources used to enhance patient satisfaction • Improved patient loyalty leading to repeat business
• Principle 2—Leadership 　• Leaders establish unity of purpose and the organization's direction should create and maintain an internal environment in which people can become fully involved in the organization's achievement of objectives.	• People understand and are motivated by the organization's goals and objectives • Activities are evaluated, aligned, and implemented in a unified way • Miscommunication between organization levels is minimized
• Principle 3—Engagement of people 　• People at all levels are the essence of an organization and are essential to enhancing organizational capability to create and deliver value.	• Motivated, committed, and involved people within the organization • Innovation and creativity further the organization's objectives • People are accountable for their own performance • Enhanced involvement of people in improvement activities
• Principle 4—Process approach 　• Consistent results are achieved more efficiently and effectively when activities are understood and managed as a system of interrelated processes.	• Lower costs and shorter cycle times through effective use of resources • Improved, more consistent, and predictable results through a system of aligned processes • Focused and prioritized improvement opportunities
• Principle 5—Improvement 　• Successful organizations have an ongoing focus on improvement. Continual improvement is essential in creating new opportunities.	• Performance advantage through improved organizational capabilities • Focus on root cause analysis, followed by prevention and corrective action • Consideration of incremental and breakthrough improvements
• Principle 6—Evidence-based decision making 　• Effective decisions based on the analysis and evaluation of data and information are more likely to produce desired results.	• Improved decision-making processes • Increased ability to demonstrate effectiveness of past decisions • Increased ability to review, challenge, and change opinions and decisions
• Principle 7—Relationship management • An organization and its suppliers are interdependent, and a mutually beneficial relationship enhances the ability of both to create value.	• Increased capability to create value for both parties by sharing resources and managing quality-related risks • A well-managed supply chain that provides a stable flow of goods and services • Optimization of costs and resources

ISO. This material is reproduced from ISO Quality Management Principles with permission of the American National Standards Institute (ANSI) on behalf of the International Organization for Standardization.

TABLE 14.4 Overview of Quality Improvement Models Used in Healthcare

Model	Main Characteristics	Related Resources
TQM/CQI (Langley et al., 2009)	• A holistic management approach used to improve organizational performance • Seeks to understand and manage variation in service delivery • Emphasizes customer satisfaction as an important performance measure • Relies on teamwork and collaboration among workers to deliver technically excellent and customer/patient-centered services • Quality management science uses tools and techniques from statistics, engineering, operations research, management, market research, and psychology • TQM/CQI tools and techniques are applied to specific performance problems in the form of improvement projects • The extent to which unit-level QI projects align with larger organizational quality goals is related to their success and sustainability	Institute for Healthcare Improvement Quality Improvement Tools: https://www.ihi.org/resources/tools/quality-improvement-essentials-toolkit
Six Sigma (Henrique & Godinho Filho, 2020)	• Developed at Motorola in the 1980s • Takes its name from the statistical notation of sigma (σ) used to measure variation from the mean • Emphasizes meeting customer requirements and eliminating errors or reworking with the goal of reducing process variation • Focuses on tightly controlling variations in production processes with the goal of reducing the number of defects to 3.4 units per 1 million units produced • Process control achieved by applying **DMAIC improvement model** • DMAIC includes: defining, measuring, analyzing, improving, and controlling • Practitioners achieve mastery levels using statistical tools to measure and manage process variation (e.g., yellow belt, green belt, black belt)	Agency for Healthcare Research and Quality (AHRQ): https://www.ahrq.gov/cahps/quality-improvement/improvement-guide/4-approach-qi-process/sect4part2.html
Lean (Ahn et al., 2021)	• Sometimes referred to as the Toyota Quality Model • Focus: eliminating waste from the production system by designing the most efficient and effective system • Production is controlled through standardization and placing the right person and materials at each step of the process • Uses the PDSA improvement cycle • Statistical tools include value stream mapping and Kanban, or a visual cue, used to warn clinicians that there is a process problem • Performance measures vary from project to project and may inform the creation of new performance measures • Uses a master teacher ("Sensei") to spread the practices of Lean through the organizational culture	Institute for Healthcare Improvement: www.ihi.org/knowledge/Pages/IHIWhitePapers/GoingLeaninHealthCare.aspx

TABLE 14.4 Overview of Quality Improvement Models Used in Healthcare—cont'd

Model	Main Characteristics	Related Resources
Clinical Microsystems (Nelson et al., 2007)	• Model of service excellence developed specifically for healthcare • Clinical microsystem is considered the building block of any health care system and is the smallest replicable unit in an organization • Members of a clinical microsystem are interdependent and work together toward a common aim	Institute for Excellence in Health and Social Systems at the University of New Hampshire, Clinical Microsystems: http://www.clinicalmicrosystem.org/https://clinicalmicrosystem.org/
High Reliability Organizing Collective Mindfulness and Enactment (Weick & Sutcliffe, 2015)	• Sensitivity to operations by heightened awareness of the state of relevant systems and processes • Reluctance to simplify the reasons for problems • Recognize that work is complex with the potential to fail in new and unexpected ways • Preoccupation with failure and view near misses as opportunities to improve, rather than proof of success • Deference to expertise and the value of insights from staff with the most pertinent knowledge regarding safety over those with greater seniority • Practice resilience to prioritize emergency training to anticipate possible system failures	The Joint Commission, High Reliability Healthcare Maturity Model: https://www.jcrinc.com/products-and-services/high-reliability/ Evidence Brief: Implementation of High Reliability Organization Principles, Evidence Synthesis Program, Department of Veterans Affairs: https://www.hsrd.research.va.gov/publications/esp/reports.cfm

practices, and outcomes associated with the structure and processes. The evolution of key perspectives used to understand and manage QI in health care organizations is summarized in Table 14.5.

QUALITY IMPROVEMENT STEPS AND TOOLS

There are several steps in the QI process used to diagnose, treat, and evaluate health system performance (AHRQ, 2017a):
- Assessing health system performance by collecting and monitoring data
- Analyzing data to identify a problem in need of improvement
- Developing a plan to treat the identified problem
- Testing and implementing the improvement plan
- Monitoring improvement to institutionalize practices or discard those that do not achieve the intended outcome
- Repeating the process over and over again to optimize system performance

Several tools facilitate each step of the QI process (Table 14.6). You can use these tools to assist with collecting and analyzing data and to identify and test improvement ideas. A case example, Reducing Medication-Related Fall Risks Among Older Adults (see Box 14.7), is presented to introduce the steps of the improvement process and apply several basic QI tools used to avoid potentially inappropriate medication prescribing among older adults.

> **TIP**
>
> It is important for QI team members to understand the role and scope of practice for colleagues from different disciplines. You will be gathering data from multiple sources and perspectives. Valuing that diversity will increase your respect for the contributions of your colleagues.

Leading a Quality Improvement Team

QI is inherently an interprofessional team process and requires contributions from stakeholders with various professional perspectives to assess the potential causes of system malfunction and improvement ideas (Nelson et al., 2007). As a leader of a QI team, you should involve representatives from diverse professional groups, support staff, patients, and families. Although all professional staff, support staff, and patients should be involved throughout the improvement process, a smaller number of staff (5 to 7 members) should be part of a lead QI team responsible for planning, coordinating, implementing, and evaluating improvement efforts. To maintain a productive lead team, it is important to set a meeting schedule and use effective meeting tools such as the following (Nelson et al., 2007):

- Meeting agenda
- Meeting roles
- Ground rules
- Brainstorming
- Multivoting

Other tools that can help with project management to keep your team and activities organized and focused include action plans and Gantt charts (Nelson et al., 2007). After the lead team is assembled and processes established, the team can begin assessment of the health system. You can access helpful data assessment templates for a variety of clinical units at https://clinicalmicrosystem.org/ under the Knowledge Center tab. Additional QI tools can be accessed at the Institute for Healthcare Improvement website: https://www.ihi.org/. To access resources on how to best facilitate interprofessional

TABLE 14.5 Evolution of Quality Improvement Perspectives in Healthcare

Model	Key Features	Quality Monitoring Mechanisms
1920s–1980s QA Used to correct differences between what should be and what actually is (Chassin & Loeb, 2011)	• Uses external standards to guide quality • Quality assessed after the fact • Corrective action is punitive • The focus is on symptoms, individual failures, and compliance with standards	• Accreditation • Chart audit • Morbidity and mortality rounds
1960s–2010s Structure-Process-Outcome Framework examines system components that lead to health care quality (Donabedian, 1966/2005)	• Stresses professional responsibility for evaluating care quality • *Structure* focuses on provider and organizational characteristics • *Process* focuses on how care is delivered • *Outcome* focuses on the end results of medical care	• Accreditation • Work redesign • Benchmarking • Professional education and credentialing
1990s–2010s Total Quality Management, Lean, Six Sigma model used to continually improve services and organizational performance (Ardnt & Bigelow, 2000)	• Systems approach to improve efficiency • Incorporates clinical, financial, administrative, and patient satisfaction perspectives • Focuses on meeting actual and unanticipated patient needs • Uses statistical analysis to reduce variation in service processes • Relies on teamwork and data-based decisions	• Accreditation • Benchmarking (Hospital Consumer Assessment of Healthcare Providers and Systems [HCAHPS]) • Clinical practice guidelines • PDSA cycles • Process redesign • Lean • Six Sigma
2000s–2010s Patient Safety Systems approach to reduce harm to patients (Chassin & Loeb, 2011)	• Applies safety science methods to design health care delivery systems • Focuses on reducing or avoiding adverse events • Domains include patients, providers, care routines, system design	• Accreditation • Sentinel event reporting • National Patient Safety Goals • HRO model • Root cause analysis

TABLE 14.5 Evolution of Quality Improvement Perspectives in Healthcare—cont'd

Model	Key Features	Quality Monitoring Mechanisms
2010s–Present High Reliability Organizing (Weick & Sutcliff 2015)	HRO principles enable organizational members to make sense of complex systems, enacting principles of high reliability results in the maintenance of safety, quality, and efficiency over long periods of time. **A Culture of Safety** • Building trust and accountability, identifying unsafe conditions, strengthening systems, and assessing key activities • At all levels of the organization (e.g., people share information; seek reasons, not scapegoats; foster discretion and variation instead of uniformity) • Mindful of having open feedback, including potential failures **Developing Leadership** • Challenge the routine and complexity of the situation • Board members, CEO/managers, and lead physicians committed to the goal of zero patient harm • Commitment to teamwork, trust, and respect, even when there is disagreement **Training and Learning Opportunities** • Training all staff on robust process improvement (e.g., a blended performance improvement model aimed at improving patient safety in health care settings by integrating Six Sigma and formal change management principles) as appropriate • Provide change procedures to reflect your new understanding **Patient Safety Interventions** • Team rounds, huddles, debriefing, and guided prioritization of findings • Incorporate justice, equity, and patient centeredness • Patient and family advisory councils • Providers from different specialties attend daily safety huddles • Utilize change management strategies to promote change • Lean thinking root cause analysis to identify what is contributing to patient safety events to identify and implement solutions **Data Systems** • Track and display quality measures; involve IT specialist to develop solutions for quality problems • Open sharing of data and other information concerning safe and reliable care • Measure progress over time • Use of an improvement process platform to monitor potential problems	• Real-time data for decision making • Mindfulness practices to promote safety • Benchmarking (HCAHPS; NDNQI) • Chart audit • Evidence-based bundles • PDSA cycles • Lean • Six Sigma • Resource optimization

TABLE 14.6 QI Tools and Activities

Basic Tools and Activities	Step 1: Assess	Step 2: Analyze	Step 3: Plan and Implement	Step 4: Test and Evaluate
Data collection	X	X	X	X
Flowcharts	X	X	X	X
Cause and effect analysis		X		
Bar and pie charts	X	X		X
Run charts	X	X		X
Control charts	X	X		X
Histograms	X	X		X
Pareto charts	X	X		X
Benchmarking	X			X
Gantt charts		X		X

Based on data from AHRQ (2017a).

teamwork, visit the National Center for Interprofessional Practice and Education at https://nexusipe.org/.

> **TIP**
>
> To keep the interprofessional QI lead team engaged and on schedule, hold team meetings at least weekly and display in a visible location a timeline of QI activities such as data collection, analysis, and results of Plan-Do-Study-Act (PDSA) cycles with completion progress for each activity. Data stored in electronic health records can be used to generate reports used in clinical QI work.

Improvement Process Step 1: Assessment

In the assessment phase, the first step is to complete a structured assessment to understand more about performance patterns. The improvement team typically begins with a series of broad questions used to guide data collection. Common methods used to collect system performance data include check sheets and data sheets to understand performance patterns and surveys, focus groups, and interviews to gather information about patient and staff perceptions of system performance. Commonly collected data elements include information about the following (Nelson et al., 2007):

- Patients: What are the average age, gender, top diagnoses, and satisfaction scores?
- Professionals: What is the level of staff satisfaction? What is their skill set?
- Processes and patterns: What are the processes for admitting and discharging patients?
- Common performance metrics: What are the rates of pressure ulcers and falls with injury?

For useful data collection templates, see Workbooks at https://clinicalmicrosystem.org/knowledge-center/workbooks/ from the Institute for Excellence in Health and Social Systems at the University of New Hampshire.

> **TIP**
>
> To reduce the data collection burden related to QI projects, identify what performance data already exists in your organization before starting the assessment phase of the QI process. For example, find out if your organization is participating in Press Ganey's National Database of Nursing Quality Indicators (NDNQI) program, which collects quarterly data on pressure ulcers, infections, falls, staff satisfaction, and other quality indicators.

Improvement Process Step 2: Analysis

The next phase of the improvement process focuses on data analysis. Because QI uses a team approach to engage in problem solving, data are displayed in graphic form so all team members can see how the system is performing and generate ideas for improvements. Several tools exist to help display and analyze performance data.

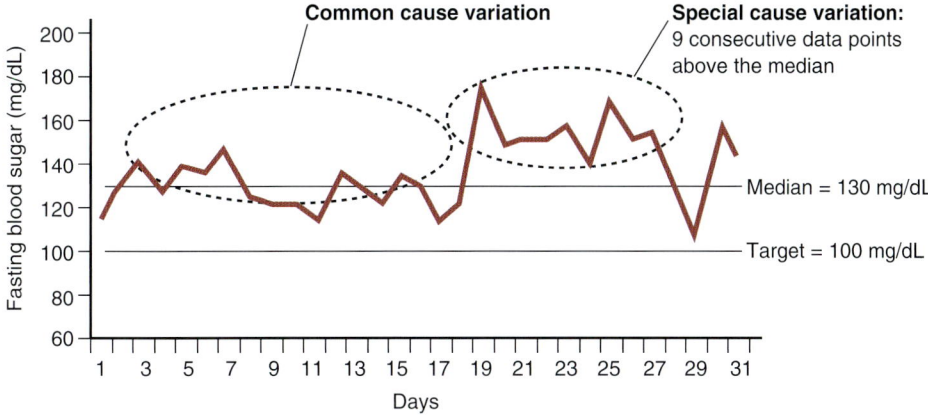

Fig. 14.1 Run Chart of Daily Fasting Plasma Glucose Levels. (From Agency for Healthcare Research and Quality (2017a).)

Trending Variation in System Performance With Run and Control Charts

If quality healthcare means that the right care is delivered to the right people in the right way, at the right time, for every person, during each clinical encounter, it is important to learn when criteria are not met and why. One method is to track performance over time and understand sources of variation in system performance, which can guide improvement activities to design a better functioning health system. Minimizing performance variation is one of the main goals of QI. There are two main types of system variation (Nelson et al., 2007, p. 346):

- **Common cause variation** occurs at random and is considered a characteristic of the system. For example, you might never leave your house in time for prompt arrival to class. In this case, you must work on better managing multiple random causes of tardiness, such as getting up late or taking too long to shower, dress, and eat, to improve your overall punctuality record.
- **Special cause variation** arises from a special situation that disrupts the causal system beyond what can be accounted for by random variation. An example might be that you usually leave your house on time for prompt arrival to class, but special circumstances such as road construction or a broken elevator delay your arrival. Once these special causes of tardiness are resolved, you will arrive to class on time.

Variations in system performance over time are commonly displayed with run charts and control charts. A **run chart** is a graphical data display that shows trends in a measure of interest; trends reveal what is occurring over time (Nelson et al., 2007). The vertical axis of the run chart depicts the value of measure of interest and the horizontal axis depicts the value of each measure running over time. A run chart shows whether the outcome of interest is running in a targeted area of performance and how much variation there is from point to point and over time. For example, a patient newly diagnosed with diabetes can record her blood glucose levels over a month using a run chart. By regularly charting blood glucose levels, the patient can reveal when blood glucose runs higher or lower than the target level of less than 100 mg/dL for the fasting plasma glucose (FPG) test. The run chart in Fig. 14.1 shows that FPG levels are consistently higher than the target, with a median FPG of 130 mg/dL; the trend of FPG readings in the first 19 days of the month is indicative of **common cause variation**. These random variations in FPG readings are likely caused by the confluence of several factors such as diet, exercise, and medication adherence. To correct the undesirable variation, the patient can assess what factors might be influencing the higher FPG values and then work with her primary care provider to develop necessary interventions to better control her blood glucose by better managing multiple causal factors. To determine whether interventions are successful, the patient and provider should continue to document blood glucose levels and then compare the median FPG values before and after interventions are implemented.

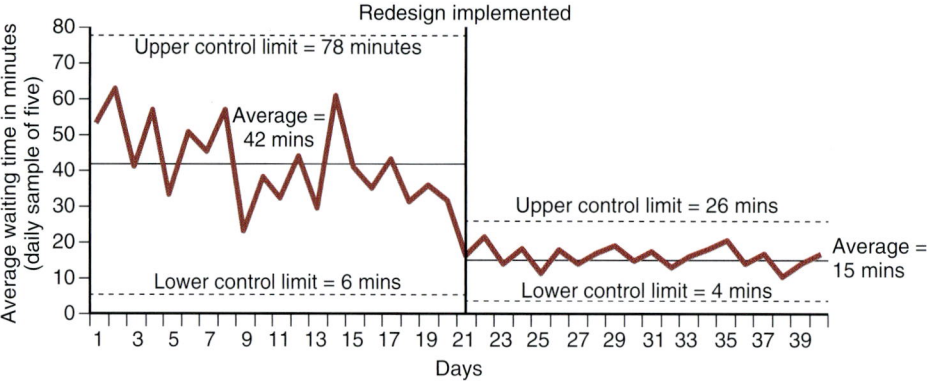

Fig. 14.2 Control Chart of Average Wait Time Before and After a Redesign. (From Agency for Healthcare Research and Quality (2017a).)

In addition, **special cause variation** in FPG is evident on days 19 to 28, where nine consecutive fasting plasma glucose (FPG) readings are above the median line. It turns out that on these days, the patient had run out of her glucose-lowering medication; this special circumstance caused increased FPG. Although various rules exist for accurately determining the presence of special cause variation, generally special cause variation is present if the following are true (Nelson et al., 2007, p. 349):

- Eight data points in a row are above or below the median or mean
- Six data points in a row are going up
- Six data points in a row are going down

Determining common and special causes of variation is important because treatment strategies for eliminating each type of variation will vary.

A **control chart** (Fig. 14.2) is also used to track system performance over time, but it is a more sophisticated data tool than a run chart (Nelson et al., 2007). A control chart includes information on the average performance level for the system depicted by a center line displaying the system's average performance (the mean value), and the upper and lower limits depicting one to three standard deviations from average performance level. The rules to detect special cause variation are the same for run and control charts, except that for control charts, the upper and lower limits are additional tools used to detect special cause variation. Any point that falls outside the control limit is considered an outlier that merits further examination.

> **TIP**
>
> Use a run chart in step two of the QI process to analyze causes of variation in fasting plasma glucose (FPG) levels from the target level of 100 mg/dL and in step four of the QI process to evaluate whether changes in diet, exercise, and medication adherence helped the patient achieve the targeted FPG.

> **TIP**
>
> The Agency for Health Research and Quality (AHRQ), the American Nurses Credentialing Center (ANCC) Magnet Recognition Program, and the Institute for Healthcare Improvement (IHI) offer toolkits and resources for clinical leaders on how to create graphs to visualize performance on key quality indicators that are easy to read and interpret.

Graphs

Graphs commonly used to understand system performance are displayed in Fig. 14.3, and include pie charts, bar charts, and histograms (see Chapter 10). Selecting the appropriate chart depends on the type of data collected and the performance pattern the improvement team is trying to understand. A bar chart is used to display categorical-level data. A pareto diagram is a special type of bar chart used to understand the frequency of factors that contribute to a common effect. It is used to display the Pareto Principle, sometimes referred to as the 80-20 Rule, or the Law of the Few (AHRQ, 2017b), which states that 80% of variation in a problem originates with 20%

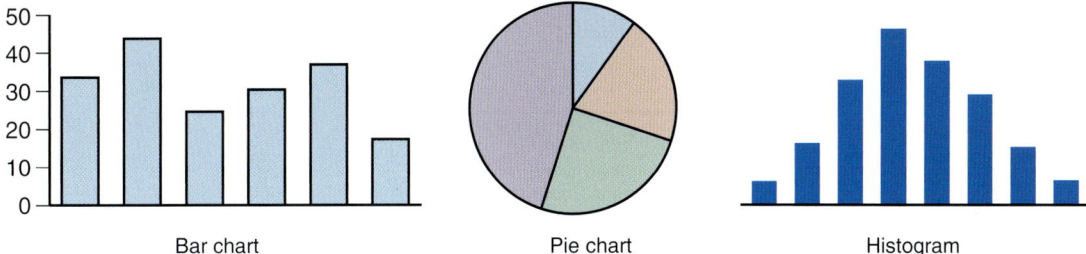

Fig. 14.3 Examples of Bar Chart, Pie Chart, and Histogram. (From Agency for Healthcare Research and Quality (2017a).)

of cases. In a pareto diagram, the bars are displayed in descending order of frequency. A histogram is another type of bar chart used for continuous-level data to show the distribution of the data around the mean, commonly called the bell curve.

Cause and Effect Diagrams

More sophisticated visual data displays include **cause and effect diagrams** used to identify and treat the causes of performance problems. Two common tools in this category are the fishbone or Ishikawa diagram and the tree diagram (AHRQ, 2017a). The **fishbone diagram** facilitates brainstorming about potential causes of a problem by grouping causes into the categories of environment, people, materials, and process (Fig. 14.4). Fishbone diagrams can be used proactively to prevent quality defects, including errors, and retrospectively to identify factors that potentially contributed to a quality defect or error that already has occurred. An example of when a fishbone diagram is used retrospectively is during **root cause analyses (RCAs)** to identify system design failures that caused errors.

An RCA is a structured method used to understand sources of system variation that lead to errors or mistakes, including sentinel events, with the goal of learning from mistakes and mitigating hazards that arise as a characteristic of the system design (U.S. Department of Veterans Affairs, 2023). An RCA is conducted by a team that includes representatives from nursing, medicine, management, QI, or risk management, and the individual(s) involved in the incident (sometimes including the patient or family members in the discovery process), and it emphasizes system failures while avoiding individual blame (U.S. Department of Veterans Affairs, 2023). An RCA seeks to answer three questions to learn from mistakes:

- What happened?
- Why did it happen?
- What can be done to prevent it from happening again?

Because the RCA is viewed as an opportunity for organizational learning and improvement, the most effective RCAs include a change in practice or work system design to lessen the chances of similar errors occurring in the future. Thus, it is important for QI leaders to integrate the findings of RCAs to systematically optimize system performance to reduce avoidable errors, system failures, and quality problems.

A tree diagram is particularly useful for identifying the chain of causes with the goal of identifying the root cause of a problem. For example, consider medication errors. The improvement team could use the **Five Whys** method to establish the chain of causes leading to poor glycemic control:

- Question 1: Why did the patient get the incorrect medicine?
  Answer 1: Because the prescription was wrong.
- Question 2: Why was the prescription wrong?
  Answer 2: Because the nurse practitioner had incomplete information when writing the prescription.
- Question 3: Why did the nurse practitioner have incomplete information when writing the prescription?
  Answer 3: Because the patient's chart was incomplete.
- Question 4: Why wasn't the patient's chart complete?
  Answer 4: Because the medical assistant had not entered the latest laboratory report.
- Question 5: Why hadn't the medical assistant charted the latest laboratory report?
  Answer 5: Because the laboratory technician telephoned the results to the receptionist, who forgot to tell the patient care assistant.

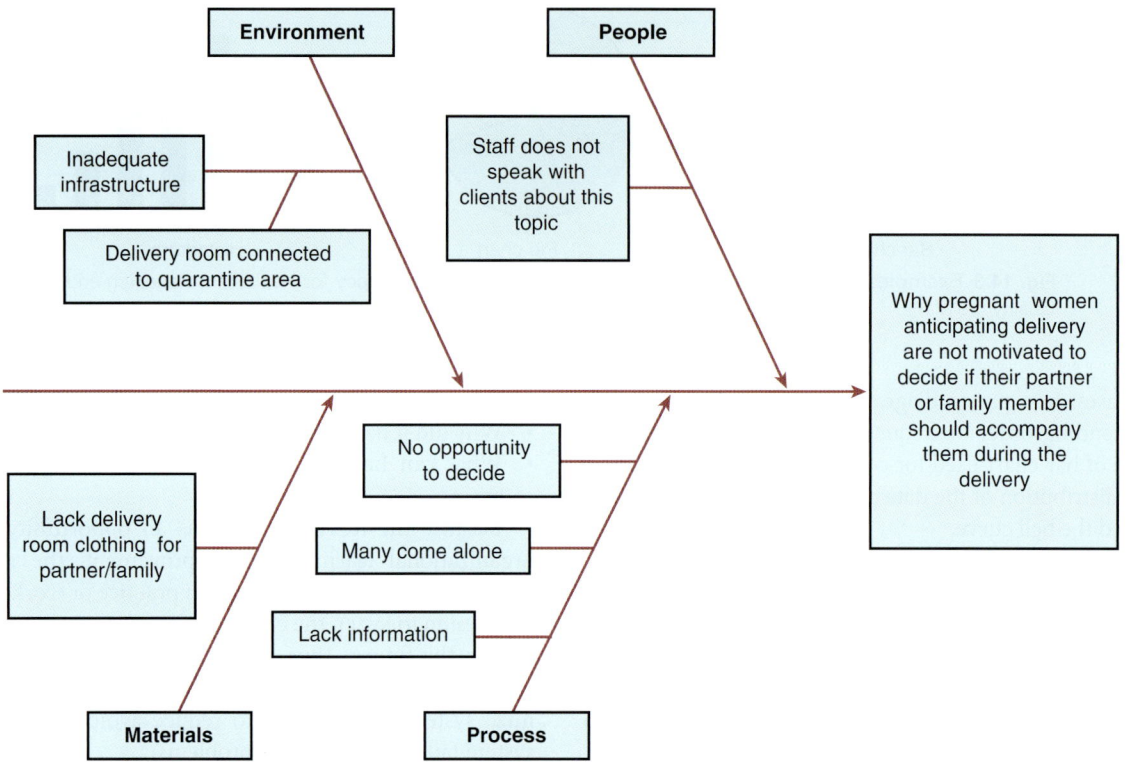

Fig. 14.4 Fishbone Diagram. (Adapted from Agency for Healthcare Research and Quality (2017a).)

In this case, using the Five Whys technique suggests that a potential solution for avoiding wrong prescriptions in the future might be to develop a system for tracking laboratory reports (AHRQ, 2017a).

Flowcharting

A flowchart depicts how a process works, detailing the sequence of steps from the beginning to the end of a process (AHRQ, 2017a). Several types of flowcharts exist, including the simplest (high level), a detailed version (detailed), and one that also indicates the people involved in the steps (deployment or matrix). Fig. 14.5 shows an example of a detailed flowchart that can be used to do the following:
- Understand processes
- Consider ways to simplify processes
- Recognize unnecessary steps in a process
- Determine areas for monitoring or data collection
- Identify who will be involved in or affected by the improvement process
- Formulate questions for further research and improvement

When you are flowcharting, it is important to identify beginning and end points of a process and then make a record of the actual, not the ideal, process. To obtain an accurate picture of the process, perform direct observation of the process steps and communicate with people who are directly part of the process to clarify all the steps.

Improvement Process Step 3: Develop a Plan for Improvement

By identifying potential sources of variation, the improvement team can pinpoint problem areas in need of improvement. The next phase is to treat the performance problem. This phase involves developing and testing a plan for improvement. A simple yet powerful model for developing and testing improvements is the Model for Improvement (Langley et al., 2009). It begins with three questions to guide the change process and focus the improvement work (Langley et al., 2009):

1. **Aim.** What are we trying to accomplish? Set a clear aim with specific measurable targets.

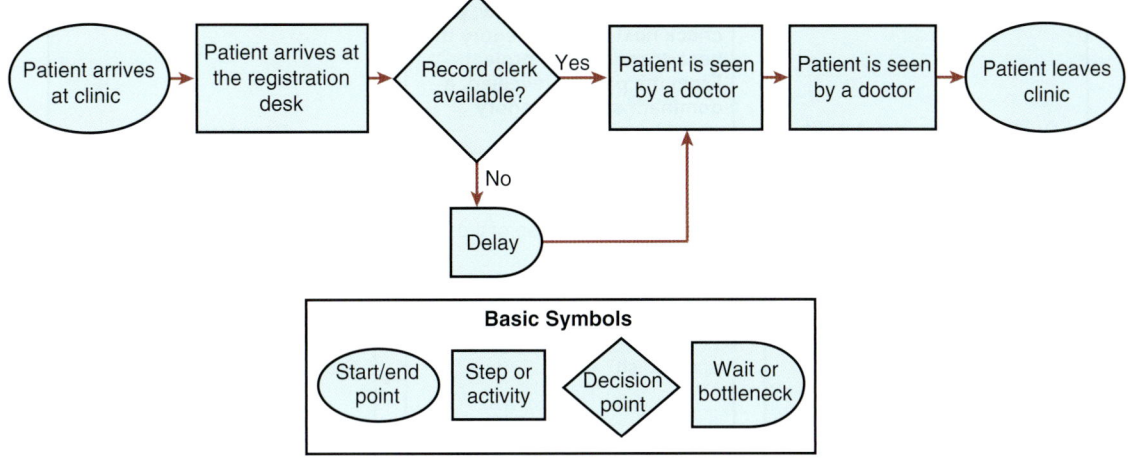

Fig. 14.5 Detailed Flow Chart. (Modified from Agency for Healthcare Research and Quality (2017a).)

2. **Measures.** How will we know that the change is an improvement? Use qualitative and quantitative measures to support real improvement work to guide change progress toward the stated goal.
3. **Changes.** What changes can we make that will result in an improvement? Develop a statement about what the team believes it can change to cause improvement.

The change ideas reflect the team's hypotheses about what could improve system performance. There are several ways in which change ideas can be generated. These ideas can be identified from the root causes of the performance problems that are evident during cause and effect and process analyses using fishbone diagrams, the Five Whys, and flowcharting tools in the analysis step of the improvement process. Another approach is to select common areas for change associated with the goals and philosophy of QI. Common change topics, also referred to as themes for improvement, include the following (Nelson et al., 2007):

- Eliminating waste
- Improving work flow
- Optimizing inventory
- Changing the work environment
- Managing time more effectively
- Managing variation
- Designing systems to avoid mistakes
- Focusing on products or services

Change ideas also can come from the evidence provided by your review of the available literature. This is where your EBP skills will be most helpful. You will need to critically appraise research studies and QI studies of interventions that can be applied to remedy the identified problem. To help you decide whether a journal article is a research study or a QI study, see the critical decision tree in Fig. 14.6. Because QI studies capture the experiences of an organization or unit, the results of these studies usually are not generalizable. To promote knowledge transfer and learning from others' improvement experiences, the Standards for Quality Improvement Reporting Excellence, or **SQUIRE 2.0 guidelines**, were developed to promote the publication and interpretation of this type of applied research (SQUIRE, 2020). The SQUIRE 2.0 guidelines are presented in Table 14.7; The Quality Improvement Minimum Quality Criteria Set (QI-MQCS) appraisal tool includes sixteen domains to critically assess the QI-specific features of publications reporting QI studies in health care settings (Hempel et al., 2015). The QI-MQCS is intended as a resource for reviewers, assisting in synthesizing the vast evidence on QI interventions, and provides a framework for critical appraisal in this complex research area. The SQUIRE 2.0 guidelines and the QI-MQCS are useful tools that enable researchers, clinicians, and quality managers to identify high-quality publications to improve the study design and improve confidence in QI research to adopt empirically validated practices into local quality improvement programs.

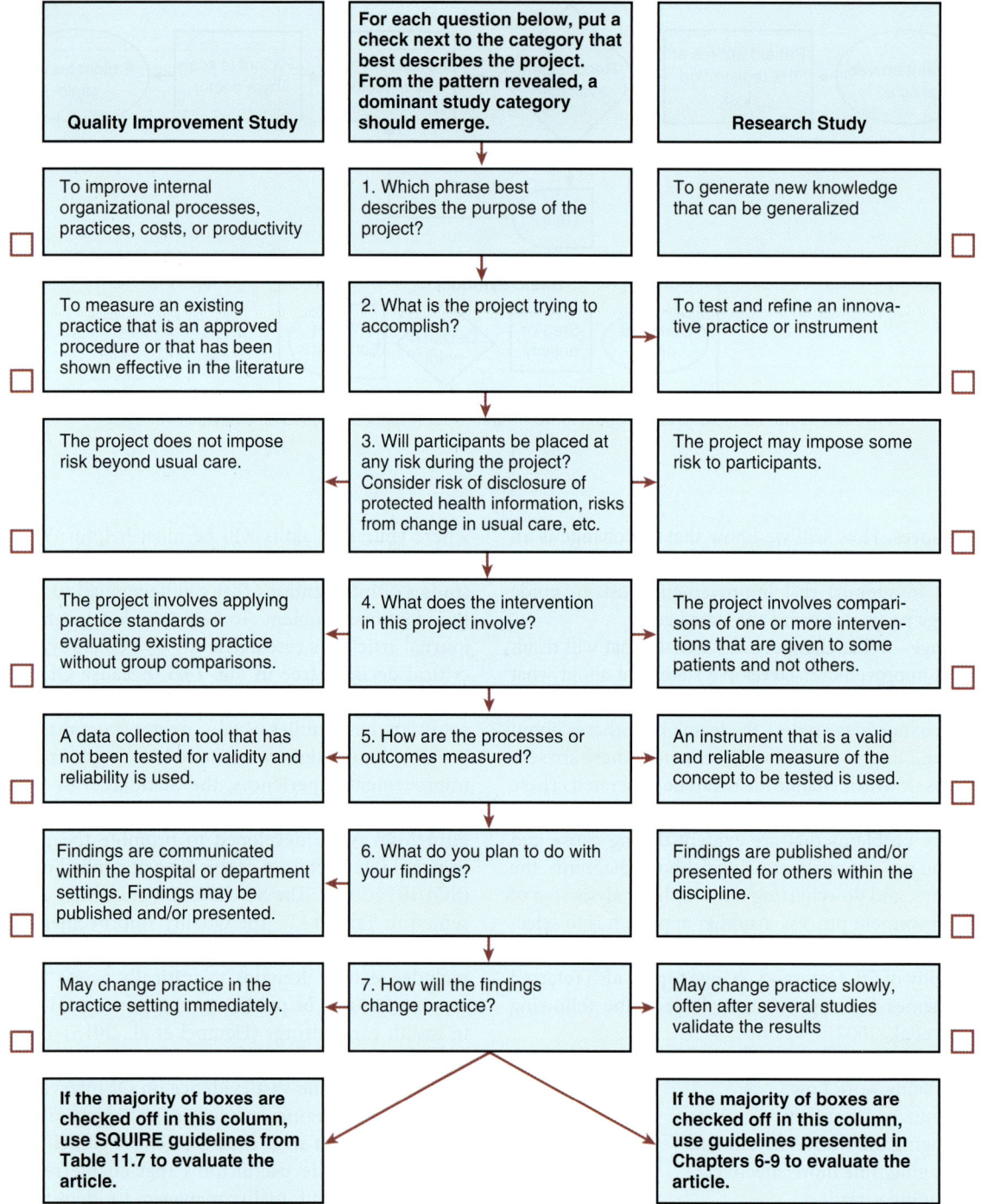

Fig. 14.6 Differentiating QI from Research Projects. (Modified from King (2008) and Bass and Maloy (2020).)

TABLE 14.7 Revised SQUIRE Guidelines Standards for QI Reporting Excellence (SQUIRE 2.0)

Title and Abstract

Title	Indicate that the manuscript concerns an initiative to improve healthcare (broadly defined to include the quality, safety, effectiveness, patient centeredness, timeliness, cost, efficiency, and equity of healthcare).
Abstract	a. Provide adequate information to aid in searching and indexing. b. Summarize all key information from various sections of the text using the abstract format of the intended publication or a structured summary, such as background, local problem, methods, interventions, results, or conclusions.

Introduction—Why did you start?

Problem description	Nature and significance of the local problem
Available knowledge	Summary of what is currently known about the problem, including relevant previous studies
Rationale	Informal or formal frameworks, models, concepts, and/or theories used to explain the problem, any reasons or assumptions that were used to develop the intervention(s), and reasons why the intervention(s) was expected to work
Specific aims	Purposes of the project and of this report

Methods—What did you do?

Context	Contextual elements considered important at the outset of the intervention(s)
Intervention(s)	a. Description of the intervention(s) in sufficient detail so that others can reproduce it/them b. Specifics of the team involved in the work
Study of intervention(s)	a. Approach chosen for assessing the impact of the intervention(s) b. Approach used to establish whether the observed outcomes were due to the intervention(s)
Measures	a. Measures chosen for studying processes and outcomes of the intervention(s), including rationale for choosing them, their operational definitions, and their validity and reliability b. Description of the approach to the ongoing assessment of contextual elements that contributed to success, failure, efficiency, and cost c. Methods employed for assessing completeness and accuracy of data
Analysis	a. Qualitative and quantitative methods used to draw inferences from the data b. Methods for understanding variation within the data, including the effects of time as a variable
Ethical considerations	Ethical aspects of implementing and studying the intervention(s) and how they were addressed, including, but not limited to, formal ethics review and potential conflict(s) of interest

Results—What did you find?

Results	a. Initial steps of the intervention(s) and their evolution over time (e.g., timeline diagram, flow chart, or table), including modifications made to the intervention during the project b. Details of the process measures and outcomes c. Contextual elements that interacted with the intervention(s) d. Observed associations among outcomes, interventions, and relevant contextual elements e. Unintended consequences such as unexpected benefits, problems, failures, or costs associated with the intervention(s) f. Details about missing data

Continued

TABLE 14.7 Revised SQUIRE Guidelines Standards for QI Reporting Excellence (SQUIRE 2.0)—cont'd

Discussion—What does it mean?	
Summary	a. Key findings, including relevance to the rationale and specific aims
	b. Particular strengths of the project
Interpretation	a. Nature of the association between the intervention(s) and outcomes
	b. Comparison of results with findings from other publications
	c. Impact of the project on people and systems
	d. Reasons for any differences between observed and anticipated outcomes, including the influence of context
	e. Costs and strategic tradeoffs, including opportunity costs
Limitations	a. Limits to the generalizability of the work
	b. Factors that might have limited internal validity, such as confounding, bias, or imprecision in the design, methods, measurement, or analysis
	c. Efforts made to minimize and adjust for limitations
Conclusions	a. Usefulness of the work
	b. Sustainability
	c. Potential for spread to other contexts
	d. Implications for practice and further study in the field
	e. Suggested next steps
Other information	
Funding	Sources of funding that supported this work; role, if any, of the funding organization in the design, implementation, interpretation, and reporting

Note: See www.squire-statement.org/ for more information on publishing QI studies.
Reproduced with permission: SQUIRE 2.0 (Standards for Quality Improvement Reporting Excellence), http://www.squire-statement.org

Improvement Process Step 4: Test and Implement the Improvement Plan

Improvement changes identified in the planning phase are tested using the **Plan-Do-Study-Act** (PDSA) **Improvement cycle**, which is the last step of the improvement model (Langley et al., 2009)) depicted in Fig. 14.7. The focus of PDSA is experimentation using small, rapid tests of change. Actions involved in each phase of the PDSA cycle are detailed in Fig. 14.7. In this step, you evaluate the success of the intervention in bringing about improvement. It is important for the team to monitor intended and unintended changes in system performance, patient and staff perceptions of the change, and ideally, cost of the change. Also, in this phase of the improvement process, it is useful to track the stability and sustainability of the new work process by monitoring system performance over time. Results data should be presented in graphic data displays (explained earlier in the chapter) and compared with baseline performance.

To promote successful implementation of your improvement interventions, you should consider using the following evidence-based implementation strategies (Powell et al., 2015, pp. 8–10):

- Practice facilitation: A process of interactive problem solving and support that occurs in a context of a recognized need for improvement and a supportive interpersonal relationship
- Educational outreach visit: When a trained person meets with providers in their practice setting to educate them about a clinical innovation with the intent of changing the providers' practices
- Educational meetings and workshops: Meetings targeted toward different stakeholder groups to teach them about a clinical innovation
- Goal setting: Establish goals to guide improvement efforts. Measure and manage performance against the stated goal(s) to engage stakeholders, mobilize action, and reward changes in practice over time

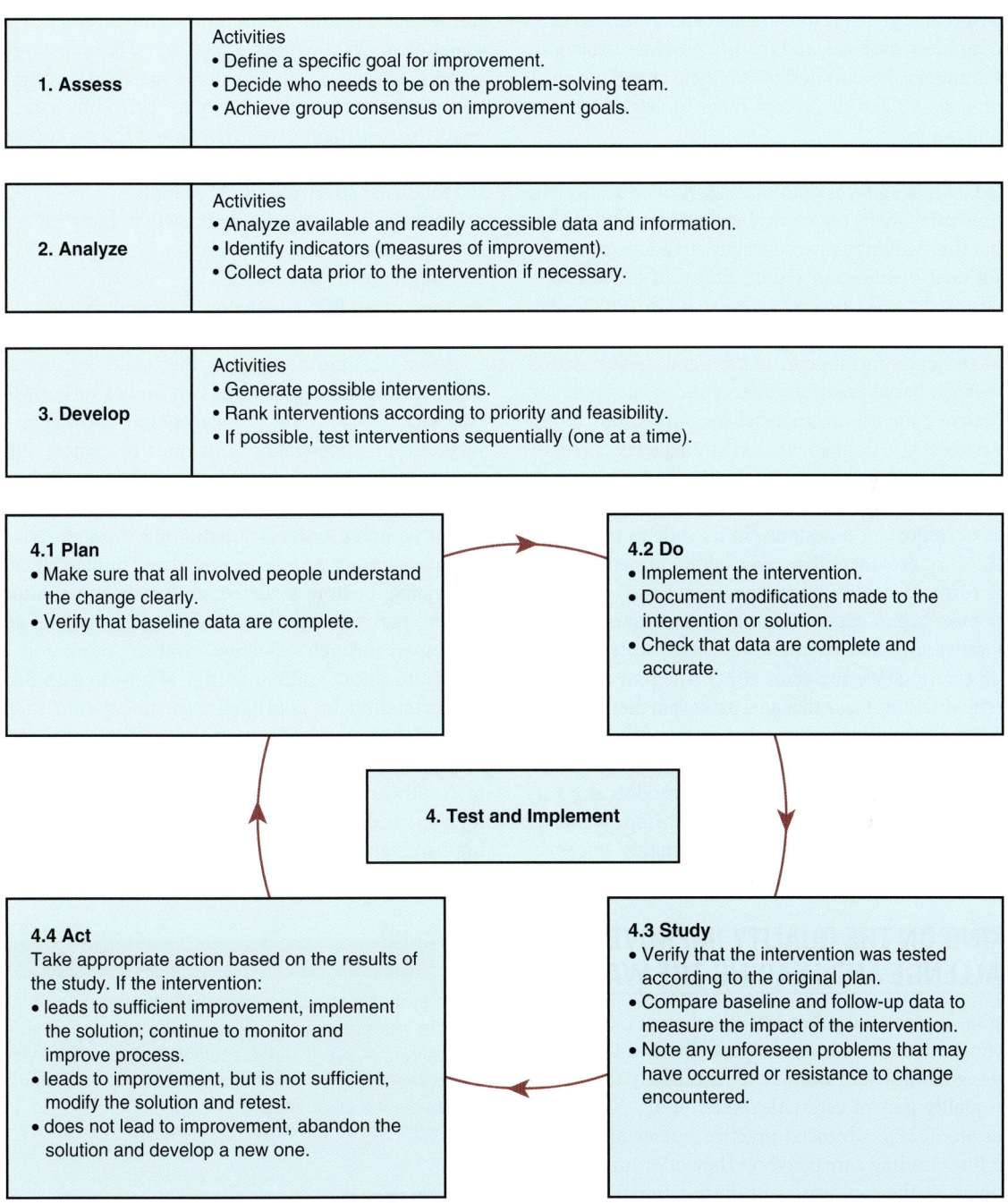

Fig. 14.7 Summary of the QI Process. (Modified from Agency for Healthcare Research and Quality (2017a).)

- Audit and feedback: Collecting and summarizing clinical performance data over a specified time period and giving it to clinicians and administrators to monitor, evaluate, and modify provider behavior
- Reminders: Systems designed to help clinicians recall information and/or prompt them to use the clinical innovation
- Local opinion leaders: Informing providers identified by colleagues as opinion leaders or educationally influential about the clinical innovation in the hope that they will influence colleagues to adopt it

National Institutes of Health Office of Disease Prevention (n.d.) and University Research Co. (2023) offer additional resources and information on evidence-based strategies for implementation and dissemination of evidence-based practices, interventions, and policies.

Evidence for use of financial incentives and multiple versus single implementation strategies is currently mixed. In the decade since the passage of the Affordable Care Act, the health care system has reached a series of important milestones in its shift to paying for value. More providers than ever before are engaged in some form of quality-linked payment, and a smaller cadre have begun experimenting with advanced forms of population-based payment and large-scale practice transformation (Werner et al., 2021). The past decade of experimentation shows that alternative payment models (APMs) as currently implemented are not driving large-scale, systemic change. Careful study of the lessons from both successful and underperforming models suggests that properly designed APMs can yield improvements in value through cost reductions and quality improvements (Werner et al., 2021).

TAKING ON THE QUALITY IMPROVEMENT CHALLENGE AND LEADING THE WAY

Hospital leaders and other key stakeholders agree that enabling clinicians to lead and participate in QI is vital to strengthening our health system's capacity to provide high-quality patient care (Alexander et al., 2022; Djukic et al., 2021). Advanced practice nurses are on the front lines leading care delivery. They offer unique perspectives on the root causes of dysfunctional care and what interventions might work reliably and sustainably in everyday clinical practice to achieve best care. However, there are multiple barriers to the participation of nurse leaders in QI, including insufficient staffing, lack of leadership support and resources for their participation in QI, and not enough educational preparation for knowledgeable and meaningful QI involvement (Alexander et al., 2022; Djukic et al., 2021). For nurse practitioners, midwives, clinical nurse specialists, educators, and administrators to contribute their knowledge and expertise to patient care delivery and the organization's quality enterprise, nursing leadership must engage in the following (Berwick, 2011, p. 326):

- Setting aims and building the will to improve
- Measurement and transparency
- Finding better systems
- Supporting PDSA activities, risk, and change
- Providing resources

Several common elements that make improvement work doable are captured in two bodies of knowledge (Berwick, 2011). One is professional knowledge that includes an understanding of one's discipline, subject matter, and values of the discipline. The other is knowledge of improvement, which includes an understanding of complex systems functioning through dynamic interplay among various technical and human elements; knowledge of how to detect and manage variation in system performance; knowledge of managing group processes through effective conflict resolution and communication; and knowledge of how to gain further understanding by continual experimentation in local settings through rapid tests of change. Linking these two knowledge systems promotes continuous improvement in healthcare. This chapter provides a starting point for you to develop basic knowledge and skills for the improvement work so you can better meet the leadership challenges embedded in the roles of clinical leaders.

> **TIP**
>
> Remember that important stakeholders should be part of the interprofessional QI team, including your administrative managers and executives who provide leadership support, like time and resources, for your team to implement a QI project.

SYNTHESIS

Leading QI initiatives is proposed to be an important role for advanced practice nurses. QI initiatives aim to influence improvements in organizational settings and strive to ensure that all patients consistently receive high-quality, cost-effective, and satisfying patient-centered care. Initiatives need to align with organizational priorities that are consistent with national goals and strategies for health care quality improvement. National performance measures, public reporting systems, and accrediting organizations require health care institutions to meet local and national quality and safety standards. Health care organizations also identify those measures that best apply to their practice in acute or primary care settings. Quality improvement models such as TQM/CQI, Six Sigma, Lean, Clinical Microsystems, and the HRO model provide a guide for developing, implementing, and evaluating QI projects. Evidence provided by QI projects, coupled with national quality data, inform clinical decision making. Teamwork and collaboration across professions is fundamental to success in developing, implementing, and evaluating QI initiatives at the micro, meso, or macrosystem level. Health care leaders agree that involving clinical leaders and clinicians is essential to strengthening our health system's capacity to provide high quality patient care.

> **TIP**
>
> Critical appraisal is a systematic process used to identify the strengths and weaknesses of a research article to assess the usefulness and validity of research findings. The most important components of a critical appraisal are an evaluation of the appropriateness of the study design for the research question and a careful assessment of the key methodologic features of this design. Other factors that also should be considered include the suitability of the statistical methods used and their subsequent interpretation, potential conflicts of interest and the relevance of the research to one's own practice.
>
> There are a variety of validated tools for researchers and clinicians to appraise a range of research designs. Be sure to select the correct appraisal tool for the EBP project at hand to accurately assess the existing evidence on a particular clinical or managerial topic.

REFERENCES

2019 American Geriatrics Society Beers Criteria Update Expert Panel. (2019). American Geriatrics Society 2019 updated AGS Beer Criteria for potentially inappropriate medicate use in older adults. *Journal of the American Geriatric Society*, 67(4), 674–694.

Agency for Healthcare Research and Quality (AHRQ) (n.d.). *AHRQ Quality Indicators*. http://www.qualityindicators.ahrq.gov.

Agency for Healthcare Research and Quality (AHRQ) (n.d.). *AHRQ Quality Indicators*. About Us. https://qualityindicators.ahrq.gov/home/about.

Agency for Healthcare Research and Quality (AHRQ). (2017a). *EVIDENCE now program. Quality improvement essentials toolkit*. Provided by the Institute for Healthcare Improvement. https://www.ahrq.gov/evidencenow/tools/qi-essentials-toolkit.html.

Agency for Healthcare Research and Quality (AHRQ). (2017b). *The national quality strategy: Fact sheet*. https://www.ahrq.gov/workingforquality/about/nqs-fact-sheets/fact-sheet.html.

Agency for Healthcare Research and Quality (AHRQ). (2018). *Measuring and benchmarking clinical performance*. https://www.ahrq.gov/evidencenow/tools/primary-care-measuring.html.

Agency for Healthcare Research and Quality (AHRQ). (2022). *2022 National healthcare quality and disparities report (AHRQ Pub. No. 22-230030)*. https://www.ahrq.gov/sites/default/files/wysiwyg/research/findings/nhqrdr/2022qdr.pdf.

Ahn, C., Rundall, T. G., Shortell, S. M., Blodgett, J. C., & Reponen, E. (2021). Lean management and breakthrough performance improvement in health care. *Quality Management in Healthcare*, 30(1), 6–12.

Alexander, C. C., Tschannen, D., Hays, D., et al. (2022). An integrative review of the barriers and facilitators to nurse engagement in quality improvement in the clinical practice setting. *Journal of Nursing Care Quality*, 37(1), 94–100.

Altmiller, G., & Hopkins-Pepe, L. (2019). Why quality and safety education for nurses (QSEN) matters in practice. *The Journal of Continuing Education in Nursing*, 50(5), 199–200.

American Medical Association. (2022). *AMA STEPS Forward Playbook series: Private practice playbook—Physician payment models guide (Version 1.0)*. https://www.ama-assn.org/system/files/steps-forward-physician-payment-models-guide.pdf.

American Organization of Nurse Executives. (n.d.). *Care innovation and transformation program*. http://www.aone.org/education/cit.shtml.

Arndt, M., & Bigelow, B. (2000). The transfer of business practices into hospitals: History and implication. *Advances in Health Care Management*, 1, 339–368. https://doi.org/10.1016/S1474-8231(00)01013-2.

Aydin, C., Donaldson, N., Stotts, N. A., Fridman, M., & Brown, D. S. (2015). Modeling hospital-acquired pressure ulcer prevalence on medical-surgical units: Nurse workload, expertise, and clinical processes of care. *Health Services Research*, 50(2), 351–373.

Bass, P. F., & Maloy, J. W. (2020). How to determine if a project is human subjects research, a quality improvement project, or both. *Ochsner Journal*, *20*(1), 56–61.

Berwick, D. M. (2011). Preparing nurses for participation in and leadership of continual improvement. *Journal of Nursing Education*, *50*(6), 322–327.

Braden, B. J., & Bergstrom, N. (1994). Predictive validity of the Braden Scale for pressure sore risk in a nursing home population. *Research in Nursing & Health*, *17*(6), 459–470.

Burns, E. R., Stevens, J. A., & Lee, R. (2016). The direct costs of fatal and non-fatal falls among older adults—United States. *Journal of Safety Research*, *58*, 99–103.

Cantu, J., Gharehyakheh, A., Fritts, S., & Tolk, J. N. (2021). Assessing the HRO: Tools and techniques to determine the high-reliability state of an organization. *Safety Science*, *134*,105082.

Centers for Medicare and Medicaid Services. (n.d.). *Quality payment program overview*. https://qpp.cms.gov/about/qpp-overview.

Centers for Medicare and Medicaid Services (CMS). (2022). *What are value-based programs?*. https://www.cms.gov/Medicare/Quality-Initiatives-Patient-Assessment-Instruments/Value-Based-Programs/Value-Based-Programs.

Centers for Medicare and Medicaid Services (CMS). (2023). *CMS national quality strategy*. https://www.cms.gov/Medicare/Quality-Initiatives-Patient-Assessment-Instruments/Value-Based-Programs/CMS-Quality-Strategy.

Chassin, M. R., & Loeb, J. M. (2011). The ongoing quality improvement journey: Next stop, high reliability. *Health Affairs*, *30*(4), 559–568.

Coleman, C. (2020). Health literacy and clear communication best practices for telemedicine. *Health Literacy Research and Practice*, *4*(4), e224–e229.

Coury, J., Schneider, J. L., Rivelli, J. S., et al. (2017). Applying the Plan-Do-Study-Act (PDSA) approach to a large pragmatic study involving safety net clinics. *BMC Health Services Research*, *17*(1), 411. https://doi.org/10.1186/s12913-017-2364-3.

Cronenwett, L., Sherwood, G., Barnsteiner, J., et al. (2007). Quality and safety education for nurses. *Nursing Outlook*, *55*(3), 122–131.

Djukic, M., Fletcher, J., Witkoski Stimpfel, A., & Kovner, C. (2021). Variables associated with nurse reported quality improvement participation. *Nurse Leader*, *19*(1), 76–81. https://doi.org/10.1016/j.mnl.2020.06.009.

Donabedian, A. (1966/2005). Evaluating the quality of medical care. *The Milbank Memorial Fund Quarterly*, *44*(3), 166–206 Reprinted December 2005, 83(4), 691–729.

Dzau, V. J., Mate, K., & O'Kane, M. (2022). Equity and quality—improving health care delivery requires both. *JAMA*, *327*(6), 519–520.

Dzau, V. J., & Shine, K. I. (2020). Two decades since to err is human: Progress, but still a "chasm." *JAMA*, *324*(24), 2489–2490.

Fick, D. M., Inouye, S. K., Guess, J., et al. (2015). Preliminary development of an ultra-brief two-item bedside test for delirium. *Journal of Hospital Medicine*, *10*(10), 645–650.

Fick, D. M., & Shrestha, P. (2022). Delirium in persons with dementia: Integrating the 4Ms of age-friendly care as a set into the care of older people. *Journal of Gerontological Nursing*, *48*(10), 3–6.

Haddad, Y. K., Bergen, G., & Luo, F. (2018). Reducing fall risk in older adults. *The American Journal of Nursing*, *118*(7), 21–22.

Hempel, S., Shekelle, P. G., Liu, J. L., et al. (2015). Development of the quality improvement minimum quality criteria set (QI-MQCS): A tool for critical appraisal of quality improvement intervention publications. *BMJ Quality and Safety*, *24*(12), 796–804. https://doi.org/10.1136/bmjqs-2014-003151.

Henrique, D. B., & Godinho Filho, M. (2020). A systematic literature review of empirical research in Lean and Six Sigma in healthcare. *Total Quality Management & Business Excellence*, *31*(3–4), 429–449.

Hibbert, P. D., Thomas, M. J. W., Deakin, A., et al. (2018). Are root cause analyses recommendations effective and sustainable? An observational study. *International Journal for Quality in Health Care: Journal of the International Society for Quality in Health Care*, *30*(2), 124–131.

Husser, E. K., Fick, D. M., Boltz, M., et al. (2021). Implementing a rapid, two-step delirium screening protocol in acute care: Barriers and facilitators. *Journal of the American Geriatrics Society*, *69*(5), 1349–1356.

Institute for Healthcare Improvement (IHI). (2017). *Patient safety 104: Root cause and systems analysis*.

Institute of Medicine (IOM). (1999). *To err is human: Building a safer health system: Executive summary*. The National Academies Press.

Institute of Medicine (IOM). (2001). *Crossing the quality chasm: A new health system for the 21st century: Executive summary*. National Academies Press.

Joint Commission Center for Transforming Healthcare. (2019). *Oro 2.0*. https://www.youtube.com/channel/UCS4jh7RvoMQAr2G-UnuD01g. [Accessed 5 April 2019].

King, D. L. (2008). Research and quality improvement: Different processes, different evidence. *Medsurg Nursing*, *17*(3), 167.

Knudsen, S. V., Laursen, H., Johnsen, S. P., Bartels, P. D., Ehlers, L. H., & Mainz, J. (2019). Can quality improvements improve the quality of care? A systematic review of reported effects and methodological rigor in plan-do-study-act projects. *BMC Health Services Research*, *19*(1), 683.

Langley, G. J., Moen, R. D., Nolan, K. M., et al. (2009). *The improvement guide: A practical approach to enhancing organizational performance* (2nd ed.). Jossey-Bass.

Lau, R., Stevenson, F., Ong, B. N., et al. (2015). Achieving change in primary care—effectiveness of strategies for improving implementation of complex interventions: Systematic review. *BMJ Open, 5*. https://doi.org/10.1136/bmjopn-2015-009993.

Lopez, M. (2019). Standardizing GRN roles and responsibilities: A strategy for sustaining NICHE in an academic medical center. In T. Fulmer, K. Glassman, S. Greenberg, P. Rosenfeld, M. Gilmartin, & M. Mezey (Eds.), *Nurses improving care for healthsystem elders* (pp. 95–112). Springer Publishing Company.

Lopez, M., Ma, C., Aavik, L., & Cortes, T. A. (2023). Implementing a quality improvement program to reduce falls and increase patient medication satisfaction in an academic medical center. *Geriatric Nursing, 49*, 207–211.

McDonald, L. (2017). *Florence Nightingale, nursing, and health care today*. Springer Publishing Company.

McConnell, J. K., Lindrooth, R. C., Wholey, D. R., Maddox, T. M., & Bloom, N. (2016). Modern management practices and hospital admissions. *Health Economics, 25*, 470–485.

Montero-Odasso, M., van der Velde, N., Martin, F. C., et al. (2022). World guidelines for falls prevention and management for older adults: A global initiative. *Age and Ageing, 51*(9), afac205. https://doi.org/10.1093/ageing/afac205.

Moreland, B., Kakara, R., & Henry, A. (2020). Trends in nonfatal falls and fall-related injuries among adults aged ≥65 years—United States, 2012–2018. *MMWR. Morbidity and Mortality Weekly Report, 69*(27), 875–881.

Morse, J. M. (1997). *Preventing patient falls*. Sage.

National Institutes of Health Office of Disease Prevention. (n.d.). *Dissemination and implementation research*. https://prevention.nih.gov/research-priorities/dissemination-implementation.

National Quality Forum (NQF). (2004). *National voluntary consensus standard for nursing-sensitive care: An initial performance measure set*. http://www.qualityforum.org/Publications/2004/10/National_Voluntary_Consensus_Standards_for_Nursing-Sensitive_Care__An_Initial_Performance_Measure_Set.aspx.

National Quality Forum (NQF). (2023). *National Quality Forum, about us*. https://www.qualityforum.org/About_NQF/.

Nelson, E. C., Batalden, P. B., & Godfrey, M. M. (2007). *Quality by design: A clinical microsystems approach*. Jossey-Bass.

Office of Disease Prevention and Promotion. (n.d.). *Healthy People* 2030. https://health.gov/healthypeople/priority-areas/social-determinants-health.

Pohl, J. M., Savrin, C., Fiandt, K., Beauchesne, M., Drayton-Brooks, S., & Werner, K. E. (2009). Quality and safety in graduate nursing education: Cross-mapping QSEN graduate competencies with NONPF's NP core and practice doctorate competencies. *Nursing Outlook, 57*(6), 349–354.

Powell, B. J., Waltz, T. J., Chinman, M. J., et al. (2015). A refined compilation of implementation strategies: Results from the Expert Recommendations for Implementing Change (ERIC) project. *Implementation Science, 10*(21), 1–14.

Quigley, P. A., & White, S. V. (2013). Hospital-based fall program measurement and improvement in high reliability organizations. *Online Journal of Issues in Nursing, 18*(2), 5.

Reed, J. E., & Card, A. J. (2016). The problem with Plan-Do-Study-Act cycles. *BMJ Quality & Safety, 25*(3), 147–152.

Schneider, E. C., Shah, A., Doty, M. M., Tikkanen, R., Fields, K., & Williams II, R. D. (2021). *Mirror, mirror 2021: Reflecting poorly: Health care in the U.S. compared to other high income countries*. The Commonwealth Fund. https://www.commonwealthfund.org/sites/default/files/2021-08/Schneider_Mirror_Mirror_2021.pdf.

Shartzer, A., Berenson, R., Zuckerman, R., Devers, K., & Moiduddin, A. (2021). *Common alternative payment model approaches: Reference guide January 2021*. Department of Health and Human Services, Office of Health Policy, Assistant Secretary for Planning and Evaluation. https://aspe.hhs.gov/sites/default/files/private/aspe-files/207901/common-apms-reference-guide-2021.pdf.

SQUIRE 2.0. (2020). *Revised standards for quality improvement reporting excellence SQUIRE 2.0*. http://www.squire-statement.org/index.cfm?fuseaction=Page.ViewPage&PageID=471.

University Research Co. (2023). *USAID ASSIST Project—25 essential resources for health care quality improvement*. https://www.urc-chs.com/assist-25/.

U.S. Department of Veterans Affairs. (2023). *Root cause analysis*. https://www.patientsafety.va.gov/professionals/onthejob/rca.asp.

Weick, K. E., & Sutcliffe, K. M. (2015). *Managing the unexpected* (3rd ed.). Jossey-Bass.

Werner, R. M., Emanuel, E., Phan, H. H., & Navathe, A. S. (2021). *The future of value-based payment: A roadmap to 2023*. Penn LDI- Leonard Davis Institute of Health Economics, University of Pennsylvania.

Yen, P. H., & Leasure, A. R. (2019). Use and effectiveness of the teach-back method in patient education and health outcomes. *Federal Practitioner: For the Health Care Professionals of the VA, DoD, and PHS, 36*(6), 284–289.

KEY POINTS

- There is much room for improvement in the quality of care in the United States.
- The quality of healthcare is evaluated in terms of its effectiveness, efficiency, access, safety, timeliness, and patient centeredness.
- As the largest group of health professionals, nurse leaders play a key role in leading QI efforts in clinical settings.
- Accreditation, payment, and performance measurement are external incentives used to improve the quality of care delivered by hospitals and health professionals. Examples of accrediting organizations focusing on health care quality in care delivery organizations include the Joint Commission, the National Committee for Quality Assurance, the Council on Accreditation, the American Nurses Credentialing Center, and the American College of Surgeons.
- The Quality Payment Program and HEDIS are sources of standardized measures to assess and improve the quality of care delivered in the United States.
- Standardized measures such as influenza vaccination rates are used to compare performance across clinical practices and organizations.
- Health care payers use quality performance measures such as 30-day readmission rates as a basis for paying hospitals and providers.
- QI is both a philosophy of organizational functioning and a set of statistical analysis tools and change techniques used to reduce variation.
- The major approaches used to manage quality in healthcare are TQM/CQI; Lean; Six Sigma; the Clinical Microsystems model; and the HRO model.
- The defining characteristics of QI are a focus on patients/customers; teams and teamwork to improve work processes; and use of data and statistical analysis tools to understand system variation.
- QI uses benchmarking to compare organizational performance and learn from high-performing organizations.
- QI tools, techniques, and principles are applied to clinical performance problems in the form of improvement projects, such as using a presurgical checklist to prevent wrong-side surgeries, a national patient safety goal.
- Practice-level improvement projects should align with national improvement priorities to promote the sustainability of local projects.
- There are four major steps in the QI process: assessment, analysis, improvement, and evaluation.
- Patient safety focuses on designing systems to remove factors known to cause errors or adverse events.
- Barriers exist that impede the leadership role of nurses in QI, including insufficient staffing, lack of leadership support, and clinical leaders' unfamiliarity with QI principles and practices.

15

Planning for Success

Marita G. Titler and Eileen P. Magri

LEARNING OUTCOMES

After reading this chapter, you should be able to do the following:
- Apply the Translating Research Into Practice Model in implementing evidence-based practices (EBPs).
- Analyze the attributes of an EBP topic that impact adoption.
- Compare and contrast roles of the EBP team in implementation.
- Describe the importance of quality improvement (QI) as a foundation for EBP implementation.
- Apply the principles of implementation derived from Rogers's Diffusion of Innovation Theory.
- Identify organization and system factors that influence implementation of EBPs.
- Develop an action plan for implementation of an EBP.
- Analyze three ethical issues in EBP.
- Compare and contrast the definitions, intent, and requirements for Institutional Review Board (IRB) approval for QI, EBP, and research.

KEY TERMS

Action plan
Implementation
Translating Research Into Practice Model

Implementation is the core of EBP. Implementation is defined as the processes and strategies used to promote the uptake and use of EBPs by clinicians, consumers, and policy makers. Attending to the details of implementation requires attention, without which there is little chance that the EBPs will be used by clinicians and patients. Implementation at times can seem messy, iterative, and nonlinear. It requires tenacity, commitment, and relationship building. The Implementation Section of this text book (Part III: Implementation) is designed for you and your team to be successful in implementing EBPs in your community, organization, and/or primary care site. This chapter provides a model, principles, and considerations when planning for implementation to guide you and your team. Chapters 16 and 17 provide specific implementation strategies and provide examples for each. If a practice change is warranted to align health care practices with current evidence recommendations, you and your team will need to develop an action plan to implement the practice changes. An action plan, described in a later section, is a written outline that details the goals/objectives, work to be achieved, person/group responsible for the work, and the designated date for completion of the work. Implementation goes beyond writing and disseminating evidence-based standards of practice; it requires interactions among direct care providers to champion and foster evidence adoption, leadership support, and system changes.

OVERVIEW OF AN IMPLEMENTATION MODEL

The Translating Research Into Practice (TRIP) Model is an implementation model based on Rogers's (2003) seminal work on diffusion of innovations, and is useful in guiding selection of strategies for promoting adoption of EBPs. According to this model (Fig. 15.1), adoption of EBPs is influenced by four key areas:
- The *nature of the innovation* (e.g., the type and strength of evidence, the clinical topic) and
- the manner in which the innovation is *communicated*
- to *members* (clinicians)
- and the social *system* (organization, patient care unit).

Successful implementation requires implementation strategies that address these areas within a context of participative, planned change (Titler et al., 2016; Titler, 2018).

The Institute for Healthcare Improvement (IHI) describes a process that emphasizes innovation, rapid-cycle testing, and spread to determine if improvement is occurring. The Model for Improvement requires that an aim be established with measurable goals within a defined period of time. The strategy includes rapid-cycle testing or Plan-Do-Study-Act (PDSA) cycles to identify early success or the need to review the process (IHI, 2023). PDSA cycles allow for small tests of change to be integrated into implementation before moving to full adoption of the proposed change. Integrating PDSA cycles into the implementation strategies ensures that workflows will support the planned change.

> **TIP**
> Planning for successful implementation starts with topic selection and continues throughout all steps of the EBP process. If the topic is not a priority for your setting or organization, you will encounter difficulties with implementation no matter how strong the evidence.

THE EVIDENCE-BASED PRACTICE TOPIC

Successful implementation is influenced by the EBP topic. Ideas for your topic may have come from several areas, such as problem- and/or knowledge-focused triggers, new practice standards, regulatory requirements, or the strategic plan of the organization (see Chapters 5 and 6). Topics tend to reveal themselves in a particular setting based on unexpected patient outcomes. In selecting a topic, it is essential that you and your team consider how the topic fits with the priorities of your practice agency (e.g., community setting, health system, primary care practice) to garner support from leaders and the necessary resources for successful implementation. Opportunity to bring practice in line with national benchmarks as demonstrated by trending quality data supports the need for change.

It is imperative that your topic has an evidence base determined by the critical appraisal and a synthesis of the evidence. Otherwise, it is not EBP. All team members should be highly knowledgeable about the strength and quality of the evidence for your topic, the rationale for selecting it, and the QI data that demonstrates the opportunities to improve the quality of care. For example, urinary tract infections (UTIs)

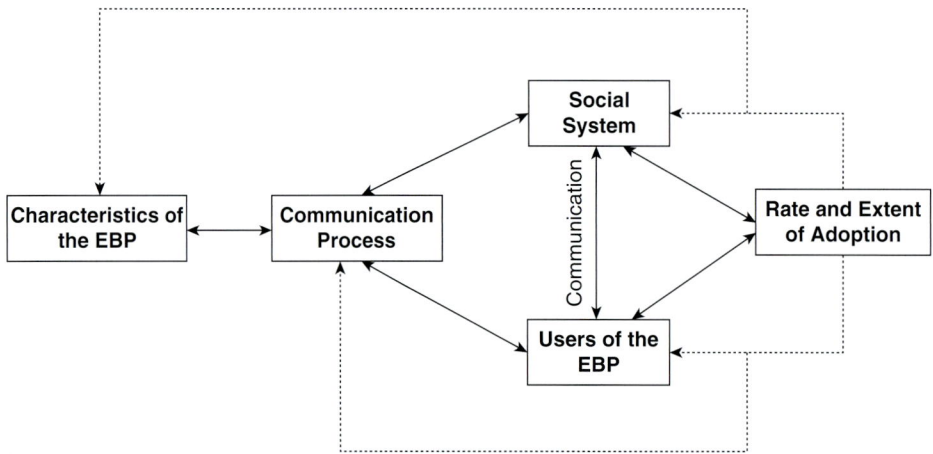

Fig. 15.1 Translating Research Into Practice Model. *EBP,* Evidence-based practice. (From Titler, 2018.)

account for approximately 40% of all hospital-acquired infections annually, with fully 80% of these hospital-acquired UTIs attributable to indwelling urethral catheters. It is well established that the duration of catheterization is directly related to risk for developing a UTI. With a catheter in place, the daily risk of developing a UTI ranges from 3% to 7% (IHI, 2023). Magtoto (2022) evaluated the best available evidence in the literature for prevention of UTIs from indwelling catheters. The critical appraisal and synthesis support recommended EBPs (Box 15.1).

Among the 10 hospital-acquired conditions selected by the Centers for Medicare and Medicaid Services, catheter-associated UTI received a high priority due to its high cost and high volume, and because it can be reasonably prevented through application of accepted evidence-based prevention guidelines (IHI, 2023).

Based on your clinical question as outlined in Chapter 5, the purpose of your EBP project should be clear including the problem, patient population, the processes and outcomes of care to be addressed, and the setting (e.g., inpatient unit(s), clinic(s), or community setting). It is important to share the purpose statement with all key stakeholders and keep it visible during implementation to prevent "scope creep"—that is, expanding the project beyond what is realistic and needed for successful implementation.

> **TIP**
>
> **Example of EBP Purpose Statement**
>
> The purpose of this EBP project is to implement practices to prevent catheter-associated urinary tract infection (CAUTI bundle) in hospitalized adults and thereby reduce CAUTI rates, morbidity, mortality, and hospital length of stay. CAUTI prevention practices include: avoid unnecessary use of indwelling catheters, use indwelling catheter alternatives, use aseptic catheter insertion, early removal of catheter ("stop orders").

BOX 15.1 Program Recommendations and Examples of Interventions to Prevent Catheter-Associated Urinary Tract Infection

Recommendation	Example of Intervention
Primary	
Conducting daily assessment of the presence of and need for an indwelling urinary catheter	Conducting daily nursing rounds to review urine-collection strategies, including indications for continued urinary-catheter use
Avoiding use of an indwelling urinary catheter by considering alternative urine-collection methods	Promoting the use of condom catheters, bladder scanners, intermittent straight catheterization, and accurate measurement of daily weight (all in lieu of indwelling urinary catheters)
Emphasizing the importance of aseptic technique during catheter insertion and proper maintenance after insertion	Developing or updating the catheter-insertion policy to include all the proper steps, developing competencies for health care workers who insert catheters, and considering periodic audits of catheter placement
Additional	
Providing feedback to the units regarding urinary-catheter use and catheter-associated UTI rates	Providing nurses and physicians with data on urinary-catheter use, with monthly feedback on use and catheter-associated UTIs
Addressing any identified gaps in knowledge of urinary management processes	Conducting an evaluation for gaps in knowledge of infectious and noninfectious consequences of urinary-catheter use; developing tailored educational materials to fill identified gaps; using multiple venues for education, including bedside and electronic; incorporating education into annual competency testing for nurses; and using multiple venues for physicians (formal presentations and meetings, with one-to-one discussions for physicians with high use)

From Saint et al., 2016.

The attributes of the EBP topic that influence implementation are (Table 15.1):
- Relative advantage
- Compatibility
- Complexity
- Trialability
- Observability (Rogers, 2003)

EBPs with more of these attributes, except complexity, will be more readily adopted in practice. However, having a new practice adopted is difficult even when it has these obvious advantages.

> **TIP**
> Attributes of the EBP topic as perceived by users and stakeholders are neither stable features nor sure determinants of EBP use.

The Team

EBP work is a team effort requiring representatives from various disciplines guided by the nature of the EBP topic and clinical question. For example, a team working on

TABLE 15.1 Attributes of EBP Topics and Implementation

Attributes of EBP Topic	Description	Examples of Implementation Strategies*
Relative Advantage	Degree to which an EBP is perceived as being better than the practice it supersedes. Cost and social status motivation aspects of new ideas or EBPs are elements of relative advantage. Early adopters and early majority are more status-motivated than the late majority and laggards.	Direct or indirect financial payment incentives may be used to support adopting an EBP. This strategy is actualized by CMS's value-based payment programs. Performance gap assessment. Benchmarking with other organizations.
Compatibility	Degree to which an innovation is perceived as consistent with the existing values, norms, past experiences, and needs of potential adopters. If an EBP is compatible with patients' and clinicians' needs, uncertainty will decrease and the rate of adoption of will increase.	Naming the EBP is an important part of compatibility. What the EBP is called should be meaningful to clinicians. Name the EBP project to clearly reflect the focus. Consider adopting an EBP market icon that reflects the EBP.
Complexity	Degree to which an EBP is perceived as relatively difficult to understand and use. Complexity is negatively correlated with the rate of adoption. Excessive complexity is a potential obstacle in its adoption.	Break complex EBP topics into conceptual parts and implement components sequentially rather than simultaneously. Narrow the selected topic so implementation is manageable. Use quick reference guides and decision aides.
Trialability	Degree to which an EBP can be tried on a limited basis. The more an EBP can be tried, the faster its adoption. Reinvention—modification of the EBP may occur during the trial and thereby create faster adoption.	Plan for piloting the change in practice as part of implementation.
Observability	Degree to which the impact of an EBP are visible to others. Role modeling and peer observation is key.	Audit and feedback. Opinion leaders and change champions.

*See Chapters 16 and 17 for discussion of implementation strategies.
CMS, Centers for Medicare and Medicaid Services.

evidence-based acute pain management should be interprofessional and include pharmacists, nurses, advanced practice nurses, physicians, and psychologists with expertise in pain management. A team working on EBPs for family presence during resuscitation may include a social worker, chaplain, psychologist, staff nurses, nurse manager, advanced practice nurse, physician(s), and a family member.

Know your team members. Planning for implementation requires that all team members participate in some component of implementation. Each team member has something to contribute. Some team members may be best skilled at teaching their peers about the EBPs to be implemented and the evidence base for each. Others may be best at managing or negotiating organizational system changes. Still others may be best suited to influence the thinking and actions of their peers using a point-of-care coaching approach. Implementation is about relationships that foster questioning, respect, and trust. Thus, planning for implementation requires that, as team members, you know one another's strengths, passions, and biases.

An essential element of planning for successful implementation is your team's clarity about the following:
- Rationale for deciding to change practice (Box 15.2)
- Specific EBPs to be implemented

Following evidence synthesis, your team sets forth EBP recommendations with an evidence grade for each (see Chapter 4). These EBP recommendations need to be converted into practice statements for your setting. This is necessary so that individuals in your setting know (1) that the practices are based on evidence, and (2) the type and evidence grade used in development of the practices.

QUALITY IMPROVEMENT AS A FOUNDATION FOR IMPLEMENTATION

QI is an essential foundation for EBP implementation (see Chapter 14). Planning for implementation success requires selecting:
- Quality metrics and data sources for evaluating the impact of implementing the EBPs
- Methods for display of quality metrics
- Methods for communicating the quality metrics to staff over time

Selected metrics are collected, analyzed, and presented in a dashboard prior to, during, and upon completion of implementation. These metrics are integrated into the organization's QI program to support and evaluate sustainability of the EBPs, and the need for implementation "boosters" over time. The use of dashboards provides real-time data to track and trend progress. For example, if the focus of your EBP project is to implement evidence-based CAUTI prevention practices that mitigate UTIs in patients with indwelling bladder catheters, the CAUTI rates would be expected to decline over time—that is from prior to implementation, during implementation, and following implementation. Therefore, utilizing the national benchmark data related to CAUTI rates, prior to implementation, during the implementation process, and following implementation can ensure sustainability of the improvement. If CAUTI rates start trending upward following implementation, you will want to determine why this is happening, and correct the problem, which may be that clinicians have become lax in continuing to use the EBPs that were implemented. See Chapter 14 for more information and illustrations of QI.

PRINCIPLES OF IMPLEMENTATION

Implementation is a dynamic, iterative process influenced by all steps of EBP described in Chapter 3 (see Table 3.4). Key principles for implementation (Rogers, 2003) are:
- Decision makers move from knowledge about an innovation (e.g., EBPs) through implementation and confirmation (see Table 15.2).
- Clinicians do not adopt EBPs at the same time.

BOX 15.2 Examples: Rationale for Changing Practice

- The evidence is relevant to our practice with opportunities to improve the quality of care.
- A significant number of studies, EBP guidelines, systematic reviews, and other evidence sources are available.
- Evidence sources reflect or include study subjects and/or study sample characteristics similar to our patient population.
- There is a consistency across evidence sources regarding practices that are supported by research findings and other types of evidence.
- Our current practice is not aligned with the evidence.
- Our QI data on [insert here] suggest we have opportunity to improve quality of care in this area.
- The benefit for our patient population outweighs the risk of harm.

TABLE 15.2 Stages of Adoption

Stage of Decision Process	Description	Examples of Implementation Strategies*
Knowledge	Decision makers (individuals or unit) are exposed and gain an understanding of the EBP. Individuals learn about the existence of the evidence for the practice and seek information about the EBP: "what?," "how?," and "why?"	Educate users about the EBP including the strength and evidence grade. Include key stakeholders in evidence appraisal and synthesis.
Persuasion	Decision makers form a favorable or unfavorable attitude toward the EBP. While the knowledge stage is more cognitive (knowing)-centered, the persuasion stage is more affective (feeling)-centered. The degree of uncertainty about the effectiveness of the EBP and the social reinforcement from colleagues and peers affect an individual's opinions and beliefs about the EBP. Close peers' subjective evaluations that reduce uncertainty about the EBP impact are usually more credible to the individual.	Use opinion leaders and change champions.
Decision	Decision makers engage in activities that lead to a choice to adopt or reject the EBP. If individuals can try the EBP, it is usually adopted more quickly, because most individuals first want to try applying the EBP in their own situation and then come to an adoption decision.	Pilot the change on a small scale. Plan for pilot as part of implementation.
Implementation	When an EBP is put into use. Uncertainty about the impact of the EBP on outcomes can still be a problem at this stage. Assistance from change agents and others to reduce the degree of uncertainty about the consequences of the EBP is helpful.	Use opinion leaders and change champions. Use audit and feedback. Use educational outreach and point-of-care coaching.
Confirmation	Individuals seek reinforcement for the EBP decision already made but may reverse the decision if exposed to conflicting messages. Individuals tend to seek supportive messages that confirm his or her decision. Individuals may reject the EBP because he or she is not satisfied with its performance.	Discuss audit and feedback of process and outcome data.

*See Chapters 16 and 17 for discussion of implementation strategies.
From Rogers, 2003.

- Time for implementation varies depending on the nature and complexity of the innovation or EBPs.
- When 30% to 40% of individuals adopt the new idea (e.g., early adopters), there is a natural take-off in the rate of adoption.

Individuals fall into different adopter categories:
- Innovators
- Early adopters
- Early majority
- Late majority
- Laggards

Within each category, individuals are similar in terms of their innovativeness—the degree to which they are earlier in adopting new ideas or willingness to change their practice as compared to others. The percentage of individuals differs across adopter categories (see Table 15.3).

Time for EBPs varies by their overall complexity; however, each implementation plan should identify a clear aim and time period for rapid-cycle testing with the end goal of sustainability. For example, EBPs that are complex (e.g., implementing CAUTI prevention bundles that target patients with indwelling bladder

TABLE 15.3 Description of Adopter Categories and Percentage in Each

Adopter Category	Description
Innovators	Innovators (2.5%) are willing to experience new ideas and are able to cope with uncertainty. They are venturesome and bring new ideas into organizations from the outside. They are respected by other members of the social system because of their sense of venturesome and close relationships to others outside the organization.
Early Adopters	Compared to innovators, early adopters (13.5%) are more limited to the boundaries of the local setting. Others come to them to get advice or information about the new idea. As role models, their subjective evaluations about the EBPs reach other clinicians through their interpersonal networks. Early adopters put their stamp of approval on a new idea by adopting it, and thus decrease the uncertainty about it.
Early Majority	Although the early majority (34%) have a good interaction with other clinicians, they do not have the leadership influence that early adopters have. However, their interpersonal networks are still important in the adoption process. They are deliberate in adopting a new idea and are neither the first nor the last to adopt it. Their decision to adopt a new idea usually takes more time than it takes innovators and early adopters. The early majority comprises about 1/3 for all members of a social system.
Late Majority	The late majority (34%) wait until most of their peers adopt the innovation and then they feel safe to adopt it. They are skeptical about the new idea and its impact, but peer pressure may lead them to adoption. Interpersonal networks of close peers usually persuade the late majority to adopt the new idea.
Laggards	Laggards (16%) have the traditional view and are more skeptical about new ideas than the late majority. Their interpersonal networks mainly consist of others from the same category. They first want to make sure that an idea works before they adopt. They tend to make decisions about adoption after looking at whether the idea is successfully adopted by others. Their process of adopting is relatively long.

catheters) require a longer time period for implementation as compared to simpler ones (e.g., screening for annual flu vaccines for hospitalized older adults).

Organization and system factors are important considerations when implementing EBPs. Thus, you need to:

1. Explicate how your EBPs support the mission, vision, strategic agendas, and organizational targets for improving quality of care (e.g., preventing hospital-acquired infections; improving the patient experience).
2. Be strategic in engaging key leaders early in the EBP work and keep them informed of the progress. Leaders include the chief nursing officer, chief medical officer, chair of service lines, a faculty member from an academic partnership, and/or nurse managers of units as well as the clinical staff at the bedside where the EBPs will be implemented. In community settings such as primary care practices, the size and complexity of the primary care medical home (PCMH) will influence who the organizational leader will be, ranging from the PCMH director to the PCMH manager.
3. Call on the expertise of individuals within your organization, such as QI leaders and advanced practice nurses (APNs). QI leaders can provide guidance on quality metrics and available benchmark data needed to evaluate the impact of the EBP. APNs, nurse practitioners, clinical nurse specialists, and unit-level champions can provide leadership for many EBP steps, including acquisition and critical appraisal of the evidence, integration of evidence into the local practice standards, and communicating with key stakeholders.
4. Engage organizational and departmental committees in the EBP work. Consider the shared governance committees and unit/clinical practice councils you will need to interact with to make changes in practice. Consult with the chairs of these committees throughout the process and keep them informed of your progress.

5. Share progress at predetermined intervals (monthly, quarterly) to all key stakeholders. Data can be displayed through electronic dashboards, departmental High Reliability Organization (HRO) boards, and meeting minutes.
6. Market messages about the EBP widely across the organization. Content of messages and methods of communication should be customized for types of recipients and will differ according to the EBP steps. For example, if the focus is to implement EBPs to prevent hypothermia in premature infants, your marketing message may be: "It is not 'hot' to be cool." If your project is to improve physical activity of community-dwelling older adults, your message may be "Mobile for Life."

> **TIP**
>
> Consider the context of implementation when planning. What is the nature of the practice culture with respect to questioning practice, leadership styles, innovativeness, and commitment to quality of care?

Although there is no one right way to implement a practice change, there are several common myths and realities regarding implementation that warrant consideration (Table 15.4). These are essential to address in planning for success.

ACTION PLANS

Action plans assist with EBP implementation. An **action plan** is a written document developed collectively by the EBP team and other key stakeholders that promotes collective buy-in for the plan. The action plan identifies key drivers that support the interventions. The importance of an action plan is that it:

- Provides a good idea about the overall scope of the work, and course of action
- Makes the work more intentional
- Breaks the EBP process into actionable steps
- Fosters clear communication of who is responsible for what steps and projected dates of achievement
- Helps prevent duplication of effort
- Makes it easier to stay focused and make midcourse corrections as needed
- Can be reviewed and updated as the EBP processes move forward
- Can serve as a timeline
- Takes into account the need for sustaining the EBP change

Key components of an action plan are the objectives, action steps, individual(s) or group responsible for each action item, due date for each action item, and progress. The EBP purpose statement is documented on the action plan and used to develop the objectives. Action items to meet each objective are set forth (Box 15.3).

> **TIP**
>
> Include dates on the action plan when it was developed and updated.

ETHICAL CONSIDERATIONS FOR EVIDENCE-BASED PRACTICE

Ethical issues are embedded in EBP processes and include (Hunt et al., 2021):
- Critical appraisal and synthesis of the evidence
- Development of EBP recommendations
- Shared decision making
- Assuring availability of resources

Knowledge is ranked and classified in a hierarchical approach. The language of EBP has traditionally mirrored that of empiricism, that is, use of findings from quantitative studies, with evidence from randomized controlled trials (RCTs) (see Chapter 8) and systematic reviews (see Chapter 10) being regarded as the most reliable and valid. More recently, experts have argued that qualitative approaches may be more applicable for some health care practices (Rycroft-Malone et al., 2012). Most qualitative research is based on in-depth explorations with smaller, more purposefully selected samples and seeks to understand the meaning that patients and families place on how their problems and health care treatments are experienced (see Chapter 11). Practice is complex, and qualitative approaches provide valuable insights for clinicians. In-depth qualitative studies call attention to health care processes that are valuable in helping clinicians deliver practices in real-world situations. Qualitative research findings can provide important insights that quantitative studies may not address. While not generalizable in the traditional sense, in-depth, qualitative data is referred to in the qualitative literature as "metaphoric generalizable," and is essential for learning about the lived experiences of diverse populations of patients

TABLE 15.4 Myths and Realities of Implementation

Components of TRIP Model	Myths	Realities and Suggestions for Implementation
Nature of the EBP topic	The evidence is strong, and clinicians will change practice if we show them the evidence. An EBP standard will change practice. Clinicians care about the EBP topic.	• Characteristics of the topic influence adoption: relative advantage, compatibility, complexity, trialability, and observability. • Engage clinicians in topic selection. • Demonstrate improvement opportunities using local QI and benchmarking data. • Explicate the relationship to strategic initiatives and QI targets. Keep discussions patient centered. • EBP recommendations need localization to fit the practice setting: develop local EBP standards. • Engage clinicians in localization of EBP recommendations. • Creation of local EBP standards is essential but alone will not change practice. • Use quick reference guides, decision aides, and clinical reminders.
Communication	Clinicians stay abreast of the latest evidence. Clinicians learn about new evidence by reading journals and other evidence sources. We just need to educate clinicians about the EBP for effective implementation.	• Explosion of evidence makes it difficult to stay abreast of the latest evidence. • Most clinicians learn about the evidence from a trusted colleague. • Education is necessary but not sufficient to change practice. • Interactive education is more effective than didactic education. • Communication factors that influence adoption include interpersonal communication channels, methods of communication, and social networks of users. • There is a simple way to package information that, under the right circumstances, can be irresistible and spur us to action. • Use opinion leaders, change champions, and educational outreach, and display key messages at the site of care delivery.
Users of the EBP	Clinicians will adopt EBPs at about the same pace. I just have to get those resistors on board. If I build it, they will come (a.k.a.: If I tell clinicians about the EBPs, they will implement them). Clinicians have been educated about the EBPs—they should follow them.	• Clinicians vary in their rate of adoption of EBPs. • Focus on adoption by innovators, early adopters, and early majority. • Implementation of a new practice requires changing how things are done and affects multiple individuals from multiple specialties and their interrelationships. • Implementation requires partnerships and collaboration. • Use performance gap assessment, audit and feedback, and trying the change in practice (pilot).
Social system	One size fits all. Practice cultures in our organization are similar across units/clinics. Changing practice is the nurse manager's responsibility.	• Context matters—practice cultures differ within organizations. • Organizational factors affecting adoption include a learning culture, leadership, and capacity to evaluate the impact of the EBP during and following implementation. • Effective implementation needs both a receptive climate and a good fit with intended users' needs and values. • Performance criteria for all professional roles should include EBP. • The governance structure needs to explicate the committees/groups responsible for advancing EBP work. • Human resources with expertise in EBP are necessary (e.g., APNs). • Although unit-level leadership is important, all clinicians are responsible for EBP. • Engage key leaders early and often. • Provide short bulleted updates for key leaders.

BOX 15.3 Action Plan

EBP project purpose statement: The purpose of this EBP project is to implement EB CAUTI risk reduction/prevention practices that target patients with indwelling bladder catheters and thereby decrease CAUTI rates in three adult medical units—7C, 3W, and 4D. The EB CAUTI bundle of care addresses risk of infection, additional hospitalized days, morbidity, and mortality.

Objective	Action Steps	Responsible Person	Completion Date	Progress
Educate clinicians about the EBP	Decide key educational content.	Jane Smith	June 2023	Completed
	Design educational methods.	Jane Smith		
	Develop education materials.	Jane Smith		
	Schedule and deliver the education	Gary Jones		
Develop EBP documents for the units	Select key elements needed at the point of care.	Suzy Jordan Name/group	June 2023	In progress
	Decide on use of Quick Reference Guides (QRG), decision aides, clinical reminders			
Integrate EBP content into organizational standards	Work with Standards Committee to update CAUTI prevention standards.	Name/group Name/group	Date Date	
	Work with Information Technology (IT) to update electronic health record documentation.			
Decide on core outcome measures to track over time for evaluation	Meet with QI chair to determine available data.	Name/group Name/group EBP team	Date Date Date	
	Note outcomes used from reviewed studies.			
	Select outcome metrics.			

Developed January 15, 2023; updated on: September 5, 2024

---

and families (Streubert & Carpenter, 2011). For example, a study using qualitative content analysis explored the experience of women choosing to continue to express milk after a perinatal loss specifically for donation to a nonprofit milk bank governed by the Human Milk Banking Association of North America. Lactation occurs after birth regardless of the infant's survival. Findings from the study identified themes: an outlet to grieve, a meaningful life, still a mother, a positive from a negative, support and recognition, letting go and moving on, and finding my way. Expressing and donating milk helped the mothers with the grieving process. The practice implication of this study identified a call to action for health care providers to include lactation and milk donation in perinatal loss programs (Paraszczuk, et al., 2022). Thus, in critical appraisal, synthesis of evidence, and development of EBP recommendations, it is essential that we are transparent about (1) methods used to acquire the evidence; (2) types of evidence appraised and synthesized; and (3) inclusiveness of both qualitative and quantitative studies in making practice recommendations (Gough et al., 2020).

Scientific evidence is central to EBP and may overshadow other important values, such as patient autonomy and choice. If EBP becomes the most important factor in health care delivery, the focus on patient/family empowerment and autonomy may be at risk. For instance, research may show a specific medication or treatment approach to be most effective, yet a patient may wish to handle his/her problem in a manner that is more consistent with their personal values, health beliefs, or strengths. While EBP does not call for clinicians to ignore the wishes of patients and families, clinicians may inadvertently become overzealous in "pushing" certain interventions. In our zeal to be objective and informed, we may forget that clinical decision making, at its core, is a patient-centered, ethical matter. Social determinants of health influence a patient's ability to continue with recommended interventions (see Fig. 25.3 in Chapter 25). For example, patients who have congestive heart failure and are advised to maintain a low-sodium diet, may be unable to have access to recommended food choices due to financial challenges and may need to decide whether to pay rent or purchase healthy food. When clinicians are educating patients and advising certain interventions, the social support systems in the community need to be evaluated to ensure optimal compliance. Shared decision making is an important component of EBP (see Chapter 18). We have an ethical obligation to share with patients and families the choices for health care treatments in a manner that they understand and relate to their current situation.

Organizations and agencies must allocate sufficient resources for staff to fully implement all phases of the EBP process. If agencies and the professionals they employ choose to embrace an organizational culture that values EBP, then EBP, in its breadth and complexity, stands to be more fully embraced—especially with respect to those elements that may require organizational realignment. By doing so, organizations are providing ethical agency responsiveness to patients, families, and communities they serve.

One concern that rises with EBP is the question of IRB approval. EBP does not require IRB approval; it is a type of QI with a definition and intent that differs from research (Table 15.5) (Bass III & Maloy,

TABLE 15.5 Differentiating QI, EBP, and Conduct of Research

	QI	EBP	Conduct of Research
Definitions	A process by which individuals work together within a specified local setting to improve systems and processes of healthcare with the intention to improve health outcomes.	Conscientious and judicious use of current best evidence in conjunction with clinical expertise, patient values, and circumstances to guide health care decisions.	A systematic investigation, including research development, testing, and evaluation, designed to develop or contribute to generalizable knowledge.
Intent	Improve health care processes, quality, and safety in a local clinical setting.	Improve quality and safety within the local clinical setting by applying evidence in health care decisions.	Contribute to and/or generate new knowledge that can be generalized.
Approaches and Methods	Plan-Do-Check-Act (PDCA) Plan-Do-Study-Act (PDSA) LEAN Six Sigma Continuous Quality Improvement (CQI) Total Quality Management (TQM)	Multiple models for EBP. Common steps: • Topic selection • Team formation • Critical appraisal and evidence synthesis • Implementation • Evaluation: processes and outcomes	Scientific research designs and methods: Quantitative: RCTs; quasi-experimental; observational cohort Qualitative: ethnography, grounded theory, phenomenology
Sample	Convenience sample. Size relatively small yet large enough to note change over time.	Convenience sample. Size relatively small yet large enough to note change over time.	Sample varies based on research questions. Size based on estimates of adequate power (power analysis) or saturation.
Data Analysis	Descriptive statistics, run charts, Statistical Process Control (SPC) charts.	Descriptive statistics, run charts, SPC charts.	Descriptive and inferential statistics to address study aims.
Impact	Improved quality and safety in local setting.	Improved quality and safety in local setting.	Generalizable knowledge.
Dissemination	Within the local setting. May publish in clinical or QI journals but doing so does not indicate this is research.	Within the local setting. May publish in clinical or QI journals but doing so does not indicate this is research.	Expected to publish in peer-reviewed scientific journals & present peer-reviewed papers at scientific meetings.
IRB	Does not meet the definition of research; some organizations require that QI projects be submitted to the IRB to ensure IRB is not required. IRB review varies by organizational IRB expectations.	Does not meet the definition of research; some organizations require that EBP projects be submitted to the IRB to ensure IRB is not required. IRB review varies by organizational IRB expectations.	IRB review and approval required. The IRB may rule the study as exempt depending on the nature of the study.

2020; Kawar et al., 2023; Hockenberry, 2014). However, some organizations recommend submitting EBP projects to the IRB to ensure IRB review is not required. For example, the University of California, San Diego (UCSD) Human Research Protections Program (HRPP) has determined that many projects involving EBP and QI are not likely to meet the definition of "research" stated in the Department of Health and Human Services Regulations for the Protection of Human Subjects at 45 CFR Part 46, Subpart A, and would, therefore, be excluded from IRB review. However, such projects require review and certification from the HRPP director that the project is not research, and no IRB review is required (Box 15.4) (https://irb.ucsd.edu/researchers/qi_rchsd.html). Therefore, check the procedures in your setting to determine what may be expected regarding IRB review for QI and EBP projects.

> **TIP**
>
> Implementation is a process, not an event.

SYNTHESIS

Now that you have been introduced to the principles and considerations of implementation, you and your team will need to plan for implementation. Remember that implementation is a dynamic, iterative process that takes time and commitment from you and your team. All EBP work is important, but implementation is most critical for people, patients, and health care systems to benefit from all the work you have invested in setting forth EBP recommendations to improve quality of care and health outcomes that are sustainable over time. What will you and your team do to plan for success and realize the benefits of promoting use of EBPs in your setting?

BOX 15.4 Procedures for Submitting EBP and QI Projects to the HRPP

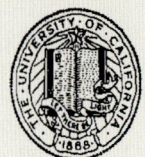

University of California, San Diego Human Research Protections Program
Fact Sheet
EBP/QA/QI Projects

The UCSD Human Research Protections Program (HRPP) has determined that many projects involving evidence-based practice (EBP), quality assurance (QA), and quality improvement (QI) are not likely to meet the definition of "research" stated in the Department of Health and Human Services Regulations for the Protection of Human Subjects at 45 CFR Part 46, Subpart A, and would, therefore, be excluded from IRB review. However, such projects will require review and certification from the HRPP director that the project is not research and no IRB review is required.

These regulations define "research" as "a systematic investigation, including research development, testing and evaluation, designed to develop or contribute to generalizable knowledge."

The UCSD HRPP Standard Operating Policies and Procedures define generalizable knowledge as "Activities designed (with intent) to collect information about some individuals to draw general conclusions about other individuals that are predictive of future events and that can be widely applied as expressed in theories, principles, and statements and that enhance scientific or academic understanding."

In order for a project to be certified as not research, the following must be true:

1. Implementing the practice outlined in the project will not incur patient harm.
2. The practice change outlined in the project is not new or novel and has been published elsewhere.
3. The practice outlined in the project will be implemented in a project location.
4. All staff and affected patients in the project location will be expected to participate in the project.
5. The project is not testing issues or adding research questions that go beyond common practice.
6. The project will not randomize patients into different intervention groups.
7. The project will not deliberately delay interpretation of data.
8. The project will not deliberately delay or abbreviate feedback to those who would benefit from the findings to enhance likelihood of publication.
9. The project has no funding support from an outside organization with a commercial interest in the use of the results.

> **BOX 15.4 Procedures for Submitting EBP and QI Projects to the HRPP—cont'd**
>
> To obtain certification, the following procedures must be done:
> 1. Complete the *EBP/QA/QI Project: Standard Application for Review Facesheets* (all questions in section 3 must be answered "Yes").
> 2. Submit the Facesheets via the web to the HRPP office.
> 3. Once the HRPP project number has been obtained, upload the signed Facesheets and the *Project Narrative* using *e-IRB services*.
> 4. If the project is certified as not research, certification will be emailed to the Investigator.
> 5. If the project is determined to be research, a letter will be emailed to the Investigator noting the determination and providing additional information regarding "re-submitting" the project for convened IRB or expedited review.
>
> For questions as to whether a project is human subjects research, please contact the Director of the Human Research Protections Program.
> Version date: 7/1715

From the University of California, San Diego.

KEY POINTS

- Successful implementation is influenced by the EBP topic.
- Five attributes of the EBP topic influence implementation of the EBPs: relative advantage, compatibility, complexity, trialability, and observability.
- Planning for implementation requires that all team members participate in some component of implementation.
- Sustainability strategies should be considered throughout your EBP project.
- Implementation planning necessitates selecting (1) quality metrics and data sources for evaluating the impact of implementing the EBPs, (2) methods for display of quality metrics, and (3) methods for communicating the quality metrics to staff over time.
- Implementation is a dynamic, iterative process.
- Time for implementation varies depending on the nature and complexity of the innovation or EBP.
- EBP topics that are complex require a longer time period for implementation as compared to simpler topics.
- Principles of organizational functioning are important considerations when implementing EBPs.
- Key components of an implementation action plan are the objectives, action steps, individual(s) or group responsible for each action item, due date for each action item, and progress.
- EBP is a type of QI with a definition and intent that differs from research.
- Some organizations require submission of EBP projects to the IRBs to ensure IRB review is not required.

REFERENCES

Bass, P. F., III, & Maloy, J. W. (2020). How to determine if a project is human subjects research, a quality improvement project, or both. *Ochsner Journal, 20*(1), 56–61.

Gough, D., Davies, P., Jamtvedt, G., Langlois, E., Littell, J., Lotfi, T., et al. (2020). Evidence synthesis international (ESI): Position statement. *Systematic Reviews, 9*, 155.

Hockenberry, M. (2014). Quality improvement and evidence-based practice change projects and the Institutional Review Board: Is approval necessary? *Worldviews on Evidence-Based Nursing, 11*(4), 217–218.

Hunt, D. F., Dunn, M., Harrison, G., & Bailey, J. (2021). Ethical considerations in quality improvement: Key questions and a practical guide. *BMJ Open Quality, 10.* : Article e001497. https://doi.org/10.1136/bmjoq-2021-001497

Institute of Healthcare Improvement (IHI). (2023). *Science of improvement.* https://www.ihi.org/about/Pages/ScienceofImprovement.aspx.

Kawar, L. N., Aquino-Maneja, E. M., Failla, K. R., Flores, S. L., & Squier, V. R. (2023). Research, evidence-based practice and quality improvement simplified. *Journal of Continuing Education in Nursing, 54*(1), 40–48.

Magtoto, L. S. (2022). *Urinary tract infection (catheter related): Prevention strategies.* JBI EBP Database. JBI-ES-2881-3.

Paraszczuk, A., Candelaria, L., Hylton-McGuire, K., & Spatz, D. (2022). The voice of mothers who continue to express milk after their infant's death for donation to a milk bank. *Breastfeeding Medicine*, *17*(8), 660–665. https://doi.org/10.1089/bfm.2021.0326

Rogers, E. M. (2003). *Diffusion of innovations*. The Free Press.

Rycroft-Malone, J., McCormack, B., Hutchinson, A., DeCorby, K., Bucknall, T., Kent, B., et al. (2012). Realist synthesis: Illustrating the method for implementation research. *Implementation Science*, *7*, 1–10.

Saint, S., Greene, M. T., Krein, S. L., Rogers, M. A., Ratz, D., Fowler, K. E., et al. (2016). A program to prevent catheter-associated urinary tract infection in acute care. *The New England Journal of Medicine*, *374*(22), 2111–2119. https://doi.org/10.1056/NEJMoa1504906

Shuman, C. J., Liu, J., Montie, M., Galinato, J. G., Todd, M. A., Hegstad, M., et al. (2016). Patient perception and experiences with falls during hospitalization and after discharge. *Applied Nursing Research*, *31*, 79–85.

Streubert, H. J., & Carpenter, D. R. (2011). *Qualitative nursing research: Advancing the humanistic imperative*. Wolters Klower Health.

Titler, M. G., Conlon, P., Reynolds, M. A., Ripley, R., Tsodikov, A., Wilson, D. S., et al. (2016). The effect of a translating research into practice intervention to promote use of evidence-based fall prevention interventions in hospitalized adults: A prospective pre-post implementation study in the U.S. *Applied Nursing Research*, *31*, 52–59.

Titler, M. G. (2018). Translation research in practice: An introduction. *OJIN: The Online Journal of Issues in Nursing*, *23*(2). Manuscript 1.

16

Launching Implementation

Marita G. Titler and Alice M. Nash

LEARNING OUTCOMES

After reading this chapter, you should be able to do the following:
- Describe the translation research model as a guide for implementation.
- Compare and contrast implementation strategies that address the characteristics of the clinical topic and practices to be implemented.
- Compare and contrast implementation strategies that address communication.
- Describe strategies to address sustainability of evidence-based practices.

KEY TERMS

Change champion
Clinical decision support
Diffusion of Innovation
Heterophily
Homophily
Opinion leader
Quick reference guides

Chapter 15 presented an overview of the Translating Research into Practice (TRIP) model (see Fig. 15.1) and the influence of Rogers's (2003) **Diffusion of Innovation (DOI)** on the development of the TRIP model. The components of the TRIP model include characteristics, communication process, social system, users, and adoption of the innovation. Communication processes are central connectors among all individual components. DOI is a broad framework explaining the adoption of many types of innovations by various groups or populations. TRIP is the application of the broad framework of DOI to the more focused translation of innovative evidence-based practices (EBPs) in healthcare (Titler, 2018). The users of EBPs, such as nurses and physicians, are members of social systems in health care organizations of diverse types. Adoption of EBPs occurs at the individual, unit, and organizational levels. Throughout the stages of adoption defined by Rogers (knowledge, persuasion, decision, implementation, and confirmation), interventions designed to improve the adoption of the EBP and overcome barriers to implementation address the attributes of the EBP topic and communication (see Tables 15.1 and 15.2). The influence of Rogers is observed particularly in that communication is critical for successful implementation in all phases of the process (Rogers, 2003). Likewise, the TRIP model stresses the importance of communication during the implementation stage of an EBP project to sustain the practice change. This chapter focuses on implementation strategies that address attributes of the EBP clinical topic and communication affect adoption. Implementation strategies to address users of the EBP and the social system are presented in Chapter 17.

The field of **translation science** is concerned with research focused on the development and testing of implementation strategies that promote adoption of EBPs (Titler, 2018). Research on the effectiveness of implementation strategies has grown substantially (Cassidy et al., 2021; McHugh et al., 2022; Perry et al., 2019). Those involved in EBP implementation can apply findings from these studies to promote effective use of EBPs. Implementation strategies should be clearly labeled, congruent with labels used in the field (e.g., audit and feedback), and conceptually defined (McHugh et al., 2022). Considerations when selecting implementation strategies include specifying (1) who or what are the targets of each implementation strategy and at what level (individuals, teams, organization, or system), (2) the stakeholder(s) who will deliver the implementation strategy, (3) the actions or processes that make up the strategy, (4) the sequence of the strategy in relation to others and across stages of implementation, and (5) dose of the strategy (e.g., the frequency of audit and feedback) (Rudd et al., 2020).

> **TIP**
>
> Effective communication strategies by interprofessional team members, using targeted messages for specific stakeholder groups at the individual, unit, and organization levels, maximize adoption of an EBP.

IMPLEMENTATION STRATEGIES THAT ADDRESS CHARACTERISTICS OF THE CLINICAL TOPIC

The attributes of the proposed practice change are important considerations leading up to the decision to implement new EBPs. The focus of the TRIP model is implementation in the context of a social system, often an organization. In an organization, the adoption decision may be optional, collective, or authority driven. The importance of stakeholder acceptance cannot be overlooked for the sustainability of the new practice at the sharp end of care. Once the decision has been made to adopt a new practice, the characteristics of the EBP clinical topic (e.g., complexity) influence adoption, and several implementation strategies are described in the following section to address these characteristics:

- Quick reference guides
- Clinical decision support
- Key messages at the point-of-care delivery
- Quick Response (QR) codes

Quick reference guides. Quick reference guides give targeted, concise information designed to help practitioners perform specific tasks. A variety of quick reference guide formats are helpful, depending on their intended use. For example, laminated checklist cards for clinicians help ensure that all components of an EBP are addressed. Badge cards are another example for use by individuals. They can be used to address a number of characteristics of the EBP topic. For example, staff nurses may have some awareness of new evidence but lack knowledge about the relative advantage of a specific practice, or they may be uncertain about the mechanism of action. If the new EBP is complex, quick reference guides can be used as an adjunct to detailed instruction to reduce any miscommunication or lack of consistent implementation. Quick reference guides are useful when it involves a procedure or treatment modality specific to a certain condition or infrequently implemented, or requires equipment that is high risk and low volume.

The characteristics of good reference guides include clarity, accuracy, and accessibility. Careful editing is needed to distill the necessary information for clinicians. Good reference guides may include tables or graphics and text. For example, one side of the guide may include a table of critical laboratory values, the other an algorithm for EBP treatments. When you are developing these guides, it may be useful to consult with a graphic specialist to ensure proper fonts are used and that tables, diagrams, and logos are well-placed and easy to read (Grudniewicz et al., 2015; Versloot et al., 2015).

In addition to design considerations, it is also essential that quick reference guides be visible and available at the point of care. The aim is to offer easily accessible information as a supplement to longer policies or references. For example, if the quick reference guide is about medication management, it may be printed on brightly colored paper, laminated, and found in the medication room. Information can also be delivered via a quick response (QR) code that is easily accessible from the clinician's organization-sanctioned smartphone. The QR code is easily accessible and readily available for information delivery at the point of care.

A recent study by Sharara and Radia (2022) on the use of the QR code demonstrated successful dissemination of data to patient, as these codes are instantly recognizable and universally readable by most smartphone cameras.

Clinical decision support tools. The use of clinical decision support tools by clinicians and patients is rapidly increasing. Frequently they are used to reduce the complexity of the EBP by offering a visual representation of the processes involved, or to illustrate the compatibility of new practices in the users' context. For example, a clinical decision support tool is often designed in the form of an algorithm that can help illustrate the compatibility of a new practice in the context of the organization, if it is designed with the current clinician workflow in mind. The relative advantage of the practice may be clarified by showing how the EBP reduces uncertainty about clinical decisions. It is important that decision support tools do not add complexity or confusion to an EBP. There are many well-developed clinical decision support tools, tested and available for use, often via toolkits or imbedded into the electronic health record (EHR), which is an advantage for organizations planning to implement EBPs.

Good decision support tools are like quick reference guides in that they must be clear, accurate, and to the point. Well-designed aids tested by research are available to clinicians when they are interacting with patients. Decision support tools provide information about evidence supporting the practice and the pros and cons of various options. The clinician may use the tools to confirm his or her own recommendations, influence patients, or converse with them about their preferences and values (Wyatt et al., 2014). Whether used for shared decision making or as a guide to EBP treatment algorithms, decision aids should be user friendly, accessible, and designed to support the clinician in choosing best practice. Decision aids utilized in critical care events can reduce errors caused by stress or loss of memory and can overcome team communication problems (Wen & Howard, 2014).

Clinical decision support is a core function of EHRs (Institute of Medicine, 2003). A variety of tools can be embedded in the EHR, including alerts, reminders, orders, care plans, and electronic surveillance systems (Lytle et al., 2015; Manaktala & Claypool, 2017). Empirical support for the effectiveness of clinical decision support embedded in EHRs is mixed (Institute of Medicine, 2011), and research involving nurses and patient outcomes is limited. Electronic clinical decision support has small to modest effects on clinician behavior and appears to be more effective than alerts alone when included as a component of multifaceted implementation strategies (Arditi et al., 2012; Kahn et al., 2013).

Two examples from the American Heart Association illustrate diverse types of clinical decision support use. First, the atherosclerotic cardiovascular disease (ASCVD) risk calculator for cardiovascular disease was developed through multiple research studies related to predicting disease. Based on research evidence, guidelines were developed and the calculator tool was devised. The risk calculator is freely available online for use by clinicians and the public. Based on input parameters, including age and comorbidities such as hypertension or diabetes, the tool can be used to help patients understand their risk for cardiovascular disease and various options that may reduce that risk. The risk calculator can be embedded in the EHR and is easily accessible at the point of care (American Heart Association, 2017).

On the other hand, guidelines for Advanced Cardiac Life Support (ACLS) include well-designed algorithms used as decision tools in cardiac arrest situations or for treatment of arrhythmias. In these cases, it is helpful if providers can practice using them in simulated experiences ahead of time to avoid treatment delays, for example, when trying to access the tools via cellphone apps (American Heart Association, 2015). Piloting the usefulness of clinical decision support tools is an effective way for organizations to overcome this type of problem. Guidelines, algorithms, and training materials are available online at https://cpr.heart.org/en/cpr-training-supplies.

Key EBP messages at the point-of-care delivery. There are a multitude of ways in which key messages or reminders about an EBP can be delivered at the point of care. Some examples include signs, posters, and infographics. In some cases, they may be built into the EHR used by staff throughout the day. Health information technologies are designed to improve clinical decision making and provide a platform for integrating evidence-based knowledge into care delivery (Office of the National Coordinator for Health Information Technology [ONC], 2023). Others can be incorporated into patient education materials. Key messages are useful for reducing complexity. It is not always possible, but distilling the essence of the EBP to a few key points that can be accessed by staff on badge cards, unit-based signs, or QR codes can be very effective when designed correctly. Displaying posters or infographics on patient care units to highlight visual displays of progress in process or outcome measures explicitly addresses the relative advantage of the new practice by illustrating its value. Selection of key message tools to ease adoption includes consideration of the knowledge of end users, the context in which the tools will be used, and their design and usability. A form of key message known as the "visual abstract" has been used to disseminate research studies and may also be effective for sharing results of practice changes on patient care units or on organizational websites (Ibrahim et al., 2017). Open-source tutorials are available for guidance in developing these tools. For examples, see https://www.surgeryredesign.com/resources/ (Ibrahim, 2017).

In summary, EBP implementation strategies that address various attributes of the specific EBP being implemented are effective in speeding the rate and extent of adoption. Selection of these implementation strategies to facilitate adoption includes consideration of the users (clinicians) and practice context of the organization.

> **TIP**
> Be creative when designing reference guides and key messages. Consult with colleagues in information technology, marketing, or graphic design departments to improve usability of these tools.

IMPLEMENTATION STRATEGIES THAT ADDRESS COMMUNICATION

In this section, the focus is on communication strategies to promote EBP adoption. The following implementation strategies are discussed:
- Mass media
- Opinion leaders
- Change champions
- Education of clinicians
- Educational outreach (academic detailing)

According to Rogers (2003, p. 5), communication is defined as "a process in which participants create and share information with one another to reach a mutual understanding." Information moves via "channels," including mass media, interpersonal (usually face-to-face), and interactive communication routes such as the internet and social media. The channels are connectors among the people involved in the project. The transfer of ideas occurs most often among people who are similar or **homophilous**. **Heterophily** means the opposite; the individuals have different attributes (e.g., professional groups, education, practice specialties). These concepts are important for implementation because although it is easier to communicate with similar people, unless there is some degree of difference, obtaining current information about innovations is unlikely (Rogers, 2003). The use of various communication channels throughout an implementation project depends on the implementation stage and desired outcomes.

Mass media. Before we get to specifics about interpersonal and interactive communication, it is important to discuss the role of mass media in implementing EBP. The primary outlets of mass media are television, radio, print, and internet sources. News and information are delivered in a directional message from one to many. The recent and rapid growth of social media platforms such as Facebook and Twitter has led to the increasing use of interactive mass media, where the communication channels are bidirectional but lack the closeness of an interpersonal or face-to-face exchange (Rogers, 2003). Researchers, professional organizations, and government agencies are among the many groups using mass media to send informational messages to stakeholder groups and the public at large. The amount of information available through mass media is staggering and can cause individuals to feel bombarded and to withdraw from media consumption. On the other hand, Rogers (2003) and other diffusion researchers suggest that some individuals are particularly adept at translating knowledge gleaned from mass media into useful practices worthy of adopting to solve problems or make improvements in structures or processes. Often, such individuals are among the first to know about innovations such as new EBP guidelines through their attendance at conferences or by reading journals or following experts on Twitter, for example. People in this category are known as early adopters. They can be both the target of mass media campaigns and active seekers of the latest information.

Opinion leaders. When early adopters are regarded by their peers as credible sources of information, they may have a great deal of influence on the adoption of

EBPs. Several attributes contribute to the development of these individuals as **opinion leaders**. The definition of opinion leadership, according to Rogers (2003), is "the degree to which an individual is able informally to influence other individuals' attitudes or overt behavior in a desired way with relative frequency" (p. 300). Opinion leaders tend to have greater exposure to mass media and bring innovative ideas from the media and other groups to their own social networks (Anderson & Titler, 2014; Bunger et al., 2023). They are widely connected with other individuals and groups, and are accessible to their followers, who are usually members of their own peer groups. Opinion leader influence is a balance between being too innovative or heterogeneous and keeping the homophily within the group that leads to credibility and trust in their judgment and evaluation of new clinical practices. Opinion leaders are visible and important for communicating via interpersonal networks that EBP innovations are compatible with community norms. Because of their visibility, opinion leaders also influence adoption by addressing the observability of new EBPs (Rogers, 2003).

The identification and use of opinion leader strategies to influence the speed of adoption of various innovations has been the topic of research for many decades, not only in healthcare but in sociology, politics, and marketing, to name just a few (Cullen et al., 2022; Flodgren et al., 2019; King & Summers, 1970; Rogers & Cartono, 1962). Four methods are useful in identifying opinion leaders. First, the sociometric method involves asking respondents to name people they would go to for advice if they were uncertain about an innovation such as a new EBP. This works best with a high response rate because there are usually few opinion leaders in a group or context. This method has the advantage of obtaining the viewpoint of the followers. A second method for finding opinion leaders is by using key informants or individuals who are knowledgeable about the local context—for example, unit managers, or educators. In the self-designating method, individuals identify themselves as being influential or sources of information for their peers. Finally, the observation method involves collection of observed communication behavior. Although valid, this method is best when employed in small systems and is rarely used because the other methods are similar in validity and more convenient (Rogers, 2003). It is important to be aware that opinion leaders often are identified as such based on their specific knowledge domains and expertise. Because opinion leaders reside in a changing local context, it is possible that their ability to influence others may change over time (Cassidy et al., 2021; Seers et al., 2018; Flodgren et al., 2019).

Opinion leader influence is achieved in a variety of ways including word of mouth and interpersonal communication through extensive personal networks (Flodgren et al., 2019; Valente & Davis, 1999). Recruiting opinion leaders for specific implementation projects should include knowledge about their expertise on a given topic and the extent to which they favor a given practice change. Obtaining opinion leaders' buy-in is essential; they must be willing to take part in the project. Opinion leaders often influence their peers by being role models for new practices, visibly demonstrating compatibility of the EBP with local norms (Rycroft-Malone et al., 2018). Opportunities for interpersonal communication between opinion leaders and their peers can take many forms, including several of the education strategies discussed in the following section.

Change champions. The term champion is sometimes used interchangeably with opinion leader, but there are conceptual differences as well as similarities (Shea, 2021). Similarities include that both have individual, informal social influence roles that are internal to an organization or system and rely on ongoing relationships. Opinion leaders evaluate new practices and are influential based on their expertise relative to their domains, such as a patient care unit or specialty practice. Their innovativeness may be slightly greater than that of their peers, but it is still within boundaries relative to the group. Champions, however, actively advocate for practice change. Their influence is based on persuasion within their personal and organizational networks and is often project specific (Shea, 2021).

Similarly, Rogers (2003) contends that the role of a champion in organizational change is like that of the opinion leader except that the opinion leader is more effective in less complex or optional adoption situations. Although organizations may allow some degree of individual innovation decisions, often such choices are collective or authority driven. His definition of a champion is "a charismatic individual who throws his or her weight behind an innovation, thus overcoming indifference or resistance that the new idea may provoke in an organization" (p. 414). A study by Bonawitz and colleagues (2020) found six key attributes of champions that contribute to success in promoting implementation: *influence* (e.g., formal authority, informal authority, institutional savvy), *ownership* (e.g., took personal responsibility for implementation success), *physically present* at the point-of-care delivery where change is occurring (e.g., embedded in the unit/clinic), *grit* (e.g., tenacity/resilience to overcome setbacks), *persuasiveness* (e.g., inspiring, convey enthusiasm, "contagious" passion), and *participative style* (e.g., collective action and decision making, others felt heard and important, address concerns with empathy and understanding). Expert consensus notes that identifying and preparing champions is one of the more important and feasible implementation strategies (Shea, 2021).

Champions can come from all levels of an organization. Important qualities include being in key linking positions (for example, middle managers); understanding the various interests of stakeholders; and finally, having interpersonal communication and negotiation skills. Change champions often have a role in organizing and brokering change because of their advocacy and personal network relationships (Rogers, 2003).

Education. Education of clinicians about the EBPs is necessary but not sufficient to change practice. Printed educational materials and didactic continuing education alone have a minimal impact on changing practice behaviors (Forsetlund et al., 2021; Giguere et al., 2020). It is essential, however, that clinicians delivering the EBPs have the knowledge and skills, including the evidence base regarding the EBPs to be implemented. In some cases, if the change is not overly complex and fits the current workflow well, a mass media-style announcement, lecture, or self-study module may be appropriate as an educational approach. For larger projects involving meaningful change, it is more likely that a formal gap analysis or audit of current practice should be conducted to address the knowledge and skills required to understand the evidence, overcome barriers, and perform the required practice. Opinion leaders and champions may need to devise individual or committee education as a means of obtaining buy-in from organizational leadership, not only for the implementation decision, but also so that adequate resources are included in the planning and execution of the change. Involving stakeholders, including potential opinion leaders and champions, in educational material development, resources, and point-of-care tools, may be initially costly but will pay off later as part of a "train the trainer" approach, where early learners can go on to teach others in classroom settings or in the practice area. Individual mentoring and coaching are useful educational strategies in ongoing development of staff skills. Many of the interventions that address the characteristics of the innovation, mentioned previously, are useful adjuncts for learning in addition to printed materials, training videos, and slide presentations (Cassidy et al., 2021).

Educational outreach/academic detailing. Multiple studies have demonstrated the effectiveness of educational outreach, also known as academic detailing, in improving the practice behaviors of clinicians (Avorn, 2010; Institute of Medicine, 2011; Wilson et al., 2016). Educational outreach involves interactive face-to-face education of

> **TIP**
>
> Explore government agency and professional organization websites for comprehensive toolkits that provide bundled resources useful for strategies addressing the characteristics of clinical topics as well as communication strategies.

individual practitioners in their practice settings by an individual (usually a clinician) with expertise in a particular topic (e.g., cancer pain management). Academic detailers can explain the research foundations of the EBP recommendations and respond convincingly to specific questions, concerns, or challenges that a practitioner might raise. An academic detailer also might deliver feedback on provider or team performance with respect to a selected EBP recommendation (e.g., frequency of pain assessment). In planning for implementation, you should identify the individual who will perform the educational outreach and the frequency with which this will be done. For example, with implementation of patient-specific fall prevention practices, an expert on fall prevention rounded every five to six weeks on each of the patient care units that were implementing this practice. Rounding was done in conjunction with the opinion leaders and change champions to identify areas for improvement and address questions and issues they encountered while implementing the EBPs (Titler et al., 2016; Wilson et al., 2016).

In summary, traditional mass media communication, interactive media, and interpersonal communication are all extremely important when implementing EBPs. Opinion leaders and champions facilitate the translation of new ideas to members of their peer groups and organizational leaders through their social network connections, enthusiasm, expertise, and credibility. Once the implementation decision is made, individuals in these roles encourage and support the engagement of key stakeholders, including staff, organizational leadership, and interdisciplinary practice partners. As credible experts, opinion leaders and champions are important resources in developing educational materials, modeling new EBPs, and providing effective feedback to peers.

SUSTAINABILITY

Guided by the TRIP model, implementation planners should consider sustainability of the EBP from the very beginning of the project. Building the evidence base for sustainability is currently a high priority for implementation scientists (Hall et al., 2022; Moore et al., 2017; Wiltsey Wiltsey Stirman et al., 2012). In a recent review, Moore and colleagues (2017) arrived at a " definition of sustainability that includes five constructs: (1) after a defined period of time, (2) the program, clinical intervention, and/or implementation strategies continue to be delivered and/or (3) individual behavior change (i.e., clinician, patient) is maintained; (4) the program and individual behavior change may evolve or adapt while (5) continuing to produce benefits for individuals/systems" (p. 7). Among the potential influences on sustainability are the innovation characteristics, context, capacity, and implementation strategies such as education and integration with organizational governance structures (Hall et al., 2022; Shuman et al., 2017; Wiltsey Stirman et al., 2012).

SYNTHESIS

Remember that when planning for implementation of EBPs, it is important to consider the characteristics of the clinical topic so you can select effective strategies that align with your goals. Is the new practice a minor adjustment to an existing clinical guideline? If so, your plan may include an email announcement and a new point-of-care message in an EHR. On the other hand, if the EBP change is new, complex, or potentially controversial, involving influential clinicians who can function as opinion leaders or change champions will contribute greatly to the success of implementing and sustaining EBPs.

KEY POINTS

- The implementation phase of EBP projects is challenging. Translation science and the Diffusion of Innovations model aid in designing and implementing EBPs that have an increased likelihood of sustainability.
- The characteristic of an innovation (EBP) accounts for up to 87% of the variance in the rate of adoption and is therefore most important in ensuring successful implementation.
- Quick reference guides, clinical decision support tools, and key messaging are strategies that address the characteristics of the EBP.
- Interpersonal communication strategies require additional resources but are unquestionably more effective than the use of mass media.
- Opinion leaders and change champions help translate EBPs into the local context through advocacy, persuasion, and extensive personal relationship networks.

REFERENCES

American Heart Association. (2015). American heart association guidelines for cardiopulmonary resuscitation and emergency cardiovascular care: Part 7, adult advanced cardiac life support. https://eccguidelines.heart.org/index.php/circulation/cpr-ecc-guidelines-2/part-7-adult-advanced-cardiovascular-life-support/.

American Heart Association. (2017). *ASCVD risk calculator*. http://static.heart.org/riskcalc/app/index.html#!/baseline-risk.

Anderson, C. A., & Tilter, M. G. (2014). Development and verification of an agent-based model of opinion leadership. *Implementation Science, 9*(136).

Arditi, C., Rege-Walther, M., Wyatt, J. C., Durieux, P., & Burnand, B. (2012). Computer-generated reminders delivered on paper to healthcare professionals; effects on professional practice and health care outcomes. *Cochrane Database of Systematic Reviews, 12*, CD001175.

Avorn, J. (2010). Transforming trial results into practice change: The final translational hurdle: Comment on impact of the ALLHAT/JNC7 dissemination project on thiazide-type diuretic use. *Archives of Internal Medicine, 170*(10), 858–860.

Bonawitz, K., Wetmore, M., Heisler, M., Dalton, V. K., Damschroder, L. J., Forman, J., et al. (2020). Champions in context: Which attributes matter for change efforts in healthcare? *Implementation Science, 15*, 62.

Bunger, A. C., Yousefi-Nooraie, R., Warren, K., Cao, Q., Dadgostar, P., & Bustos, T. E. (2023). Developing a typology of network alteration strategies for implementation: A scoping review and iterative synthesis. *Implementation Science, 18*, 10.

Cassidy, C. E., Harrison, M. B., Godfrey, C., Nincic, V., Khan, P. A., Oakley, P., et al. (2021). Use and effects of implementation strategies for practice guidelines in nursing: A systematic review. *Implementation Science, 16*(102).

Cullen, L., Hanrahan, K., Edmonds, S. W., Reisinger, H. S., & Wagner, M. (2022). Iowa implementation for sustainability framework. *Implementation Science, 17*, 1.

Flodgren, G., O'Brien, M. A., Parmelli, E., & Grimshaw, J. M. (2019). Local opinion leaders: Effects on professional practice and healthcare outcomes. *Cochrane Database of Systematic Reviews* (6), CD000125.

Forsetlund, L., O'Brien, M. A., Forsen, L., Reinar, L. M., Okwen, M. P., Horsley, T., et al. (2021). Continuing education meetings and workshops: Effects on professional practice and health care outcomes. *Cochrane Database of Systematic Reviews* (9), CD003030.

Foy, R., Sales, A., Wensing, M., et al. (2015). Implementation science: A reappraisal of our journal mission and scope. *Implementation Science, 10*, 51.

Gagliardi, A. R., Marshall, C., Huckson, S., James, R., & Moore, V. (2015). Developing a checklist for guideline implementation planning: Review and synthesis of guideline development and implementation advice. *Implementation Science, 10*(1), 19.

Giguere, A., Zomahoun, H. T. V., Carmichael, P. H., Uwizeye, C. B., Legare, F., Grimshaw, J. M., et al. (2020). Printed educational materials: Effects on professional practice and healthcare outcomes. *Cochrane Database of Systematic Reviews, 8*, CD 004398.

Grudniewicz, A., Bhattacharyya, O., McKibbon, K. A., & Straus, S. E. (2015). Redesigning printed educational materials for primary care physicians: Design improvements increase usability. *Implementation Science, 10*, 156.

Hall, A., Shoesmith, A., Doherty, E., et al. (2022). Evaluation of measures of sustainability and sustainability determinants for use in community, public health, and clinical settings: A systematic review. *Implementation Science, 17*, 81.

Ibrahim, A. M., Lillemoe, K. D., Klingensmith, M. E., & Dimick, J. B. (2017). Visual abstracts to disseminate research on social media: A prospective, case-control crossover study. *Annals of Surgery, 266*(6), e46–e48.

Ibrahim, A. M. (2017). *Visual abstract open source primer*. https://www.surgeryredesign.com/.

Institute of Medicine. (2011). *Clinical practice guidelines we can trust*. National Academies Press.

Institute of Medicine. (2003). *Key capabilities of an electronic health record system: Letter report*. National Academies Press.

Kahn, S. R., Morrison, D. R., Cohen, J. M., Emed, J., Tagalakis, V., Roussin, A., et al. (2013). Interventions for implementation of thromboprophylaxis in hospitalized medical and surgical patients at risk for venous thromboembolism. *Cochrane Database of Systematic Reviews* (7), CD008201.

King, C. W., & Summers, J. O. (1970). Overlap of opinion leadership across consumer product categories. *Journal of Marketing Research, 7*(1), 43–50.

Lytle, K. S., Short, N. M., Richesson, R. L., & Horvath, M. M. (2015). Clinical decision support for nurses: A fall risk and prevention example. *CIN: Computers, Informatics, Nursing, 33*(12), 530–537; quiz E531.

Manaktala, S., & Claypool, S. R. (2017). Evaluating the impact of a computerized surveillance algorithm and decision support system on sepsis mortality. *Journal of the American Medical Informatics Association, 24*(1), 88–95.

McHugh, S., Presseay, J., Luecking, C. T., & Powell, B. J. (2022). Examining the complementarity between ERIC compilation of implementation strategies and the behaviour change technique taxonomy. *Implementation Science, 17*, 56.

Moore, J. E., Mascarenhas, A., Bain, J., & Straus, S. E. (2017). Developing a comprehensive definition of sustainability. *Implementation Science, 12*(1), 110.

Perry, C. K., Damschroder, L. J., Hemler, J. R., Woodson, T. T., Ono, S. S., & Cohen, D. J. (2019). Specifying and comparing implementation strategies across seven large implementation interventions: A practical application of theory. *Implementation Science, 14*(32).

Rogers, E. M. (2003). *Diffusion of innovations* (5th ed.). Free Press.

Rogers, E. M., & Cartono, D. G. (1962). Methods of measuring opinion leadership. *Public Opinion Quarterly, 26*(3), 435–441.

Rudd, B. N., Davis, M., & Beidas, R. S. (2020). Integrating implementation science in clinical research to maximize public health impact: A call for the reporting and alignment of implementation strategy use with implementation outcomes. *Implementation Science, 15*, 103.

Rycroft-Malone, J., Seers, K., Eldh, A. C., et al. (2018). A realist process evaluation within the Facilitating Implementation of Research Evidence (FIRE) cluster randomized controlled international trial: An exemplar. *Implementation Science, 13,* 138.

Seers, K., Rycroft-Malone, J., Cox, K., et al. (2018). Facilitating Implementation of Research Evidence (FIRE) cluster randomized controlled international trial to evaluate two models of facilitation informed by the Promoting Action on Research Implementation in Health Services (PARIHS) framework. *Implementation Science, 13,* 137.

Sharara, S., & Radia, S. (2022). Quick response (QR) codes for patient information delivery: A digital innovation during the coronavirus pandemic. *Journal of Orthodontics, 49*(1), 89–97.

Shea, C. M. (2021). A conceptual model to guide research on the activities and effects of innovation champions. *Implementation Research and Practice* (2), 1–13.

Shuman, C. J., Xie, J., Herr, K., & Titler, M. G. (2017). Sustainability of evidence-based acute pain management practices for hospitalized older adults. *Western Journal of Nursing Research, 40*(12), 1749–1764.

The Office of the National Coordinator for Health Information Technology (ONC). (2023). *Clinical decision support.* https://www.healthit.gov/topic/safety/clinical-decision-support.

Titler, M. G., Conlon, P., Reynolds, M. A., Ripley, R., Tsodikov, A., Wilson, D. S., et al. (2016). The effect of a translating research into practice intervention to promote use of evidence-based fall prevention interventions in hospitalized adults: A prospective pre-post implementation study in the U.S. *Applied Nursing Research, 31,* 52–59.

Titler, M. G. (2018). Translation research in practice: An introduction. *OJIN: The Online Journal of Issues in Nursing, 23*(2), Manuscript 1.

Valente, T. W., & Davis, R. L. (1999). Accelerating the diffusion of innovations using opinion leaders. *Annals of the American Academy of Political and Social Science, 566,* 55–67.

Versloot, J., Grudniewicz, A., Chatterjee, A., Hayden, L., Kastner, M., & Bhattacharyya, O. (2015). Format guidelines to make them vivid, intuitive, and visual: Use simple formatting rules to optimize usability and accessibility of clinical practice guidelines. *International Journal of Evidence-Based Healthcare, 13*(2), 52–57.

Wen, L. Y., & Howard, S. K. (2014). Value of expert systems, quick reference guides and other cognitive aids. *Current Opinion in Anaesthesiology, 27*(6), 643–648.

Wilson, D. S., Montie, M., Conlon, P., Reynolds, M., Ripley, R., et al. (2016). Nurses' perceptions of implementing fall prevention interventions to mitigate patient-specific fall risk factors. *Western Journal of Nursing Research, 38*(8), 1012–1034.

Wiltsey Stirman, S., Kimberly, J., Cook, N., Calloway, A., Castro, F., & Charns, M. (2012). The sustainability of new programs and innovations: A review of the empirical literature and recommendations for future research. *Implementation Science, 7,* 17.

Wyatt, K. D., Branda, M. E., Anderson, R. T., et al. (2014). Peering into the black box: A meta-analysis of how clinicians use decision aids during clinical encounters. *Implementation Science, 9,* 26.

17

Implementation Strategies for Stakeholders

Mary Margaret Brennan and Linda Zieman

LEARNING OUTCOMES

After reading this chapter, you should be able to do the following:
- Describe the facilitators and barriers to evidence-based practice (EBP).
- Analyze the role of leaders in EBP implementation.
- Analyze the influence of the practice context on implementation of EBPs.
- Describe the purposes of conducting an environmental scan as an implementation strategy.
- Perform a performance gap assessment, audit, and feedback as implementation strategies.
- Assess the level of power and interest for relevant stakeholders.
- Discuss use of meetings with stakeholders as an implementation strategy.
- Apply tools to assess various components of the practice context.
- Prioritize essential elements of meetings with key leadership stakeholders.
- Develop action steps for piloting EBP in practice settings.
- Describe the importance of revisions in standards of practice and documentation systems as part of implementation.
- Identify examples of recognitions and rewards for EBP implementation and their importance.

KEY TERMS

Auditing and feedback
EBP culture
EBP implementation climate
Environmental scan
Facilitators and Barriers
Frameworks
Implementation
Leadership
Organizational context
PDSA cycle
Performance gap assessment
Piloting the change
Recognition and rewards
Stakeholder meetings
Stakeholders
Standards of practice and documentation systems
Training programs

Implementing evidence-based practice (EBP) is a complex, iterative process that involves multiple disciplines and their relationships in the provision of healthcare based on the best available evidence. The implementation process is a nonlinear, cyclical process and takes time, depending on the complexity of the EBP quality improvement (QI) initiatives being implemented. Merely increasing staff knowledge about EBP and using passive dissemination strategies will not work. In Chapter 16, you learned about implementation strategies that address the *nature of the EBPs* (e.g., fall prevention, acute pain management in older adults) and *communication* with key clinicians. An important element to include is the partnership of PhDs and doctors of nursing practice (DNPs). Both PhDs and DNPs are doctorally prepared experts and share complementary skills that support EBP implementation. This collaboration can positively impact the quality and outcomes of EBP implementation (Cowan & Munro, 2019; Cygan & Reed, 2019).

In this chapter, you will learn about implementation strategies that address users of EBPs and organizational cultures where they work (see Fig. 15.1, Chapter 15). Implementation strategies are described, and suggested methods for actualizing them are provided.

Implementation strategies have been described as approaches that successfully increase the adoption, integration, implementation, sustainability, and advancement of evidence-based outcomes (Powell et al., 2019). Implementation strategies can be integrated throughout different phases of the EBP process, from preimplementation to implementation and postimplementation. These strategies are critical to ensure success of evidence-based healthcare, although there is a dearth of research to support which implementation strategies are most effective. Bringing evidence to practice and promoting optimal outcomes is challenging and technically and psychologically complex, requiring several different, but necessary, interactive processes. Implementation strategies should be well defined, specific regarding the different elements of a strategy, precise enough to allow for reproducibility when appropriate in a similar unit or practice setting, and evidence based (Proctor et al., 2013).

The Expert Recommendations for Implementing Change (ERIC) (Powell et al., 2015) group of experts conducted a Delphi study to compile a list of accepted implementation strategies and their conceptual definitions necessary for testing different strategies. A list of 73 separate, discrete, and nonranked strategies were identified for use in research, practice, and QI projects (Table 17.1). While leadership is not specifically defined as a strategy in this list, many of the strategies speak to the active leadership role involved in implementing EBP, such as building a coalition among different stakeholders, conducting local discussion practices with stakeholders, creating a local learning collaborative, mandating change, and modeling and simulating change (Powell et al., 2015). Additional strategies included: (a) identifying barriers and facilitators; (b) collecting and monitoring performance data through audit and providing feedback for ongoing evaluation and modification of the EBP-QI process; (c) conducting cyclical small tests of change; (d) running educational sessions to teach participants the knowledge, skills, attitudes, and application of EBP; and (e) creating a formal blueprint for implementing EBP-QI. In the chapter, we will elaborate on some of the most commonly used implementation strategies in nursing.

BARRIERS AND FACILITATORS TO IMPLEMENTATION OF EVIDENCE-BASED PRACTICE

Knowing the facilitators and barriers to EBP is critical for ensuring successful EBP health outcomes (Joy et al., 2015; Mathieson et al., 2018). Facilitators were defined as those strategies that assist and support each of the phases of the EBP process once the project has been initiated (Mathieson et al., 2018). Effective implementation strategies were described as innovations that were "easy to use" and "time-saving" (Mathieson et al., 2018, p. 7). A "bottom-up approach" was an important facilitator in contrast to a "top-down approach," which was deemed unsuccessful due to the lack of ownership experienced by the nurse (Mathieson et al., 2018, p. 7). Educational programs targeted to the innovation were helpful if delivered prior to the EBP as was email and telephone support for nurses during the EBP process. Professional development of key EBP knowledge and skill sets helped facilitate EBP. The strategic allocation of roles within the EBP team was integral to success, ensuring that nurses with the appropriate expertise were hired or appointed into key positions to monitor the EBP process, collect data, and provide support.

BARRIERS TO EVIDENCE-BASED PRACTICE

There are several barriers that hinder or impede the process of EBP. Barriers are described as the opposite of facilitators and disrupt the EBP process. In the systematic review performed by Mathieson and colleagues (2018), only 6 of the 22 studies integrated a theory when designing an implementation project. Few authors used a theoretical framework when selecting an intervention, directing the implementation process, or analyzing the results. Selecting a theoretical framework provides a unifying structure to help guide and direct improvement efforts so that the intended results will be achieved. Insufficient education regarding the EBP process was reported as another barrier and contributed to a lack of confidence in using EBP. Other barriers included the

TABLE 17.1 ERIC Discrete Implementation Strategy Compilation (n = 73)

Strategy	Definitions
Access new funding	Access new or existing money to facilitate the implementation
Alter incentive/allowance structures	Work to incentivize the adoption and implementation of the clinical innovation
Alter patient/consumer fees	Create fee structures where patients/consumers pay less for preferred treatments (the clinical innovation) and more for less-preferred treatments
Assess for readiness and identify barriers and facilitators	Assess various aspects of an organization to determine its degree of readiness to implement, barriers that may impede implementation, and strengths that can be used in the implementation effort
Audit and provide feedback	Collect and summarize clinical performance data over a specified time period and give it to clinicians and administrators to monitor, evaluate, and modify provider behavior
Build a coalition	Recruit and cultivate relationships with partners in the implementation effort
Capture and share local knowledge	Capture local knowledge from implementation sites on how implementers and clinicians made something work in their setting and then share it with other sites
Centralize technical assistance	Develop and use a centralized system to deliver technical assistance focused on implementation issues
Change accreditation or membership requirements	Strive to alter accreditation standards so that they require or encourage use of the clinical innovation. Work to alter membership organization requirements so that those who want to affiliate with the organization are encouraged or required to use the clinical innovation
Change liability laws	Participate in liability reform efforts that make clinicians more willing to deliver the clinical innovation
Change physical structure and equipment	Evaluate current configurations and adapt, as needed, the physical structure and/or equipment (e.g., changing the layout of a room, adding equipment) to best accommodate the targeted innovation
Change records systems	Change records systems to allow better assessment of implementation or clinical outcomes
Change service sites	Change the location of clinical service sites to increase access
Conduct cyclical small tests of change	Implement changes in a cyclical fashion using small tests of change before taking changes system wide. Tests of change benefit from systematic measurement; and results of the tests of change are studied for insights on how to do better. This process continues serially over time, and refinement is added with each cycle
Conduct educational meetings	Hold meetings targeted toward different stakeholder groups (e.g., providers, administrators, other organizational stakeholders, and community, patient/consumer, and family stakeholders) to teach them about the clinical innovation
Conduct educational outreach visits	Have a trained person meet with providers in their practice settings to educate providers about the clinical innovation with the intent of changing the provider's practice
Conduct local consensus discussions	Include local providers and other stakeholders in discussions that address whether the chosen problem is important and whether the clinical innovation to address it is appropriate
Conduct local needs assessment	Collect and analyze data related to the need for the innovation

Continued

TABLE 17.1 ERIC Discrete Implementation Strategy Compilation (n = 73)—cont'd

Strategy	Definitions
Conduct ongoing training	Plan for and conduct training in the clinical innovation in an ongoing way
Create a learning collaborative	Facilitate the formation of groups of providers or provider organizations and foster a collaborative learning environment to improve implementation of the clinical innovation
Create new clinical teams	Change who serves on the clinical team, adding different disciplines and different skills to make it more likely that the clinical innovation is delivered (or is more successfully delivered)
Create or change credentialing and/or licensure standards	Create an organization that certifies clinicians in the innovation or encourage an existing organization to do so. Change governmental professional certification or licensure requirements to include delivering the innovation. Work to alter continuing education requirements to shape professional practice toward the innovation
Develop a formal implementation blueprint	Develop a formal implementation blueprint that includes all goals and strategies. The blueprint should include the following: (1) aim/purpose of the implementation; (2) scope of the change (e.g., what organizational units are affected); (3) time frame and milestones; and (4) appropriate performance/progress measures. Use and update this plan to guide the implementation effort over time
Develop academic partnerships	Partner with a university or academic unit for the purposes of shared training and bringing research skills to an implementation project
Develop an implementation glossary	Develop and distribute a list of terms describing the innovation, implementation, and stakeholders in the organizational change
Develop and implement tools for quality monitoring	Develop, test, and introduce into quality monitoring systems the right input—the appropriate language, protocols, algorithms, standards, and measures (or processes, patient/consumer outcomes, and implementation outcomes) that are often specific to the innovation being implemented
Develop and organize quality monitoring systems	Develop and organize systems and procedures that monitor clinical processes and/or outcomes for the purpose of quality assurance and improvement
Develop disincentives	Provide financial disincentive for failure to implement or use the clinical innovations
Develop educational materials	Develop and format manuals, toolkits, and other supporting materials in ways that make it easier for stakeholders to learn about the innovation and for clinicians to learn how to deliver the clinical innovation
Develop resource sharing agreements	Develop partnerships with organizations that have resources needed to implement the innovation
Distribute educational materials	Distribute educational materials (including guidelines, manuals, and toolkits) in person, by mail, and/or electronically
Facilitate relay of clinical data to providers	Provide as close to real-time data as possible about key measures of process/outcomes using integrated modes/channels of communication in a way that promotes use of the targeted innovation
Facilitation	A process of interactive problem solving and support that occurs in a context of a recognized need for improvement and a supportive interpersonal relationship
Fund and contract for the clinical innovation	Governments and other payers of services issue requests for proposals to deliver the innovation, use contracting processes to motivate providers to deliver the clinical innovation, and develop new funding formulas that make it more likely that providers will deliver the innovation

TABLE 17.1 ERIC Discrete Implementation Strategy Compilation (n = 73)—cont'd

Strategy	Definitions
Identify and prepare champions	Identify and prepare individuals who dedicate themselves to supporting, marketing, and driving through an implementation, overcoming indifference or resistance that the intervention may provoke in an organization
Identify early adopters	Identify early adopters at the local site to learn from their experiences with the practice innovation
Increase demand	Attempt to influence the market for the clinical innovation to increase competition intensity and to increase the maturity of the market for the clinical innovation
Inform local opinion leaders	Inform providers identified by colleagues as opinion leaders or "educationally influential" about the clinical innovation in the hopes that they will influence colleagues to adopt it
Intervene with patients/consumers to enhance uptake and adherence	Develop strategies with patients to encourage and problem solve around adherence
Involve executive boards	Involve existing governing structures (e.g., boards of directors, medical staff boards of governance) in the implementation effort, including the review of data on implementation processes
Involve patients/consumers and family members	Engage or include patients/consumers and families in the implementation effort
Make billing easier	Make it easier to bill for the clinical innovation
Make training dynamic	Vary the information delivery methods to cater to different learning styles and work contexts, and shape the training in the innovation to be interactive
Mandate change	Have leadership declare the priority of the innovation and their determination to have it implemented
Model and simulate change	Model or simulate the change that will be implemented prior to implementation
Obtain and use patients/consumers and family feedback	Develop strategies to increase patient/consumer and family feedback on the implementation effort
Obtain formal commitments	Obtain written commitments from key partners that state what they will do to implement the innovation
Organize clinician implementation team meetings	Develop and support teams of clinicians who are implementing the innovation and give them protected time to reflect on the implementation effort share
Place innovation on fee-for-service lists/formularies	Work to place the clinical innovation on lists of actions for which providers can be reimbursed (e.g., a drug is placed on a formulary, a procedure is now reimbursable)
Prepare patients/consumers to be active participants	Prepare patients/consumers to be active in their care to ask questions, and specifically to inquire about care guidelines, the guidance behind clinical decisions, or about available evidence-supported treatments
Promote adaptability	Identify the ways a clinical innovation can be tailored to meet local needs and clarify which elements of the innovation must be maintained to present fidelity
Promote network weaving	Identify and build on existing high-quality working relationships and networks within and outside the organization, organizational units, teams, etc. to promote information sharing, collaborative problem solving, and a shared vision/goal related to implementing the innovation
Provide clinical supervision	Provide clinicians with ongoing supervision focusing on the innovation. Provide training for clinical supervisors who will supervise clinicians who provide the innovation

Continued

TABLE 17.1	ERIC Discrete Implementation Strategy Compilation (n = 73)—cont'd
Strategy	Definitions
Provide local technical assistance	Develop and use a system to deliver technical assistance focused on implementation issues using local personnel
Provide ongoing consultation	Provide ongoing consultation with one or more experts in the strategies used to support implementing the innovation
Purposely reexamine the implementation	Monitor progress and adjust clinical practices and implementation strategies to continuously improve the quality of care
Recruit, designate, and train for leadership	Recruit, designate, and train leaders for the change effort
Remind clinicians	Develop reminder systems designed to help clinicians recall information and/or prompt them to use the clinical innovation
Revise professional roles	Shift and revise roles among professionals who provide care, and redesign job characteristics
Shadow other experts	Provide ways for key individuals to directly observe experienced people engage with or use the targeted practice change innovation
Stage implementation scale up	Phase implementation efforts by starting with small pilots or demonstration projects and gradually move to a system-wide rollout
Start a dissemination organization	Identify or start a separate organization that is responsible for disseminating the clinical innovation. It could be a for-profit or nonprofit organization
Tailor strategies	Tailor the implementation strategies to address barriers and leverage facilitators that were identified through earlier data collection
Use advisory boards and workgroups	Create and engage a formal group of multiple kinds of stakeholders to provide input and advice on implementation efforts and to elicit recommendations for improvements
Use an implementation advisor	Seek guidance from experts in implementation
Use capitated payments	Pay providers or care systems a set amount per patient/consumer for delivering clinical care
Use data experts	Involve, hire, and/or consult experts to inform management on the use of data generated by implementation efforts
Use data warehousing techniques	Integrate clinical records across facilities and organizations to facilitate implementation across systems
Use mass media	Use media to reach large numbers of people to spread the word about the clinical innovation
Use other payment schemes	Introduce payment approaches (in a catch-all category)
Use train-the-trainer strategies	Train designated clinicians or organizations to train others in the clinical innovation
Visit other sites	Visit sites where a similar implementation effort has been considered successful
Work with educational institutions	Encourage educational institutions to train clinicians in the innovation

From Powell et al., 2015.

restructuring of the organization, which was felt to take time and focus away from EBP processes. Organizational changes that shifted resources away from the EBP process were perceived as threatening the EBP implementation process.

Leadership as an Implementation Strategy

Leadership has been defined as applying influence over another individual or group to bring about a certain effect, such as EBP (Elsheikh et al., 2023). In organizations committed to EBP, leadership is thought to be a critical factor in establishing an EBP **culture and** an EBP **climate**. According to the Agency for Healthcare Research and Quality (AHRQ, 2018) recommendations, administrative leadership must create a vision to foster successful EBP integration into the organization. AHRQ (2018) provides the following recommendations for leaders when implementing EBP:

- Provide an environment that allows all members to feel safe expressing ideas for improvement.
- Establish a nonpunitive environment and acknowledge that human errors occur in complex systems. Discussing near-misses and errors in a blame-free environment helps establish a psychologically safe environment that allows everyone to flourish.
- Establish a learning community.
- View learning as an organizational value and recommend leaders provide opportunities for members to learn on the job.
- Identify EBP champions who are excited about EBP and who can help unleash this passion in others.
- Determine that EBP measures of effective implementation are reviewed periodically to ensure that EBP goals are being met.
- Ensure that all members have time to implement EBP and provide nonclinical time for team members to accomplish this priority.

Several nursing studies have explored the role nursing leaders play in the effective implementation of EBP. Titler (2010) described a variety of high-level, executive administrative nursing leadership responsibilities to facilitate EBP that include:

- Creating an organizational mission, vision, and strategic plan that incorporates EBP.
- Implementing performance expectations for staff that include reviewing the evidence.
- Integrating the work of EBP into the governance structure of the health care system.
- Establishing explicit expectations that nurse leaders will create microsystems that value and support clinical inquiry.
- Using motivational techniques to inspire, educate, and role model.

A descriptive study was performed involving nursing leaders, executives, and managers from the United States, Canada, Australia, and Sweden (Kitson et al., 2021) who were queried about the strategies they use to promote EBP. Some of their recommendations included:

- Establish an EBP culture and help the staff learn how to use evidence.
- Interact with nursing staff to determine how the evidence would help their practice.
- Role model EBP and lead by example.
- Communicate consistently about the necessity of EBP.

Leaders will need to communicate their vision throughout the organization and deploy leadership behaviors such as role modeling, training, periodic review, and feedback to ensure active participation by all members of the health care team. Stetler et al. (2014) explored key leadership behaviors and discovered nursing leaders use strategic thinking in "planning-organizing-aligning" as an important factor when facilitating EBP in the organization (p. 224). Additional essential behaviors included EBP goal setting and EBP infrastructure support (Stetler et al., 2014, p. 224). Additionally, Stetler found that functional behavior such as inspiring, inducing, cajoling, and intervening actively helped promote EBP within the organization.

Leaders must also distribute power among other leaders (AHRQ, 2018). Several studies have determined that middle managers, those individuals who report to the executive leadership and who supervise others, have an important role in promoting the success of improvement efforts. Clavijo-Chamorro and colleagues (2022) conducted a meta-synthesis to assess nurse managers' perspectives on the different organizational elements that help promote EBP in their practice settings. Three main factors were delineated, including effective teamwork, effective organizational structures, and transformational leadership. Effective teamwork involved collaboration and communication. Organizational structures included engaging all members of the team in collecting evidence to develop EBP policies and procedures, carrying out auditing, and communicating results of EBP initiatives with staff. Transformational behaviors included role modeling evidence-based interventions and implementing policies that reflected evidence-based care. Nurse managers empowered the nurses in their units by encouraging nurses to express their ideas about how to improve practice. Nurses were encouraged to serve on different EBP committees on their local units and on hospital-wide committees. In one of the qualitative interviews, a nurse manager reflected on the level of trust that had developed between the nurse manager and the nursing staff:

I'm just now starting to really reap the benefits of having very active committees, my staff experts . . . they drive their own work environment . . . . I can't be in the committees—if they want me to go and answer some questions I will. But I pretty much have said, I trust you . . . . I know what your capabilities are, you don't need a unit coordinator to be sitting in these committees because you all are the experts.

Kueny et al., 2015, as cited in Clavijo-Chamorro et al., 2022, p. 576.

While leaders need to implement a series of technical strategies to advance implementation efforts, leaders need to harness the power of stakeholders to promote behavior change to implement the changes they want. The Institute of Healthcare Improvement (Hilton & Anderson, 2018) developed a framework to advance the psychology of change that complements the technical strategies associated with evidence-based QI methods (Fig. 17.1). The "Psychology of Change" is defined as "the science and art of human behavior as it relates to transformation" (Hilton & Anderson, 2018, p. 6). In this model, individuals within an organization use their personal knowledge, skills, and experiences, individually and collectively, to advance the evidence-based initiative. The central component of this model is to promote the individual's and groups' collective "agency," defined as the "ability to act with purpose" (Hilton & Anderson, 2018, p. 8). As depicted in Fig. 17.1, there are five important components to this framework, including: (a) unleashing intrinsic motivation of the stakeholders; (b) co-designing people-driven change with stakeholders; (c) co-producing in authentic relationships with stakeholders; (d) distributing power; and (e) adapting in action (Hilton & Anderson, 2018, p. 8). Overall, this model is person centered and inclusive and invites all individuals to use their inherent power to collaborate on the development and advancement of EBP.

To develop a culture of EBP, it is important to promote psychological safety within the organization. Psychological safety is defined as the "belief that the team is safe for interpersonal risk taking" and that individuals will not face retribution for openly discussing their beliefs or when discussing their mistakes (Edmundson, 1999, p. 354). In order to promote change, innovation, and EBP, leaders will need to develop a culture of psychological safety and encourage members to speak up honestly about the current process or processes and convey their ideas about how the process can be improved. In the absence of psychological safety, team members may be reluctant to speak up and challenge the status quo, or may fear retribution for expressing ideas that are unpopular. According Hilton and Anderson (2018), there are several ways to promote a psychologically safe environment including:

- Soliciting feedback from all team members
- Motivating all individuals to speak up and participate

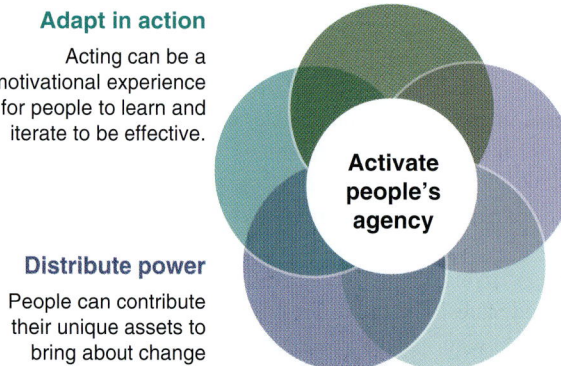

Fig. 17.1 Psychology of Change Framework.

- Fostering listening, teaching, and learning from all members
- Celebrating failures and missteps as necessary steps toward eventual improvement

Implementation Leadership Scale

Leadership behaviors can be assessed using the Implementation Leadership Scale (ILS). This is a 12-item scale that measures the extent to which leaders enact behaviors that support EBP implementation (0 = not at all to 4 = great extent) (Aarons et al., 2014a; Torres et al., 2018). There are two versions of the ILS, one for staff to report their perceptions of supervisors' leadership and another for supervisors and leaders to assess themselves. The leadership characteristics that are assessed include the following:

- Proactive
- Knowledgeable
- Supportive
- Perseverant

> **TIP**
>
> A preliminary study conducted by Williams and colleagues (2020) revealed that when leaders in a pediatric mental health clinic used the specific leadership characteristics measured by the ILS, improvements in the EBP implementation climate were seen, leading to an improvement in the use of EBP psychotherapy techniques within the organization.

> **TIP**
>
> Consider using the ILS to assess leadership behaviors of nurse managers, clinical nurse leaders, directors of clinical services, and/or advanced practice nurses.

SOCIAL SYSTEM

Leadership is critical in developing systems and organizational structure to facilitate EBP. Prior to implementation, there are several conditions that must be in place to support or facilitate EBP. Clearly, the social system or context of care delivery is important when implementing EBPs (Squires et al., 2015).

Implementation strategies to address the social system are based on the following principles:

- Building relationships among and across disciplines
- Garnering initial and ongoing support of key senior leaders and middle managers
- Providing rewards and recognition for staff who align practices with the evidence
- Ensuring that organizational practice standards and documentation systems support the ongoing use of the EBPs

These principles are essential for ongoing sustainability of the practice change after implementation. Implementation strategies that target the social system are the following:

- Conducting an environmental scan
- Meeting with key leadership stakeholders
- Revising practice standards and documentation systems
- Providing recognition and rewards

Potential **users of EBP** are also called members of a social system (e.g., nurses, physicians, clerical staff, patients, families) who influence how quickly and widely EBPs are adopted. To be effective in an increasingly complex health care system, *users* of EBP, specifically nurses, and members of a social networking system must have the skills to engage in EBP to improve patient care (Hilton & Anderson, 2018). A recent meta-analysis composed of eight randomized controlled trials was conducted to assess the effectiveness of social networking strategies to address health behavior changes and determined these networks were associated with improvements, although significant heterogeneity was noted (Laranjo et al., 2015). Implementation strategies targeted at users include the following (Titler et al., 2016):

- Leadership
- Auditing and feedback
- Performance gap assessment
- Piloting the EBP initiative
- Soliciting stakeholder experiences and perspectives
- Eliciting patient values and preferences
- Regular meetings among the implementation team members to address challenges and recognize successes
- Feedback from the members of the social system to identify opportunities to optimize EBP

Organizational Capacity and EBP

Organizational capacity is important in building an EBP culture (Stetler et al., 2009). Capacity is described as the necessary structures, resources, and workforce staff necessary to implement EBP interventions (Brownson et al., 2018). Capacity building is defined as delivering activities that help build a sustainable EBP organization

(Brownson et al., 2018). According to the Evidence-Based Practice Society (2024), capacity is defined as the characteristics that help develop the organization's EBP goals such as collaborative relationships, motivations, knowledge, attitudes, and skills. Components of organizational capacity for EBP include the following:

- Strong leadership
- Clear strategic vision
- Good managerial relations
- Visionary staff in key positions
- A climate conducive to experimentation and risk-taking
- Effective data-capture systems

An organization may be generally amenable to innovations but not ready or willing to assimilate a particular EBP. Elements of system readiness include the following (Ramanadhan et al., 2022):

- Use specific implementation strategies
- Identify targeted outcome measures to assess improvements
- Develop reliable and validated tools to measure outcomes
- Support and advocacy for equity issues
- Dedicated time and resources
- Capacity to evaluate the impact of the EBP during and after implementation

Organizational Context

Context for EBP implementation traditionally has been defined as the physical setting, with little attention paid to the dynamics of the practice environment (May et al., 2016). Organizational context refers to the characteristics of the physical setting of implementation and the dynamic practice factors in which implementation processes occur (May et al., 2016; Squires et al., 2015). A broader definition can divide context into three different components: (a) the macro level, or the political-economic forces that shape policies; (b), the meso level, including factors such as the culture, or the climate, factors that impact employees' actions and behaviors; and (c) the micro level that refer to the local unit's policies, procedures, and processes (Li et al., 2018). Contextual factors that impact implementation include the following:

- Organizational capacity for EBP (Kueny et al., 2015; Li et al., 2018; Yamada et al., 2017)
- Leadership support (Aarons et al., 2014a, 2014b; Jun et al., 2016; Li et al., 2018; Richter et al., 2016)
- Practice climates for use of EBPs (Jacobs et al., 2014; Yamada et al., 2017)
- EBP competencies of staff and nurse managers (Melnyk et al., 2014; Shuman et al., 2018)
- Monitoring, feedback, and evaluation (Li et al., 2018)
- When performing a context assessment, you will need to do the following:
  - Select concepts that you believe will impact implementation and that are important to assess (e.g., climate, leadership, competencies)
  - Select tools that are aligned with the concepts
  - Be thoughtful about how the results of the assessment will be incorporated into implementation
  - Select methods for sharing the results of the assessment and deciding who will receive them

> **TIP**
>
> Be selective when choosing assessment tools; refrain from measuring all concepts, and consider the length of the tool.

Culture of EBP

Organizational culture influences effective EBP implementation. Organizations that have adopted the principles and behaviors of a High Reliability Organization (HRO) are apt to have the tools in which EBP can be most successful. AHRQ (2023) defines HROs as those "that operate in complex, high-hazard domains for extended periods without serious accidents or catastrophic failures." The implementation of EBP is important to mitigate safety and quality risks in health care organizations for these reasons. The principles of high reliability include preoccupation with failure; sensitivity to operations; deference to expertise; and commitment to resilience (AHRQ, 2023). The behaviors that support these principles include that everyone makes a personal commitment to safety; everyone is accountable for clear and complete communication; and everyone supports a questioning attitude (AHRQ, 2023).

When assessing organizational readiness for EBP implementation and the strategy therein, it is imperative to consider organizational culture. Peter Drucker was renowned for his quote, "Culture eats strategy for breakfast." What he and other leadership gurus have found is that "the culture is the secret sauce that keeps employees motivated and clients happy" (Engel, 2018). The improved engagement and resultant outcome successes that result from a positive organizational culture cannot be understated.

The reality is that strategy and culture should work in tandem and be complementary. A strategic EBP plan without cultural alignment will not be as successful and may fail entirely. A strong culture of staff empowerment and engagement is needed to achieve strategic success. In healthcare, this association improves staff experience, patient experience, and organizational sustainability. A strong culture of engaged staff improves not only the work environment, but also clinical outcomes tied to the EBP implementation.

EBP Implementation Climate

EBP implementation climate is described as "employees' shared perceptions of the policies, practices, procedures, and behaviors that are rewarded, supported and expected in order to facilitate effective EBP implementation and its use" (Aarons et al., 2014b, p. 258). Some research reveals that a strong organizational climate for EBP is associated with a collective commitment to EBP by employees (Ehrhart et al., 2014; Williams et al., 2020). Clinicians working within this kind of a practice environment are thought to exhibit more skillful use of EBP (Williams et al., 2020).

To create an EBP climate, Schein (2010, as cited in Aarons et al., 2014b) has proposed a multilevel model designed for leadership to convey their EBP vision to their teams. The model includes six "embedding mechanisms" (Aarons et al., 2014, p. 6) for leaders to implement:

1. Leaders convey what they assess, measure, and improve as EBP.
2. Leaders manage critical incidents and crises related to EBP.
3. Leaders allocate resources for EBP.
4. Leaders' role model, mentor, and educate EBP.
5. Leaders recognize EBP initiatives and distribute rewards.

> **TIP**
>
> In an observational, repeated, cross-sectional design (Williams et al., 2022) conducted over 7 years in community mental health agencies, a strong organizational climate for EBP predicted improved compliance with evidence-based approaches to cognitive behavioral training. The design and structure of the organization was organized around the dissemination of EBP. Mechanisms such as EBP policies and partnerships among providers, researchers, and policy makers help facilitate EBP reimbursement and payment systems, electronic information systems, and clinical decision support.

Environmental Scan

An **environmental scan** is a systematic process used to collect information necessary to organize and support organizational change. The entire organization is usually examined, and data are collected from both the external environment, such as the political, technological, sociocultural aspects affecting the organization, and the internal environment, such as staff, budget, electronic health care data, and administrative leadership (Charlton et al., 2021). Environmental scans can be performed as part of a strategic plan or as a prerequisite to employing an EBP-QI initiative to improve a particular aspect of healthcare. An environmental scan can be performed to understand the organization's mission, vision, and values and to articulate how the EBP project contributes to and aligns with meeting these organizational goals.

A scoping review of 96 studies was conducted to determine the nature and extent of environmental scans used in health services delivery research (Charlton et al., 2021). A thematic analysis revealed that most of the environmental scan studies were conducted to collect evidence, to inform decision making, and to guide strategic planning. The authors determined that there was a lack of consistent terminology to describe environmental scans and this gap may have contributed to a lack of conceptual clarity and confusion regarding whether or not to conduct an environmental scan. Based on this research, a working definition of an environmental scan (ES) was developed:

> *Within a health services delivery context, an ES is a type of inquiry that involves the collection and synthesis of existing information and/or the pursuit of new evidence to inform decision making and help shape future response(s) to existing and emerging policy and service delivery issues and opportunities.*

"Drawing information from any source within the internal and/or external environments of an organization, and an environmental scan is often conducted to examine the current landscape of services, practice, and/or policies; identify needs, service barriers, gaps and priorities; inform planning, policy, and program design; inform QI and patient safety initiatives; and identity successful strategies, models, and innovations to inform system transformation" (Charlton et al., 2019, p. 7).

Environmental scans are used to review the governance structure and to identify senior leaders in various disciplines with whom you will need to interact with for

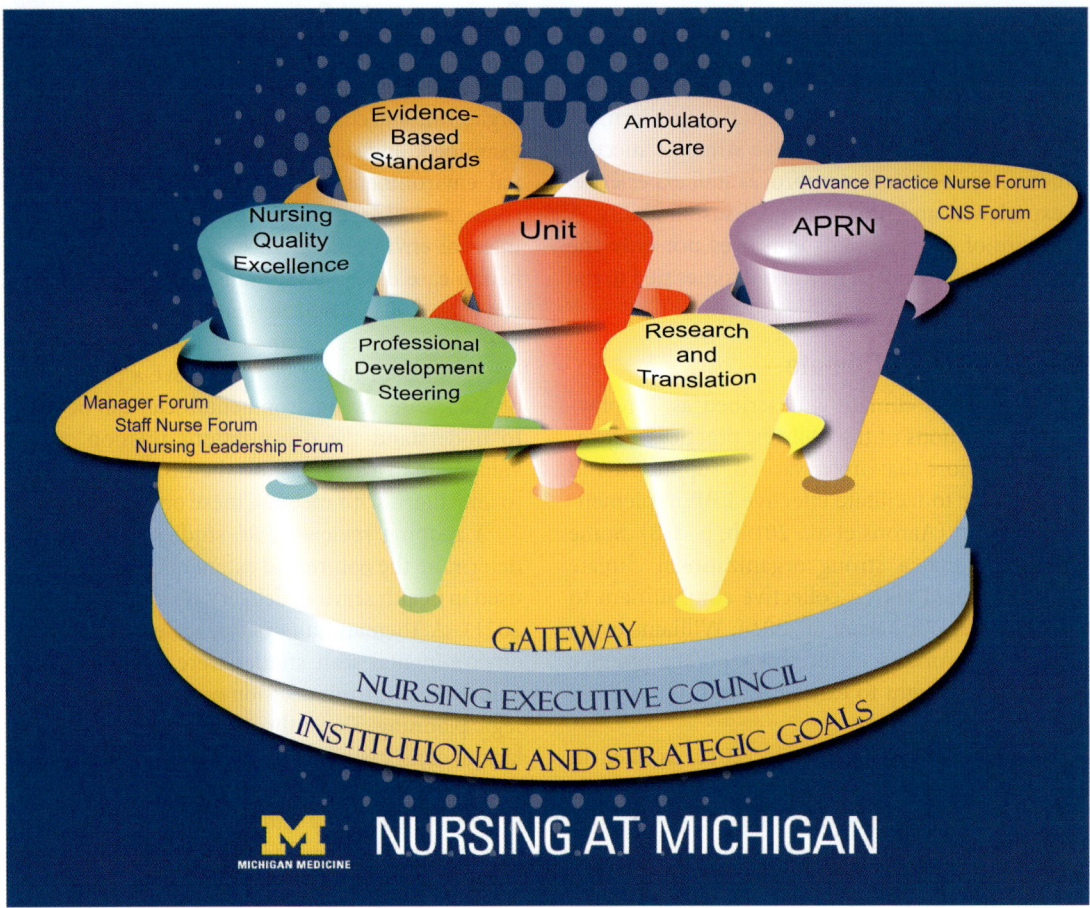

Fig. 17.2 Structure of a Nursing Quality Committee, Standards Committee, and Research Committee in the Department of Nursing Governance at the University of Michigan Health System. Committees are depicted by cones (e.g., Nursing Quality Excellence Committee). (From the University of Michigan Health System.)

implementation. Specifically, you will want to understand the functions and roles of the various committees or councils that compose the governance structure and evaluate which ones you need to work with for implementation. For example, the department of nursing governance may include a nursing quality committee, a standards committee, and a research committee (Fig. 17.2 for an example from the University of Michigan). You will want to meet with the chairs of each to engage their expertise and seek guidance on what processes may be required to institutionalize the work of your team. The **standards committee** can guide the team on revising existing standards to align with the evidence base and understanding the steps necessary to have the revised standards approved. The **nursing quality committee** can assist with quality performance indicators for performance gap assessment, audit and feedback, and evaluation. The **research and EBP committee** may have members with expertise regarding EBPs that are the focus of your project and thus may serve as consultants.

Context Assessment

Your environmental scan may include an assessment of key context factors that impact implementation, such as unit climate and leadership behaviors for EBP implementation. A variety of tools with good reliability and validity are available for assessment and are summarized in Table 17.2. Two scales are discussed for illustrative purposes: the Implementation Climate Scale and the

TABLE 17.2 Examples of EBP Assessment Tools

Name of Tool	What It Measures	Number of Items	Scores	References
Implementation Climate Scale (ICS)	Staff perceptions of the extent to which a unit or practice setting prioritizes and values EBP	18 items Likert scale: 0 = not at all to 4 = very great extent	Total score and 6 subscale scores: Focus; Educational Support; Recognition; Rewards; EBP Selection; Openness	Ehrhart et al., 2014
Work Environment for EBP Scale	Staff perceptions of the values and resources available to support EBP	8 items Likert scale: Strongly agree to strongly disagree	Total score No subscales	Pryse et al., 2014
Absorptive and Receptive Capacity Scale (ARCS)	Staff perception about organizational processes to use knowledge (evidence) in practice	14 items Likert scale: 1 = lack of routine processes to 5 = good processes in place	Total score and 5 subscale scores: Questioning culture; Acquiring New Knowledge; Knowledge Sharing; Knowledge Use; Vision, Culture, and Leadership	Burton, 2017
Implementation Leadership Scale (ILS)	Staff perceptions regarding the extent to which leaders enact behaviors that support EBP implementation	12 items Likert scale: 0 = not at all to 4 = great extent	Total score and 4 subscale scores: Proactive, Knowledgeable, Supportive, and Perseverant Leadership	Aarons et al., 2014a; Torres et al., 2018
Nursing Leadership for EBP Scale	Staff perceptions about the behaviors of their managers who support EBP	10 items Likert scale: Strongly agree to strongly disagree	Total score No subscales	Pryse et al., 2014
Implementation Citizenship Behavior Scale (ICBS)	Behaviors employees perform that exceed their expected job tasks to support implementation of EBPs	6 items Likert scale: 0 = not at all to 4 = frequently if not always	Total score and 2 subscale scores: Helping Others, Keeping Informed	Ehrhart et al., 2015
Nurse Manager EBP Competency Scale	Self-assessment of level of competency for EBP knowledge and skills	16 items Likert scale: 0 = not competent to 3 = expertly competent	Total score and 2 subscale scores: EBP Knowledge, EBP Activity	Shuman et al., 2018
RNs EBP Competency Scale	Assessment of RNs' abilities in selected aspects of EBP	13 items	Total score No subscale scores	Melnyk et al., 2014
APN EBP Competency Scale	Assessment of APNs' abilities in all aspects of EBP	24 items	Total score No subscale score	Melnyk et al., 2014
Organizational Readiness for Implementing Change (ORIC) Instrument	Assessment of an organization's readiness for implementing change	12 items Likert scale: 1 = disagree to 5 = agree	Total score and 2 subscale scores: Change Commitment, and Change Efficacy	Shea et al., 2014

RN, Registered nurse; *APN*, advanced practice nurse.

Implementation Leadership Scale. Findings from context assessments provide insights for tailoring implementation strategies such as educational approaches and fostering leadership behaviors that promote EBP.

EBP Climate Scale

The Implementation Climate Scale (ICS) is a reliable and valid instrument to measure the unit climate for EBP implementation (Ehrhart et al., 2014). It is short (18 items) and evaluates the extent (1 = slight to 4 = very great) to which the unit or setting prioritizes and values EBP in six areas:

- Focus on EBP
- Educational support for EBP
- Recognition for EBP
- Rewards for EBP
- Selection of staff for EBP knowledge and experience
- Selection of staff for openness (flexible, adaptable, open to new interventions)

All items are anchored to a specific unit or practice setting as a point of reference.

You should treat individual responses as confidential, and results should be aggregated for reporting. Comparing certain assessment measures (e.g., ILS, ICS) across units is helpful to guide implementation, but units should be blinded. For example, ICSs for units can be reported, and when discussing EBP implementation with a specific unit, staff would be informed which one is their unit (A, B, C, or D).

The ICS suggests that the unit climate for EBP implementation in Unit D is quite positive, whereas the climate of Unit C is not as positive. You should consider how these results can guide the tailoring of implementation.

In summary, an EBP implementation climate should:
- Develop EBP policies to institutionalize EBP practices, procedures, and behaviors
- Recruit EBP champions to promote EBP and dissemination
- Provide support and rewards for EBP practice for all stakeholders
- Develop EBP electronic information systems
- Implement and use EBP clinical decision support systems

Performance Gap Assessment

Performance gap assessment (PGA) is defined as the baseline practice performance that provides information on the state of existing practices at the beginning of a practice change. This aspect of an implementation strategy engages clinicians in discussions about practice issues and formulation of strategies to promote alignment of their current practices with EBP recommendations. Specific practice indicators selected for PGA are derived from EBP recommendations for the specified topic, such as pain assessment every 4 hours for acute pain management (Titler et al., 2009). Studies have demonstrated improvements in performance when

> **TIP**
>
> As part of a quality improvement project to improve nursing physical assessments, Fontenot and colleagues (2022) performed a gap analysis to determine the existing physical assessment competencies of nurses in a large academic medical hospital. The initial survey queried nurses about the barriers they experienced when performing a full physical assessment. A follow-up survey was sent to the leadership asking how important it was for nurses to perform a physical assessment and recognize a change in a patient's status. The second phase of the gap analysis involved selecting one to two nurses randomly from each unit and observing their physical examinations. The results revealed that nurses prioritized other responsibilities over physical assessments such as the patient's hygiene, administering medications, and drawing labs. Twenty-five percent of nursing leaders believed that a physical examination was not a priority for nurses and was primarily the physician's responsibility (Table 17.3). A comprehensive QI project was implemented to improve the physical assessment competencies of nurses. The following measures were tracked: (a) completeness of the physical exam; (b) use of equipment to assist with physical assessment, including a stethoscope and a pen light; (c) appropriate timeliness of documentation; and (d) accuracy of the physical assessment. The results of the gap assessment are depicted in the following table prior to the QI implementation and revealed that only 78% of nurses performed a thorough physical examination. Fewer than 50% used a pen light. Ninety-one percent of nurses used a stethoscope. Fewer than 70% of nurses documented their findings within a 4-hour period, and fewer than 70% documented their findings accurately. See the post-QI results, which revealed significant improvements in the accuracy of documentation as well as the completeness of the physical assessment (see Table 17.3).

PGA is part of multifaceted implementation strategies (Titler et al., 2016). The following steps are a guide for using PGA:
- Select the practice performance indicators to use (e.g., acute pain assessment every 4 hours).
- Illustrate the current state of practice using these indicators.
- Select a venue for discussing the gap between the current practice indicators and recommendations based on evidence.
- Engage clinicians in a dialogue about improving practices to align with the evidence.

IMPLEMENTATION STRATEGIES

Leaders are instrumental in creating the necessary foundations for implementing EBP. Once the foundation has been established, and an evidence-practice gap has been identified as a target for improvement, there are several important implementation strategies that can be initiated. The following strategies can assist with specific EBP initiatives once deployed to help achieve the desired outcomes.

Stakeholders

Stakeholders are described as individuals or groups who share a concern, interest, and/or involvement in the design, implementation, evaluation, and outcomes of an EBP initiative or EBP-QI project (Silver et al., 2016). Identifying stakeholders who are central to the improvement goal both within and outside of the organization is a critical step in formulating a team. Stakeholders may have various roles internal to the organization, such as administrative leadership roles or direct care roles. Alternatively, stakeholders may have a role external to the organization, ensuring or requiring an organization's performance or outcome of a project, such as accreditors or regulatory officials. Stakeholder teams involved in an EBP-QI project are usually composed of interprofessionals and may include diverse professionals such as nurses, nurse managers, case managers, nurse practitioners, directors of a service, physicians, pharmacists and social workers, registrars, administrators, and professional organizations, to name a few.

Stakeholder mapping is a tool used to graphically depict or diagram the relationships among the different stakeholders along with their relationships to the project. There are several tools that can be used to draw, diagram, or visually depict these relationships. In a hypothetical scenario depicting the different constituents critical to the EBP-QI process, Silver and colleagues (2016) used a snowflake diagram to reflect the multidisciplinary stakeholders' involvement in the EBP

TABLE 17.3 Average Completeness of Physical Assessments Throughout Methodist Proficient Assessment Competency (MPAC)

	Pre-MPAC $n = 179$	Post-MPAC $n = 1,391$	p
Completeness of assessment			
Percentage of components completed	78%	94%	< 0.001
Equipment to perform assessment			
Used a penlight/pupilometer	87 (48.6%)	1202 (86.9%)	< 0.001
Used a stethoscope	166 (92.7%)	1379 (99.2%)	< 0.001
Timeliness of documentation			
Documentation completed within 4 hours of assessment	116 (67.4%)	1205 (94.7%)	< 0.001
Accuracy of documentation			
Actual assessment corresponded to documentation	102 (64.2%)	1200 (90.6%)	< 0.001

From Fontenot et al., 2022.

project. The different stakeholder roles were delineated and may include the team lead, or the individual who oversees and manages the daily operations for the program. The author noted that nurses and physicians can both serve as the team lead. The team may include technical experts, those individuals who possess expertise in their respective professions and should be recruited to participate in the improvement teams. The clinical/systems leaders are the hemodialysis managers who are responsible to test the changes initiated by the technical experts. The improvement advisors, or persons with QI expertise, will advise the team leader and experts on QI initiatives and how to interpret results and coordinate improvement efforts based on those results. The executive sponsor, the person who holds the leadership authority for obtaining resources, might be the head of nephrology or chief nursing officer of the hospital system.

The diagram in depicts the scope and variety of professionals necessary to implement a home dialysis center, including nephrologists, program directors, nursing staff, and patient support groups. Each constituent or organization has a different role but is part of a collective to ensure the success of the project. While stakeholder mapping depicts the different stakeholders, it does not reflect the different levels of power and interest relative to each stakeholder.

A stakeholder matrix is a tool to help define and differentiate the levels of interest and power among the stakeholders. Power reflects the stakeholder's level of power or authority within the organization and interest is reflected as the stakeholder's level of concern or the degree to which the project impacts the stakeholder. The matrix is composed of four quadrants, with the level of power ranging from low to high on the Y axis or vertical line, and the level of interest from low to high power on the X axis or horizontal line. Stakeholder roles are plotted in each of the four quadrants depending on their level of interest and their level of power relative to the EBP project. Project leads can use this tool to focus their attention and efforts on the stakeholders with the most power and interest to ensure the successful implementation of the project.

In this hypothetical scenario, an interest/power matrix was developed to reflect the different level of interest and power among the stakeholders (Silver et al., 2016).

As seen in stakeholders such as nephrologists, clinical managers, and funding organizations, with high power and high interest on the upper right quadrant, possess significant decision-making authority and will need to be kept apprised of the project's progress. While the interest of the patients, nurses, social workers, and caregivers were high, their level of power to promote the development of a home dialysis program was lower. It is not uncommon to find physicians and administrators holding powerful positions to facilitate change; however, it is important for leaders to promote the power of patients, health care professionals, and caregivers as they are often associated with providing the care or receiving the care and should have an active, strong voice in the process.

> **TIP**
>
> Mapping stakeholders and assessing the level of their power/interest in decision making will help the EBP leader focus their attention on the key stakeholders who can advance the EBP project.

Stakeholder Meetings

Regular interprofessional stakeholder meetings among opinion leaders, change champions, staff and leaders of the EBP project are essential to track the process of implementation, provide guidance, address questions that arise, solve ongoing challenges, and share implementation strategies that are working (Titler et al., 2016). You should (a) decide who will participate in these meetings; (b) select a regular meeting time and date (e.g., first Tuesday of the month at 1 p.m.); (c) determine the length and location of the meeting (recommend 30 to 60 minutes); and (d) set forth and distribute a meeting agenda that includes:

- What issues have arisen
- Questions about the EBPs or implementation approaches
- Report on action items from the previous meeting
- Plan for follow-up of action items from the current meeting
- Verbal summary of the meeting followed by meeting minutes

Meetings With Key Leadership Stakeholders

As a leader of the EBP project, you and your selected team members will want to initially meet with the chief nurse executive (CNE) to describe the project and overall goals related to quality and safety to ensure alignment with the nursing strategic plan and objectives. This initial meeting should include a discussion of the current practice, the gap in alignment with EBPs, and practice sites for implementation. You will want to include data about current practice indicators and a beginning synthesis of the evidence to illustrate EBPs that need to be modified. You should also articulate how this work aligns with the organization's mission, vision, and strategic agenda. The purpose of this meeting is to garner support to proceed with the project and the overall implementation plan. The CNE is likely to provide recommendations for involvement of key stakeholders, additional members to consider for the implementation team, units for implementation, and individuals to serve as opinion leaders. A subsequent meeting(s) with the CNE may be warranted to provide follow-up information. Ongoing methods of communication with the CNE should be established (e.g., email updates, face-to-face meetings, quarterly reports).

Conversely, the EBP project may be driven by the CNE to address a quality-of-care issue. It is still important to meet with the CNE to understand his or her perspective and be clear about the focus of the project, as well as level of prioritization among organizational goals and the nursing strategic plan.

Meetings With Other Disciplines

After meeting with the CNE, you and your EBP team will need to meet with key leaders from other disciplines who will be impacted by the EBP changes. It is helpful to have the CNE or their designee attend these meetings to illustrate his or her support for the project. A workplace culture that provides clear communication of EBP goals or regulatory changes and senior leader support is essential for the successful promotion of EBP (Kueny et al., 2015). They can be structured as one gathering of all senior leaders or individual meetings with each senior leader. The meetings should include the following:

- Data that illustrate opportunity for improvement such as the PGA report
- A summary of the EBPs to be implemented, including references
- The role of each discipline in promoting and facilitating implementation of the EBPs
- Planned implementation strategies
- An evaluation plan
- Summary of the implementation timeline and action plan
- What is working well

For example, when implementing evidence-based fall prevention practices targeted to patient-specific fall risk factors, consider meeting with the CNE (or designee), the chief medical officer (CMO) (or designee), directors of pharmacy and physical therapy services, and the director of quality improvement.

Nurse Manager Meetings

Nurse managers (NMs) of practice sites (e.g., ambulatory care clinic, patient care unit) where EBPs will be implemented are assets to EBP implementation and are keys to success. These individuals have different titles depending on the site of implementation, but they are characterized as licensed registered nurses who are direct supervisors of staff nurses on the unit or in a clinical practice, and who have responsibility and accountability for unit-level or practice operations, including budget, resource allocation, staffing, and quality of care. Engaging with NMs early in the planning and implementation process is essential to ensure their support for implementation and include their knowledgeable recommendations. One strategy to engage with NMs is an organizational meeting to discuss:

- An overview of the project
- The EBPs
- Timeline and rationale for the practice change
- Commitment to implementation
- The role of NMs in implementation

NMs can foster implementation by role modeling the EBPs, providing visible feedback and support to staff who are aligning their practices with the evidence base, providing resources such as time for change champions to attend meetings and do EBP work, including EBP as part of staff evaluations, and creating enthusiasm among staff for improving care based on evidence. These meetings usually take 60 to 90 minutes, depending on the group size. Meeting as a collective group of NMs provides opportunities for rich dialogue and discussion.

In addition to the NM, clinical leaders such as clinical nurse specialists (CNSs) are essential to all aspects of the EBP process, including implementation. They have specific education, knowledge, and expertise dealing with EBPs, EBP implementation, and the data analyses therein. CNSs may work directly with staff or engage unit-based educators or change agents to implement and evaluate EBP.

EBP Leader Meetings

As the leader of an EBP project, you will need to ensure that everyone participates in meetings and has a voice at the table. Meeting minutes and accountability for actions after the meeting are important to engage participants and move the project forward. For example, monthly meetings to implement fall prevention practices and mitigate patient-specific fall risk factors addressed challenges in education of nursing assistants, strategies to make each patient's fall prevention interventions visible, and strategies to modify prescribed medications to avoid use of high-risk drugs that contribute to falls. Participants shared the approaches they used to meet these challenges, such as a structured education session for nursing assistants, use of white boards in patients' rooms to list their specific fall prevention interventions, review of medications by a clinical nurse leader, and discussions with physicians to modify medication orders.

Academic Partners

Partnerships between health care organizations and their academic partners can be extremely helpful in EBP by helping with benchmarking and researching current best practices. This partnership can continue through the implementation and analysis of outcomes data. Linking academia with practice allows bilateral exchange of information and incorporation of best practices into academic curricula.

> **TIP**
> As recipients of health care practices, patients and families should be incorporated into the implementation processes. Patient-centered EBP is discussed in Chapter 18.

Educational Programs

Providing an educational program for nurses helps facilitate the acceptance and implementation of EBP. Training programs considered most successful were of longer duration (3 hours to 2 weeks) and provided ongoing support at regular intervals throughout the implementation period (Joy et al., 2015; Kapp, 2013). One study used telephone and email reminders periodically to support nurses throughout the testing process (Kapp, 2013).

> **TIP**
> Vaajoki and colleagues (2023) conducted a pre-post study to determine if an online educational program would help nurses learn different EBP skills to implement in practice. The intervention was composed of 50 hours of teaching and close to 60 hours of independent studying over an 8-month period. Nurse participants followed the sequential steps of EBP, including developing a PICOT question, searching for best available evidence, critically appraising the evidence, applying the evidence in their clinical practice, evaluating the change, and then integrating the evidence into policy at their institution. Results revealed a statistically significant increase in the participants' self-perceptions of their attitudes toward EBP and their work based on EBP. They noted improvements in their abilities to apply EBP skills in practice.

Piloting the Change

Piloting the change is a critical component of a successful EBP implementation. A pilot test represents an opportunity for EBP designers, leaders, and frontline clinicians to conduct a trial run and test the initiative on a smaller scale and in one location before widespread implementation (AHRQ, 2022; Laures & Fowler, 2020). Conducting early pilot tests provides the EBP team with an opportunity to use the process, obtain users' responses, address early challenges and provide feedback to the designers and leaders of the process. This feedback can be used to address problems and modify or adapt the process as needed. Piloting an initiative helps guarantee successful adoption and implementation on a broader scale.

Plan-Do-Study-Act (PDSA) provides a cylical framework for implementation and testing change. Planning involves designing an intitative. Do involves the act of implementation. Study involves monitoring the results.

Act involves integrating the successful parts of the initiative. Multiple PDSA cycles may be implemented until the intended results are achieved. PDSA is a framework used to implement and test an EBP-quality improvement initiative.

> **TIP**
>
> Friesen and colleagues (2017) conducted a mixed-methods pilot study to determine the effectiveness of an EBP educational program and system approach to EBP for nurses prior to implementation of the program hospital wide. The researchers used the Evidence-Based Practice Implementation Scale (EBPI) and Evidence-Based Practice Beliefs Scale (EBPB) to assess nurses who were early adopters and recruited them to participate in an educational program in EBP. The results of a pre-test/post-test program revealed a statistically significant increase in EBPI and an increase in EBPB, which was not significant. Focus group participants revealed that the education was helpful and noted that keeping the process streamlined and easy to use helped nurses implement EBP in practice. They also noted that encouraging nurses to participate was a challenge, however, once the nurses became involved, there was less resistance.

Recommendations for pilot testing include:
- Selecting the time frame for the pilot. Usually, this represents a shorter period, such as a week.
- Selecting the unit for the pilot if the EBP is targeted to multiple units in a health system. Pilot tests are often usually implemented on one unit to evaluate and modify as needed.
- Selecting implementation strategies for the pilot. Usually, the same implementation strategies designed for the EBP initiative can be used for the pilot test, albeit on a smaller scale.
- Selecting performance measures for evaluation. The performance measures are usually the ones that will be used.
- Eliciting feedback from clinicians who implemented and used the EBP.
- Revising the implementation plan based on the pilot.

Frameworks

Selecting a **framework** to guide and structure the EBP process is a necessary implementation strategy when incorporating EBP processes to advance change. Refer to Chapter 4 for a thorough review of different EBP-QI frameworks that may be used addressing practice gaps and implementing EBP improvements.

Auditing and Feedback

Auditing and feedback is described as an implementation strategy designed to motivate health care professionals to improve their clinical practices. An audit is a professional review that compares an individual or groups' performance in meeting standards of care against the optimal performance of that standard. Audits are performed periodically at regular intervals and help provide necessary feedback on progress toward meeting evidence-based standards. Audits help track measurement of performance indicators. Information from audits can be used for aggregating data into reports, communicating that data, and discussing the findings with health care practitioners on a regular basis *during the practice change* (Reynolds, 2020). This strategy helps staff see how their efforts to improve care and patient outcomes are progressing throughout the implementation process. Staff feedback on changes impacting workflow must be examined and modified if needed to optimize care and workflow.

While audit and feedback are prevalent, there is minimal research documenting its effectiveness. Ivers and colleagues (2012) conducted a Cochrane review of 140 studies where audit and feedback were used as a primary component of an evidence-based initiative and found a small improvement in practice. Another mixed-methods systematic review (Dufour et al., 2019), which included 31 studies investigating the effect of audit and feedback on nursing performance, discovered that some nurses viewed the feedback negatively and were concerned that the reports could be used in a punitive fashion. Many nurses noted that more explanation of the purpose and EBP processes could ameliorate the negative perspectives of this strategy. Staff feedback on changes impacting workflow must be examined and modified if needed to optimize care and workflow.

The following action steps should be considered when using audit and feedback strategies:
- Selection of the performance indicators to audit
- Selection of the data source (e.g., electronic medical records, observation, patients, and family members) and methods for auditing (frequency, selection of records, or observation time points)
- Deciding who will do the audits

- Designing methods for data displays
- Deciding who will receive the reports
- Deciding on frequency and methods for dissemination of reports (e.g., paper or electronic such as website or email)
- Determining how feedback reports will be shared with staff (e.g., verbally, display in the practice setting, monthly staff meetings)

> **TIP**
>
> Audit and feedback reports are more effective when they are disseminated regularly and are used to actively discuss practice with staff rather than passive dissemination to selected individuals. Discussing the results with staff in a nonpunitive, psychologically safe culture may help staff understand the importance of receiving feedback to foster improvement in health care outcomes. Incorporating patient and family feedback is also helpful when examining these data.

Standards of Practice and Documentation Systems

It is important that written **standards of practice** (e.g., policies, procedures, clinical pathways) **and documentation systems** support the use of EBPs. Clinical information systems may need revision to support practice changes; documentation systems that fail to readily support the new practice thwart change (see Chapter 16). For example, if staff members are expected to reassess and document pain intensity within 30 minutes after administration of an analgesic, documentation systems must reflect this practice standard and easily fit within current workflows if possible. It is the role of leadership to ensure that organizational documents and systems are flexible and supportive of EBPs.

Recognition and Rewards

As you plan for implementation, you will need to decide how staff will be recognized and rewarded for their work. **Recognition and rewards** are important to acknowledge staff's investment in delivery of EBP. When considering rewards and recognition, appreciating the perspective of the staff is essential. There are now four generations practicing together (Hendricks & Cope, 2013), so these generational differences must be identified and supported to engage diverse teams. According to Stevanin and colleagues (2018), "generational differences in nurses' job attitudes, emotional, practice and leadership factors should be considered to enhance workplace quality." Recognition can be achieved through organizational publications such as newsletters, personal thank-you notes from the nurse manager and EBP team, highlighting the work at system-level QI meetings, and nominating individuals or teams for practice excellence awards offered by the health system, the clinical practice, or professional organizations.

Many health systems have recognition programs for nurses through events such as an annual recognition day or celebration dinner. For example, you may want to solicit nominations for an annual EBP Nurse of the Year Award for individuals who exemplify excellence in nursing practice through implementing EBPs to improve quality of care. Additional opportunities to have staff present this work at a meeting via podium or poster presentations may exist in your organization.

Recognition also can be achieved by nominations for awards offered by professional organizations. For example, the Association for Pediatric Hematology/Oncology Nurses presents an annual EBP Excellence Award to a member who demonstrates high-quality contributions to EBP in the nursing care of children and their families. The recipient of this award receives a $250 honorarium, recognition at the annual conference awards luncheon and through a press release, and an announcement sent to the recipient's employer. The Center for Nursing at the Foundation of the New York State Nurses Board of Trustees recognizes excellence in implementing nursing research in the practice setting through an Evidence-Based Practice Award (Center for Nursing, 2023). It is given to an individual or group using research-based evidence to make a practice change that results in demonstrated improvement in outcomes for patients, families, staff, community, or the organization. The Eastern Nursing Research Society has an EBP Award for an individual or group using research-based evidence to make a practice change that results in demonstrated improvement in health outcomes.

Rewards can be achieved through bonus payments, salary increases, and educational funds to be used at the discretion of the individual, team, or unit. For example, an individual or team who has been instrumental in implementing EBPs may receive financial support to attend a regional or national conference to present their work. Different options should be offered based on the generational differences within your unit, service line, or organization.

SYNTHESIS

Now that you are informed about multiple implementation strategies, you and your team can decide which strategies to use and formulate a reasonable timeline for implementation. Use the action plan (see Chapter 15) to guide your work, the time frame for each implementation strategy, and the individual(s) who will take the lead in enacting each implementation strategy. Be creative in imparting information to others and consider how you and your team can continuously engage stakeholders at all levels of the organization. Implementation can be the most fun and rewarding component of EBP. Enjoy the journey and keep a journal of lessons learned to use in your future work.

KEY POINTS

- To facilitate EBP, the organization's social systems, culture, and climate need to have necessary EBP structures in place.
- Leadership is integral to the successful implementation of EBP.
- A performance gap assessment is used at the beginning of implementation to engage clinicians in discussions about deficiencies in performance.
- Auditing and feedback require decisions about performance indicators, methods of data display, and frequency and methods for distributing reports to clinicians.
- Use audit and feedback reports during implementation to discuss practices with clinicians.
- Piloting the EBPs as a part of implementation has a positive effect on adoption.
- Plan-Do-Study-Act (PDSA) cycles may be used to implement the EBP on a smaller scale for a short test period to receive feedback about the effectiveness of the initiative. Modifications can be made immediately and the next **PDSA cycle** can be implemented to test the modifications.
- Perform an environmental scan to assess strengths and challenges.
- Engage senior leaders in implementation.
- Know your governance structure and how you will interact with each committee or group.
- Plan for recognition and rewards.

REFERENCES

Aarons, G. A., Ehrhart, M. G., & Farahnak, L. R. (2014a). The Implementation Leadership Scale (ILS): Development of a brief measure of unit level implementation leadership. *Implementation Science*, 9(1), 45.

Aarons, G. A., Ehrhart, M. G., Farahnak, L. R., & Sklar, M. (2014b). Aligning leadership across systems and organizations to develop a strategic climate for evidence-based practice implementation. *Annual Review of Public Health*, 35, 255–274.

Agency for Healthcare Research and Quality (AHRQ). (2018). Key driver 6: Nurture leadership and create a culture of continuous learning and evidence-based practice. https://www.ahrq.gov/evidencenow/tools/keydrivers/nuture-leadership.html.

Agency for Healthcare Research and Quality (AHRQ). (2022). *Developing and pilot testing change: Implementing the medication reconciliation process. Medications at transitions and clinical handoffs (MATCH) Toolkit for medication reconciliation.* Rockville, MD: Agency for Healthcare Research and Quality. https://www.ahrq.gov/patient-safety/setting/hospital/match/chapter-4.html.

Agency for Healthcare Research and Quality (AHRQ). (2023). High reliability. https://psnet.ahrq.gov/primer/high-reliability.

Brown, R. E. (2020). Empowering nurses with an online roadmap for evidence-based practice. *Journal of Hospital Librarianship*, 20(4), 309–322. https://doi-org.proxy.library.nyu.edu/10.1080/15323269.2020.1819748.

Brownson, R. C., Fielding, J. E., & Green, L. W. (2018). Building capacity for evidence-based public health: Reconciling the pulls of practice and the push of research. *Annual Review of Public Health*, 39, 27–53. https://doi.org/10.1146/annurev-publhealth-040617-014746.

Burton, C. (2017). The Absorptive and Receptove Capacity Scale (ARCS) [personal correspondence with Burton, C. J.

Center for Nursing. (2023). *Rona F. Lewin evidence-based practice Award*. Foundation of NYS Nurses, Inc. Center for Nursing at the Foundation of New York State Nurses, Inc. https://cfnny.org.

Charlton, P., Doucet, S., Azar, R., Nagel, D., Boulos, L., Luke, A., … Montelpare, W. (2019). The use of the environmental scan in health services delivery research: A scoping review protocol. *BMJ Open*, *11*(11), 1–12. https://doi.org/10.1136/bmjopen-2019-029805. e029805.

Charlton, P., Kean, T., Liu, R. H., Nagel, D. A., Azar, R., Doucet, S., et al. (2021). Use of environmental scans in health services delivery research: A scoping review. *BMJ Open*, *11*, 1–12. https://doi: 10.1136/bmjopen-2021-050284.

Clavijo-Chamorro, M. Z., Romero-Zarall, G., Gomez-Luque, A., Lopez-Espuela, F., Sanz-Martos, S., & Lopez-Medina, L. M. (2022). Leadership as a facilitator of evidence implementation by nurse managers: A metasynthesis. *Western Journal of Nursing Research*, *44*(6), 567–581.

Cowan, L., Hartjes, T., & Munro, S. (2019). A model of successful DNP and PhD collaboration. *Journal of the American Association of Nurse Practitioners*, *31*(2), 116–123. https://doi.org/10.1097/JXX.0000000000000105. PMID: 30589755.

Cygan, H., R., & Reed, M. (2019). DNP and PhD scholarship: Making the case for collaboration. *Journal of Professional Nursing*, *35*(5), 353–357. https://doi.org/10.1016/j.profnurs.2019.03.002. PMID: 31519337.

Dufour, É., Duhoux, A., & Bolduc, J. (2019). Measured and perceived effects of audit and feedback on nursing performance: A mixed methods systematic review protocol. *Systematic Reviews*, *8*(38), 1–6. https://doi.org/10.1186/s13643-019-0956-1.

Edmundson, A. (1999). Psychological safety and learning behavior in work teams. *Administrative Science Quarterly*, *44*(2), 350–383. http://www.jstor.org/stable/2666999. https://web.mit.edu/curhan/www/docs/Articles/15341_Readings/Group_Performance/Edmondson%20Psychological%20safety.pdf.

Ehrhart, M. G., Aarons, G. A., & Farahnak, L. R. (2014). Assessing the organizational context for EBP implementation: The development and validity testing of the Implementation Climate Scale (ICS). *Implementation Science*, *9*(1), 157.

Ehrhart, M. G., Aarons, G. A., & Farahnak, L. R. (2015). Going above and beyond for implementation: The development and validity testing of the Implementation Citizenship Behavior Scale (ICBS). *Implementation Science*, *10*, 65–54.

Elsheikh, R., Le Quang, L., Nguyen, N. Q. T., Van, P. T., Hung, D. T., Makram, A. M., et al. (2023). The role of nursing leadership in promoting evidence-based nursing practice. *Journal of Professional Nursing*, *48*, 93–98. ISSN 8755-7223.

Engel, J. E. (2018). Why does culture "Eat strategy for breakfast"? *Forbes*. https://www.forbes.com/sites/forbescoachescouncil/2018/11/20/why-does-culture-eat-strategy-for-breakfast/?sh=5fb307671e09.

Fontenot, N. M., Hamlin, S. K., Hooker, S. J., Vazquez, T., & Chen, H.-M. (2022). Physical assessment competencies for nurses: A quality improvement initiative. *Nursing Forum*, *57*(4), 710–716. https://doi.org/10.1111/nuf.12724.

Friesen, M. A., Brady, J. M., Milligan, R., & Christensen, P. (2017). Findings from a pilot study: Bringing evidence-based practice to the bedside. *Worldviews in Evidence-Based Nursing*, *14*(1), 22–34. https://doi:10.1111/wvn.12195.

Hendricks, J. M., & Cope, V. C. (2013). Generational diversity: What nurse managers need to know. *Journal of Advanced Nursing*, *69*(3), 717–725. https://doi-org.proxy.library.nyu.edu/10.1111/j.1365-2648.2012.06079.x.

Hilton, K., & Anderson, A. (2018). *Institute for healthcare improvement psychology of change framework to advance and sustain improvement. IHI white paper. Version 1.* Boston, MA: Institute for Healthcare Improvement. https://www.ihi.org/resources/white-papers/ihi-psychology-change-framework. [Accessed 23 June 2023].

Ivers, N., Jamtvedt, G., Flottorp, S., et al. (2012). Audit and feedback: Effects on professional practice and healthcare outcomes. *Cochrane Database of Systematic Reviews*, *6*, CD000259.

Jacobs, S. R., Weiner, B. J., & Bunger, A. C. (2014). Context matters: Measuring implementation climate among individuals and groups. *Implementation Science*, *9*(46), 1–14. https://doi.org/10.1186/1748-5908-9-46.

Jamtvedt, G., Flottorp, S., & Ivers, N. (2019). Audit and feedback as a quality strategy. In R. Busse, N. Klazinga, D. Panteli, et al. (Eds.), *Improving healthcare quality in Europe: Characteristics, effectiveness and implementation of different strategies* (p. 10). European Observatory on Health Systems and Policies (Health Policy Series, No. 53.). https://www.ncbi.nlm.nih.gov/books/NBK549284/.

Joy, H., Bielby, A., & Searle, R. (2015). A collaborative project to enhance efficiency through dressing change practice. *Journal of Wound Care*, *24*(312), 314–317.

Jun, J., Kovner, C. T., & Stimpfel, A. W. (2016). Barriers and facilitators of nurses' use of clinical practice guidelines: An integrative review. *International Journal of Nursing Studies*, *60*, 54–68.

Kapp, S. (2013). Successful implementation of clinical practice guidelines for pressure risk management in a home nursing setting. *Journal of Evaluation in Clinical Practice*, *19*, 895–901.

Kitson, A. L., Harvey, G., Gifford, W., Hunter, S. C., Kelly, J., Cummings, G. G., et al. (2021). Nursing leaders promote evidence-based practice implementation at point-of-care: A four-country exploratory study. *Journal of Advanced Nursing*, *77*(5), 2447–2457. https://doi.org/10.1111/jan.14773.

Kueny, A., Shever, L., Lehan Mackin, M., & Titler, M. G. (2015). Facilitating the implementation of evidence-based practice through contextual support for nursing leadership. *Journal of Healthcare Leadership, 7*, 29–39.

Laranjo, L., Arquel, A., Neves, A. L., Gallagher, A. M., Kaplan, R., Mortimer, N., et al. (2015). The influence of social networking sites on health behavior changes: A systematic review and meta-analysis. *Journal of the American Medical Informatics Association, 22*(1), 243–256. https://doi.org/10.1136/amiajnl-2014-002841.

Laures, E., & Fowler, C. (2020). The power of the pilot. *Journal of PeriAnesthesia Nursing, 35*(5), 543–547. https://doi.org/10.1016/j.jopan.2020.02.009.

Li, S.-A., Jeffs, L., Barwick, M., & Stevens, B. (2018). Organizational contextual features of evidence-based practices across healthcare settings. *Systematic Reviews, 7*(72), 1–19. https://doi.org/10.1186/s13643-018-0734-5.

Mathieson, A., Grande, G., & Luker, K. (2018). Strategies, facilitators and barriers to implementation of evidence-based practice in community nursing: a systematic mixed-studies review and qualitative synthesis. *Primary Health Care Research & Development, 20*(e6), 1–11. https://doi.org/10.1017/S1463423618000488.

May, C. R., Johnson, M., & Finch, T. (2016). Implementation, context and complexity. *Implementation Science, 11*(1), 141.

Melnyk, B. M., Gallagher-Ford, L., Long, L. E., & Fineout-Overholt, E. (2014). Practice competencies for practicing registered nurses and advanced practice nurses in real-world clinical settings: Proficiencies to improve healthcare quality, reliability, patient outcomes, and costs. *Worldviews on Evidence-Based Nursing, 11*(1), 5–15.

Meyers, D. (2024). Becoming an evidence-based organization: Five key components to consider. http://ebpsociety.org/blog/education/10=91-evidence-based-management-principles-processes. [Accessed 21 August 2023].

Powell, B. J., Fernandez, M. E., Williams, N. J., Aarons, G. A., Beidas, R. S., Lewis, C. C., et al. (2019). Enhancing the impact of implementation strategies in healthcare: A research agenda. *Frontiers in Public Health, 7*, 3. https://doi.org/10.3389/fpubh.2019.00003.

Powell, B. J., Waltz, T. J., Chinman, M. J., Damschroder, L. J., Smith, J. L., Matthieu, M. M., et al. (2015). A refined compilation of implementation strategies for implementing changes (ERIC) project. *Implementation Science, 10*(21), 1–14. https://doi.org/10.1186/s13012-015-0209-1.

Proctor, E., Powell, B., & McMillen, J. C. (2013). Implementation strategies: Recommendations for specifying and reporting. *Implementation Science, 8*(139), 1–11. https://doi.org/10.1186/1748-5908-8-139.

Pryse, Y., McDonald, A., & Schafer, J. (2014). Psychometric analysis of two new scales: The evidence-based-practice nursing leadership and work environment scales. *Worldviews on Evidence-Based Nursing, 11*(4), 240–247. https://doi.org/10.1111/wvn.12045.

Ramanadhan, S., Mahtani, S. L., Kirk, S., Lee, M., Weese, M., Mita, C., et al. (2022). Measuring capacity to use evidence-based interventions in community-based organizations: A comprehensive, scoping review. *Journal of Clinical Translational Science, 6*(1), e92, 1–15. https://doi.org/10.1017/cts.2022.426.

Reynolds, S. (2020). Using audit and feedback to improve compliance with evidence-based practices. *American Nurse, 15*(10), 16–19.

Richter, A., von Thiele Schwarz, U., Lornudd, C., Lundmark, R., Mosson, R., & Hasson, H. (2016). iLead—A transformational leadership intervention to train healthcare managers' implementation leadership. *Implementation Science, 11*(1), 108.

Shea, C. M., Jacobs, S. R., Esserman, D. A., Bruce, K., & Weiner, B. J. (2014). Organizational readiness for implementing change: A psychometric assessment of a new measure. *Implementation Science, 9*(7), 1–15. https://doi.org/10.1186/1748-5908-9-7.

Shuman, C. J., Ploutz-Snyder, R., & Titler, M. G. (2018). Development and testing of the NM EBP Competency Scale. *Western Journal of Nursing Research, 40*(2), 175–190.

Silver, S. A., Harel, Z., McQuillan, R., Weizman, A. V., Thomas, A., Chertow, G. M., et al. (2016). How to begin a quality improvement project. *Clinical Journal of the American Society of Nephrology, 11*(5), 893–900. https://doi.org/10.2215/CJN.11491015.

Squires, J. E., Graham, I. D., Hutchinson, A. M., et al. (2015). Identifying the domains of context important to implementation science: A study protocol. *Implementation Science, 10*(1), 135.

Stetler, C. B., Ritchie, J. A., Rycroft-Malone, J., & Charns, M. P. (2014). Leadership for evidence-based practice: Strategic and functional behaviors for institutionalizing EBP. *Worldviews Evidence-Based Nursing, 11*(4), 219–226. https://doi.org/10.1111/wvn.12044. Epub 2014 Jul 1.

Stetler, C. B., Ritchie, J. A., Rycroft-Malone, J., Schultz, A. A., & Charns, M. P. (2009). Institutionalizing evidence-based practice: An organizational case study using a model of strategic change. *Implementation Science, 4*(78), 1–19.

Stevanin, S., Palese, A., Bressan, V., Vehviläinen-Julkunen, K., & Kvist, T. (2018). Workplace-related generational characteristics of nurses: A mixed-method systematic review. *Journal of Advanced Nursing, 74*(6), 1245–1263. https://doi.org/10.1111/jan.13538.

Titler, M. G. (2010). Translation science and context. *Research and Theory for Nursing Practice, 24*(1), 35–55.

Titler, M. G., Conlon, P., Reynolds, M. A., et al. (2016). The effect of translating research into practice intervention to promote use of evidence-based fall prevention interventions in hospitalized adults: a prospective pre-post implementation study in the U.S. *Applied Nursing Research*, *31*, 52–59.

Titler, M. G., Herr, K., Brooks, J. M., et al. (2009). Translating research into practice intervention improves management of acute pain in older hip fracture patients. *Health Services Research*, *44*(1), 264–287.

Torres, E. M., Ehrhart, M. G., Beidas, R. S., Farahnak, L. R., Finn, N. K., & Aarons, G. A. (2018). Validation of the Implementation Leadership Scale (ILS) with supervisors self-ratings. *Community Mental Health Journal*, *54*(1), 49–53.

Vaajoki, A., Kvist, T., Kulmala, M., & Tervo-Heikkenen, T. T. (2023). Systematic education has a positive impact on nurses' evidence-based practice: Intervention study results. *Nurse Education Today*, *120* Article 105597.

Williams, N. J., Becker-Haimes, E. M., Schriger, S. H., & Beidas, R. S. (2022). Linking organizational climate for evidence-based practice implementation to observed clinician behaviors in patient encounters: A lagged analysis. *Implementation Science Communication*, *13*(1), 64. https://doi.org/10.1186/s43058/s43058-022-00309-v.

Williams, N. J., Wolk, C. B., Becker-Haimes, E. M., & Beisas, R. S. (2020). Testing a theory of strategic implementation leadership, implementation climate, and clinician's use of evidence-based practice. *Implementation Science*, *15*, 10. https://doi.org/10.1186/s13012-020-0970-7.

Yamada, J., Squires, J. E., Estabrooks, C. A., Victor, C., & Stevens, B. (2017). The role of organizational context in moderating the effect of research use on pain outcomes in hospitalized children: A cross sectional study. *BMC Health Services Research*, *17*(1), 68.

18

Patient-Centered Evidence-Based Practices

Amy Lynn Msowoya and Elizabeth Anna Fair

LEARNING OUTCOMES

After reading this chapter, you should be able to do the following:

- Apply principles of evidence-based practice that are relevant to patient-centered care.
- Discuss the evidence for, principles of, and assessment of shared decision making and patient activation.
- Compare patient activation and real-world strategies to activate patients across levels of health literacy and numeracy.
- Describe the value of evidence-based shared decision making.
- Identify strategies to engage individuals, families, and communities in the shared decision-making process.
- Identify real-world strategies to incorporate shared decision making into clinical practice.

KEY TERMS

Contextual barrier	Patient activation	Shared decision making
Health literacy	Patient engagement	Shared decision-making aid
Health numeracy	Patient portal	

This chapter provides a unique perspective on using innovative, evidence-based strategies to engage individuals, families, and communities as partners. The goal is to advance a self-care agenda, using patient activation, health literacy, shared decision-making aids, and virtual health modalities in a post-COVID health care landscape. Putting the patient, family, and community at the center of all care decisions is at the core of evidence-based practice (EBP). In the EBP process, it is essential to address patients' values, characteristics, and contextual factors that are important to them. If patients' concerns are ignored or not addressed, how will they be able to experience their best outcomes? Although this is important at the individual and family levels, it is also valuable when considering the larger scale health concerns of communities or organizations. For administrators, educators, and policy-leading clinicians, this topic is of vital importance because it impacts resource utilization, provider satisfaction, and clinical and financial outcomes for which they are accountable, such as satisfaction and readmission rates (Miller & Reihlen, 2023). By keeping EBP person centric, the filter for interpreting and applying evidence is the contextual world in which that patient lives to achieve health. Strategies to engage patients in their care are therefore applied with the awareness of how the evidence supports such strategies. Matching strategies for engagement that not only addresses individuals of all levels of health understanding but also targets how involved they want to (or believe they can) be in their care becomes necessary when behavior change or self-management is the goal. This chapter builds on the content in previous chapters that addresses the "doing" of EBP by emphasizing considerations for applying that evidence *with* individual patients and groups, not *to* them. Evidence-based strategies to address patient characteristics that impact understanding, ways to engage them deeper in their care, and the evidence-based methods that are necessary to create tools to promote working *with* patients are addressed in this chapter.

CLINICAL SCENARIO

Try to imagine the following scenario: You're a patient sitting in a hospital bed, and you've just been told that you have cancer. Provider A walks into your room, and after saying hello, starts rattling off a description of the latest treatment options available for your condition. You can only comprehend the word "cancer," yet this provider keeps talking at you. Too afraid to ask questions of someone you perceive as much smarter than yourself, you sit there, silently overwhelmed by the amount of information being discussed, and feel even more out of control of your situation and health as the conversation ends and Provider A asks you to make a choice as to which treatment you want to undertake. Do you think this doesn't happen? Guess again.

Let's look at an alternative approach to this same situation. You're there, sitting in your hospital bed, and Provider B has just told you that you have cancer and asks what is most important to you with regard to your future health. The provider asks if you have any questions right now and recommends that you reach out to anyone you want to share this news with before having to make a treatment decision. Provider B also leaves you with a piece of paper called a shared decision-making aid, with a link to your patient portal website, and tells you that the clinical team will be available to answer any questions you may have to help you make a decision about treatment when you're ready.

Which provider would you feel has *you* at the center of their mindset? Odds are you'd say Provider B because that person has just shown you an example of person-centered care. Patient centricity and involvement in healthcare guides clinicians to provide evidence-based care based on outcomes that patients and their families feel matter. In giving up their own centricity, providers can feel more professionally fulfilled by managing patient health instead of patient flow.

> **TIP**
>
> Effective communication by interprofessional teams is an essential feature of providing high-quality patient-centered care. The Interprofessional Education Collaborative (IPEC) Competencies stress the importance of effective communication between and among health professionals as a key element of engaging patients, families, and communities as partners in achieving their health care goals (see https://www.ipecollaborative.org/ipec-core-competencies for further details).

PATIENT ENGAGEMENT AND EMPOWERMENT THROUGH SHARED DECISION MAKING

In the current climate of direct-to-consumer advertising and the mainstay of health promotion campaigns telling patients to "ask your provider" about potential illnesses and treatments, patients are encouraged and, in some respects, expected to fully understand their treatment options and evaluate their own preferences and beliefs to make informed decisions and truly engage in their health decision making (Tietbohl & Bergen, 2022). This is a task easier said than done. Emotional forces, lack of knowledge, organizational constraints, autonomy, family forces, racial and cultural beliefs, among other factors, all can influence patient decision making (Street et al., 2017). See Chapter 28 for a further in-depth discussion of the importance of acknowledging and identifying factors of diversity, equity, and inclusion in healthcare and EBP. This puts health care providers in a difficult position, namely how to provide guidance and direction for questioning patients without exercising paternalistic control, in a way that makes decisions *with* patients instead of *for* them. This opens the door for EBPs to develop, which empower patients through patient engagement and shared decision making.

Patient engagement is an umbrella term for the cultural change aimed at actively involving patients in their care and supporting them on an informational, emotional, and behavioral level (Bonetti et al., 2022). **Shared decision making** is defined as the process by which patients and clinicians partner to make informed health decisions that benefit the patient. It encourages patients to evaluate their own knowledge and beliefs about treatment options before talking to their providers (Rose et al., 2016). Similarly, it requires providers to clarify patient values and concerns as they talk *with* their patients, not simply *to* them. This fosters effective, open dialogue between the patient and provider and keeps the focus on the patient. The risk of not engaging the patient is too great, since it puts clinicians at risk of making a "silent misdiagnosis" by not addressing a patient's preferences for care (Street et al., 2017). Given that patients must implement many health care decisions and deal with the financial, emotional, and quality of life implications of those decisions on their own (such as whether to fill prescriptions, attend follow-up visits, or monitor blood pressures), shared decision making between the patient and provider should be the norm rather than the exception. Although barriers do exist to implementing shared decision making, the information presented here is intended to reduce the impact of those barriers and support you in implementing patient-centered EBPs in real time within the constraints of actual clinical practice. This industry-wide shift toward shared decision making between the provider and patient has started the "era of participatory medicine," and nursing professionals are in a strategic role to promote these efforts because the concept of relationship-based care has always been a cornerstone of the nursing care paradigm (Bonetti et al., 2022).

EVIDENCE TO SUPPORT SHARED DECISION MAKING

Shared decision making gained traction in the health care industry with shifts in payment models from a fee-for-service payment structure to a pay-for-performance structure based on value (Lu et al., 2022). In the emerging value-based delivery system, there is increased focus on providing quality care at lower cost for populations. Proper utilization of shared decision-making interventions has the potential to decrease overall health care costs while increasing the quality of healthcare delivered and promoting better health (Institute for Healthcare Improvement (IHI), 2023). When the U.S. Congress authorized creation of the Patient-Centered Outcomes Research Institute (PCORI), a nongovernmental, nonprofit, independent organization in 2010, its mission was to sponsor high-quality research that addressed the questions that concerned stakeholders (e.g., patients, caregivers, clinicians, policy makers). Quickly, the goal of helping consumers make informed health decisions was followed by funding streams to promote the study of methods, instrumentation, and decision-making models. The current national priorities for research within this institute focus on increasing the evidence for existing interventions and emerging innovations in health, enhancing infrastructure to accelerate patient-centered outcomes research, advancing the science of dissemination, implementation and health communication, achieving health equity, and accelerating progress toward an integrated learning health system (PCORI, 2022).

Although some organizations state that value is determined through subjective goals stated by the patient, others argue that solid research must support the value of an intervention for use in a clinical situation. Patient-centered shared decision making bridges these two extremes by including patients as partners so that the best evidence-based treatment plans for their lifestyles and clinical situations is created *with* them and not *for* them. Recently, the PCORI has been awarded nearly $4 billion in funding for more than 2,000 research studies and related projects, with a total of 483 of these studies being complete and published. This work demonstrated that while the research interest in shared decision making and patient empowerment and engagement is great, the need for nursing and other health care professionals to partner with patients to complete these studies and expand the available body of literature is just as great.

SHARED DECISION-MAKING AIDS

Many Americans are familiar with components of the Patient Protection and Affordable Care Act (ACA) of 2010, such as the creation of health insurance exchanges, but few realize the benefit of some of the more minor provisions. One such provision that was explicitly written into the ACA was the promotion of shared decision making and the use of patient decision support interventions such as decision aids to improve patient knowledge (Lu et al., 2022; Alston et al., 2014). **Shared decision-making aids** are defined as evidence-based documents or tools that portray health care options; give information about risks, benefits, and outcomes for the options; assist patients in clarifying their values; and incorporate clinical judgment and counseling (Kijewski, 2016). These are intended to be used to complement, rather than completely replace, the counseling and education provided by nursing and health care professionals (LeRouge et al., 2021). A variety of decision-making tools are available to primary care clinicians in both online and print formats, such as the exemplar discussed in the patient scenario in this chapter. Unfortunately, even after proof of the efficacy of such tools has been shown, few clinicians and patients utilize existing decision-making tools such as patient decision aids, primarily citing a lack of access to these resources (Alston et al., 2014). More than 500 evidence-based decision aids are currently available on the internet, but they are scattered across dozens of websites and not well advertised. The Tip box provides examples of free-to-use decision aids that may be accessed online.

> **TIP**
>
> **Shared Decision-Making Aids Resources**
>
> - Wiser Choices Program at the Knowledge and Evaluation Research Unit at Mayo Clinic: https://carethatfits.org/tools/
> - Dartmouth Health Decision Making Resources for Patients: https://www.dartmouth-hitchcock.org/decision-making-help/patient-resources
> - Dartmouth Health Decision Making Resources for Healthcare Professionals: https://www.dartmouth-hitchcock.org/decision-making-help/professional-resources
> - Ottawa Hospital Research Institute: https://decisionaid.ohri.ca/index.html
> - Choosing Wisely: https://www.choosingwisely.org/

EVIDENCE-BASED METHODS TO DEVELOP PATIENT ENGAGEMENT TOOLS

One example of a method used to create an evidence-based tool for patient engagement is Oral Health Patient Facts (see Exemplar). The Oral Health Nursing Education and Practice (OHNEP) Program and the American College of Physicians (ACP) collaborated on this evidence-based project to develop a set of four user-friendly oral health literacy handouts: Oral Health and HPV; Oral Health and You; Oral Health and Older Adults; and Oral Health and Diabetes. To create and validate these tools, the EBP project team conducted a search and critical appraisal of the literature to find the best available evidence that provided a base for developing the content. Consumer focus groups were conducted for each of the target populations to identify their knowledge gaps and concerns. Based on the literature review and qualitative data from the focus groups, drafts of the four Oral Health Patient Facts handouts were developed in English and Spanish and written at a sixth-grade reading level. Handouts were reviewed by an interprofessional panel of health professional judges with content and clinical expertise in each of the target areas. Once the content validity was established, the Oral Health Patient Facts handouts were reviewed by another panel of consumers for face validity, readability, and relevance to their health issues. Feedback from content judges and consumer panelists was used by the EBP team to revise the drafts and finalize the Oral Health Patient Facts for pilot testing. The pilot study included a sample of primary care clinicians, physicians, nurse practitioners, and physician assistants who introduced the health literacy handouts to patients in their primary care settings. They used each with the appropriate patient populations to test their comfort as professionals using the Oral Health Patient Facts to engage patients in promoting shared decision making and effective self-management. Qualitative data from the pilot study showed that the tools were viewed positively. Targeted dissemination was done via a press release, email blasts, and posting on the ACP and OHNEP websites.

> **TIP**
>
> **Oral Health Patients Facts**
>
> Oral Health Patient Facts, an evidence-based oral health literacy product, was developed to address a clinical problem (see Chapter 5 for further information on developing compelling clinical questions). Clinicians had difficulty integrating oral health promotion into overall healthcare for their primary care patients. There was a lack of consumer-friendly, evidence-based oral health literacy products targeting specific patient populations at high risk for oral health comorbidities. For example, preteens, adolescents, and young adults not yet or currently sexually active often do not realize that if they contract human papillomavirus (HPV), they are at risk for oropharyngeal cancer. Immunization protects this population and decreases risk of HPV and its negative sequelae, oral cancer. Another population, those with type 2 diabetes, is at high risk for periodontal disease with potential infection and tooth loss. Effective glycemic control and education about the importance of oral hygiene in primary care practices is significantly correlated with decreasing risk for periodontal disease. Similarly, collaboration with and referral to dental colleagues for treatment of gum disease is associated with improvement of glycemic status. More information and direct download of the tools are available at https://nursing.nyu.edu/w/ohnep.

PATIENT ACTIVATION

To truly implement patient-centered EBPs, one must "meet patients where they are," tailoring strategies that address their strengths and challenges. **Patient activation** is defined as the knowledge, confidence, and skills that a patient possesses and is willing to use to make decisions about health. By assessing level of patient activation, a clinician can better understand the knowledge, confidence, and skill level patients have to be able to effectively engage in shared decision making about their care (Hibbard, 2016; Al Juffali et al., 2022). Activation is a dynamic state, not a static one, meaning that patients can progress and regress between levels of activation at various points in their lives. Patient expectations for involvement in decision making vary based on clinical setting and patient characteristics, and a good provider needs to be able to tailor shared decision-making interventions based on a patient's activation level and the type of support individuals at that activation level need.

The most common tool used to assess a patient's activation level is the Patient Activation Measure (PAM). First developed in 2005, the PAM is a validated assessment tool that objectively measures an individual's mindset about managing their own health using a 13-item scale (Hibbard, 2016; Dammery et al., 2023). The literature supports that the PAM score is a predictor of many health behaviors, such as costly service utilization of the emergency department, adherence to medication regimens, health maintenance behaviors, and self-management of chronic conditions (Al Juffali et al., 2022; Cohen, 2017; Hibbard, 2016). Individuals are classified by Levels 1 to 4. Level 1 identifies low-activated individuals, and Level 4 identifies the most activated patients. See Fig. 18.1 for a further description of the levels of patient activation described in the PAM.

Over time, it has been shown that highly activated individuals (PAM Levels 3 and 4) are more likely to seek and use information to be advocates for their own health (Hibbard, 2016). They are also more likely to participate in wellness activities like regular exercise, maintaining a healthy diet, and adhering to medical regimens because they consider themselves partners in their own health promotion. Individuals with lower PAM scores (Levels 1 and 2) are more likely to have low confidence in their ability to self-manage and tend to take a more passive approach to their health (Hibbard, 2016). PAM Level 1 and 2 patients are less likely to embrace patient support resources even when offered, and they are more likely to be overwhelmed by stressful situations due to limited problem-solving agility. It's important to remember that individuals can move between levels depending on clinical context, life situations, and efforts made to engage and empower them by the clinical team (McCormack

Level 1	Level 2	Level 3	Level 4
Disengaged and overwhelmed	**Becoming aware, but still struggling**	**Taking action**	**Maintaining behaviors and pushing further**
Individuals are passive and lack confidence. Knowledge is low, goal-orientation is weak, and adherence is poor. Their perspective: "My doctor is in charge of my health."	Individuals have some knowledge, but large gaps remain. They believe health is largely out of their control, but can set simple goals. Their perspective: "I could be doing more."	Individuals have the key facts and are building self-management skills. They strive for best practice behaviors, and are goal-oriented. Their perspective: "I'm part of my health care team."	Individuals have adopted new behaviors, but may struggle in times of stress or change. Maintaining a healthy lifestyle is a key focus. Their perspective: "I'm my own advocate."

Increasing Levels of Activation

©2018 Insignia Health. Patient Activation Measure® (PAM®) Survey Levels. All rights reserved.

Fig. 18.1 Patient Characteristics Based On and Description of Patient Activation Measure (PAM) Scores. (Adapted from Insignia Health. (2016). Patient Activation Measure (PAM) Survey Levels. http://www.insigniahealth.com/products/pam-survey.)

et al., 2016). It has been shown that even a single point increase in PAM score leads to a 2% to 3% improvement in overall health outcomes and a decrease in use of health services (Dammery et al., 2023), which again supports the IHI Quadruple Aim goals of better care, better health, and lower costs delivered by a satisfied health care workforce.

HEALTH LITERACY AND NUMERACY

Individuals with limited activation in their own care (PAM Level 1 and 2) may struggle more to participate in care decisions because they cannot comprehend or use the information being discussed, not because they have a lack of desire to do so. Health literacy is defined as an individual's ability to access, interpret, and understand *qualitative* data about their health (i.e., delivered without numbers, typically as words or pictures). Conversely, health numeracy is defined as an individual's ability to access, interpret, and understand *quantitative* data about their health (i.e., delivered with numbers or portraying numbers). Clinicians can gain insight into an individual's problem-solving ability and potential for activation by assessing the person's health literacy and health numeracy levels (Schulz et al., 2022). Health literacy and numeracy, while related, are not interchangeable concepts. When assessing an individual's health *literacy* level, one evaluates a person's ability to access, interpret, and understand qualitative data (i.e., written text) to improve health. Individuals with "adequate" health literacy can comprehend and use health information provided in written text form, including electronic media, when making health decisions. Those with "inadequate" health literacy have difficulty understanding and thereby acting on this health information, leading to an increase in the potential for health disparities and poorer health outcomes (McAnally & Hagger, 2023).

Much health information is delivered as numbers (e.g., prescription dosing recommendations, appropriate laboratory values, or target carbohydrate limits for a person with diabetes). Health *numeracy* becomes important when information is given in nontext formats such as graphs, tables, or raw numbers. Health numeracy adequacy and mathematical understanding of statistical data became all the more important during the COVID-19 pandemic, when people across the globe were exposed to large amounts of statistical data and mathematical concepts like "flattening the curve," "exponential growth," and "false negative rates" for the first time en masse (Lau et al., 2022). Box 18.1 highlights assessment of health literacy and health numeracy.

To judge health literacy and numeracy objectively, the Organization for Economic Cooperation and Development created the Program for the International Assessment of Adult Competencies (PIAAC) survey with the goal of developing a tool to assess and compare the basic literacy and numeracy skills of individuals across the globe (Rampey et al., 2016). Individuals in 24 countries participated in 2011–2012 (round 1), 9 additional countries participated in 2014–2015 (round 2), and 5 additional countries participated in 2017–2018 (round 3) (Rampey et al., 2019). The PIAAC survey built and expanded on previous international adult assessments such as the International Adult Literacy Survey and the Adult Literacy and Life Skills Survey (Rampey et al., 2016). The United States participated in all three rounds of data collection during the initial field test of the PIAAC survey. Cycle II of the PIAAC survey began in 2022, with 31 countries participating in the first round of data collection utilizing a revised survey. Results from the first two rounds of data analysis (results are combined into 2012/2014 and 2017 scoring for the U.S. data sets) offer a sobering picture of the health literacy and numeracy of the average American adult.

Participants are scored in the PIAAC survey with "proficiency levels" of 1 to 5, with "below Level 1" as the lowest level of problem solving/proficiency, and "Level 5" as the highest. Between both the 2012/2014 and 2017 data collections, there was no significant changes in the

---

BOX 18.1 Assessing Health Literacy and Health Numeracy

Clinicians can gain insight into an individual's problem-solving ability and potential for activation by assessing his or her **health literacy** and **health numeracy** levels. Health literacy and numeracy, while related, are not interchangeable concepts.
- When assessing an individual's health *literacy* level, a clinician is looking at that person's ability to access, interpret, and understand qualitative data (i.e., written text) to improve health.
- Health *numeracy* is defined as an individual's ability to access, interpret, and understand quantitative data (i.e., nontext formats, raw numbers, computational data, graphs, tables).

percentages of adults performing at each proficiency level, so the 2017 data will be used as representative of the average American population. The percentages of adults performing at the lowest levels (Level 1 or below) were 19% in health literacy, 29% in health numeracy, and 24% in digital problem solving. The percentages performing at the highest levels (Level 3 or above in literacy and numeracy and Level 2 or above in digital problem solving) in 2017 were 48% in literacy, 37% in numeracy, and 38% in digital problem solving (Rampey et al., 2019). Sadly, the percentage of U.S. adults reporting "fair" or "poor" health increased from 15% to 17% between 2012/2014 and 2017, and those reporting "excellent" or "very good" health decreased from 57% to 54% (Rampey et al., 2019), illuminating the urgent need for nursing and health care professionals to increase their efforts at improving health literacy and numeracy rates to support better health outcomes in the American population. (See Figs. 18.2 and 18.3 for a more detailed breakdown of the health literacy and numeracy proficiency levels of adults in the United States, respectively.)

STRATEGIES TO IMPROVE HEALTH LITERACY AND NUMERACY

Even adults with limited skills can increase engagement and have better health outcomes if their environment supports the health literacy and numeracy skills that they *do* have. Individuals may be skilled in one, both, or neither of these areas, and different strategies may need to be implemented to support a person across numerous levels of influence. Clinicians and patients can both affect change at the individual, interpersonal, organizational, community, and macro levels of influence (Cohen, 2017). Strategies to address barriers across levels of health literacy and engagement are described in Table 18.1 along with effective and evidence-based exemplars.

At the individual level, factors such as a lack of knowledge of health information and a low value placed on engagement can make it difficult to improve health literacy or numeracy. Using plain language, with no medical jargon, when communicating and offering personalized health education sessions is one type of intervention to address these challenges (McCormack et al., 2016). One way of addressing individuals with low health numeracy is to provide infographics that break down numbers and display them as pictures. Examples can be found in the March of Dimes campaign "Healthy Babies Are Worth the Wait," which educates the public about preventing premature birth (see https://www.marchofdimes.org/glue/images/HBWW-Infographic.jpg). Interpersonal barriers such as poor communication skills and lack of social support can be addressed with teach-back methods and patient and family support groups. One example of a family support resource is the network of 30 advocacy groups affiliated with the Preemie Parent Alliance (https://nicuparentnetwork.org/header-test/). They offer evidence-based education, in-person peer support, and navigation help during transitions when fragile infants are discharged from neonatal intensive care units. Another example is provided by an advocacy group to end rare diseases that affect fragile infants such as necrotizing enterocolitis (NEC), one of the 10 leading causes of infant death in the United States

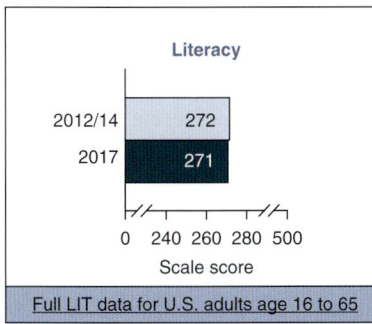
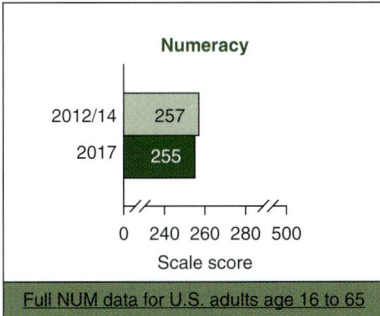
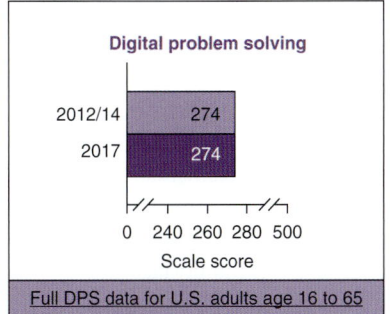

NOTE: LIT = Literacy. NUM = Numeracy. DPS = Digital problem solving. The PIAAC literacy, numeracy, and digital problem solving scales range from 0 to 500. Some apparent differences between estimates may not be statistically significant. Only statistically significant differences between years are marked with an asterisk. Users may explore other differences via the full data links and using the International Data Explorer tools.

Fig. 18.2 Average Scores on PIAAC Literacy, Numeracy, and Digital Problem Solving for U.S. Adults Age 16 to 65: 2012/2014 and 2017. (From Rampey et al., 2019.)

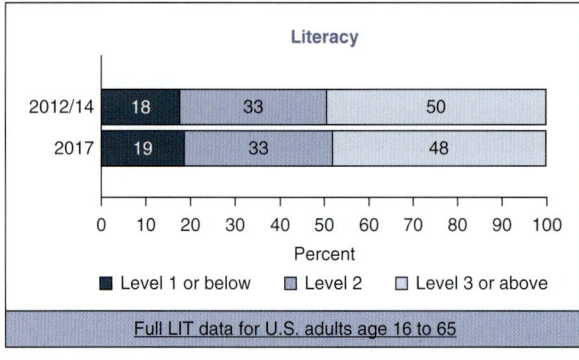
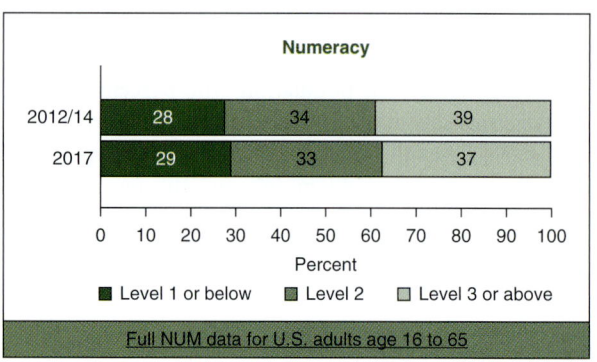
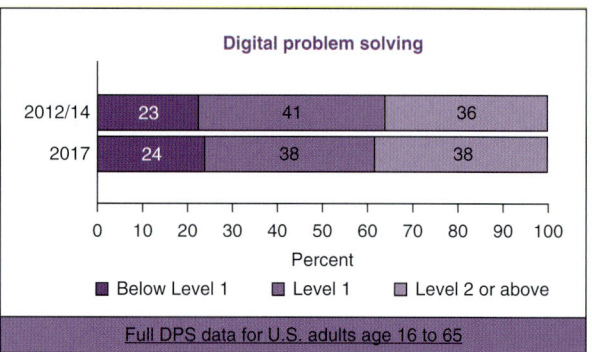

NOTE: LIT = Literacy. NUM = Numeracy. DPS = Digital problem solving. Detail may not sum to totals because of rounding. Only statistically significant differences between years are marked with an asterisk. Users may explore other differences via the full data links and using the International Data Explorer tools. In literacy and numeracy, higher, middle, and lower performance are denoted by "Level 3 or above," "Level 2," and "Level 1 or below," respectively. In digital problem solving, these are denoted by "Level 2 or above," "Level 1," and "Below level 1."

Fig. 18.3 Percentage Distribution of U.S. Adults Age 16 to 65 at Selected Levels of Proficiency on PIAAC Literacy, Numeracy, and Digital Problem Solving: 2012/2014 and 2017. (From Rampey et al., 2019.)

(www.necsociety.org, https://babyloss-awareness.org/organisations/). Groups that are organized around and promote EBPs can vet their information by engaging with clinical and research advisory board members, as is the case with the NEC Society. Table 18.2 provides examples of multilevel strategies to improve health literacy and numeracy.

The physical layout of a building and signage, although seemingly unimportant, can have a great effect on the organizational factors of system integration and infrastructure planning and implementation to support health outcomes. Social marketing campaigns can support integration of public health concerns and health care systems when addressing community factors. Finally, macroenvironmental initiatives address adjustments that need to be made in public policy and legal regulations to support improved health literacy and numeracy, such as ongoing health care reforms through the Centers for Medicare and Medicaid Services (Lu et al., 2022; Cohen, 2017; Rathert et al., 2016).

MOVING FROM PATIENT-CENTERED TO PERSON-CENTERED CARE AS AN EDUCATIONAL STANDARD

Patient-centered care can be implemented by developing patient education handouts, tools, and protocols, evaluating commercial education resources such as brochures, pamphlets, books, audio, videos, resource aids, and internet materials, and selecting instructional materials appropriate for the patient's readiness to learn and preferred media delivery (Bastable, 2017). Effective patient education focuses on the concepts of "patient-centered" and "patient engagement." Different generations of both patients and providers may have different preferred learning styles and resource interaction. Older generations may engage more easily with in-person education and physical resources while younger generations may prefer online resources that can be quickly accessed at their convenience with easy clicks to the

TABLE 18.1 Barriers Against and Strategies for Patient Engagement

Barriers to Engagement	Strategies That Address Engagement Barrier
Low health literacy or health numeracy	• Ask patients what they understand about their health. • Educational materials should be understandable at the sixth-grade reading level. • Ask patients to "teach back" what you have taught them. • Ensure decision aids and shared decision-making tools have been shown to be effective in individuals with limited health literacy or numeracy.
Language	• Communicate via certified medical interpreters. • Ensure that educational materials in the patient's own language convey the appropriate meaning after translation.
Values and cultural beliefs	• Ask patients what role they want to play in decision making. If they don't decide or don't want to decide, work with family and those who are perceived to decide to make sure they all understand the health education or condition. • Encourage patients to express their values and cultural beliefs and ask questions. • Education with evaluation in cross-cultural care. • Involve family.
Time constraints	• Include patient-reported outcomes and other measures of engagement in surveys they complete when arriving at the office. • Provide time, opportunity, and safe places for patients to reflect on information and ask questions. • Reduce the need for quick decisions when possible. • Provide evidence-based decision aids and educational materials for them to take home and consider before deciding.
Clinical workflow	• Embed decision aids into the patient portal. • Use electronic patient portals to collect information before appointments. • Embed decision guidance for clinicians in their clinical workflow to assist patients in making decisions and learning about their health. • Engage patients after diagnosis, prognosis, and available treatment options have been clarified by the clinical team.
Organizational priority	• Payment models that incentivize shared decision making. • Leadership commitment to patient engagement.

Adapted from Blumenthal-Barby, 2016, p. 15.

desired information (American Association of Colleges of Nursing, 2021a).

As promoted in The Essentials: Core Competencies for Professional Nursing Education, patient-centered care is a growing educational standard in higher education, informal learning, professional development, community engagement, and in the design of learning technologies to transform growing academic–practice partnerships and delivery expectations of quality care (American Association of Colleges of Nursing, 2021). This implies providers meet the patient at their level, not the preferred level of the provider. Moving from a focus on visit-based assessments of health needs to recognizing the unique challenges and problems that face an individual over the lifespan facilitates a transition in the clinician from providing patient-centered care to person-centered care (Starfield, 2011). This is especially important in care environments like primary care, where person-focused, not disease-focused, care is provided over a longer period of time.

Health care providers should use EBP to inform their clinical decision making while also considering the unique needs and preferences of individual patients and involving patients in their own care (Engle et al., 2021). Effective strategies include using plain language and focusing on behaviors and actions, not just knowledge, but best practice combines all these elements (Bastable, 2017).

TABLE 18.2 Multilevel Strategies to Improve Health Literacy and Numeracy

Level of Influence	Influential Factors	Interventions to Address Limitations	Exemplars
Individual	Health-related knowledge; attitudes/health beliefs; values/preferences for levels of engagement; health literacy skills	• Use of plain language, best practices, and clear communication in written communications • Data visualization to communicate health information (infographics) • Clarify values by asking, "What are you concerned about today?"	U.S. "Safe Sleep" campaign to prevent Sudden Infant Death Syndrome (SIDS) uses the "A-B-C" metaphor to remind all caregivers how to prevent SIDS when they put a baby to sleep: A = alone B = [on the] back C = [in a] crib
Interpersonal	Promote communication skills and leverage social support	• Patient-centered communication • Active listening and teach back • Group health visits, patient and family support groups • Community health workers • Shared decision making	March of Dimes promotes group prenatal care courses to prevent premature birth, especially in states and populations with high premature birth rates. The Mayo Clinic has a well-validated, evidence-based suite of decision aids that are freely available to support shared decision making on topics such as selecting medications for diabetes, hypertension, and cancer treatment.
Organizational	Infrastructure planning and implementation; system integration and coordination	• Staff training, workforce enhancement • Team-based care with care coordination • Physical environment, layout, and signage • Electronic health records that integrate decision support into patient education or shared decision making • Pay-for-performance systems that value prevention and support self-management	Intermountain Healthcare in Utah links patient portals to the electronic and billing systems making patient information visible in one place. Kaiser Healthcare locates all services a patient will need in one place to support ease of access. The National Health Service in the United Kingdom is adapting the PAM to make care more patient centered and holistic. Based on level of activation, patients are enrolled in different intensities of coaching for prevention and disease management.
Community	Community-based programs; integration of public health and health care systems	• Leverage virtual and physical social networks using targeted marketing campaigns • E-health communication (i.e., applications, patient portals) • Community-based participatory research to adapt patient engagement approach to meet the needs of the target community	MedlinePlus is hosted and curated by the National Library of Medicine to provide evidence-based health information to consumers on a wide variety of topics. Regional library affiliates of the National Library of Medicine are working together to teach professional and lay people about available resources and how to use them.
Macro	Public policy; regulation; legal regulations and initiatives; accountability; reliance on evidence-based policies	• National legislation to promote reimbursement models for Medicare and Medicaid that value quality of care, outcomes, and population-based care. Clinical guidelines are vetted by professional organizations and include specific recommendations.	The Choosing Wisely campaign engages clinicians and consumers to select the best evidence-supported treatments and avoid those that have been shown to be harmful or ineffective. A clearinghouse of active guidelines is available at https://www.cdc.gov/mmwr/volumes/71/su/su7101a1.htm.

PAM, Patient Activation Measure.
Adapted from McCormack et al., 2016, p. 10.

PATIENT-CENTERED CARE STRATEGIES FOR CLINICAL PRACTICE

Healthcare in the United States today is marked by constant evolution and increasing complexity. No longer is it acceptable to say, "That's how we've always done it." Health care teams are engaged in EBP and quality improvement initiatives that consistently seek improved methods of caring for patients and optimizing health outcomes. Using a patient activation lens, we as clinicians need to be able to look at an intervention and ask ourselves:

- Who is the intervention reaching?
- Who is the intervention helping?
- What is the evidence base for this intervention for this population?

The answers to these questions allow practitioners to remain patient centered, but often unveil barriers that exist and must be addressed before an engagement strategy can be implemented in clinical practice. Barriers to patient engagement are multifactorial in nature, so strategies to overcome them should address this complexity (Sprague Martinez et al., 2018; Rose et al., 2016). For further details on these barriers and strategies to address them, see Table 18.1.

One provider-patient–focused strategy that can support person-centered care and patient engagement by moving away from limiting interactions and education to only the standard office visit is the use of a patient portal (see Chapter 24). **Patient portals** are web-based platforms that compile various evidence-based resources for patient engagement, such as decision-making aids, educational materials, and communication applications. They are typically connected to the electronic health record (EHR) used by providers to communicate health care data to the patient. They are designed to promote patient engagement and self-care. Patient portals can be tailored to the individual needs of a clinical setting and patient population (Sergeeva, 2023; Kijewski, 2016). Clinics and hospitals may choose to design a patient portal companion website or can contract for standalone portal access. EHRs also may include a patient portal to provide secure messaging and educational information. Incorporating patient portal access allows primary care practices to achieve patient engagement core measures that are required to meet Stage 2 of Meaningful Use for implementing EHRs (Mcbride & Tietze, 2016; Blumenthal & Tavenner, 2010). Omitting these features can place clinicians at risk for not meeting benchmarks in the Merit-Based Incentive Payment System, a Centers for Medicare and Medicaid Services initiative that became mandatory in early 2017. Additional virtualist skills will be required by interprofessional clinical teams as they increasingly communicate with patients in non–face-to-face encounters via telehealth modalities. Fickenscher and colleagues (2018) remind us about the importance of effective collaboration and information sharing across the professions that will require a team model of care delivery.

INDIVIDUAL BARRIERS AGAINST PATIENT-CENTERED CARE

Individual barriers are those that pertain to the intrinsic characteristics and values of the patient or provider. These barriers tie closely to personal traits that determine an individual's activation level, as discussed earlier in this chapter. Barriers such as low health literacy and lack of education can be countered by clinicians with direct patient–provider interactions (Obaremi & Olatokun, 2021; McCormack et al., 2016; Smith et al., 2015). Asking patients what they already know and understand and using teach-back methods to assess that understanding allows patients and providers to enter conversations with a more equal knowledge base. Language barriers can be mitigated by using trained interpreters and ensuring that materials are available in a patient's language of preference. Translation also can occur over the phone or be mediated with smartphone- or tablet-based applications such as *MediBabble* (NiteFloat, Inc, San Francisco, CA). Training in cross-cultural care to ensure that providers understand a patient's cultural values and encouraging patients to express those values can illuminate many otherwise missed value discussions (Okere, 2022; Hibbard, 2016). (See Chapter 28: Diversity, Equity, and Inclusion for further information and discussion.)

CONTEXTUAL BARRIERS AGAINST PERSON-CENTERED CARE

Contextual barriers are defined as challenges in the environment, health care system, clinical workflow, administrative, and patient care contexts that make engagement more difficult to accomplish (Baumann et al., 2022; Blumenthal-Barby, 2016). These barriers are often more related to system constraints and, as such, require more resources to resolve them than the individual patient and provider. One barrier cited repeatedly in the literature is a lack of time for patient–provider interactions (Blumenthal-Barby, 2016; Cohen, 2017). Providing adequate time and safe places for patients to reflect on information, such as the time that Provider B gave our patient in the opening chapter scenario, is vital to ensuring that a patient feels like a valued partner in the clinical team. Clinical workflow can be a barrier to patient engagement, if we insist that patients make quick clinical decisions and we don't engage patients throughout the clinical progression, from diagnosis and prognosis to treatment options. Finally, institutional attitudes such as payment models that support shared decision-making interventions can encourage a continued culture of person-centered care (Kissam et al., 2019; Blumenthal-Barby, 2016).

CHALLENGES TO PATIENT-CENTERED CARE IN A POST-COVID WORLD

Major world events can define a generation and shared experiences can drastically transform expectations of the health care delivery system. The COVID pandemic has challenged nearly everything about health care delivery, including the needs and experiences of patients and families to the expectations of delivery methods, communication, education, and technology associated with patient care; although the how of delivery has changed, the timeless and universal commitment to patient-centered care should not (Engle et al., 2021).

The pandemic has heightened the need for holistically approaching both team-based care and patient-centered care while highlighting the pivotal role of nurses in improving health care equity and how their well-being affects the quality, safety, and cost of the services and systems of care (Hassmiller & Wakefield, 2022). When the needs of the providers are well taken care of, they are better equipped to respond well to patient needs.

Data drives decisions. Technology adoption has been the primary vehicle connecting the provider and empowering the patient ownership over their delivery of care. COVID initiated an accelerated need to identify and interpret patient and provider needs along with the implementation of evidence-based strategies to holistically produce quality care and allocate resources amid a changing landscape of service delivery requirements. The creation, assembly, and utilization of artificial intelligence (AI) as seen in the COVID-19 Open Research Dataset (CORD-19) allowed researchers and providers to collaborate and leverage large, shared data sets used to identify and interpret needs, relationships, and opportunities of care influencing resource allocation and decision making while protecting patient privacy (Zou & Li, 2022).

As a result of these changes, there is widespread adoption of telemedicine, and the implementation of technologies that support remote patient monitoring, virtual and in-home services, and customized treatment plans (Engle et al., 2021). Examples of the technological experience may include digital test results, online appointments and check-ins, fillable patient forms, mobile apps for health data, patient portals for communication with providers, email and text reminders or notifications, delivery of care through audio or video, online prescription ordering, and the technology-based provider–patient interactions and resources continue to evolve. (See Chapter 24: Informatics for additional information and challenges that must be assessed when utilizing health technologies.)

However, not all patients and providers fully embrace these technological changes. Technological adoption spans five stages: awareness, interest, evaluation, trial, and adoption. Barriers to reaching adoption are significant and often connected to embarrassment, feeling overwhelmed, lack of time to learn and implement something new, and combating preestablished habits and behaviors of receiving care. Thus, the provider is presented with a unique challenge to ensure patients not only have access to the latest and greatest implementation of information, plans, and resources, but also know how to access, navigate, and use them for personal ongoing quality care.

The COVID-19 pandemic revealed gaps, identified opportunities, instigated deeper research, and implemented innovative technological advancements emphasizing the need for patient-centered care at all levels of system and care delivery with a strong emphasis and dependency on technological integration and adoption.

SYNTHESIS

Patient-centered care will continue to be a growing focus in the health care industry, encompassing the view that patients should be allowed to decide their own treatment courses with the support of a team of educated and invested health care providers. Proper utilization of evidence-based shared decision-making interventions has the potential to decrease overall health care costs while increasing the quality of healthcare delivered, which is why federal and organizational support for these programs has continued to grow. By assessing levels of patient activation, health literacy, and health numeracy, clinical leaders like you are better able to meet patients "where they are" and engage in productive shared decision making. Using tools such as shared decision-making aids and patient portals can decrease some of the workload of shared decision making for individual clinicians, making it easier to incorporate EBPs into existing clinical settings and patient workflows. Keeping these interventions focused on the patient and their style of engagement, especially with the increased use of virtual modalities in a post-COVID world, are key to supporting patient-centered care by all nursing and health care professionals. What are some areas in your own clinical settings where you can implement some of these practices? What new and novel ways are there to implement patient-centered, evidence-based care in your own clinical practice?

KEY POINTS

- Putting people at the center of health care decisions is the core of EBP.
- Person-centered EBP practices are important considerations for clinicians, administrators, educators, and policy-leading nurses because of the impact on clinical outcomes, resource utilization, provider and patient satisfaction, and policy.
- Shared decision making is a process by which patients and clinicians partner to make informed decisions to benefit the patient, whether the patient is an individual, family, or community.
- Evidence supports the use of shared decision-making aids that are patient engagement tools.
- Patient engagement tools should reflect the appropriate level of health literacy and health numeracy tailored to meet the needs of a specific patient or patient population.
- Level of patient activation needs to be assessed using tools like the Patient Activation Measure (PAM) to measure an individual's mindset toward being a manager of his or her own health.
- Patient portals aim to be an online strategy to promote patient engagement and self-care.
- Individual and contextual barriers can mitigate against patient engagement and activation, and need to be addressed by clinical leaders and teams through tailored evidence-based strategies that are relevant to a specific patient population.

REFERENCES

Al Juffali, L., Almalag, H. M., Alswyan, N., Almutairi, J., Alsanea, D., Alarfaj, H. F., et al. (2022). The Patient Activation Measure in patients with rheumatoid arthritis: A systematic review and cross-sectional interview-based survey. *Patient Preference and Adherence*, 16, 2845–2865. https://doi.org/10.2147/ppa.s379197

Alston, C., Berger, Z., Brownlee, S., Elwyn, G., Fowler, F. J., Jr., Hall, L. K., et al. (2014). Shared decision-making strategies for best care: patient decision aids. *IOM Roundtable on Value & Science-Driven Health Care: Learning Health System Series*. https://doi.org/10.31478/201409f.

American Association of Colleges of Nursing. (2021a). AACN's vision for academic nursing. *Journal of Professional Nursing*, 35(4), 249–259. https://doi.org/10.1016/j.profnurs.2019.06.012

American Association of Colleges of Nursing. (2021b). The essentials: Core competencies for professional nursing education. https://www.aacnnursing.org/essentials.

Bastable, S. B. (2017). Patient education practice guidelines for health care professionals. *Health Care Management Review*, 42(4), 322–330. https://doi.org/10.1097/HMR.0000000000000125

Baumann, L. A., Reinhold, A. K., & Brütt, A. L. (2022). Public and patient involvement in health policy decision-making on the health system level—A scoping review. *Health Policy*. https://doi.org/10.1016/j.healthpol.2022.07.007

Blumenthal, D., & Tavenner, M. (2010). The "Meaningful Use" regulation for electronic health records. *New England Journal of Medicine, 363*(6), 501–504.

Blumenthal-Barby, J. S. (2016). "That's the doctors job": Overcoming patient reluctance to be involved in medical decision making. *Patient Education & Counseling, 100*(1), 14–17.

Bonetti, L., Tolotti, A., Anderson, G., Nania, T., Vignaduzzo, C., Sari, D., et al. (2022). Nursing interventions to promote patient engagement in cancer care: A systematic review. *International Journal of Nursing Studies, 133*, 1–13. https://doi-org.lopes.idm.oclc.org/10.1016/j.ijnurstu.2022.104289.

Cohen, M. D. (2017). Engaging patients in understanding and using evidence to inform shared decision making. *Patient Education & Counseling, 100*(1), 2–3.

Dammery, G., Vitangcol, K., Ansell, J., Ellis, L. A., Smith, C. L., Carrigan, A., et al. (2023). The Patient Activation Measure (PAM) and the pandemic: Predictors of patient activation among Australian health consumers during the COVID–19 pandemic. *Health Expectations.* https://doi.org/10.1111/hex.13725

Engle, R. L., Mohr, D. C., Holmes, S. K., Seibert, M. N., Afable, M., Leyson, J., et al. (2021). Evidence-based practice and patient-centered care: Doing both well. *Health Care Management Review, 46*(3), 174–184. https://doi.org/10.1097/HMR.0000000000000254

Fickenscher, K., Kvedar, J., & Nichols, J. (2018). Beyond the medical virtualists: Creating capability in the health care team. *Health Affairs Blog.*

Hassmiller, S., & Wakefield, M. (2022). The future of nursing 2020–2030: Charting a path to achieve health equity. *Nursing Outlook, 70*(6 Suppl 1), S1–S9. https://doi.org/10.1016/j.outlook.2022.05.013.

Hibbard, J. H. (2016). Patient activation and the use of information to support informed health decisions. *Patient Education & Counseling, 100*(1), 5–7.

Institute for Healthcare Improvement. (2023). *The IHI triple aim*. https://www.ihi.org/Engage/Initiatives/TripleAim/Pages/default.aspx.

Kijewski, A. (2016). *Dissemination of patient decision-making aids via a web-based platform*. University of Arizona. Doctoral dissertation http://arizona.openrepository.com/arizona/bitstream/10150/621453/1/azu_etd_14868_sip1_m.pdf.

Kissam, S. M., Beil, H., Cousart, C., Greenwald, L. M., & Lloyd, J. T. (2019). States encouraging value–based payment: Lessons from CMS's state innovation models initiative. *The Milbank Quarterly, 97*(2), 506–542. https://doi.org/10.1111/1468-0009.12380

Lau, N. T. T., Wilkey, E. D., Soltanlou, M., Lagacé Cusiac, R., Peters, L., Tremblay, P., et al. (2022). Numeracy and COVID-19: Examining interrelationships between numeracy, health numeracy and behaviour. *Royal Society Open Science, 9*(3). https://doi.org/10.1098/rsos.201303

LeRouge, C., Nguyen, A. M., & Bowen, D. J. (2021). Patient decision aid selection for shared decision making: A multicase qualitative study. *Medical Care Research and Review.* https://doi.org/10.1177/10775587211012995. 107755872110129.

Lu, Y., Elwyn, G., Moulton, B. W., Volk, R. J., Frosch, D. L., & Spatz, E. S. (2022). Shared decision-making in the U.S.: Evidence exists, but implementation science must now inform policy for real change to occur. *Zeitschrift Fuer Evidenz, Fortbildung Und Qualitaet Im Gesundheitswesen, 171*, 144–149. https://doi-org.lopes.idm.oclc.org/10.1016/j.zefq.2022.04.031.

McAnally, K., & Hagger, M. S. (2023). Health literacy, social cognition constructs, and health behaviors and outcomes: A meta-analysis. *Health Psychology, 42*(4), 213–234. https://doi.org/10.1037/hea0001266

Mcbride, S., & Tietze, M. (2016). Appendix 5.1. HIMSS patient engagement framework with meaningful use categories. In *Nursing informatics for the advanced practice nurse: patient safety, quality, outcomes, and interprofessionalism.* Springer Publishing Company.

McCormack, L., Thomas, V., Lewis, M. A., & Rudd, R. (2016). Improving low health literacy and patient engagement: A social ecological approach. *Patient Education & Counseling, 100*(1), 8–13.

Miller, T., & Reihlen, M. (2023). Assessing the impact of patient-involvement healthcare strategies on patients, providers, and the healthcare system: A systematic review. *Patient Education and Counseling, 110*: Article 107652. https://doi-org.lopes.idm.oclc.org/10.1016/j.pec.2023.107652.

National Academy of Medicine. (2021). In M. Wakefield, D. R. Williams, S. L. Menestrel, & J. L. Flaubert (Eds.), *The future of nursing 2020–2030: Charting a path to achieve health equity*. National Academies Press. https://doi.org/10.17226/25982.

Obaremi, O. D., & Olatokun, W. M. (2021). A survey of health information source use in rural communities identifies complex health literacy barriers. *Health Information & Libraries Journal.* https://doi.org/10.1111/hir.12364

Office of the Federal Register, National Archives and Records Administration. (2010, December 21). *124 Stat. 119—Patient Protection and Affordable Care Act*. U.S. Government Publishing Office. [Government].

Okere, C. A. (2022). Cultural competence in nursing care. *Clinical Nurse Specialist, 36*(6), 285–289. https://doi.org/10.1097/nur.0000000000000706

PCORI. (2022, May 25). The PCORI strategic plan: National priorities for health. *PCORI.* https://www.pcori.org/about/

about-pcori/pcori-strategic-plan/pcori-strategic-plan-national-priorities-health.

Rampey, B. D., Finnegan, R., Goodman, M., et al. (2016). Skills of U.S. unemployed, young, and older adults in sharper focus: Results from the Program for the International Assessment of Adult Competencies (PIAAC) 2012/2014: First look (NCES 2016039REV) National Center for Education Statistics. https://nces.ed.gov/pubsearch/pubsinfo.asp?pubid=2016039rev.

Rampey, B., Xie, H., & Provasnik, S. (2019). *Highlights of the 2017 U.S. PIAAC results web report*. U.S. Department of Education. NCES 2020-777) https://nces.ed.gov/surveys/piaac/national_results.asp.

Rathert, C., Mittler, J. N., Banerjee, S., & McDaniel, J. (2016). Patient-centered communication in the era of electronic health records: What does the evidence say? *Patient Education & Counseling, 100*(1), 50–64.

Rose, A., Rosewilliam, S., & Soundy, A. (2016). Shared decision making within goal setting in rehabilitation settings: A systematic review. *Patient Education & Counseling, 100*(1), 65–75.

Schulz, P. J., Lindahl, B., Hartung, U., Naslund, U., Norberg, M., & Nordin, S. (2022). The right pick: Does a self-assessment measurement tool correctly identify health care consumers with inadequate health literacy? *Patient Education and Counseling, 105*(4), 926–932. https://doi-org.lopes.idm.oclc.org/10.1016/j.pec.2021.07.045.

Sergeeva, A. V. (2023). Why developers matter: The case of patient portals. *Health Informatics Journal, 29*(1): Article 14604582231152780. https://doi-org.lopes.idm.oclc.org/10.1177/14604582231152780.

Smith, S. G., Curtis, L. M., O'Conor, R., Federman, A. D., & Wolf, M. S. (2015). ABCs or 123s? The independent contributions of literacy and numeracy skills on health task performance among older adults. *Patient Education & Counseling, 98*(8), 991–997.

Sprague Martinez, L., Carolan, K., O'Donnell, A., Diaz, Y., & Freeman, E. (2018). Community engagement in patient-centered outcomes research: Benefits, barriers, and measurement. *Journal of Clinical and Translational Science, 2*(6), 371–376. https://doi.org/10.1017/cts.2018.341

Starfield, B. (2011). Is patient-centered care the same as person-focused care? *The Permanente Journal, 15*(2), 63–69. https://doi.org/10.7812/tpp/10-148

Street, R. L., Jr., Volk, R. J., Lowenstein, L., & Michael Fordis, C., Jr. (2017). Engaging patients in the uptake, understanding, and use of evidence: Addressing barriers and facilitators of successful engagement. *Patient Education & Counseling, 100*(1), 4.

Tietbohl, C. K., & Bergen, C. (2022). "I was gonna ask you": How patients use agency framing to display engagement in primary care. *Social Science & Medicine, 314*, 1–11. https://doi-org.lopes.idm.oclc.org/10.1016/j.socscimed.2022.115496.

Zou, K. H., & Li, J. Z. (2022). Enhanced patient-centricity: How the biopharmaceutical industry is optimizing patient care through AI/ML/DL. *Healthcare, 10*(10). https://doi.org/10.3390/healthcare10101997. (2227-9032).

PART IV Evaluation and Dissemination

19

Evaluation of Evidence Based-Practice

Diane Rita Maydick-Youngberg and Daniel David

LEARNING OUTCOMES

After reading this chapter, you should be able to do the following:
- Summarize the purpose of evaluating the impact of evidence-based practice (EBP).
- Select and define process and outcome measures used for EBP.
- Describe common methods used for evaluation of EBP.
- Summarize approaches to evaluate impact on outcomes (patient, clinician, or cost)
- Apply principles of quality improvement for collection, analysis, and display of evaluation data.
- Synthesize key elements to include in evaluation summaries for key stakeholders.
- Summarize the psychometric properties of strong measurement tools.
- Describe the process of adapting existing measures to be used for EBP.

KEY TERMS

Data display
Evaluation of evidence-based practice
Outcome measure

Process measure
Quality improvement

Evaluation of evidence-based practices (EBPs) is often used to demonstrate improved patient, clinician, and cost outcomes, including a health care system's return on financial investment (Connor et al., 2022; Maydick et al., 2020; McGee-Vincent et al., 2023; Seton et al., 2022; Short, 2019; Spano-Szekely et al., 2019). Additionally, health care systems must demonstrate meeting standards of EBP, national patient safety goals, affordable and value-based outcomes, and regulatory requirement. This is especially evident for organizations striving to achieve or maintain Magnet Status; the Magnet Recognition Program has strong roots in improving nursing related structures, processes, and outcomes (American Nurses Credentialing Center [ANCC], 2023, p. 54). Exemplary professional practice which focuses on excellence, collaboration, quality, safety, and best practices and a professional practice model are important components of the Magnet Recognition Program (Luzinski, 2012). The health care delivery system is integrated with the Professional Practice Model (PPM) and promotes continuous, consistent, efficient, and accountable delivery of nursing care.

The care delivery system is adapted to meet EBP standards, national patient safety goals, affordable and value-based outcomes, and regulatory requirements.

Nurses create patient care delivery systems that delineate the nurses' shared authority and accountability for evidence-based nursing practice, clinical decision making, outcomes, and performance improvement initiatives" (American Nurses Credentialing Center, 2023, p. 54). A PPM depicts the beliefs and values consistently used to demonstrate professional nursing practice within an organization.

Evaluation of implementing EBP is essential to illustrate the impact of process and outcomes. Evaluation is a structured approach to evaluate the impact of EPB implementation in practice. Evaluation is a key part of piloting the changes in practice (see Chapter 17) and when EBPs are being extended to additional practice settings. To evaluate any changes in practice it is imperative to collect and analyze data to determine whether the EBPs should be retained, modified, or eliminated. Evaluation is essential because outcomes achieved in a controlled environment when an investigator is implementing a study protocol with a homogeneous sample of participants (conduct of research efficacy) may not result in similar outcomes (implementation effectiveness) when the EBPs are implemented in a practice setting by multiple clinicians for a heterogeneous patient population (see Chapter 8). The key to effective evaluation is to demonstrate that the EBPs that are implemented improve the quality of care and do not impose negative impacts on patients, clinicians, or costs. The steps of evaluation are summarized in Box 19.1.

A good understanding of the principles of **quality improvement** (QI) provides a basis for evaluation of EBPs (see Chapters 12 and 14).

> **BOX 19.1 Steps of Evaluation for Evidence-Based Practice**
>
> 1. Identify process and outcome variables of interest.
>   *Example:* Process variable—Patients will have a fall risk assessment every 12 hours.
>   Outcome variables—Fall rates, fall injury rates, severity of fall injuries
> 2. Determine methods and frequency of data collection.
>   *Example:* Process variable—Chart audit of all patients on [name unit] 1 day a month.
>   Outcome variable—Calculated by month by quality improvement program
> 3. Determine number of baseline and follow-up patients needed for each measure as appropriate.
> 4. Design data collection forms.
>   *Example:* Process chart audit abstraction form for fall risk assessment
>   Risk or incident reports standardized in the organization for adverse events such as falls
> 5. Establish content validity of data collection forms.
> 6. Train data collectors.
> 7. Assess interrater reliability of data collectors.
> 8. Collect data at specified intervals.
> 9. Provide staff regular feedback of measures (e.g., every 3 months) to illustrate progress in achieving the practice change.
> 10. Use data to assist staff in modifying or integrating the EBP change.
> 11. Provide final evaluation to staff and senior executives.
> 12. Write final evaluation report.

> **TIP**
>
> EBP evaluation is a type of quality improvement, not conduct of research. Refrain from turning the evaluation of EBPs into a study (conduct of research). It is not necessary to have a simultaneous comparison group, calculate a sample size, or randomly select subjects; all are research methods used in the conduct of research but not necessary in EBP evaluation.

METHODS FOR EVALUATION

To evaluate the implementation of a best practice recommendation, clinicians evaluate the findings of the QI project when making decisions about changes in practice. The findings, or evidence, in combination with their clinical expertise and patients' preferences are evaluated when making decisions about practice changes.

A common approach to evaluation is a prospective pre-post implementation design. For example, McGee-Vincent and colleagues (2023) used a pre-post training implementation approach to evaluate staff training and to evaluate use of free, publicly available, evidence-informed mental health apps as a resource for veterans. It is important that baseline measures be collected before implementation to compare with the same measures at postimplementation (Titler et al., 2009). In some circumstances you may want to collect and analyze evaluation data during implementation to share with staff who are implementing the practice change.

Also, to promote sustainability of the EBPs, you should plan to evaluate at specific points in time after implementation (e.g., every 3 months) and include selected evaluation metrics in your QI program.

WHAT TO MEASURE

Evaluation must include both process and outcome measures (see Chapter 12). Process measures are derived from the "I" component of PICOT, the EBP intervention (see Chapters 5 and 8). Process of care measures are designed to evaluate staff's use of EBPs as detailed in the local EBP standard. They measure whether the EBPs demonstrated to benefit patients are followed correctly. Outcome measures are those projected to change as a result of implementing the EBPs, the "O" component of the PICOT (see Chapters 3 and 5). Outcome measures are used to evaluate whether implementation of the selected EBPs is resulting in improvements in health outcomes. They do not reflect care processes; they are the actual results of care delivered on outcomes. The "T" component of PICOT is the time or duration for data collection.

PROCESS MEASURES

When evaluating implementation of EBP, the outcome measure ideally is reflective of seamless and properly delivered care. However, how would one determine if the EBP was delivered as it was intended? The answer lies in the process measures. A process measure is defined as the measurement of steps a provider takes in order to ensure that an EBP is delivered according to recommended practice. Process of care measures are designed to evaluate staff's use of the EBPs as detailed in the local EBP standard. For example, the process measure of EBP fidelity might report if all elements of a bundle were delivered as planned. If this process measure demonstrates that the practice was not delivered as intended, it might give valuable information as to why the outcome measured was not optimal. Furthermore, it may give information as to which elements of the EBP were vital and which elements were not. Collectively, they measure whether EBPs demonstrate benefit to patients when they are followed correctly. Examples of process measures are:
- Using an interprofessional collaborative approach to prevent hospital-acquired tracheostomy pressure injury (Maydick et al., 2020).
- Reducing frequency of central line dressing changes to decrease central line-associated dislodgment and blood stream infections (CLABSIs) (Short, 2019).
- Initiating an individualized fall prevention bundle in acute care (Spano-Szekely et al., 2019).

TIP
Process Measures

When selecting process measures, think about the EBP recommendations, what practices should be changing, and the key EBPs that need to be followed to obtain the desired outcomes. Were clinicians correctly carrying out the EBPs that are embedded in the practice standard?

OUTCOME MEASURES

Outcome measures are those that are projected to change as a result of implementation of EBPs, or the "O" of PICOT, the outcome (see Chapters 16 and 17). Outcome measures are used to evaluate whether the implementation of the selected EBPs results in improvement in health outcomes (such as decreasing catheter-associated blood stream infections, hospital-acquired pressure injury, falls with injury, patient or staff satisfaction). Outcome measures do not reflect care processes; they are the actual results of care delivered on outcomes (see Chapter 14). Outcome measures may include patient outcomes (hospital-acquired pressure injuries [HAPIs], CLABSIs, and falls), but also clinician outcomes such as improvement in staff knowledge (McGee-Vincent et al., 2023) and cost outcomes such as cost reductions (Spano-Szekely et al., 2019). Examples of outcome measures are:
- Decreased incidence of tracheostomy-related pressure injuries (Maydick-Youngberg et al., 2020).
- Decreased central line dislodgment and CLABSI in the neonatal intensive care unit (NICU) (Short, 2019).
- Decreased fall rates and cost savings related to in-person observation (Spano-Szekely et al., 2019).
- Increased use of mobile mental health apps by multidisciplinary staff to reach veterans and bridge gaps by providing resources to those not engaged in mental health treatment (McGee-Vincent et al., 2023).

> **TIP**
>
> **Outcome Measures**
>
> The Magnet Model, derived from the 14 forces of magnetism, consists of five components: transformational leadership, structural empowerment, exemplary professional practice, new knowledge and innovation and improvements, and empirical outcomes. Empirical outcomes include such topics as organizational support for nurses' continuous professional development, registered nurse satisfaction, nursing-sensitive clinical indicators, patient satisfaction data related to nursing care, and advancing nursing research. Organizations awarded Magnet Recognition are required to demonstrate structures and processes that improve measurement of outcomes related to these five components. Outcome measures such as trended data (pre- and postintervention time frames) are examples of empirical outcomes that may be trended and reported (ANCC, 2023).
>
> Measuring outcomes is essential to evaluating whether the implementation of the EBPs results in outcomes similar to or better than those in the studies that formed the basis of your EBP standard. One must be cautious not to measure outcomes alone without also measuring process of care. Improving outcomes requires improvement of care processes. When outcomes do not improve, there is a tendency to jump to the conclusion that EBPs are not working if the desired outcome was not achieved. However, there may be too much variability in the way EBPs were implemented (process measures), and thus the impact on outcomes may be limited. You will not know this if you do not measure both processes of care and outcomes.

All measures, both process and outcomes, require clear conceptual and operational definitions for calculations of the measures. Evaluation of EBPs examines clinically meaningful changes in process and outcomes. There is no clear answer to how much data will be needed to evaluate the practice change associated with EBPs. Implementation of EBPs is not "research" so you do not have to conduct a power calculation or do random assignment. The preferred number of patients (N), patient days, or visits is somewhat dependent on the nature of practice setting, type of EBP being implemented, and the size of the patient population affected by the practice change.

Patient Outcome Examples

An implementation of a central line maintenance bundle for dislodgement and infection prevention in the NICU (Short, 2019) provided evidence for a practice change for central line maintenance for nontunneled central lines. Infection and dislodgement for both tunneled and nontunneled lines were examined in order to have a control and intervention group. Before implementing a change in practice using a central line maintenance bundle, 19 total incidences of central line dislodgments and 5 central line infections were noted. Postintervention, there was one total dislodgment and four central line infections. Prior research had shown that frequent dressing changes using a chlorhexidine patch decreased rates of infection. However, the author concluded that skin breakdown and risk of dislodgement for NICU infants outweighed the benefit of decreased infection. Although this was a QI project, the authors suggest further investigation.

Maydick and colleagues (2020) demonstrated the following common approach for evaluation using a prospective pre-post implementation design. Briefly, an increase in tracheostomy-related pressure injuries was noted, a literature search was conducted, followed by critical appraisal and synthesis of the literature; the existing literature led to best practice recommendations using a bundled approach for prevention of tracheostomy-related pressure injury. The authors used a pre-post implementation approach to evaluate improvements in tracheostomy-related pressure injury. The authors collected baseline measures (patients with tracheostomy-related pressure injuries) prior to implementing practice changes; data of the same measures were collected postimplementation for evaluation. Prior to the intervention there were 104 patients with tracheostomy and 4 incidents of pressure injury; postimplementation there were 38 individuals with a tracheostomy and 1 incident of pressure injury. Use of a bundle for prevention of injury has continued over time and the protocol is now standardized. Use of a fenestrated foam dressing, suture removal by day 7, and maintenance of a neutral head position may lead to reducing tracheostomy-related pressure injury in vulnerable patients (Maydick et al., 2020). Given that HAPIs are not reimbursable by many third-party payors, including the Centers for Medicare and Medicaid Services (CMS), the hospital avoids the cost of pressure injury treatment but assumes the cost of the preventive interventions. Ideally, the cost of delivering the EBP is compared with the overall benefits in the face of no cost savings or cost reductions.

Clinician Outcome Examples

McGee-Vincent and colleagues (2023) conducted a national QI project to develop, disseminate, and evaluate multidisciplinary staff training. The goal of the training was to increase use of free, publically available, evidence-informed mental health apps as a resource for veterans. Staff across the Veterans Administration (VA) service in the United States received instruction about the apps' features and limitations and how to introduce them to veterans. Satisfaction and effectiveness of the training was measured by pre- and posttraining surveys to assess changes in knowledge, skills, and intention to use the apps with veterans. Training included educational modules delivered via a live, web-based format. Participants (n = 1,110) represented 34 disciplines from 19 VA sites. Posttraining app knowledge scores and confidence in their ability to show veterans how to downland and use VA mental health apps improved. Participants were satisfied with the training, and most reported their intention to recommend the apps to veterans and to other VA staff to share with veterans (MaGee-Vincent et al., 2023).

Seton and colleagues (2022) developed an EBP project to evaluate an interactive pressure injury (PI) education program for frontline hospice staff and evaluated staff outcomes including knowledge and practice. Baseline PI incidence and prevalence data was collected, interviews were conducted with key leaders, and a literature review was conducted. Analysis of the existing literature led to development of the PI education intervention for staff followed by collection of data (staff PI knowledge after attending the workshop). The authors concluded that staff knowledge and practice improved.

Cost Outcomes

Cost outcomes are estimated health care costs that may be affected by implementing EBPs. Cost outcomes can be addressed in three ways. *First*, by evaluating the potential cost savings of an EBP using selected outcome measures such as additional costs of care delivery associated with adverse events such as HAPIs, falls, CLABSI, or catheter-associated urinary tract infection (CAUTI). Some hospital-acquired conditions are not reimbursed by CMS; thus, avoidance provides additional cost saving depending on the nature of the condition. A *second* approach focuses on cost reductions with the use of EBPs. Cost reduction focuses on cost reduction in delivery of care. For example, an average direct cost of implementing evidence-based acute pain management practices for older adults hospitalized with a hip fracture was $17,714 (Brooks et al., 2009; Titler et al., 2009). Use of evidence-based acute pain management practices reduced the cost of an average inpatient stay by about $1,500 per patient. Given this estimated cost reduction, it would only take the treatment of 12 patients with acute pain for the evidence-based acute pain management practices to reduce costs. Therefore, a hospital treating 100 older adults with acute hip fracture could expect an overall *net* cost reduction of $132,286 ($150,000 −$17,714) from implementing the evidence-based acute pain management practices (Brooks et al., 2009). A *third* approach is evaluating the benefits of an EBP intervention on outcomes in relationship to the cost of delivering the evidence-based intervention. A cost–benefit analysis requires that the cost of delivering the intervention be compared with the overall benefits in the face of no cost savings or cost reductions.

> **TIP**
>
> When evaluating the cost benefit of making a practice change, you, as a team leader, need to think "out of the box." That kind of decision often involves stakeholders who are from the finance department of your organization. If the practice change involves supplies or equipment, representatives from the purchasing department also may need to be included in evaluating the cost benefit of making a practice change.

DATA SOURCES

Sources for process and outcome data can include staff and/or patient reports, medical records, or clinical observations. During the data collection phase it is important that data collection instruments are easy to use, short, concise, and easy to complete, and have content validity. The focus must be on collecting the most essential data. Individuals collecting data must be trained on data collection methods and be assessed for interrater reliability to ensure consistency and fidelity to the data collection methods.

Data are something to be measured; they are a way to obtain information in order to quantify an attribute or construct; for example, descriptive statistics provide information about the population being studied. Numbers may be assigned to objects to help us characterize quantities of the same attribute or construct. Data sources to consider for your project may be available as part of internal QI or infection control programs in your practice setting. For example, if you are implementing EBPs to reduce CAUTIs, you will need to obtain data related to CAUTI. This may be obtained from the nursing quality or infection control departments. Most health care organizations collect data for falls, HAPIs, CLABSIs, CAUTIs, infection rates, medication errors, readmissions, and emergency department visits. It is advisable to meet with key stakeholders early in the planning process to determine what data are available and how you may use them in your evaluation.

Depending on the size of the practice and length of implementation, the team may want to collect and analyze evaluation data during implementation to share with staff who are implementing the practice change(s). To promote sustainability of the EBP changes you should plan to evaluate at strategic time points after implementation (i.e., every 3 months) and include selected evaluation metrics in your QI program.

Changing Measurement During a QI Project

When using the Plan-Do-Study-Act concept, the QI team may test improvement strategies in a controlled manner to measure results of the change strategy and drive further improvement. For example, in some situations clinicians may observe no benefit or even harm. Testing or measuring small changes in a controlled manner is a way to evaluate the practice changes and further improve or to determine the need for additional practice changes to prevent harm. Spano-Szekely and colleagues (2019) utilized small test of change during implementation of a fall prevention program. They used a staged implementation plan and evaluated the effectiveness of each intervention, and built on successes with additional interventions (Spano-Szekely et al., 2019).

Psychometrics

The terms psychometrics, reliability, and validity produce great consternation in developing EBP scholars. Each term helps those that evaluate EBP make a decision if the instrument used for evaluation meets a threshold of quality such that the outcomes reported are reflective of performance. We will refer to surveys, tests, and questionnaires as instruments or measures. The term psychometrics is used to describe the rigor of an instrument. Why is this important? Simply put, when one reports their findings to evaluate practice, it is helpful to use well-accepted instruments that produce consistent results and measure what they claim to measure.

Primarily, there are two psychometric components to consider—reliability and validity. To demonstrate these concepts, let's consider a metaphorical example. If one were to use a tool to hammer a nail into wood, the most effective way to do so is to use the right tool for the job. An appropriately sized hammer that delivers consistent force to the nail head would be better than, say, an irregularly sized rock that may be used for generic smashing with variable results or a sledge hammer that may be more appropriate for different types of hammering. While these concepts may seem extreme or even a bit ridiculous, they describe qualities of psychometrics—reliability and validity. Let's take a closer look.

Reliability refers to the variability of recorded results from the measure. A measure with sound reliability can be used repeatedly with similar results. For example, if Adrian uses an instrument to measure a patient's level of depression and gets a score, will Carmen get the same score if the same instrument is used on the same patient? This is an example of *interrater reliability*. The higher the interrater reliability, the higher the consistency of scores between raters. The metric used to describe interrater reliability is called "κ" or "kappa" and refers to the percentage of time raters are in agreement. An instrument with a kappa of 0.75 is considered to have excellent interrater reliability. Instruments with a lower reliability score may still be used. However, care must be taken when considering the implications of the results or the limitations of the findings. Another type of reliability is called *internal consistency*. This type of reliability is the correlation of the individual questions within a measure and the overall score. A well-developed instrument will consist of only "good questions" that contribute to consistent measurement of a construct. As an instrument is being developed, researchers will remove elements that lower internal consistency or possibly add questions that provide a more consistent and accurate measure of the construct. The metric frequently used to describe internal consistency is called "α" or "Cronbach's alpha" and is a measure of internal consistency within a test. A measurement tool with a Cronbach's alpha of 0.7 or higher is considered to have strong internal consistency. A third test of reliability is *test-retest reliability*. This type of reliability demonstrates that a test would result in a similar measurement after a latency of a specified period time. In summary, there are different ways to identify if an instrument is reliable. Using a reliable instrument to evaluate EBP is an effective way to convey that your findings stem from an accurate measurement that produces consistent results.

Validity refers to the characteristic that an instrument measures what it intends to measure. What does this mean? Let us consider the expression, "a broken clock correctly measures the time twice a day." If we were to consider the broken clock in terms of reliability described above, it would have great consistency. Regardless of the passing of time, the broken clock provides reliable information that does not waiver whether read by two people or at different times of the day—fantastic reliability. However, is that broken clock a valid measure of time? Of course not. It does not measure what it intends, namely the time of the day. Alternatively, a sun dial may be an accurate measure of time during daylight hours but does not provide a valid measure of time during the night time. While these examples may seem facetious, they do provide the context to understand the psychometric property of validity.

There are four types of validity used to describe the psychometric properties of EBP measures.

Face validity is a subjective term that descriptively states that an instrument appears to measure what it intends. This subjective term is used to convey a general confidence that an instrument will provide effective measurement of a construct. Face validity may be declared on the basis of the opinion of experts, nonpsychometric descriptions of the measurement in academic literature, consensus of a focus group or comparisons to similar measures. For example, Teike Luthi and colleagues (2020) use a panel of experts to identify potential questions to be included on an instrument that distinguish between an individual with general care needs and one with palliative care needs. Using a panel of experts to describe what are and are not important elements to measure provides modest support that questions in an instrument may be used to evaluate a phenomenon. In essence, face validity establishes that knowledgeable people accept this form of measurement as valid.

Construct validity is an objective metric that reports if an instrument measures what it intends. There are similarities between construct and face validity; however, construct validity uses objective reportable metrics described in psychometric reports. There are three common methods used to establish construct validity. *Convergent validity* testing looks at the relationship between the measure of interest and other measures that are similar. Additionally, psychometricians may investigate *discriminant validity* testing to complement *convergent validity* testing and demonstrate that different measures do not measure similar constructs. For example, Shahnawaz and Rehman (2020) developed a Social Network Addiction Scale. After establishing test-retest reliability, they demonstrated convergent validity with an established loneliness scale and divergent validity with a life satisfaction scale. The authors use psychometric data to establish the relationship with problematic internet and social media use, which is distinct from more general feelings of dissatisfaction.

Content validity is an objective metric that reports if an instrument measures all aspects of a construct that it claims to measure. If there are certain aspects of a construct that are omitted, it threatens the validity of what the instrument claims to measure. Objective measures of content validity may be reported with a content validity index, which is a calculated metric based on agreement between experts. An example of this can be found in a patient care safety checklist for nurses caring for infants in NICUs developed by Manzo and colleagues (2023). Using multiple rounds of evaluation with a team consisting of 43 expert nurses, they included items on the measure meeting a threshold content validity index of 0.9 or greater. Through reporting this metric, users have psychometric support for using a checklist that includes expert-established aspects of safety.

Criterion validity is a measure of how well an instrument predicts a past, current, or future outcome compared to an established standard. A measure with strong criterion validity would be a strong indicator that there is a relationship between the measurement tool and the outcome one wishes to measure. A common example of this are standardized tests for academics, which have been thought to be an indicator of how well a student performs on tests in the academic setting. It is worth noting that the association between standardize testing and student performance on tests is only one metric of success. Care must be taken not to overstate that the criterion validity established in standardized testing and student performance on tests supersedes other holistic measures, which academic settings view as equally important (Newman et al., 2022).

Adapting Measures for Practice

The EBP environment of healthcare is dynamic whereas the psychometric properties of instruments are determined in a rigorously controlled setting. Even measures with strong psychometric properties are context dependent. Each evaluation is done in a specific context with a discrete population. An instrument that is valid to measure outcomes in one setting may not necessarily have the same reliability and validity in another. Furthermore, when questions are added or removed from an instrument, the psychometric properties change. For a person seeking to evaluate an EBP outcome, there are three options.

1. Use a psychometrically sound measure in the same context it was developed.
2. Create a measure that reflects the pragmatic context in which you are seeking to measure.
3. Adapt a measure with strong psychometric properties.

Option 1 is very limiting. EBP is context dependent. It is unreasonable to assume that the context or population in which the initial measure was standardized will represent the context or population of wherever the EBP evaluation will be performed. Flexibility is needed to support the evaluation of EBP. Option 2 is also a dangerous choice. Creating new instruments is a common attempt at establishing a context-specific evaluation. This is no easy task to do without extensive psychometric training and lengthy preliminary evaluation to ensure the measurement is psychometrically sound. Furthermore, without using established instruments, one risks multiple disappointing fates: (a) an evaluation that fails to detect the successful adoption of EBP, (b) an evaluation that reports a meaningful adoption of EBP when one is not present, and (c) an evaluation that truthfully reports a meaningful adoption of EBP that is not accepted by those judging the findings due to lack of confidence in the quality of the measure.

Adapting a measure (option 3) offers an alternative that addresses the limitations of using an instrument only in its prescribed setting (option 1 limitation: restricted context) or creating a new measurement that is untested (option 2 limitation: unsound psychometrics). The process of adapting an instrument must be done with caution. The following information should be reported when describing the methodology of evaluation.

1. Present a description of the instrument including the number of questions, the structure of the questions, scoring, and the psychometric properties.
2. Describe the context in which the initial instrument was validated.
3. Report that this initial instrument was adapted.
4. Report the reasons for adaption and conditions in which the adaption occurred.
5. Describe any preliminary evaluation that describes the face validity of the instrument.
6. Report the outcome with the adapted measure.
7. Discuss the limitations of adapting the measure.

These steps provide a transparent acknowledgment that an instrument is being used in a context in which it was not initially validated, yet provides information in which to conduct a meaningful evaluation with thoughtful consideration for how the adaption impacts the interpretation of the findings.

> **TIP**
>
> Health care organizations have multiple measures that are routinely used to improve quality of care. You can improve efficiency in evaluation by meeting with members of the health care system who are responsible for monitoring these measures. For example, you will want to meet with the person(s) responsible for reporting core measures required by the CMS and then determine which measures might be useful for your evaluation. If your organization contributes to national QI data sets such as the National Database of Nursing Quality Indicators, it is important to understand the QI measures your organization reports and their data definitions (Press Ganey, 2024).

ANALYSIS AND DISPLAY OF DATA

Evaluation measures are analyzed by comparing measures from pre- to postimplementation. Descriptive statistics such as frequencies, means, and rates are commonly used in the analyses. Descriptive statistics provide information about the population studied and can be used to describe or summarize elements of the sample group. In some circumstances, depending on the type of data you use, inferential statistics such as tests of differences, including t test, chi-square, analysis of variance (ANOVA), correlation, regression analysis, and odds ratio, may be used to examine differences from pre- to postimplementation (see Chapter 13). These statistics should be used with caution as they are generally research and hypothesis driven.

You may decide to observe similarities or differences between groups. For example, the *comparison group* would be a group of participants whose scores or outcomes are used to evaluate the outcomes of the group of primary interest; it is a term often used in lieu of control group when the study is not a randomized experiment.

Additionally you may decide to see if there are any *relationships* among the variables. This is a way to describe the bond or connection between two or more variables.

You will also report any *observation period*, which is defined as the collection of information or measures by directly watching and recoding behavior or characteristics within a time frame (see Chapter 10).

Statistical Process and Control Charts

When evaluation data is collected at different time points such as before, during, and after implementation, uses of statistical process control charts are helpful to visualize trends over time. You can display data as a run chart or a control chart. A run chart is a graphical **data display** that shows trends for a measure occurring over time.

A control chart is a graphical display of data plotted in timely increments. Control charts have a central line or average, an upper line for an upper limit, and a lower line for the lower limit. Historical data are used to determine upper and lower limits. Use of these upper and lower limits to compare current data allows the reader to draw conclusions in regards to variation (i.e., Is it consistent or out of control?). Further information can be found at the American Society for Quality (https://asq.org/).

Studying data over time offers key stakeholders results of the EBP results.

> **TIP**
>
> Communicating through displays: As mentioned earlier, using control charts or other graphics provides the reader with a visual display of change over time in response to implementation of the EBP and the results.

EVALUATION SUMMARY FOR KEY STAKEHOLDERS

Presentation of the EBP work should be summarized and presented to key stakeholders, including executive leadership and members of the interprofessional team. Essential elements of the report should include: project leadership and team members, background information and purpose of the project, state of the science and current standards for EBP, changes that were implemented, locations where implementation occurred, detailed strategies for implementation, impact on outcomes, limitations, and recommendations for further work. The use of process control charts to illustrate improvements can be included to highlight outcomes (Fig. 19.1, Table 19.1, and Box 19.2).

SYNTHESIS

Evaluation is essential to demonstrate the impact of EBP implementation on processes of care and patient outcomes. It is imperative that you use both process and outcome measures in the evaluation. Standardizing definitions of measures is required to compare measures over time and across different units of practice. You should include fiscal outcomes as part of evaluation when possible. Evaluation data may be measured using descriptive statistics to summarize and describe the sample groups; and by comparing measures from pre- to postimplementation. Descriptive statistics such as frequencies, means, and rates are commonly used in the analyses. Descriptive statistics provide information about the population studied and can be used to describe or summarize elements of the sample group. Tests of differences such as *t* test, chi-square, ANOVA, correlation, regression analysis, and odds ratio may be used to examine differences from pre-to postimplementation. Keeping the results in mind that these tests are generally used in research studies to guide hypothesis testing. A summary of the evaluation is warranted and the design should be based on the key stakeholder groups who will receive the information.

> **TIP**
>
> Evaluation demonstrates the impact of your work on improving quality of care. It is essential to illustrate how your work improved patient or clinician outcomes, addresses cost, and supports strategic initiatives such as meeting national benchmarks, core measures for regulatory agencies, and quality of care.

Upon completion of an EBP study and evaluation of the results you should be highlighting the results and discuss the implications of the EBP study. You should also discuss the results and how they do or do not improve care and whether they support a practice change that aligns with the population and setting studied. Lessons learned and recommendations for future EBP studies should be provided. Sharing information with stakeholders and others will substantiate the success of any proposed practice changes.

Directions: The following template is a guide to assist you with the report of your EBP work. It should be customized to your project.

Title of the Project Here
Date of the Report Here

Purpose of the EBP project: [Describe the purpose of the EBP project guided by your PICO]

Rationale: [Describe the rationale for this work. What is the clinical problem to be addressed by this work? Include QI data to support the work if available]

Team Leader(s): [Names, credentials and titles of the leader or co-leaders of the project]

Team Member(s) [Names, credentials, and titles of the team members]

Patient Population: [Describe the nature of the patient population that is the focus of your project]

Practice Sites: [Name the units, clinics, or other practice sites that were the focus of the project. Names, and credentials of the nurse managers of practice sites]

Disciplines involved in the practice change: [Types of clinicians involved in the EBP project such as physicians, nurses, respiratory therapists, etc.]

Time Frame: Summarize the time frame for the project. [May include critique and synthesis of the evidence (dates); formulation and approval of EBP standard (dates); implementation (dates); evaluation (dates)]

Synthesis of the Evidence and Practice Recommendations: [Describe in one to two paragraphs the synthesis of the evidence that supported the project. Set forth practice recommendations used to formulate the EBP standard. Evidence tables can be appended to this report]

EBP Standard and Approval Process: [Describe the EBP standard that was implemented and the governance committee(s) that approved the standard. The EBP standard can be appended to this report]

Implementation Strategies: [List and briefly describe the strategies used for implementation. Some are listed under this section as prompts. Only include those that you used for implementation]

Fig. 19.1 Template for Reporting an EBP Project to Key Stakeholders. *EHR,* Electronic health record; *QI,* quality improvement; *PICO,* population, intervention, comparison or control, outcome.

- Education of clinicians – [Describe who was educated, the educational methods used, and the focus of the education.]

- Performance gap assessment – [Describe the baseline data that illustrated a gap between the practice and the evidence. Describe how these data were shared with clinicians]

- Clinical decision support such as quick reference guides, pocket cards, or algorithms. Include any decision support or reminders added to the EHR [briefly describe each, may append copies of each]

- Key reminders or messages at the point-of-care delivery such as posters or infographics

- Opinion leadership – [Names of opinion leaders and their role]

- Change champions – [Names and their role]

- Educational outreach (academic detailing) – [Describe how this was done and by who (e.g. rounds made on units every two weeks by the NAME)]

- Audit and feedback – [Describe what practices were audited, how the data were shared with clinicians (e.g., posters, etc.), and how often it was shared (e.g., every 6 weeks over 6 months).

- Piloting – [If the change in practice was piloted, describe the practice site and length of the pilot as well as lessons learned and any revisions made in the EBP standard and/or implementation strategies]

- Meetings – [Describe frequency of meetings of the team]

- Engagement of key leaders – [Describe the names and roles of key organizational leaders who you met with to garner initial support and methods used to keep them appraised of your work. Address the involvement and support of nurse managers of the practice sites where the EBPs were implemented]

- Modification of documentation systems – [Describe any modifications made to the clinical documentation system. If no changes were made but you have recommendations for modification of the documentation system, include them here]

- Recognition and rewards – [Describe activities used to recognize and reward staff]

Evaluation: [List the process and outcome measures used for evaluation. Include the definitions of each. Summarize the impact on each measure from pre- to postimplementation. Append data displays (e.g., statistical process control charts, run charts) and indicate the beginning and end of the implementation phase]

Sustainability: [Indicate what measures will be integrated into QI program and what measures are taken to assure sustained improvements in practice]

Lessons Learned: [Briefly describe the lessons learned and how these lessons may be applied to future implementation of EBPs]

Plans for Dissemination: [Describe plans for presentations at conferences and/or publications. List any presentations that have occurred to date]

Reference List: [Provide a list of references as an appendix]

Fig. 19.1, cont'd

TABLE 19.1 Evaluation of Evidence-Based Practice Form

Purpose of the EBP Project:

Evaluation Focus:

Measures/Metrics (Process, Outcome, Knowledge, Fiscal)	Operational Definition	Data Source	Frequency of Data Collection	Aggregate Data Every _____ by time (e.g., month) _____ variable (e.g., unit; clinic; patient population)	Data Feedback to _____ (who) every _____ (frequency)	Modifications in Practice	Other Actions	Frequency of Submission to Quality Improvement
Process:								
Patient Outcomes:								
Clinician Knowledge:								
Fiscal Outcomes:								

TABLE 19.2 Examples of Process and Outcome Measures

Outcome Measures	Conceptual Definition	Operational Definition	Calculation
Fall rates	Number of patient falls, defined as unplanned descent to the floor, on a designated unit	Number of falls per 1,000 patient days	Number of falls × 1,000 divided by number of inpatient days
Severity of fall injury	Minor, moderate, major, or death	Minor: Needs application of dressing, ice, cleaning of wound, limb elevation, or topical medicine Moderate: Results in suturing, steri-strips, fracture, or splinting Major: Results in surgery, casting, or traction Death: Death as a result of fall	For fall events, proportion in each category represented as a percentage
NICU admission temperature	Number of NICU admissions with hypothermic, normothermic, and hyperthermic rectal temperatures	Normal temperature 36.5–37.5; Hypothermic < 36.5; Hyperthermic > 37.5 Proportion of NICU admissions with normothermia, hypothermia, hyperthermia	Number of normothermic infants upon admission to NICU divided by total number of NICU admissions
Nurses' knowledge regarding pain management	Pre- and posttest scores on knowledge assessment test regarding pain management via an educational test	Number/percentage of correct answers	For each nurse, the number of correct responses divided by the number of test items

Process Measures	Conceptual Definition	Operational Definition	Calculation
Delivery of fall prevention interventions targeted to patient-specific risk factor	Frequency and type of fall prevention interventions implemented to mitigate a patient-specific fall risk factor	Delivery of a fall prevention intervention targeted to a specified type of risk factor (e.g., mobility, elimination) for each patient day in which the risk factor was present	Rate per 100 patient days: Number of times per 100 patient days when a fall prevention intervention was implemented to mitigate a specific type of risk. Example: Of the 1,333 patient days of mobility risk factors, fall prevention interventions targeted to mobility were delivered 88/100 patient days.
Rate of applying the polyethylene bag for thermal management (decrease heat loss) to very low birth weight infants immediately after birth	For each premature birth, the number of times the polyethylene bag for thermal management is applied	Application of the polyethylene bag for thermal management for each premature delivery	Number of infants with application of the polyethylene bag divided by the number of premature births. Example: Out of 50 premature deliveries, the polyethylene bag was applied 44 times. 44/50 = 0.88

NICU, Neonatal intensive care unit.

BOX 19.2 Guidelines for the EBP Evaluation Form in Table 19.1

- Measures/metrics—This column should include process, outcome, and knowledge measures. Serious consideration also should be given to including fiscal outcomes. Be selective of the indicators you choose. Group indicators into categories: Process, Outcome, Knowledge, and Cost.
- Be clear about the operational definition of each metric—how you will measure each. If you are using a rate (e.g., fall rate), define the numerator and denominator. See Table 19.2 for examples.
- Define the data source for each indicator. If you need to collect data, the form should include directions specific enough for each individual collecting information to do so in the same manner.
- Define how frequently each indicator will be collected. Examples are daily for 1 week per month or 1 day per month for 6 months. Include dates.
- Define how data will be aggregated. For example, data collected daily for 1 week per month could be aggregated by day (e.g., Monday, Tuesday, Wednesday...) over 3 months for each unit.
- Define who will receive the data and frequency.
- Define what modifications are needed in practice, if any, and what additional actions are needed. This should include continuing to monitor specified indicators over time.
- Define frequency of time submitting a report to quality improvement program (e.g., annually; every 6 months).

KEY POINTS

- Approaches for evaluation differ; one approach is a prospective pre-post implementation design.
- Evaluation methods include both process and outcome measures.
- Process and outcome measures should be defined prior to making assumptions about EBP implementation.
- Process measures reflect the staff's use of the EBPs and whether the proposed EBPs are followed correctly.
- Be clear about the outcome being measured (patient, clinician, cost).
- Use well-accepted, reliable, and validated instruments that produce consistent results and measure what they claim to measure.
- Patient outcomes: did the selected EBP result in improved patient outcomes?
- Clinician outcomes may include improved knowledge and/or competency.
- Financial outcomes may include cost savings, cost reduction, and cost benefit.
- When presenting cost savings include costs of the comparison measure (i.e., use of virtual constant observation in lieu of in-person constant observation; the costs of both virtual constant observation equipment and cost of in-person constant observation personnel should be clearly defined for evaluation).
- Data sources include staff and/or patient self-reports, medical records, clinical observations, and those available in QI program data/dashboards (e.g., CLABSI, HAPI, falls, patient and/or staff satisfaction).
- Data analysis may include descriptive statistics (frequencies, means, or rates commonly used in analysis), comparisons, relationships, and inferential statistical analysis.
- Display of data is an important component of illustrating the effect of the EBP on processes and outcomes.
- Run charts and control charts are useful to illustrate data over time.
- An evaluation summary report should be prepared and shared with key stakeholders.

REFERENCES

American Nurses Credentialing Center (ANCC). (2023). *2023 Magnet application manual*. American Nurses Credentialing Center.

American Society for Quality. *Quality resources*. https://asq.org/quality-resources.

American Society for Quality. (2024). *Excellence through quality*. ASQ. Available at: https://asq.org. (Accessed: 23 October 2024).

Brooks, J., Titler, M. G., Ardery, G., & Herr, K. (2009). The effect of evidence-based acute pain management practices on inpatient costs. *Health Services Research*, *44*(1), 245–263.

Connor, L., Dean, J., McNett, M., Tydings, D. M., Shrout, A., Gorsuch, P. F., et al. (2023). Evidence–based practice improves patient outcomes and healthcare system return on investment: Findings from a scoping review. *Worldviews on Evidence-Based Nursing*, *20*(1), 6–15.

Luzinski, C. (2012). Exemplary professional practice the core of a magnet organization. *The Journal of Nursing Administration*, *42*(2), 72–73. https://doi.org/10.1097/NNA.ob013e318243352a.

Manzo, B. F., Silva, D. C. Z., Fonseca, M. P., Tavares, I. V. R., de Oliveira Marcatto, J., da Mata, L. R. F., et al. (2023). Content validity of a safe nursing care checklist for a neonatal unit. *Nursing in Critical Care*, *28*(2), 307–321.

Maydick-Youngberg, D., Liao, J., Francis, K., & Kaplan, S. (2020). An evidence-based interprofessional collaborative practice approach to decrease tracheostomy related pressure injury. *MedSurg Nursing*, *29*(3), 189–191.

McGee-Vincent, P., Mackintosh, M. A., Jamison, A. L., Juhasz, K., Becket-Davenport, C., Bosch, J., et al. (2023). Training staff across the veterans affairs health care system to use mobile mental health apps: A national quality improvement project. *JMIR Mental Health*, *10*, e41773. https://mental.jmir.org/2023/1/e41773.

Newman, D. A., Tang, C., Song, Q. C., & Wee, S. (2022). Dropping the GRE, keeping the GRE, or GRE-optional admissions? Considering tradeoffs and fairness. *International Journal of Testing*, *22*(1), 43–71.

Press Ganey. (2024). *Nursing quality (NDNQI), Resources for NDNQI Nursing Quality Indicators Database*. Available at: https://info.pressganey.com/ndnqi. (Accessed: 23 October 2024).

Scton, J. M., Hovan, H. M., Bofie, K. M., Murray, M. M., Wasil, B., Banks, P. G., et al. (2022). Interactive evidence-base pressure injury education program for hospice nursing: A quality improvement approach. *Journal of Wound, Ostomy, and Continence Nursing*, *49*(5), 428–435. https://doi.org/10.1097/WON.0000000000000911.

Shahnawaz, M. G., & Rehman, U. (2020). Social networking addiction scale. *Cogent Psychology*, *7*(1): Article 1832032.

Short, K. L. (2019). Implementation of a central line maintenance bundle for dislodgement and infection prevention in the NICU. *Advances in Neonatal Care*, *19*(2), 145–150. https://doi-org.ezproxy.med.nyu.edu/10.1097/ANC.0000000000000566.

Spano-Szekely, L., Winkler, A., Waters, C., Dealmeida, S., Brandt, K., Williamson, M., et al. (2019). Individualized fall prevention program in an acute care setting: An evidence-based practice improvement. *Journal of Nursing Care Quality*, *34*(2), 127–132. https://doi.org/10.1097/NCQ.000000000000344

Teike Lüthi, F., Bernard, M., Beauverd, M., Gamondi, C., Ramelet, A. S., & Borasio, G. D. (2020). IDentification of patients in need of general and specialised PALLiative care (ID-PALL©): Item generation, content and face validity of a new interprofessional screening instrument. *BMC Palliative Care*, *19*, 1–11.

Titler, M. G., Herr, K., Brooks, J., Xie, X.-J., Ardery, G., Schilling, M., et al. (2009). Translating research into practice intervention improves management of acute pain in older hip fracture patients. *Health Services Research*, *44*(1), 264–287.

20

Nursing Scholarship

Alice M. Nash, Mary Jo Vetter, and Kathleen Evanovich Zavotsky

LEARNING OUTCOMES

After reading this chapter, you should be able to do the following:
- Define nursing scholarship.
- Differentiate between scholarship of discovery, scholarship of teaching, scholarship of practice, and scholarship of integration.
- Discuss nursing scholarship as it relates to clinical practice.
- Relate principles of scholarship to the academic setting.
- Discuss alternate forms of scholarship.

KEY TERMS

Alternate form of scholarship
Clinical practice scholarship
Magnet Recognition Program
Nursing scholarship
Scholarship of application
Scholarship of discovery
Scholarship of integration
Scholarship of teaching

Nursing scholarship has been evolving since Florence Nightingale first laid the foundation by communicating and publishing her knowledge of nursing as she continually questioned the status quo. The definition of scholarship continues to change over time as nurses seek to improve patient and health system outcomes through research and evidence-based practice (EBP). Early, traditional definitions focused on scholarship as knowledge development within an academic environment where scholars were supported in scientific endeavors to advance the profession and meet societal health needs (Riley et al., 2002). At this time, scholarship was evaluated in terms of research productivity and publication. Developments leading to increased complexity of the health care environment and nursing education prompted the need for a new definition that recognized nursing as a discipline that exists in both the academic and practice environment simultaneously. The seminal work of Boyer (1990) reconsidered scholarship in broader terms that capture scholarly endeavors in more creative ways. As a practice discipline, nursing adopted Boyer's view that a scholar should work in four interrelated areas of scholarship in the pursuit of knowledge that responds to both human and societal needs. Looking beyond the scholarship of discovery of new knowledge through theory development, empirical research, and systematic investigation, three additional areas of scholarship were identified as relevant to nursing: integration, application, and teaching. The scholarship of integration creates connectiveness across disciplines and encompasses reciprocal research, teaching, and community engagement at the local, regional, national, and global levels to impact program development, knowledge dissemination, funding, and health policy. The scholarship of application or practice scholarship encompasses promoting competency in all aspects of nursing service delivery and involves the assessment of patient care outcomes, measurement of quality indicators, development of practice protocols, evaluation of systems of care, and the analysis of innovative models of care. The **scholarship of teaching** supports the development of educational environments that embrace diverse learning styles and focuses on the learner's needs in developing effective teaching and evaluation methods, program evaluation, and professional role modeling (American Association of Colleges of Nursing [AACN], 1999).

Building on Boyer's work, the American Association of Colleges of Nursing (AACN) advanced a definition of nursing scholarship as "those activities that systematically advance teaching, research, and the practice of nursing through rigorous inquiry that (1) is significant to the profession, (2) is creative, (3) can be documented, (4) can be replicated or elaborated, and (5) can be peer-reviewed through various methods" (1999, p. 3). As a more holistic model of nursing scholarship in the professional discipline of nursing continued to move forward, several assumptions served as foundational tenets (Riley et al., 2002):

1. All nurses share the obligation to take part in generating scholarship.
2. Nursing scholarship is setting related, but it is not setting dependent; both academic and practice-oriented individuals produce scholarship that is critical to the discipline's growth.
3. Nursing scholarship is dynamic and presents limitless opportunities to generate and use knowledge from conceptual, empirical, practice, and service sources.
4. Nursing scholarship is inseparably linked to the evolution of nursing as a professional practice discipline.

Multiple landmark reports from the Institute of Medicine issued since 1999 have propelled all health professions toward building a safer, high-quality, high-value health care system that values equitable access to care for diverse populations. Subsequently, AACN (2018) set forth an updated conceptualization of nursing scholarship as informing science, enhancing clinical practice, influencing policy, and impacting best practices for educating nurses as clinicians, scholars, and leaders. Scholarship in contemporary practice is typically interprofessional and requires a high level of teamwork emphasizing the integration of scholarly endeavors across institutional missions. **Nursing scholarship** is now defined as the generation, synthesis, translation, application, and dissemination of knowledge that aims to improve health and transform healthcare (AACN, 2018). It involves the communication and impact of knowledge generated through multiple forms of inquiry, which is communicated both in the profession and throughout the health care system.

A concept that is related to the scholarship of application is that of **clinical practice scholarship**, which is an approach that enables evidence-based nursing and the development of best practice to meet the needs of patients efficiently and effectively. Clinical scholars are curious, critical thinkers who reflect on practice and develop a culture of sharing their work with the broader nursing, health care, and general community. They integrate theoretical and experiential knowledge from the analytic observation of patients and seek to advance nursing knowledge and ensure the quality of the profession's essential service to humankind. Clinicians perceive personal attributes of vision and passion to be essential elements of clinical scholarship as they are required to challenge, shift, and redefine clinical practice in response to new research evidence. It is expected that clinical scholars disseminate to larger audiences and share their knowledge with the public through expert consultation, publication, and evidence translation to promote practice change. Clinical scholarship must be practice directed and involves partnership with colleagues conducting research to focus their combined efforts on improving care delivery (Wilkes et al., 2013).

Health care organizations play an important role in promoting nursing scholarship as clinical nurses identify gaps in practice and research that need to be addressed in the care setting. As the role of nursing continues to grow in healthcare, the engagement of frontline nurses in EBP, quality improvement (QI), and clinical research should be the rule, not the exception. Practicing nurses are in a unique position to inform scholarly projects and implement practice change when empowered with the necessary resources and support to overcome barriers and leverage facilitators to clinical inquiry (Whalen et al., 2020). By designing rigorous projects from the conception of the idea through implementation, evaluation of outcomes, and dissemination, clinical nurses can structure initiatives to ensure criteria are met for scholarship. The support needed for clinical nurses to have their work documented, peer reviewed, and disseminated internally and externally includes a wide variety of organizational resources (Limoges & Acorn, 2016) (Table 20.1).

TABLE 20.1 Resources to Support Clinical Scholarship

Resources and Strategies

Access to knowledgeable clinical leaders and subject matter experts with experience in clinical scholarship to inspire and guide other nurses

Educational programs and structures that support identification of clinical, operational, quality, fiscal, and ethical issues in need of attention

Ongoing tracking of scholarly projects underway in the organization to promote collaboration and reduce duplication of effort

Library access and assistance with literature search, documentation of the search strategy, critical appraisal, and synthesis of available evidence

Support for defining a data collection approach that includes identifying storage methods that are organized and retrievable to support project outcomes and conclusions

Data management, display, and statistical analysis support

Internal peer review support to provide insight into the external processes that scholarly work will be subjected to

Strategies to support identification of rigorous dissemination channels by means of journal publication and oral presentation

Writing support, including preparation and editing of abstracts, manuscripts, posters, and presentation materials

Recognition and reward strategies that make clinical scholarship efforts visible to nursing and interprofessional colleagues

Budget allocation for reimbursement of expenses related to dissemination at conferences and other venues

Access to expert consultation regarding Institutional Review Board requirements

From Limoges & Acorn, 2016.

ACADEMIC IMPLICATIONS

The Essentials: Core Competencies of Professional Nursing Education (AACN, 2021) has identified scholarship for the discipline as a domain of competency that is essential to nursing practice at both entry and advanced levels of preparation. Nursing professionals are called on to advance the scholarship of nursing, integrate best evidence into practice, and promote the ethical conduct of scholarly activities. Educating the nursing workforce of the future requires a proactive response to the ever-changing landscape of higher education and demands of employers, students, and the public. Academic institutions are expected to adapt curricula, teaching strategies, and learning assessment to ensure nursing knowledge, skills, and values embrace change and innovation through lifelong learning (AACN, 2019).

The role of academic nursing in an increasingly complex learning and practice environment has changed since the release of AACN's report: *Advancing Healthcare Transformation: A New Era for Academic Nursing* (2016). The report recommended six actions: embrace a new vision for academic nursing, enhance the clinical practice of nursing, partner in preparing future nurses, partner in the implementation of accountable care, integrate nursing research into clinical practice, and implement a plan to promote a new era for academic nursing. Academic and practice leaders are encouraged to advocate for strategies that expand the role of academic nursing in clinical practice. As full partners in health care delivery, the mission of a school of nursing should be connected to that of the practice environment. Academic nursing now encompasses the integration of practice, education, and research with a commitment to inquiry, generating new knowledge for the discipline, connecting practice with education, and leading scholarly pursuits that improve health and healthcare. The integration of scholarly endeavors across institutional missions requires alignment between practice and academia who work together to demonstrate the synergistic expertise and knowledge contributed by scholars from both settings. Opportunities abound as alternative forms of scholarship that capture the depth and breadth of contemporary clinical inquiry activities are increasingly embraced as important contributions in advancing the science of nursing (Ramirez et al., 2022).

NURSING IMPLICATIONS

In health care delivery settings, the expectation is for all clinicians who are at the sharp end of patient care practice based on the most up-to-date evidence. Nursing practice is not only regulated and guided by local state boards of nursing and the nurse practice act but by many regulatory agencies that oversee the care delivered in various settings. Regulatory bodies can help promote and protect professional integrity and evaluate competency and training (Cassiani et al., 2020). Many regulatory bodies such as the Joint Commission, Centers for Medicare and Medicaid Services, local departments of health, and the Occupational Safety and Health Administration provide frameworks, bundles of care, and standards to ensure that the latest evidence and care provided is based on the current science. Collaborative relationships between regulatory and health care organizations are necessary for ensuring patient safety standards are maintained and nurses are practicing with knowledge and competence. The safe and competent care of a patient who is at risk for suicide is an example of a standard of care that is often examined during a regulatory survey to ensure best practice measures are maintained to prevent injury or harm. Health care organizations can be held accountable through financial penalties and loss of accreditation if deficiencies related to patient safety are found.

In addition to responsibilities to regulatory agencies, there are many other organizations that help drive health care organizations to strive for best outcomes for patients. Many of these organizations offer accolades and award recognition, which showcase positive patient outcomes in the aggregate achieved through quality nursing care. Examples of these rankings and honors given to organizations that meet and/or exceed the specific safety criteria include: Five-Star Quality Rating by the Centers for Medicare and Medicaid Services, Best Hospitals Honor Roll by the *U.S. News and World Report*, Top Performers Vizient Awards, and the Gold Seal of Approval by the Joint Commission. The goal to meet the elements of these rigorous awards requires demonstration of scholarly activities through interdepartmental collaboration. These public accolades are very important to consider in a competitive health care environment. Referring practitioners and patients make important health care decisions based on data that is available to them via the internet and savvy advertising (DeAngelis, 2016).

The American Nursing Credentialing Center (ANCC) **Magnet Recognition Program**, which showcases nursing excellence and scholarship, is the platform many organizations strive to achieve. This program was conceptualized in 1983 and continues to evolve well into the 21st century. The Magnet Recognition Program designates organizations worldwide where nurses and nursing leaders successfully align strategic goals to improve the organization's patient outcomes. The Magnet Recognition Program provides a roadmap to nursing excellence, which benefits organizations. To the nursing profession, Magnet Recognition fosters education and development through every career stage, which leads to greater autonomy at the bedside. To patients, it means the very best care, delivered by nurses who are supported to be the very best that they can be (ANCC, 2022).

Achieving this designation is coveted as the requirements are rigorous and the journey takes a good deal of planning and commitment for health care organizations to analyze gaps and transform culture. The Magnet designation process clearly integrates the need for organizations to mobilize scholarly resources. In order to create and transform a nursing culture, the organization, including the senior nurse leaders, must support scholarly practice.

In Beal and Riley's (2019) qualitative study they examined the best practices of Magnet-designated hospitals as it relates to scholarly nursing practice. The study participants consisted of 32 senior nursing leaders from across the country. The overarching theme reported was that the organization creates and sustains a core culture supportive of scholarly nursing practice. They also reported some subthemes that include expectations for professional development, resources that support scholarly nursing practice, and the power of the senior nurse leader. The researchers conducted a crosswalk of the findings with the AACN (2016) and National Academies of Science, Engineering, and Medicine (NASEM, 2016) reports, which are clearly supported. The authors concluded that when the nursing culture embraces a scholarly nursing practice environment, it is more linked to an organization that supports nursing and its senior nursing leadership.

In Magnet-designated organizations, evidence of scholarly practice should be evident in all levels of nursing. One mechanism with which to ensure that scholarship is integrated in organizations is through the implementation of robust clinical ladder/professional advancement programs. In the work done by DeMarco and Pasadino (2018), the value of integrating scholarly work being conducted through a clinical ladder structure are clearly demonstrated. They discuss the benefits to the nurses and the organization at large. The ladder incorporates methodology for implementation and evaluating the QI process, patient-centered care, new knowledge, informatics, safety, and education, which has proven to improve retention and overall participation in the promotion process in that organization.

Scholarship in clinical practice has tremendous implications for nurses and healthcare. Nurse leaders are expected to consider initiatives and projects that involve nurses as well as other disciplines. This collaboration helps enrich projects and ensure alignment with the organization and overall with the nursing profession.

PARTNERSHIP IMPLICATIONS

The opportunities for partnership in EBP and healthcare are many and can be very far reaching. Just like in all opportunities for partnership, it is critical to show that there is joint benefit to both parties. This topic of partnership is elaborated on in greater detail in Chapters 1 and 22, and in this section, we will focus on the scholarly benefits specifically as it relates to nursing science and EBP overall.

The advantages of developing inter- and intraprofessional partnerships in nursing are many. Nurse leaders will be called on to develop and lead multidisciplinary teams through projects that have far-reaching implications. The multidisciplinary projects can involve research, EBP, or QI.

It is through the relationships that form during team projects that lifelong professional partners for future work are created. Some projects can be long term, short lived, successful, and perhaps not successful. It is important as the project evolves to take time to reflect on the scholarly opportunities that includes internal and external dissemination. Depending on the scope of the project, it can provide opportunities to continue to develop yourself and your team (Taberna et al., 2020; Epstein, 2014; Rosell et al., 2018).

An example of a project that can show multidisciplinary scholarly partnership includes working on a hospital-wide safe patient handling (SPH) EBP initiative. SPH is a major complex undertaking that has many implications for both patient and staff safety.

The work surrounding this is clearly multidisciplinary in nature. The work group and/or stakeholders include administrators, employee health/wellness staff, physical and occupational therapists, clinical nurses, doctorally prepared nurses, clinical nurse specialists, advanced practice nurses, educators, and physicians. The project completion time could be more than 12 months. This time would include the planning, implementation, and evaluation process. The outcomes to report would be patient- and staff-centered and multidisciplinary in nature, and provide scholarship opportunities outside of nursing. Venturing outside of the discipline of nursing enables professional networking to help broaden clinical perspectives toward a shared vision for addressing health care outcomes.

FUTURE CONSIDERATIONS

The future of nursing scholarly work continues to evolve. With the ongoing development of the internet there are opportunities that enable nurses to communicate across the globe. While keeping in mind that all information available on the internet is not scholarly, the footprint for reaching large audiences and various disciplines, patients, and families is possible (Vukušić Rukavina et al., 2021; Casella et al., 2014; Peck, 2014; National Council of State Boards of Nursing [NCSBN], 2018).

Social media venues, for example, are a great outlet for professionals to collaborate, share the results of scholarly work, and increase our intra- and interprofessional network. Blogs, chat rooms, and podcasts are another medium to help disseminate opinions, share stories, and recruit for research studies and other scholarly works. While the reach is vast, it is important to keep in mind that information posted is not peer reviewed nor vetted and should be used with caution (NCSBN, 2018).

When engaging in these modern communication mediums, it is also important to keep in mind the changing way nurses interact today. Technology creates a blurry line between the social and professional boundary (Casella et al., 2014). In some respects, this medium allows for more creativity and freedom of expression, but we need to seek guidance from employers and professional organizations to ensure that we are not compromising the profession of nursing, placing your employment and licensure at risk, or negatively impacting the perception of the health care profession (Casella et al., 2014; NCSBN, 2018).

The National Council of State Boards of Nursing (2018) published a document to help guide nurses on the use of social media. They recommend that nurses must understand the guidelines and be mindful that there are risks, particularly related to patient privacy. The instant nature of this communication mode does not encourage reflection, and it carries with it a burden once posted that is discoverable by a court of law even following deletion. The recommendations for nurses when utilizing social media include the following: Be aware, be cognizant of feelings and behavior, be observant of the behavior of other professionals, and always act in the best interest of the patient (NCSBN, 2018).

SYNTHESIS

Nursing scholarship will continue to evolve with the profession and through the advancement of technology. It is important as professional nurses to remain actively involved and engaged to ensure that the needs of the profession and those of patients and families within complex health care systems are safely met. It is important to the future of the nursing profession for the practice environment, in collaboration with academic partners, to develop rigorous scholarship to drive health and healthcare forward.

KEY POINTS

- Collaboration between academic and practice settings is essential to advance rigorous scholarship across disciplines and institutional missions to improve health and healthcare.
- In increasingly complex and dynamic health care environments, nurses must be educationally prepared to demonstrate practice competencies that are valuable across the lifespan in multiple settings serving diverse populations.
- Nursing scholarship is valued in both academic and practice settings as evidenced by requirements for professional advancement, organizational certification of excellence, and compliance with regulatory standards.
- In a rapidly expanding technological environment, the products of scholarship will continue to evolve and diversify with the goal of improving health and healthcare.

REFERENCES

American Association of Colleges of Nursing. (2016). *Advancing healthcare transformation—A new era for academic nursing*. Washington DC: ANCC.

American Association of Colleges of Nursing (AACN). (2019). AACN's vision for academic nursing. *Journal of Professional Nursing, 35*, 249–259. https://doi.org/10.1016/j.profnurs.2019.06.012

American Association of Colleges of Nursing (AACN). (2018). *Defining scholarship for academic nursing task force consensus position statement*. AACN.

American Association of Colleges of Nursing (AACN). (1999). *Position statement on defining scholarship for the discipline of nursing*. AACN.

American Association of Colleges of Nursing (AACN). (2021). *The essentials: Core competencies for professional nursing education*. AACN.

American Nurses Credentialing Center (ANCC). (2022). *Magnet Recognition Program Application Manual*. Silver Spring, MD: ANCC.

Beal, J. A., & Riley, J. M. (2019). Best organizational practices that foster scholarly nursing practice in Magnet® hospitals. *Journal of Professional Nursing, 35*(3), 187–194. https://doi.org/10.1016/j.profnurs.2019.01.001

Boyer, E. (1990). *Scholarship of the professorate*. Carnegie Foundation.

Casella, E., Mills, J., & Usher, K. (2014). Social media and nursing practice: Changing the balance between the social and technical aspects of work. *Collegian, 21*(2), 121–126. https://doi.org/10.1016/j.colegn.2014.03.005

Cassiani, S. H. B., Lecorps, K., Rojas Cañaveral, L. K., da Silva, F. A. M., & Fitzgerald, J. (2020). Regulation of nursing practice in the region of the Americas. *Pan American Journal of Public Health, 44*, e93. https://doi.org/10.26633/RPSP.2020.93

DeAngelis, C. D. (2016). How helpful are hospital rankings and ratings for the public's health? *The Milbank Quarterly, 94*(4), 729–732. https://doi.org/10.1111/1468-0009.12227

DeMarco, K., & Pasadino, F. (2018). Transforming a nurse practice advancement program for the new millennium. *Nurse Leader, 16*(4), 234–239. https://doi.org/10.1016/j.mnl.2018.05.010

Epstein, N. E. (2014). Multidisciplinary in-hospital teams improve patient outcomes: A review. *Surgical Neurology International, 5*(Suppl. 7), S295–S303. https://doi.org/10.4103/2152-7806.139612

Limoges, J., & Acorn, S. (2016). Transforming practice into clinical scholarship. *Journal of Advanced Nursing, 72*(4), 747–753. https://doi.org/10.1111/jan.12881

National Academies of Sciences, Engineering, and Medicine. (2016). *Assessing Progress on the Institute of Medicine Report The Future of Nursing*. Washington, DC: The National Academies Press. https://doi.org/10.17226/21838.

National Council of State Boards of Nursing (NCSBN). (2018). *A nurse's guide to the use to the use of social media*. https://www.ncsbn.org/public-files/NCSBN_SocialMedia.pdf.

Peck, J. (2014). Social media in nursing education: Responsible integration for meaningful use. *Journal of Nursing Education, 53*(3), 164–169. https://journals.healio.com/doi/full/10.3928/01484834-20140219-03.

Ramirez, J., Ro, K., Lin, Y., Thomas, A., DeNysschen, M., Smart, A., et al. (2022). Exploring alternative forms of scholarship for nurse educators' success. *Journal for Professional Nursing, 43*, 68–73. https://doi.org/10.1016/j.profnurs.2022.09.001

Riley, J., Beal, M., Levi, J., & McCausland, P. (2002). Revisioning nursing scholarship. *Journal of Nursing Scholarship, 34*(4), 383–389.

Rosell, L., Alexandersson, N., Hagberg, O., & Nilbert, M. (2018). Benefits, barriers and opinions on multidisciplinary team meetings: A survey in Swedish cancer care. *BMC Health Services Research, 18*, 249. https://doi.org/10.1186/s12913-018-2990-4

Taberna, M., Gil Moncayo, F., Jané-Salas, E., Antonio, M., Arribas, L., Vilajosana, E., et al. (2020). The multidisciplinary team (MDT) approach and quality of care. *Frontiers in Oncology, 10*, 85. https://doi.org/10.3389/fonc.2020.00085

Vukušić Rukavina, T., Viskić, J., Machala Poplašen, L., Relić, D., Marelić, M., Jokic, D., & Sedak, K. (2021). Dangers and benefits of social media on e-professionalism of health care professionals: Scoping review. *Journal of Medical Internet Research, 23*(11), e25770. https://doi.org/10.2196/25770.

Whalen, M., Baptiste, D., & Maliszewski, B. (2020). Increasing nursing scholarship through dedicated human resources: Creating a culture of nursing inquiry. *The Journal of Nursing Administration, 50*(2), 90–94.

Wilkes, L., Mannix, J., & Jackson, D. (2013). Practicing nurses' perspectives of clinical scholarship: A qualitative study. *BMS Nursing, 12*(21).

21

Dissemination

Carl A. Kirton and Althea L. Mighten

LEARNING OUTCOMES

After reading this chapter, you should be able to do the following:

- Apply the principles of dissemination in sharing evidence-based practice projects.
- Compare and contrast types of dissemination and advantages of each type.
- Use the Reach, Effectiveness, Adoption, Implementation, and Maintenance (RE-AIM) framework to guide inclusion of essential components in dissemination reports.
- Develop a plan for publishing your work in a peer-reviewed journal.
- Discuss barriers to dissemination and strategies to overcome the same.

KEY TERMS

Active dissemination	Implementation fidelity	Sustainability
Barrier to dissemination	Implementation science	
Dissemination venues	Passive dissemination	

Communicating and disseminating the results of an evidence-based practice (EBP) change is an important phase of any of EBP model used to conduct your doctor of nursing practice project. As a clinical leader, it is an expectation that you will disseminate your results to the staff nurses on a nursing unit and at shared governance councils (e.g., nurse practice quality improvement councils) and/or to interprofessional colleagues on a hospital-wide quality improvement council. You may be asked to present your findings at a local or national conference or prepare your findings for journal publication. The purpose of this chapter is to apply principles of dissemination for sharing your EBP project with the professional community and internal stakeholder groups.

Dissemination: Dissemination can be described as the purposeful act of widely spreading information and ideas across a variety of contexts and settings. In healthcare, the intent is to spread knowledge and evidence-based interventions across specific public health or clinical practice audiences (Agency for Healthcare Research and Quality [AHRQ], 2017; Mauricio, 2022). For our purposes, dissemination is the spreading of the methods and results of an EBP project to potentially relevant audiences such as the nursing staff, interprofessional clinical team, academic community, patients, or policy makers. The intent is to spread the project, the methods for implementation, and the impact on care delivery—both process and outcomes. Communicating the results of your work is an important part of EBP. Widespread dissemination of your EBP project can assist others in considering whether to use all or part of your project in their practice settings. Sharing your work engages others to help advance clinical practice and optimize patient care. You will want to incorporate dissemination into your action plan (see Chapter 15, Box 15.3) and your key stakeholder summary (see Chapter 19, Fig. 19.1). Research on dissemination provides insights on how to package, transmit, and share your EBP work with other professionals nationally and with key stakeholders locally (U.S. Department of Health and Human Services Program announcement number PAR-22–105, https://grants.nih.gov/grants/guide/pa-files/PAR-22-105.html).

PRINCIPLES OF DISSEMINATION

Principles of dissemination are important to guiding your plans for sharing your EBP project. These include considering the following:
- The intended audience
- The primary objective(s) of dissemination
- Types of dissemination

INTENDED AUDIENCE

As you analyze your evaluation data (see Chapter 19), you will want to reflect on who needs to be informed about your work—both internal and external audiences. For example, internal audiences include clinicians (nurses, physicians, clinical pharmacists, social workers) where the project was implemented; leaders such as nurse managers, chairs of service lines, chief nurse executives, chief medical officers, and chief executive officers; and selected governance councils or committees such as the organization and nursing department quality improvement committee. External audiences to consider are clinicians within your geographical region, members of national professional societies, and public policy makers. Examples include professional societies (e.g., Sigma Theta Tau International), specialty organizations (e.g., Oncology Nursing Society), interdisciplinary meetings (e.g., American Geriatric Society Annual Conference), and regional research meetings (e.g., Eastern Nursing Research Society annual conference). It is important to identify the intended audience because objectives, methods, and venues for dissemination need to be tailored to the intended audience. For example, busy clinical leaders in your organization are more likely to read short two-page executive summaries with details appended rather than a 15-page project report.

PRIMARY OBJECTIVES OF DISSEMINATION

After identification of the intended audience, you and your team will want to determine the primary objectives for disseminating information to the group. For example, objectives for dissemination to staff nurses on the unit where the EBP projects are implemented may be to illustrate how their contributions have improved processes of care delivery and outcomes, and to discuss strategies for ongoing sustainability of the EBP improvements. In contrast, an objective for dissemination to key senior leaders may be to illustrate improvements in both quality and cost. In considering your audience, identify the one or two key messages and lessons learned that you want to convey. It is important for you and your team to discuss the primary objectives(s) for dissemination to each specified audience, as this will guide the key messages that you want to convey. Essential elements to consider in your EBP project reports are discussed in a subsequent section of this chapter.

TYPES OF DISSEMINATION

Dissemination methods have conceptually been categorized as passive and active. Passive dissemination is a one-way communication process such as publishing or posting information with the expectation that the intended audience will access and use the information. Passive dissemination is not as effective as active dissemination, which is real-time interaction with the intended audience to impart key messages or information (AHRQ, 2017; Eljiz et al., 2020). In active dissemination, bidirectional communication and multiple conversations are used to discuss EBPs and rationale for their use.

Passive dissemination is popular and generally inexpensive in terms of material cost and requires a minimal amount of labor, expense, and effort. This strategy is generally a one-way process of communication using a top-down approach (e.g., clinical leader to staff). For example, Underwood (2015) implemented a unit-based protocol aimed at reducing the number of catheter-associated urinary tract infections (CAUTIs) in a neurosurgical and neurological intensive care unit. The staff received didactic education on the proper maintenance and care of urinary catheters. At the end of the training session, each staff member signed a document indicating awareness of the EBPs and agreed to the principles to prevent CAUTIs. Posters were placed in the unit to remind staff of urinary catheter removal practices. These are examples of passive dissemination strategies. As you plan for dissemination, consider the effectiveness of reaching staff nurses and interprofessional team members about the results of the EBP project by sending them an email with an attached report, displaying a poster in the unit or on the unit's community page, presenting in grand rounds/High Reliability Organizing huddles or rounding in the unit at various times of day and days of the week with the intent of interacting with the staff to illustrate in a graph the results of the project and thanking them for their contributions. Which method do you believe would be more effective?

DISSEMINATION VENUES

As you reflect on the methods and impact of your EBP project, you will want to consider the various venues for dissemination. These include traditional scholarly methods (e.g., poster presentations, oral presentations, and publications) and newer methods such as using various social media platforms.

Scholarly presentations are a key component of dissemination of EBP findings. These presentations are opportunities to share findings and recommendations with audiences local to your health care organization or setting as well as to wider audiences at professional conferences (Golash-Boza, 2022). Scholarly presentations typically involve the use of slides or other visual information displays as a supplement to the information being provided orally. It is important that slides and other visuals be clear, easy to see, and easy to understand. Many organizations provide templates for slide decks that meet these criteria. Visual displays (e.g., slides, poster boards) should not be crowded with text; rather, they should communicate the main ideas, and details should be provided orally by the presenter (Golash-Boza, 2022). Graphs or charts may be important to include but should be clearly understandable and large enough to be easily interpreted. Many professional organizations typically have guidelines for scholarly presentations available at their websites. It is important that presenters become familiar with the guidelines as appropriate.

TRADITIONAL METHODS

Poster Presentations

A poster presentation is a story board of key information. Posters generally are prepared for scientific meetings. Posters are displayed throughout the meeting or at designated times, they can also be displayed electronically, accompanied by a brief recorded oral presentation. Conference organizers will inform you of attendance requirements, but it is advantageous to have one or more members of the EBP team present to showcase your work. Because it is a summary of your work, conference participants will have questions about specific components; sometimes you will answer questions in real time at in-person poster sessions, and other times, with virtual posters, you will respond to inquiries by email or by posting your response. Presenting a poster is a social and interactive experience. The design and layout of your poster is important, because this will draw people to your work. There are many excellent online tutorials that will help you create effective and appealing posters.

> **TIP**
>
> Online resources and tutorials for creating effective poster presentations:
> https://www.youtube.com/watch?v=OyGf3awMfaQ
> https://www.youtube.com/watch?v=Hlzk6FGrHow
> https://www.youtube.com/watch?v=1RwJbhkCA58
> https://designcenter.uiowa.edu/creating-effective-posters#heading771
> https://www.brightcarbon.com/blog/effective-academic-posters-powerpoint/
> https://colinpurrington.com/tips/poster-design

Oral Presentation

An oral presentation requires you to present your work in front of a live (or virtual) audience. The hardest part of doing an oral presentation is anticipating your audience and tailoring your presentation to that audience. Does your audience consist of individuals who know nothing about your topic or subject matter and have some level of curiosity or is your audience individuals who know a great deal about the subject matter and are interested in your perspective on the subject matter? Is your audience interprofessional or solely nursing?

Oral presentations are generally timed, for about 15 to 20 minutes. Always tailor your presentation so that the audience has 5 minutes to critique or ask questions about your work. Use of presentation slides program such as PowerPoint or Google Slides to augment your presentation is common practice. Because of the limited time frame and the number of presentations to be heard in a day, the audience generally wants the speaker to get to the point. Don't burden your talk with conceptually or methodically complex discussions. In preparation for your talk, define your central message and do your best to develop a summary of your work and its impact that you can state in 25 words or less (your "elevator speech"), preferably in words that your intended audience will understand. You should practice your presentation, being mindful of the time allocation for your talk. If you are new to presenting, this tutorial will walk you through the dos and don'ts of effective presentations: https://www.youtube.com/watch?v=N5t3NTix1hw.

As you develop your presentation, think about the template you will use for your presentation. Some templates that are available may overwhelm the information you wish to present, so feel free to modify them. For example, templates designed for reporting research studies are not likely to be useful for presenting an EBP project. Box 21.1 is an example of a template for presentations on EBP projects.

> **BOX 21.1 Template for Presenting EBP Projects**
>
> Description of the problem, patient population, and clinical setting context
> EBP purpose statement
> Synthesis of the evidence on the clinical topic being implemented
> EBPs to be implemented
> Implementation strategies
> Evaluation (process and outcome measures)
> Lessons learned
> Strategies for sustainability of the practice change

Publications

Preparing your work for publication is time consuming and can be a tedious process. Publishing in a peer-reviewed journal adds a high level of credibility to your work and makes it available to a larger audience than oral or poster presentations can reach. Your work will be indexed in a large database, searchable by anyone with access to it (see Chapter 6). Every journal has "information for authors" listed on its website or in the journal. It is essential that you follow these submission requirements to ensure that you meet the journal's technical requirements for publication. Many journals require that authors of EBP guidelines use the SQUIRE 2.0 guidelines. SQUIRE stands for Standards for Quality Improvement Reporting Excellence. The SQUIRE guidelines provide a framework for reporting new knowledge about how to improve healthcare. They are intended for reports that describe system-level work to improve the quality, safety, and value of healthcare (see https://www.squire-statement.org/). Your manuscript should be reviewed by those with expertise in publishing before submission to the journal. It is likely that your manuscript will undergo multiple revisions before it is ready for submission.

With publication, having subject matter experts review and comment on your work is a cornerstone of the peer review process. Once these comments are sent to you, it is important to respond to each one in a collegial, nondefensive manner. Providing corrections and clarifications moves your manuscript one step closer to publication. Having your work published is an enormous professional accomplishment, because you will have contributed to the body of work in your professional discipline.

Publication is also an important vehicle for promoting replication of your project. Success in reaching your goals or targets may happen in one unit or department, but you may not be able to achieve the same results in other practice settings. Because EBP projects are not controlled experiments, many variables can be at play and affect results. However, encouraging replication of your work through publication or presentation helps confirm that the findings of your original work are accurate and applicable in different situations, and can serve as a resource to others who may be experiencing the same or similar issues.

SOCIAL MEDIA METHODS

Social media are potentially novel ways of enabling teams to communicate and disseminate their EBP findings. Traditional dissemination methods are slow in communicating and changing practice. The use of social media as a dissemination method is growing rapidly and gaining popularity. Social media are not simply a one-way avenue for a stream of information, but a two-way engaging process that allows for feedback, criticism, and conversation (Almutairi et al., 2022). Social media platforms are constantly evolving. These tools can be broadly classified into four major categories. These categories are not mutually exclusive. Most sites perform some level of each of these functions:

- Social networking (Facebook, X, Threads)
- Professional networking (LinkedIn, ResearchGate, Google Scholar, SlideShare)
- Media sharing (Instagram, YouTube, Flickr)
- Blogs and microblogs (X, Pinterest, WordPress)

Social Networking Site: Social networking sites are the most popular type of social platform and allow people to connect to each other through meaningful social relationships and patterns of interaction, such as relationships with family members, friends, and neighbors. Most social networks permit a limited number of characters or figures so the clinicians using these sites must communicate relevant and important information that encourages the reader to continue to engage and explore further (Lee et al., 2021).

Professional Networking: Professional networking differs from using a social networking site in that these sites specifically focus on building relationships and connecting with individuals who have similar professional interests or goals. It can also provide professional benefits such as job opportunities or mentorship. Over time, these sites have been used to announce professional accomplishments such as promotions, awards, and publications. ResearchGate is a professional network site specifically designed for scholarly dissemination, which reports to having well over 160 million publications posted to its site.

Media Sharing: YouTube and Vimeo are two popular video-sharing websites where users can upload, share, and view videos. Online video has become a major platform for dissemination of multimedia information. These tools can be effective dissemination tools for evidence-based findings. Gaining popularity is the use of a podcast to disseminate EBP initiatives and outcomes achieved. A podcast is an audio program that can be streamed or downloaded from the internet. Globally, there are more than 400 million podcast listeners. Because of this high listenership, there are over 2 million independent podcasts with tens of millions of episodes between them (Marshall, 2023). Podcasts provide the listener with direct access to the individual conducting the EBP project, allowing the listener to ask questions and clarify information. It has the added benefit of being recorded and can be listened to by anyone interested in the topic at any point in time.

Blogs and Microblogs: A blog is a website that contains a log or diary of information, specific topics, or opinions. A microblog is a smaller version a blog website that contains succinct thoughts or sentences. Blogs generally are designed to give career advice, education, or information about trending news, including an overview or recent discussion of importance. They can also be used as an relevance source of information dissemination.

IMPLEMENTATION SCIENCE AND DISSEMINATION OF EVIDENCE-BASED PRACTICE PROJECTS

Implementation science is an interprofessional discipline that explores the systematic uptake of EBPs and interventions in order to translate evidence more effectively and efficiently into practice (Boehm et al., 2020) (see Chapter 4). Implementation science supports the delivery of high-quality and effective healthcare by systematically assessing multilevel factors that contribute to implementation of a practice or process. Although implementation science shares common aims and features with quality improvement initiatives, implementation science uses more robust evaluation methods and is oriented to produce generalizable knowledge that can be applied outside of a particular study context (Boehm et al., 2020). As a research discipline, implementation science is theory driven and can employ a variety of frameworks to support the assessment and evaluation of EBP implementation. Some of the most commonly used implementation science frameworks are the Consolidated Framework for Implementation Research (CFIR); Reach, Effectiveness, Adoption, Implementation, and Maintenance (RE-AIM) framework; and Promoting Action on Research Implementation in Health Services (PARIHS) framework (refer to Table 21.1). Whereas these frameworks can be used to identify the essential elements to be included in the dissemination of your work to internal and external audiences, the RE-AIM framework seems to be more commonly used (Holtrop et al, 2021).

TABLE 21.1 Comparison of Selected Implementation Science Frameworks

Implementation Science Framework	Reach, Effectiveness, Adoption, Implementation, and Maintenance Framework (RE-AIM) Glasgow et al. (1999)	Consolidated Framework for Implementation Research (CFIR) Damschroder et al. (2009)	Promoting Action on Research Implementation in Health Services Framework (PARIHS) Kitson et al. (1998)
Purpose	Describes and evaluates the impact of an intervention based on five factors across individual and organizational levels	Comprehensive framework for understanding factors that influence implementation and evaluating intervention effectiveness	Framework to understand and analyze successful implementation of quality improvement interventions as a function of three core components
Components	Five factors: 1. Reach: individual-level measure of participation in an intervention and factors influencing participation 2. Effectiveness: individual-level measure assessing positive and negative outcomes of an intervention 3. Adoption: organization-level measure evaluating proportion and representativeness of sites and settings that adopt intervention 4. Implementation: organization-level measure of extent to which intervention is delivered as intended 5. Maintenance: individual- and organizational-level measure of extent to which intervention is sustained	Five major domains: 1. Intervention Characteristics: attributes of the intervention that influence implementation 2. Outer Setting: social, political, and economic contexts in which organization functions 3. Inner Setting: structural, political, and sociocultural contexts in which intervention is being implemented 4. Characteristics of Individuals: attributes of individuals that inform adoption or rejection of intervention and implementation 5. Implementation Process: how intervention is being implemented and factors that influence the process of implementation Each domain comprised of multiple constructs	Three core components: 1. Context: setting or environment where intervention occurs 2. Evidence: knowledge supporting intervention 3. Facilitation: process used to support stakeholders to change knowledge, attitudes, skills, etc. to successfully implement intervention
Applications for Nursing Practice	Planning and evaluation of quality improvement and/or evidence-based practice interventions	Planning and evaluation of quality improvement and/or evidence-based practice interventions	Planning and evaluation of quality improvement and/or evidence-based practice interventions

The RE-AIM framework, illustrated in Fig. 21.1, provides a guide for these essential elements. It originally was designed to plan and evaluate implementation of evidence-based public health programs or interventions (Glasgow et al., 1999; Gaglio et al., 2013). Today, RE-AIM is used in the planning stages for implementation in diverse areas of healthcare (e.g., health promotion, disease prevention, disease management) and settings (e.g., communities, hospitals, primary care, schools) as well as *reporting* results of implementing

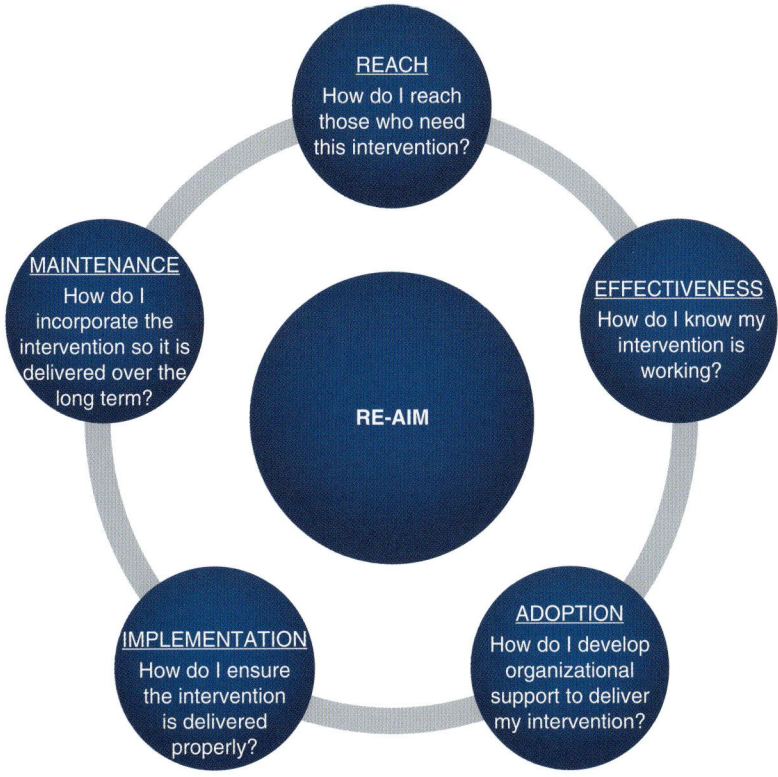

Fig. 21.1 The RE-AIM Framework. RE-AIM elements: planning and evaluating questions (see www.reaim.org for more information).

EBPs (Gaglio et al., 2013). RE-AIM focuses on five RE-AIM dimensions:
- Reach
- Effectiveness
- Adoption
- Implementation
- Maintenance (Gaglio et al., 2013)

Table 21.2 defines each of the RE-AIM dimensions and important elements to include in your EBP project presentation or publication. Table 21.3 provides a description of sections to consider in publications and presentations of EBP projects with links to the RE-AIM framework dimensions.

> **TIP**
>
> Disseminating the findings of your team's EBP or quality improvement project to internal and external audiences involves collaboration with other departments in your organization to develop targeted messaging for each stakeholder group to maximize adoption and sustainability of the initiative.

PEER REVIEW AND DISSEMINATION

Dissemination of scholarly work regardless of type, venue, or setting is subject to peer review. In this context, peer review is viewed as an organized process for assessing a body of work for quality, relevance and accuracy (American Nurses Credentialling Center [ANCC], 2021; Foster et al., 2019).

Abstract Submission

In order to present your scholarly work at an academic conference or submit a manuscript for publication in an academic journal, you will need to first develop and submit an abstract that provides an overview of your EBP improvement initiative. Most journals or professional organizations have specific requirements for abstract submission to their journal or conference, so always be sure to look for instructions regarding format, structure, and word count for any abstract you plan to submit. Generally, abstracts follow a similar template to

TABLE 21.2 RE-AIM Dimensions to Consider When Preparing Presentations or Publications

RE-AIM Dimension	Definition	Questions to Consider
Reach	Participants or intended users of the EBP change (e.g., staff nurses). This should include the number and representativeness of those participating in the EBP change and the setting (see Chapters 15 and 17).	Who were the users (e.g., types of clinicians) of the EBPs? Did the users include multiple disciplines? What were the characteristics of the users? What settings were targeted for implementation?
Effectiveness	Impact of EBPs on outcomes. Effectiveness can be measured at the individual, unit, or organizational level (see Chapters 14 and 19).	Did implementation of the EBPs improve outcomes? What outcomes were improved? Were there any negative effects of implementing the EBPs? If so, what were they?
Adoption	Uptake or participation rate of using the new EBPs Fidelity to the EBPs or interventions Proportion of patients who received the EBPs Fidelity is the degree to which the EBPs are delivered as intended (See Chapter 19)	Were EBPs adopted by the end users? What were the processes of care measures that reflect adoption? Were the EBPs being carried out as intended (fidelity to the clinical intervention), or were some components of the EBPs not followed?
Implementation	Strategies used to promote adoption of the EBPs (e.g., education, audit, and feedback)* Strategies used to ensure ongoing use of the EBPs (e.g., modification of documentation systems) (See Chapters 16 and 17)	What implementation strategies were used to promote use of the EBPs? When were they done? If done repeatedly, how often (e.g., every 4 weeks for 6 months)? How long was the implementation phase (e.g., 6 months)?
Maintenance	Sustainability—Continued use of the EBPs after implementation Sustained use of the EBPs for 6 months after implementation (See Chapter 16)	What process and outcome measures were sustained after implementation? What strategies were used to promote sustained use and integration of the EBPs into routine care? Are practices now embedded into daily workflow?

*Modified from RE-AIM.
EBP, Evidence-based practice; *RE-AIM*, Reach, Effectiveness, Adoption, Implementation, and Maintenance.

manuscripts using an Introduction, Methods, Results, and Discussion (IMRAD) format (Modesitt et al., 2022). Some abstracts will also include an "Implications for Practice" section in addition to or in lieu of the Discussion section. Abstracts should clearly communicate what you did, how you did it, and why it matters. Unless otherwise noted, it is not necessary to include references or citations in an abstract.

Peer Review of Abstract

Abstracts and manuscripts undergo a rigorous peer review process following submission. For abstracts submitted for a conference poster or podium presentation, peer review typically entails the conference committee and other volunteer members of the relevant professional organization reading submitted abstracts and evaluating them using a set of criteria

TABLE 21.3 Sections to Consider in Publications and Presentations of EBP Projects

Section of Paper or Presentation	Description	Relationship to RE-AIM Dimensions
Background and rationale	Description of the clinical topic, why it is important, rationale for using an EBP approach	
Purpose of the EBP project	Formulated from PICOT. Describes project's purpose, including problem and patient population, evidence-based intervention, and the outcomes to be achieved	Reach Effectiveness
Synthesis of the evidence base	Describes the synthesized evidence used to formulate the EBP intervention, program, or standard	
Description of the EBPs to be implemented (clinical intervention)	Detailed description of the evidence-based clinical intervention that was implemented, including each of the component parts	Adoption
Setting	Where the EBPs were implemented	Reach
Users of the EBPs	Principal users of the EBP implemented	Reach
Design	The design used to compare the impact of implementing the EBPs	
What was measured and when (include process and outcomes)	Description of process measures, outcome measures, calculation of each measure, data sources, and when they were measured during the project	Effectiveness Adoption Maintenance (if measures are collected at time points after implementation)
Description of the users of the EBPs (characteristics, number, etc.)	Description of the clinicians who used the EBPs; description of the patient population who were recipients of the EBPs.	Reach
How the EBPS were implemented; implementation strategies used; length of time for implementation	Describe specific strategies used for EBP implementation, how often each was done, and when completed (e.g., beginning of implementation, during implementation, etc.); describe or illustrate tools used for implementation such as decision-support algorithms, etc.	Implementation
Results	Describe the impact of EBP implementation on outcomes and processes before and at the end of implementation and at follow-up time periods after implementation is completed	Effectiveness Adoption Maintenance
Discussion	Discuss how your results compare to the synthesized evidence base mentioned previously and to other EBP projects	
Lessons learned	Description of what you learned during this project considering what went well, what challenges you encountered, and what you would recommend for others interested in implementing similar EBPs	

EBP, Evidence-based practice.

(Foster et al., 2019). These criteria may vary by conference or organization and may not be made publicly available. Peer reviewers are responsible for assessing the submitted abstracts for relevance to stated conference objectives and quality of the project.

Manuscript Submission

Manuscripts describing nursing research or EBP projects generally follow the IMRAD format described above. The manuscript introduction should provide an overview of relevant background information and extant literature for the project and clearly state the study purpose and objectives (Modesitt et al., 2022). Gaps in the existing evidence base should be identified, and authors should clearly describe how the study or project purpose will address these evidence gaps.

The Methods section should succinctly describe how the project was conducted, including the theoretical framework guiding the study, methodology used, and data collection and analysis procedures. The authors should clearly state whether Institutional Review Board approval was needed to conduct the project. The Methods section should also specify whether any applicable reporting guidelines, such as the SQUIRE checklist for quality improvement and EBP projects (Ogrinc et al., 2016), were used to guide the project and manuscript (Modesitt et al., 2022).

In the Results section, study findings or changes in outcomes related to the EBP project should be communicated. Authors may choose to include tables or graphs to facilitate communication of these results and provide additional details regarding study findings and outcomes. Only include the most important results in the text of the manuscript—it is not necessary to repeat the information contained in graphs or tables.

The Discussion section should explain and provide context for the results, connecting them back to the original research question and evidence gap (Modesitt et al., 2022). Authors can think of this section as the "so what?" portion of the manuscript, where they can discuss what the results mean, why they matter, and what the implications are for nursing practice and further research.

Manuscript submission for publication in an academic journal can be a lengthy process. Peer-reviewed journals often have specific requirements for formatting, word length, and content. Journal websites usually have a separate page or document that provides specific instructions for authors to guide the development and submission of manuscripts. It is strongly recommended that authors refer to these instructions when preparing their manuscript for submission to prevent immediate rejection by the journal editor.

Some authors choose to identify a preferred journal for publication prior to beginning manuscript development and draft the manuscript to the specifications of that journal, while others choose to write the manuscript first and revise subsequent drafts based on the journal selected for submission (Johnson, 2011). Significant revisions may need to be made to the manuscript drafts in order to satisfy journal-specific submission requirements. To help reduce the formatting burden related to in-text citations and references, the use of a reference management software can be most beneficial (see Chapter 6). Examples of commonly used reference management systems include EndNote, Zotero, and RefWorks. These systems enable authors to easily change a document's citation and reference style if needed.

A brief note on authorship: journals usually have specific guidelines to follow regarding authorship. The International Committee of Medical Journal Editors (ICMJE) recommendations defining the role of authors and contributors is one of the most commonly used guidelines (ICMJE, 2023). Other publishers and journals may ask for a CRediT (Contributor Roles Taxonomy) statement to be included that outlines the contributions of each author to the manuscript (Allen et al., 2019). Authorship should be discussed early during the manuscript development process, and authors should defer to specific journal requirements regarding authorship when submitting a manuscript.

Peer Review of Manuscript

Manuscript submission occurs electronically through the selected journal's submission portal. After submission, the manuscript will usually be assigned to the journal editor (or other managing editor, depending on the journal) for initial review. If the editor decides that the manuscript does not align with their journal, or if there are fatal flaws in the manuscript itself that make it unsuitable for publication, the editor may issue a "desk reject" to the authors stating that the manuscript is not a good fit for the journal (Mittacc, 2020). The authors are then free to submit the manuscript to another journal if they choose. If the editor determines that the manuscript should be sent for review, the editor must then find peer reviewers willing to read the manuscript and provide feedback. Peer reviewers are typically doctorate-prepared nurse scientists with content or subject matter expertise relevant to the journal scope and manuscript topic. The purpose of peer review is to provide constructive feedback on a manuscript to assess the quality of the manuscript both as a piece of writing and as a scholarly contribution to the discipline (Chinn, 2020). Depending on the availability of peer reviewers, it can take weeks or months to receive feedback on a submitted manuscript. Most journals will provide an estimated or average time to decision on their websites, but it may take longer for peer reviewers to provide their feedback.

Peer review feedback can take many forms depending on the journal and/or publisher. Generally, peer review feedback will contain a narrative paragraph(s) that summarize the manuscript and provide general comments on the relevance and scientific merit of the manuscript. In addition, peer reviewers read the manuscript line-by-line and provide specific feedback on each section. This feedback is given with the goal of strengthening the quality and clarity of the manuscript and can be quite detailed. Once the peer reviewers submit their feedback to the editor, the editor will share it with the manuscript authors with either a recommendation to consider submitting the manuscript to a different journal, or a recommendation to revise the manuscript based on the peer review feedback and then resubmit the manuscript to the journal (MacPhail, 2014).

Depending on the journal, there may be a specific process for authors to follow when revising and resubmitting their manuscripts. In general, it is recommended to use a peer review response table to help organize the feedback and the author's response (MacPhail, 2015). This response table is comprised of two columns: on the left, each of the reviewer's comments or suggestions in separate rows, and on the right the author's response to the feedback. Authors are not required to make all the changes recommended by the peer reviewer, but should provide a rationale or justification for why they choose not to take the reviewer's suggestion. A response table can provide structure to the author's response and serve as a reference to the author when revising the manuscript prior to resubmission (MacPhail, 2015). Again, depending on the journal, a manuscript may undergo multiple rounds of peer review prior to publication.

ANCC Magnet Standards for Dissemination

The ANCC Magnet recognition program underscores the importance of disseminating nursing research, EBP, and quality improvement projects. The ANCC Magnet Standards have specific requirements for internal (within the organization where the work was conducted) and external (outside of the organization where the work was conducted) dissemination of EBP and nursing research under the New Knowledge, Innovations, and Improvements component. Table 21.4 outlines the ANCC Magnet requirements for dissemination of nursing research or EBP project findings.

STRATEGIES TO OVERCOME BARRIERS TO DISSEMINATION

There are several barriers to dissemination of research findings and EBPs. For practicing clinicians, finding the time to work on manuscripts or submit abstracts for conferences while simultaneously meeting clinical obligations can be challenging (Graystone, 2018; Schmidt, 2018). Lack of prior experience with writing for publication can also pose a barrier to dissemination, as nurses may not feel confident in their writing abilities or know how to access resources to support them in developing and submitting their manuscripts for publication (Schmidt, 2018). Moreover, low levels of institutional support for nurse-led publications and dissemination of findings can discourage nurses from pursuing opportunities to share their work with broader audiences (Graystone, 2018; Schmidt, 2018).

Challenges may also exist related to a perceived lack of academic rigor in EBP work. Whereas manuscripts of research studies have a well-established format that clearly communicate the research methodologies used to conduct a study, manuscripts describing EBP findings may not have the same structure or elements (Dean et al., 2021). It is important to follow the guidelines required by the journal. Most journals require that EBP projects use the structured format of the SQUIRE 2.0 guidelines (see

TABLE 21.4 2023 ANCC Magnet Requirements for Dissemination

Magnet Sources of Evidence	Requirement	Notes
NK3	Provide two examples, with supporting evidence, of how clinical nurse(s) disseminated the organization's completed nursing research study to internal audiences.	Internal audiences refer to individual(s) within the applicant organization; the nursing research study must be completed and disseminated within the 48 months prior to document submission.
NK4	Provide one example, with supporting evidence, of how clinical nurse(s) disseminated the organization's completed nursing research study to external audiences.	External audiences refer to individual(s) outside of the applicant organization; the nursing research study must be disseminated within the 48 months prior to document submission but may be completed prior to the 48-month time frame.

NK, New Knowledge.
From ANCC, 2023.

https://www.squire-statement.org/). Peer review of EBP manuscripts often cites the absence of research-related concepts such as study design and sampling methods as reasons to not publish an EBP manuscript even though those concepts are not relevant to EBP methodology (Dean et al., 2021). Manuscript rejection from peer-reviewed journals on these grounds can be discouraging for authors and can pose an additional challenge to the dissemination and sharing of EBP findings.

There are many strategies to overcome these identified barriers and support clinicians in their efforts to disseminate findings. Protected time for writing and dissemination of findings can help clinicians with multiple competing priorities have the time needed to move their work forward. For inexperienced authors, the guidance and support of a writing mentor or experienced colleague can be invaluable in manuscript development. Additionally, leveraging institutional resources, including nursing research councils, writing workshops from professional organizations, and library research services, provides an opportunity for feedback and can strengthen the quality of the manuscript (Graystone, 2018; Schmidt, 2018). An EBP Practice Dissemination Guide developed by Dean and colleagues (2021) offers one potential structure for manuscript development that clearly outlines the approach and steps used in an EBP project. Clinicians can use this guide as a resource for dissemination of high-quality EBP manuscripts.

Dissemination Outside of Academic Spaces

Dissemination of EBP efforts offer an opportunity for professional development and is considered a professional obligation to the communities nurses serve (Graystone, 2018). Dissemination outside of traditional academic spaces such as professional organization conferences or professional publications is becoming increasingly necessary to support translation of research findings into practice and to educate the lay public. The use of social media to disseminate and publicize research findings is increasingly common in nursing research, particularly as individual researchers, professional organizations, and other academic health settings develop a larger social media presence (Quatrara, 2022). Manuscripts published in peer-reviewed journals can be shared on social media by the authors as well as the academic institutions where they work (Quatrara, 2022). Despite the usefulness of social media, one must be cautious of *predatory publishing*—dubious open access publishers who exist to make a profit from your work. With predatory publishing, there are alterations with established peer-review standards that jeopardize academic integrity (Milton, 2019).

Other mediums such as podcasts or blogs may also be appropriate vehicles to share findings outside of academic spaces. To avoid predatory publishing, one should consider reaching out to the public relations or marketing teams at the organizations where the work occurred to discuss opportunities to publicize their work to a broader audience (Quatrara, 2022).

Given the applicability and utility of EBP findings to clinical care, it is important that these findings be shared with participants, community partners, and other stakeholders who were involved in the EBP project or research study (George et al., 2023; Hagan et al., 2017). The Dissemination Framework developed by the Agency for Healthcare Research and Quality (AHRQ) is a tool made available to support researchers and clinicians in disseminating research findings and outcomes of EBP projects (Carpenter et al., 2005; Hagan et al., 2017). The framework is comprised of five components: (a) content, (b) end users, (c) dissemination partners, (d) communication, and (e) evaluation. Consideration of each component can guide clinicians and researchers in developing a plan to effectively disseminate findings to stakeholders and partners (Hagan et al., 2017). Potential approaches for dissemination include individual meetings with relevant stakeholders or larger events where the community of interest and research participants are invited to hear about study findings and provide feedback on how to best incorporate these findings into clinical practice (George et al., 2023; Hagan et al., 2017). Researchers and clinicians should build their dissemination plan into the study protocol and carefully consider the needs and preferences of their target audience when developing a dissemination plan (George et al., 2023). Concerted efforts to disseminate findings to participants and community partners serves to strengthen the relationships between the researcher or clinician and the larger community and can facilitate the translation of findings to clinical practice (George et al., 2023; Hagan et al., 2017).

Implications for Practice Settings

Nurses implementing EBP projects, quality improvement initiatives, or a research project should consider sharing their findings with the nursing community so that others can learn from the knowledge gained. Dissemination can occur in informal ways such as social media sites and more formal ways such as publications. Dissemination activities are an important part of the nurse's professional development as well as an important part of advancing nursing practice.

SYNTHESIS

As coordinators of interprofessional health care teams, clinical leaders like yourself use evidence to achieve positive patient and health system outcomes. Nurses in all roles are important consumers and generators of evidence. Effective dissemination of EBP work by leaders in clinical, education, or administrative roles provides an opportunity to promote the visibility of clinical leaders and the nursing profession overall. EBP innovators like you lead their communities and health care organizations to make significant and replicable evidence-based contributions to improving population health and quality of care, cost-effective health care delivery, and satisfying patient experiences.

KEY POINTS

- Dissemination is the purposive distribution of information and intervention materials to a specific public health or clinical practice audience.
- Principles of dissemination include considering the intended audience, primary objectives of dissemination, and types of dissemination.
- Passive dissemination is a one-way communication process such as publishing or posting information with the expectation that the intended audience will access and use it.
- Active dissemination fosters bidirectional communication with the intended audience.
- Traditional methods of dissemination include poster presentations, oral presentations, and publication.
- Nontraditional methods of communication include use of social media and other electronic means of communication.
- The RE-AIM framework provides a structured approach to reporting results of implementing EBPs and addresses five dimensions: Reach, Effectiveness, Adoption, Implementation, and Maintenance.
  - Reach is the intended audience or users of the EBP change.
  - Effectiveness is the impact of the EBPs on outcomes and can be measured at the individual, unit, or organizational level.
  - Adoption is the uptake or use of the EBPs by the intended clinicians and/or patients and is usually

- reflected in the process of care measures that are part of evaluation.
- Implementation is how the EBPs were put into practice—the strategies used to promote adoption of the EBPs (e.g., education, audit, and feedback) and their sustainability.
- Maintenance is the sustained use of the EBPs after implementation.
- **Implementation fidelity** measures the degree to which participants carry out the EBPs as intended.
- Sustainability occurs when a new practice becomes embedded into daily workflow.

REFERENCES

Agency for Healthcare Research and Quality (AHRQ). (2017). *Communication and dissemination strategies to facilitate the use of health-related evidence.* https://effectivehealthcare.ahrq.gov/products/medical-evidence-communication/research-protocol#:~:text=Active%20dissemination%20strategies%20involve%20active,or%20no%20spread%20of%20information.

Allen, L., O'Connell, A., & Kiermer, V. (2019). How can we ensure visibility and diversity in research contributions? How the contributor role Taxonomy (CRediT) is helping the shift from authorship to contributorship. *Learned Publishing, 32*(1), 71–74. https://doi.org/10.1002/leap.1210

Almutairi, M., Simpson, A., Khan, E., & Dickinson, T. (2022). The value of social media use in improving nursing students' engagement: A systematic review. *Nurse Education in Practice, 64,* 103455. https://doi.org/10.1016/j.nepr.2022.103455. Epub 2022 Sep 19. PMID: 36182729.

American Nurses Credentialling Center (ANCC). (2021). *2023 Magnet application manual.* ANCC.

Boehm, L. M., Stolldorf, D. P., & Jeffery, A. D. (2020). Implementation science training and resources for nurses and nurse scientists. *Journal of Nursing Scholarship: An Official Publication of Sigma Theta Tau International Honor Society of Nursing, 52*(1), 47–54. https://doi.org/10.1111/jnu.12510

Carpenter, D., Nieva, V., Albaghal, T., & Sorra, J. (2005). *Development of a planning tool to guide dissemination of research results. Advances in Patient Safety: From research to implementation. Vol. 4, programs, Tools, and products.* AHRQ. http://www.ncbi.nlm.nih.gov/books/NBK20603/.

Chinn, P. L. (2020). Becoming a peer reviewer. *Nurse Author and Editor, 30*(3), 2–3.

Damschroder, L. J., Aron, D. C., Keith, R. E., Kirsh, S. R., Alexander, J. A., & Lowery, J. C. (2009). Fostering implementation of health services research findings into practice: A consolidated framework for advancing implementation science. *Implementation Science, 4,* 50. https://doi.org/10.1186/1748-5908-4-50

Dean, J., Gallagher-Ford, L., & Connor, L. (2021). Evidence-based practice: A new dissemination guide. *Worldviews on Evidence-Based Nursing, 18*(1), 4–7. https://doi.org/10.1111/wvn.12489

Eljiz, K., Greenfield, D., Hogden, A., Taylor, R., Siddiqui, N., Agaliotis, M., et al. (2020). Improving knowledge translation for increased engagement and impact in healthcare. *BMJ Open Quality, 9,* e000983. https://bmjopenquality.bmj.com/content/9/3/e000983.

Foster, C., Wager, E., Marchington, J., Patel, M., Banner, S., Kennard, N. C., et al. & the GPCAP Working Group. (2019). Good practice for conference abstracts and presentations: GPCAP. *Research Integrity and Peer Review, 4*(1), 11. https://doi.org/10.1186/s41073-019-0070-x

Gaglio, B., Shoup, J. A., & Glasgow, R. E. (2013). The RE-AIM framework: A systematic review of use over time. *American Journal of Public Health, 103*(6), 38–46.

George, M. S., Gaitonde, R., Davey, R., Mohanty, I., & Upton, P. (2023). Engaging participants with research findings: A rights-informed approach. *Health Expectations: An International Journal of Public Participation in Health Care and Health Policy, 26*(2), 765–773. https://doi.org/10.1111/hex.13701

Glasgow, R. E., Vogt, T. M., & Boles, S. M. (1999). Evaluating the public health impact of health promotion interventions: The RE-AIM framework. *American Journal of Public Health, 89*(9), 1322–1327. https://doi.org/10.2105/ajph.89.9.1322

Golash-Boza, T. (2022). *6 tips for giving a fabulous academic presentation.* The Wiley Network. https://www.wiley.com/en-us/network/publishing/research-publishing/writing-and-conducting-research/6-tips-for-giving-a-fabulous-academic-presentation.

Graystone, R. (2018). Disseminating knowledge through publication: Magnet nurses changing practice. *The Journal of Nursing Administration, 48*(1), 3–4.

Hagan, T. L., Schmidt, K., Ackison, G. R., Murphy, M., & Jones, J. R. (2017). Not the last word: Dissemination strategies for patient-centered research in nursing. *Journal of Research in Nursing: JRN, 22*(5), 388–402. https://doi.org/10.1177/1744987117709516

Holtrop, J. S., Estabrooks, P. A., Gaglio, B., Harden, S. M., Kessler, R. S., King, D. K., et al. (2021). Understanding and applying the RE-AIM framework: Clarification and resources. *Journal of Clinical and Translational Science, 5,* 1–10. https://www.cambridge.org/core/journals/journal-of-clinical-and-translational-science/article/understanding-and-applying-the-reaim-framework-clarifications-and-resources/6EC2598C1C83F65FE5495A220A8A500E.

International Committee of Medical Journal Editors (ICMJE). (2023). *ICMJE | recommendations | defining the role of authors and contributors.* https://www.icmje.org/recommendations/browse/roles-and-responsibilities/defining-the-role-of-authors-and-contributors.html.

Johnson, A. M. (2011). *Charting a course for a successful research career: A guide for early career researchers* (2nd ed.). Elsevier. https://www.monash.edu/__data/assets/pdf_file/0003/1017543/20120227-ecr-guide.pdf.

Kitson, A., Harvey, G., & McCormack, B. (1998). Enabling the implementation of evidence-based practice: A conceptual framework. *Quality in Health Care, 7*(3), 149–158. https://doi.org/10.1136/qshc.7.3.149

Lee, G., Choi, A. D., & Michos, E. D. (2021). Social media as a means to disseminate and advocate cardiovascular research: Why, how, and best practices. *Current Cardiology Reviews, 17*(2), 122–128. https://doi.org/10.2174/1573403X15666191113151325

MacPhail, T. (2014). The revise and resubmit series, part 1: Coping with criticism. *Chronicle of Higher Education Community.* https://community.chronicle.com/news/830-the-revise-and-resubmit-series-part-1-coping-withcriticism.

MacPhail, T. (2015). The revise and resubmit series, part 3: Techniques for easier and faster revisions. *Chronicle of Higher Education Community.* https://community.chronicle.com/news/920-the-revise-and-resubmit-seriespart-3-techniques-for-easier-and-faster-revisions.

Marshall, N. (2023). Podcasting is growing for a reason—don't miss out on that growth. *Forbes.* https://www.forbes.com/sites/forbesagencycouncil/2023/01/17/podcasting-is-growing-for-a-reason-dont-miss-out-on-that-growth/?sh=64d1270342a7.

Mauricio, B. P. (2022). Nursing research, dissemination of knowledge and its potential contribution to the practice. *Investigación Y Educación Y Enfermería, 40*(3), e01. https://doi.org/10.17533/udea.iee.v40n3e01

Milton, C.L. (2019). Predatory publishing in nursing. *Nursing Science Quarterly, 32*(3), 180–181. https://doi.org/10.1177/0894318419845400.

Mittacc, S. (2020). *Tips for publishing in nursing journals.* Elsevier Connect. https://www.elsevier.com/connect/tips-for-publishing-in-nursing-journals.

Modesitt, S. C., Havrilesky, L. J., Previs, R. A., Alejandro Rauh-Hain, J., Michael Straughn, J., Bakkum-Gamez, J. N., et al. (2022). Ridiculously good writing: How to write like a pro and publish like a boss. *Gynecologic Oncology Reports, 42,* 101024. https://doi.org/10.1016/j.gore.2022.101024

Ogrinc, G., Davies, L., Goodman, D., Batalden, P., Davidoff, F., & Stevens, D. (2016). SQUIRE 2.0 (standards for quality improvement reporting excellence): Revised publication guidelines from a detailed consensus process. *Journal of Nursing Care Quality, 31*(1), 1–8. https://doi.org/10.1097/NCQ.0000000000000153

Quatrara, B. (2022). Digital dissemination platforms. *American Nurse.* https://www.myamericannurse.com/digital-dissemination-platforms/.

Schmidt, K. L. (2018). Dissemination of best practices. *Journal for Nurses in Professional Development, 34*(1), 1. https://doi.org/10.1097/NND.0000000000000417

Underwood, L. (2015). The effect of implementing a comprehensive unit-based safety program on urinary catheter use. *Urologic Nursing, 35*(6), 271–279.

PART V Evidence-Based Practice Innovation in Healthcare

22

Doctorally Prepared Nurses: Synergy for Professional Power

Debra Albert, Kathleen Evanovich Zavotsky, and Mary Jo Vetter

LEARNING OUTCOMES

After reading this chapter, you should be able to do the following:

- Discuss the history of the development of the doctorally prepared nurse.
- Differentiate academic preparation and competencies of the doctorate of philosophy, doctorate of education, and doctorate of nursing practice.
- Identify practice opportunities for doctorally prepared nurses.
- Review the impact that collaboration with doctorally prepared nurse has on healthcare.
- Identifies the scholarly opportunities that academic–practice partnerships can create for doctorally prepared nurses.
- Reviews the future implications for synergy between doctorally prepared nurses in practice and healthcare.

KEY TERMS

Academic–practice partnership
Collaboration
Dissemination
Evidence-based practice
Professional power
Synergy

The definition of **synergy** according to the Merriam-Webster's Dictionary (Merriam-Webster, 1999) is the interaction or cooperation of two or more organizations or substances to produce a combined effect greater than the sum of their separate effects. This definition is important to keep in mind as we discuss the opportunities that doctorally prepared nurses have related to **evidence-based practice** (EBP) and healthcare.

As we enter the 21st century there continues to be challenges for nurses in ensuring that our health care system is guided by the latest evidence. One of the opportunities that can guide us is to capitalize on the relationships between well-educated, doctorally prepared nurses. Doctoral nursing education degrees include the doctorate of nursing practice (DNP), doctorate of education (EdD), and doctorate of philosophy (PhD). While not all health care organizations have access to doctorally prepared nurses, when faced with the opportunity to leverage their expertise, we should take complete advantage of all that they have to offer. Doctorally prepared nurses have the opportunity to work synergistically to help advance the science of nursing and break down silos that exist in both practice and academic settings. The best way to accomplish this is by focusing on shared goals to help move nursing forward and improve healthcare, and by addressing critical contemporary issues such as nurse wellness and social determinants of health (SDOH) in the communities that we serve. Each doctorally prepared nurse has a unique skill set and should be respected for their academic and clinical contributions (see Table 22.1). This chapter will demonstrate that there is professional **professional power** in developing doctoral nurse synergy through focusing on improving health care outcomes and advancing the science of the profession.

HISTORY OF DOCTORALLY PREPARED NURSES

Reflecting on our nursing history enables us to move forward as a profession. Similar to the overall history of nursing, the development of the doctorally prepared nurse is rich in lessons learned that will help guide our future. Stevenson and Woods (1985) describe the historical phases of doctoral programs in nursing. The first phase took place between 1900 and the 1940s, when the EdD became available. It was during this phase that there was focus on developing academic education for nurses in colleges and universities. The second phase began between 1940 and 1960 when nurses were enabled to obtain a doctoral degree within the disciplines of the social and basic sciences, which did not include the specialty of nursing. The third phase took place between 1960 and 1970 when a doctoral degree was offered with nursing as a minor. The fourth phase took place during the 1970s with the development of the PhD and the doctorate of nursing science. It was this evolution that helped set the stage for nursing to be viewed as a respected profession and the rigor in nursing science began to evolve.

In the late 1970s, a new clinical doctorate in nursing was developed at the Frances Payne Bolton School of Nursing at Case Western Reserve University, which was the doctorate of nursing (ND). This was developed in order to help mirror other scientific disciplines minimum education requirement for entry into practice such as medicine and veterinary medicine. As the available doctorates developed there was debate about how the ND degree would serve the profession (Carter, 2013). Thirty years later in 2001, as an early response to the call from the Institute of Medicine (IOM, 2001) report to reform health care education to better meet the needs of the complexity in our health care system, the University of Kentucky developed the doctorate of nursing practice (DNP) program. This degree was developed to guide the education of the advanced practice nurses that are educated in order to better meet the complex needs of patients in healthcare.

The American Association of Colleges of Nursing (AACN) soon after developed the *Essentials of Doctoral Education for Advanced Nursing Practice* (AACN, 2006) In 2021, AACN embraced a new vision for professional nursing achieved through competency-based education delivered across the trajectory of nursing preparation with entry-level baccalaureate expectations and advanced-level graduate expectations defined.

TABLE 22.1	Key Differentiating Points of Doctoral Degrees: PhD, EdD, and DNP		
	DNP	**EdD**	**PhD**
Focus	Nursing Practice/Clinical Leadership	Education	Research
Clinical hours required for degree	Yes	No	No
Final degree requirement	Capstone	Dissertation	Dissertation
Average time to completion	2-4 years	4-7 years	4-7 years
Job opportunities	Leader, Translational Scientist, Advanced Practitioner; Academia	Specializes in education that addresses real world problems; Academia	Academia, ANCC Magnet Organizations as a Nurse Scientist, Research Laboratories

DNP, Doctorate of nursing practice; *EdD*, doctorate of education; *PhD*, doctorate of philosophy.

The framework, created with input from those involved in care delivery, seeks to bridge the gap between practice and academia to empower the profession far into the future. In addition, AACN (2022) published a position statement that outlines the preferred vision for education of the research-focused doctorate in nursing. These recommendations will continue to evolve to mirror the challenges faced in healthcare. Regardless of degree, doctoral education is critical to generate and integrate evidence that will shape the health and well-being of diverse populations across the globe. Strong, innovative academic–practice partnerships (APPs) are a key to the success of nursing education and are paramount to address the needs of our complex health care system (AACN, 2021).

DOCTORAL NURSE OPPORTUNITIES

The opportunities for doctorally prepared nurses have continued to evolve in order to meet the complex needs of healthcare and the patients and systems we serve. We will discuss some of the contemporary opportunities available. These include leadership, education, practice, and research/EBP that can be utilized to help you plan for your future as a clinical leader and or a doctorally prepared nurse.

Leadership

Leadership skills are the foundation of our practice and are critical in creating and sustaining change in healthcare (Heinen et al., 2019). There are many education programs that promote leadership skills in nursing and it is not just limited to doctoral programs (Page et al., 2021). The doctoral programs that are most appropriate for a nurse who is pursuing an executive leadership role can include a DNP, EdD, or PhD. For the most part, the choice to pursue the degree is a professional and personal decision. Your decision should be guided by a shared vision and be in alignment with the values of the academic setting. Some of the things that should be taken into considered are the depth and breadth of the curriculum, timing, program availability, and if you are going to be able to accomplish your goals within the setting. Regardless of the doctoral preparation there is an opportunity to develop leadership skills that involve higher-level thinking, complex analysis, and process work that contributes to a deeper understanding and appreciation of the need to create synergy in the science of nursing.

Appreciating the benefit of synergy in doctorally prepared nurses is a leadership skill that must be developed and shared in order to help move the profession forward and address our complex health care needs. There are many examples of success, with the most important and fundamental being the APP. One recent example is the work being conducted at the University of Michigan. A collaborative group from both the academic and health systems setting developed a partnership to create a nurse executive fellowship based on the American Organization of Nurse Leaders (AONL) competencies. This collaborative program created curriculum, a road map, and activities that focused on developing future nurse executives with proven success (Schoville et al., 2023).

The APP requires leadership and commitment from both partners (Kennedy et al., 2022). The practice and academic partner should utilize opportunities to develop a shared vision and mutual respect for what each organization can contribute to healthcare as well any other mutually beneficial goals. When leaders establish these partnerships, it encourages nurses to return to school and advance their education, develop unique recruitment strategies and practice models, as well as promote scholarly activities including dissemination of meaningful work.

When nurse leaders in the acute care setting are interested in pursuing and/or maintaining American Nurses Credentialing Center (ANCC) Magnet designation, they are responsible for ensuring that structures and processes are in place to achieve those goals. Eligible organizations are required to ensure that empirical outcomes are achieved and maintained in all areas where nursing is practiced. This includes ensuring that key personnel (such as the DNP and EdD/PhD-prepared nurse) are working together to establish that the latest evidence is being utilized in care delivery and that interdisciplinary groups and nurses are actively engaged in research and EBP (Speroni et al., 2020). Nursing research and EBP are no longer viewed as a "nice to have" in health care settings, and they are a necessity for ANCC Magnet designation organizations (Powers, 2020). Nursing leaders are responsible for developing structures and processes that can address the research and EBP infrastructure. The best way to accomplish this is to leverage available various doctoral resources by bringing them together in order to develop seamless sustainable processes. The challenge remains for organizations that do not have doctorally prepared nurses. In those situations, leaders have to establish relationships outside of the organization, which requires time and skill.

Education

Education of nurses has been essential to the evolution of the profession (AACN, 2021; Zhang et al., 2023). In today's complex health care environment, it is important that graduates of nursing programs are on the right journey to being practice ready, which enables them to competently deliver care in alignment with their scope of practice. The journey to becoming a nurse requires a commitment to lifelong learning regardless of the specialty. In the academic setting the opportunities to create an environment that values EBP is generally where the concept is introduced through coursework designed and delivered by faculty to meet curriculum requirements set forth by academic accreditation bodies recognized by the U.S. Department of Education, including the Commission on Collegiate Nursing Education and the Accreditation Commission for Education in Nursing. As the student enters the clinical setting there is an opportunity for both the academic and practice partner to continue to develop appreciation for and skills related to EBP through policies, procedures, and project work. Once the student transitions from prelicensure to a licensed professional nurse, the EBP skills and competencies need to continue to evolve.

Practice partners often times provide tailored transition to practice opportunities such as new graduate nurse residency programs. The foundation of new graduate nurse residency programs is based on EBP principles that prepare and support the novice nurse to address complex health care needs. There are many opportunities for doctorally prepared nurses to be engaged in this process. The EdD-prepared nurse can offer expertise on curriculum development and delivery that utilizes the most current teaching methods. PhD-prepared nurses can help ensure that the latest science is being integrated into the curriculum and assist with dissemination of completed project work. The DNP-prepared nuses can help ensure that the clinical curriculum is based on the latest evidence and includes appropriate stakeholders in the delivery of the material while at the same time providing structure to the program evaluation to inform ongoing improvement in program outcomes. Each doctorally prepared nurse can ensure that there are sustainable benefits both to the individual nurse and the organization.

An additional opportunity for synergy through the APP relationship would be in response to a contemporary shortage of a specific nursing specialty that is projected to be long term, such as perioperative, emergency department, or ambulatory care nurses. Together the APP could develop a course and offer it to undergraduate nurses who would like to commit to a specialty prior to graduation. The course could be co-offered by both the practice and academic partners that include all doctorally prepared nurses. The faculty and the course would be rooted in EBP principles, practice, and project-based learning that could be used to help the transition to practice. The DNP-prepared nurse could focus on curriculum development and clinical practice supervision, while the EdD/PhD-prepared nurse could develop a longitudinal research study to follow the students as they transition. Both could work together to develop a dissemination plan that provides the foundation for future research and funding opportunities and lead the way to providing sustainable alternatives to addressing the shortage of specialty nurses.

It is through the synergy that takes place between doctorally prepared nurses in examples like this that challenges in nursing workforce recruitment and retention can be addressed. An important guiding principle to keep in mind is that developing exceptional nurses leads to exceptional healthcare. When doctorally prepared nurses come together and are respected for what each has to contribute to address a common goal, the possibilities are endless.

Practice

Nursing practice has evolved with the roles of the advanced practice nurse (APN) that includes the certified nurse practitioner (NP), the clinical nurse specialist (CNS), the certified nurse midwife (CNM), and the certified registered nurse anesthetist (CRNA). While the NP, CNM, and CNS roles require a minimum of a master's degree, by 2025 all new graduates of a CRNA program will need a DNP to practice. There is a good deal of literature supporting a requirement for a DNP as a minimum for entry into practice (McCauley et al., 2020). Regardless of what the final outcome is regarding the debate to require a DNP to practice as an APN, the opportunities to utilize doctoral collaboration to address practice issues should be centered around quality, safety, and health care outcomes. The collaboration should center around developing frameworks and processes that allow practitioners to methodically address a problem. Chapters 3 and 4 provide more details about EBP and various models of care.

Most agencies have a responsibility to report patient quality accountability data that is public facing and affects ratings in the competitive health care market. Generally, health care organizations have a mission and vision with specific quality goals that can be used to help direct the doctorally prepared nurses as they work together to address issues. Some examples of clinical practice issues are listed in Box 22.1. Together the DNP/EdD/PhD partners can review the practice issue and determine if there is enough evidence to guide change in practice or whether research is indicated to generate new knowledge to inform a practice change. While doctorally prepared nurses have knowledge specific to their educational preparation, there are areas of overlap and opportunities to bring complementary skills to bear in improving patient and health system outcomes (Melnyk, 2013). The impact that doctoral collaboration has on safety and quality outcomes has been demonstrated at the patient and system level and is a sustainable strategy for success that should be utilized regularly (Cowan et al., 2019; Murphy et al., 2015; Rivaz et al., 2021; Rosenfeld et al., 2022).

RESEARCH/EVIDENCE-BASED PRACTICE

Doctorally prepared nurses are the most qualified individuals to lead the advancement of meaningful, contemporary nursing science. Both the DNP and EdD/PhD-prepared nurse have unique skills. The EdD/PhD-prepared nurse creates new knowledge through sound research methodology, while the DNP-prepared nurse is seen as an expert in translational/implementation science. While each nurse has a unique skill set, there is no reason why the scientific process from bench to bedside cannot be done together working in intraprofessional and interprofessional teams. With healthcare continuing to become more and more complex, it is critical that well-educated nurses work together to address clinical issues in a scientific way that is sustainable. There are many examples of this goal being accomplished successfully as long as the opportunities are focused on a shared vision that includes measurable improvement in health care outcomes. Developing a shared nursing research agenda has been recommended by many professional nursing organizations (IOM, 2021; ANCC, 2021; National Institute of Nursing Research [NINR], n.d.; AACN, 2006; Cohen et al., 2021; Shirey et al., 2021).

SCIENTIFIC INQUIRY

Creating and maintaining a culture of scientific inquiry through capitalizing on nurses' professional curiosity is essential to health care outcomes. We have an obligation to develop science that addresses the environment that we practice in and the only way to do this is through doctoral nurse collaboration. As a nurse who is either considering the pursuit of a doctoral education or is already prepared, you need to seek out opportunities to develop multidisciplinary relationships. One of the most important relationships that should be pursued is with doctorally prepared nurses. It is this pursuit that will enable you to determine what stakeholders will ensure that your EBP projects are successful and sustainable (Cowan et al., 2019; Cygan, & Reed, 2019; Kennedy et al., 2022).

For those health care organizations that are ANCC Magnet designated or are on the path to excellence journey, demonstrating that clinical nurses are actively

---

BOX 22.1 Examples of Doctoral Clinical Practice Collaborative Opportunities

Workforce Trends
    Safe staffing
    Nurse engagement
Nursing-Sensitive Indicators
    Central line blood stream infections
    Catheter-acquired urinary tract infections
    Falls
    Deep vein thrombosis
Patient Experience
Age-Specific Considerations
    Pediatric
    Geriatric
    Developmental disabilities
Social Determinants of Health
Medication Administration
    Error prevention
    Patient education
Innovation/Technology
    Electronic health record documentation burden
    Remote monitoring
    Virtual nursing

involved in developing, implementing, and disseminating practice-based nursing research and EBP is an essential tenant (ANCC, 2021). The Magnet designation process provides an opportunity for all doctorally prepared nurses to be actively involved with frontline nurses to guide them in developing scientific inquiry skills. When frontline nurses are engaged in project work that involves intradisciplinary and interdisciplinary teams, they can be mentored and guided to help see the value of incorporating stakeholder engagement into their everyday practice to promote adoption of EBPs and assist in their lifelong learning.

Many health care organizations have professional advancement systems or clinical ladders. These programs were developed to help reward and recognize nurses who work at the bedside (Moore et al., 2019). Often times, these programs require demonstration of scholarly accomplishments such as research, EBP, or quality improvement (QI) project implementation, which should ideally be guided by doctorally prepared nurses. The doctorally prepared nurse can ensure that the project is based on the need to address gaps in the scientific literature or the availability of new evidence while simultaneously meeting the strategic goals of the organization and the population served. Doctorally prepared nurses are the stars of the profession, well suited to provide mentorship and build on the professional curiosity of the nurse.

Dissemination of project work in organizations and beyond is another opportunity that doctorally prepared nurses can assist with. Regardless of whether the goal is internal or external dissemination, the doctorally prepared nurse can help lead this charge. Doctorally prepared nurses are educated to possess skills relating to nursing scholarship (see Chapter 20). They can support nurses in writing abstract submissions for conferences, writing manuscripts for publication, and preparing presentations that meet author guidelines. Each of these scholarly skills takes thoughtful planning that includes including contributing team members, following complex directions, and using effective public speaking and writing skills that some nurses may not be familiar with or have the confidence to perform independently.

For those organizations that have the resources, there is benefit to building a spirited culture of scientific inquiry that encompasses networking opportunities through the development of annual scholarly nursing forums or conferences that incorporate research, EBP, and QI. An undertaking like this can often times feel overwhelming to nurses without experience, but by partnering with doctorally prepared nurses and APP colleagues, it can become a highly attended and sought-after perennial event.

ACADEMIC–PRACTICE PARTNERSHIP INFLUENCE

While affiliated academic institutions are not always readily available to all health care organizations, the advent of technology-enhanced communication has enabled doctorally prepared nurses to reach out and establish relationships with organizations nationally and internationally. When considering exploring the APP, it is important to understand that it will require commitment to a common goal along with time and planning. According to the AACN-AONL (2012) task force on APPs, effective partnerships help create systems for frontline nurses to achieve educational and career advancement, prepare nurses of the future to practice and lead, provide mechanisms for lifelong learning, and provide a structure for nurse residency programs. This relationship can also create a mechanism to advance nursing practice in order to improve healthcare. A strategic approach can include intentional and formalized relationships that are based on mutual goals, respect, and shared knowledge. Building the relationship and goal setting may be broadly defined and should include intra- and interdisciplinary partnerships, corporations, government entities, and foundations.

The first step in the process is to seek relationships in which there are shared vision and culture. If such alignment is not preexisting, working together to create that shared vision has had proven success (Robertson et al., 2021; Paton et al., 2022; Beal & Zimmerman, 2019). Developing that shared vision will take leadership skill in order to navigate this often-complex process. Regardless of your role in the institution, the opportunity should be taken to be part of the solution as a doctorally prepared nurse. This is typically a once-in-a-lifetime experience that can lead to a career-changing experience for all involved. By establishing the APP, nurses are provided with the opportunity for joint appointments, research and EBP development, scholarly dissemination, and grant funding opportunities that would otherwise not be available (see Chapter 2).

Prado-Inzerillo and colleagues (2023) describes a unique APP model, developed by DNP and PhD-prepared nurses, which was established for DNP students. Their focus is on developing nursing leaders for the future at a large academic medical center. They demonstrate through this model that they were able to influence practice, professional growth, leadership development, and projects that impacted SDOH at the local level. This program serves as a model for APPs as it has been proven to be sustainable with successful outcomes.

Powerful APPs will provide doctorally prepared nurses with the opportunity to work together to develop and translate the science that can expand our ability to plan and prepare for the changes to come in healthcare.

FUTURE OPPORTUNITIES FOR DOCTORAL SYNERGY

In order to move from silos to synergy, doctorally prepared nurses should focus on the future of healthcare and respect the contribution of each other's unique skills. There are many opportunities in which DNP/EdD/PhD-prepared nurses can partner and develop vibrant programs for our future. Some of the innovative implications that will be discussed in this section include education considerations, informatics/innovation, and opportunities in large health care systems.

Within the last 10 years several doctoral programs that offer the DNP/PhD degree in combination have been established. The purpose of these programs is to offer a dual degree that is motivated by clinical practice, education, and research. Programs like these that are continuing to evolve and should be viewed as an option for nurses looking for a way to advance the science of nursing and enhance health care outcomes (Wysocki et al., 2015).

While the future of education may look different for the doctorally prepared nurse, there are many opportunities that currently exist to build the future of the profession together. One of the greatest opportunities that we have looking forward is through innovations in informatics and technology (see Chapter 24).

The nursing specialty of informatics is one of the advances that has had major impact on healthcare and nursing, in particular, the electronic health record (EHR). The opportunities abound for doctorally prepared nurses to explore and refine implementation strategies and electronic documentation requirements needed to produce meaningful, actionable data to inform clinical practice. The impact nursing informatics can have on scientific development in healthcare is limitless. One concept that must be explored is that of documentation burden in the EHR and how it is perceived by a nursing workforce with generational differences that influence perceptions of care. All disciplines as well as patients and families rely on the EHR to stay informed about specific details of health and health care delivery. As nurses, we must be part of continued innovation in technology-enhanced care and be prepared with evidence to ensure that functionality and usability is meeting the needs of our providers, patients, and families. DNP/EdD/PhD partners can serve on committees, conduct project work and rigorous research studies to formally evaluate technological processes and impact to nursing practice. Nurses' perception of the time they spend engaged with patients is very important to our practice. Thus, we must remain attuned to the concern that the evolution of the EHR may have a negative impact on that critical relationship (Moy et al., 2021; Strudwick et al., 2022).

Innovations in healthcare will continue to evolve in order to help meet the needs of patients and families. As nurses, we are on the front line and have to ensure that the technology is utilized appropriately to enhance care delivery while at the same time keeping in mind how it will affect the overall patient experience, safety, and quality of care. Currently there is movement to utilize virtual care encounters, remote physiological monitoring, and other telehealth options to care for patients both in and outside of the acute care setting (Schuelke et al., 2019; Cloyd & Thompson, 2020). Considerations related to the evolution of health care technology can be complex. Ethical dilemmas may arise when access to care is improved for some but not equitably for those who lack internet access or devices. Attention must be given to confidentiality, data security, and meeting established standards of care during a virtual encounter. DNP/EdD/PhD-prepared nurses need to be at the forefront in technological advancement to ensure that new knowledge is being generated and the best evidence is being implemented to protect patient rights, ensure high-quality health outcomes and data generated in EHRs are used to identify and prevent hospital-acquired conditions and clinical errors, empower patient and family decision making, and positively influence the overall patient experience.

Currently, many hospitals are merging to create large health care systems with thousands of nurses on staff who need professional development and its impact on patients and families (Russo et al., 2018; Attebery et al., 2020). This provides an opportunity for doctorally prepared nurses and APPs to focus on program development in order to meet the future needs of nurses and healthcare. One example is the establishment of acute care academies, residencies, and fellowships that help introduce both research and EBP to frontline nurses. Research/EBP succession planning programs like these could be helpful in cultivating professional curiosity in care settings. Structured processes can be used to guide nurses through their clinical nursing research and translational science interests by honing in on and mentoring the development of those skills. Programs like this will help prepare nurses for doctoral work and ensure that they are well equipped to address contemporary issues as we move into the future (Kim et al., 2017).

SYNTHESIS

This chapter makes it clear that the opportunities for doctoral collaboration in nursing are unlimited. There is an opportunity now and, in the future, to create and develop strategies that are contemporary, that help guide us while focusing on health care outcomes. Reflecting back on the definition of synergy, that the whole is better than the sum of its separate parts, this principle can be used to guide us in determining the benefits of doctorally prepared nurses working together and not in silos. It is through this synergy that we will enable continuation of the development of professional power required to move healthcare forward.

KEY POINTS

- Collaboration between doctorally prepared nurses can impact the future of health care outcomes.
- There are numerous roles for doctorally prepared nurses in healthcare.
- The impact that doctorally prepared nurses have on nursing is broad and multifaceted.
- The APP can be leveraged to promote doctorally prepared nurse collaboration.
- Both academic and practice accreditation bodies promote doctoral nurse collaboration to influence positive outcomes in both organizations.
- There is professional power when doctorally prepared nurses focus on common goals that focus on health care outcomes.

REFERENCES

American Association of Colleges of Nursing (AACN). (2006). *The essentials of doctoral education for advanced nursing practice.* AACN. https://www.aacnnursing.org/portals/42/publications/dnpessentials.pdf.

American Association of Colleges of Nursing (AACN). (2017). *Nursing research.* https://www.aacnnursing.org/News-Information/Position-Statements-White-Papers/Nursing-Research.

American Association of Colleges of Nursing (AACN). (2021). *The essentials: Core competencies for professional nursing education.* AACN. https://www.aacnnursing.org/Portals/0/PDFs/Publications/Essentials-2021.pdf.

American Association of Colleges of Nursing (AACN). (2022). *The research-focused doctoral program in nursing pathways to excellence.* https://www.aacnnursing.org/Portals/0/PDFs/Position-Statements/Pathways-Excellence-Position-Statement.pdf.

American Association of Colleges of Nursing-American Organization of Nurse Leaders (AACN-AONL). (2012). *Guiding principles.* https://www.aonl.org/system/files/media/file/2020/12/AACN-AONL-academic-practice-partnerships.pdf.

American Nurses Credentialing Center (ANCC). (2021). *Magnet application manual.* Silver Springs, Maryland: ANCC.

Attebery, T., Hearld, L., Carroll, N., Szychowski, J., & Weech-Maldonado, R. (2020). Better together? An examination of the relationship between acute care hospital mergers and patient experience. *Journal of Healthcare Management, 65*(5), 330–343. https://doi.org/10.1097/JHM-D-19-00116

Beal, J. A., & Zimmermann, D. (2019). Academic-practice partnerships: Update on the national initiative. *JONA: The Journal of Nursing Administration, 49*(12), 577–579. https://doi.org/10.1097/NNA.0000000000000817

Carter, M. (2013). The evolution of doctoral education in nursing. In S. DeNisco, & A. Barker (Eds.), *Advanced practice nursing: Evolving roles for the transformation of the profession* (pp. 27–35). Jones and Bartlett Publishers.

Cloyd, B., & Thompson, J. (2020). Virtual care nursing: The wave of the future. *Nurse Leader, 18*(2), 147–150. https://doi.org/10.1016/j.mnl.2019.12.006. ISSN 1541-4612.

Cohen, C. C., Barnes, H., Buerhaus, P. I., Martsolf, G. R., Clarke, S. P., Donelan, K., et al. (2021). Top priorities for the next decade of nursing health services research. *Nursing Outlook, 69*(3), 265–275. https://doi.org/10.1016/j.outlook.2020.12.004

Cowan, L., Hartjes, T., & Munro, S. (2019). A model of successful DNP and PhD collaboration. *Journal of the American Association of Nurse Practitioners, 31*(2), 116–123.

Cygan, H. R., & Reed, M. (2019). DNP and PhD scholarship: Making the case for collaboration. *Journal of Professional Nursing : Official Journal of the American Association of Colleges of Nursing, 35*(5), 353–357. https://doi.org/10.1016/j.profnurs.2019.03.002

Heinen, M., Oostveen, C., Peters, J., Vermeulen, H., & Huis, A. (2019). An integrative review of leadership competencies and attributes in advanced nursing practice. *Journal of Advanced Nursing, 75*(11), 2378–2392. https://doi.org/10.1111/jan.14092

Institute of Medicine (IOM). (2001). *Crossing the quality chasm: A new health system for the 21st century*. National Academies Press.

Institute of Medicine (IOM). (2021). *The future of nursing 2020–2030: Charting a path to achieve health equity*. National Academies Press. https://doi.org/10.17226/25982.

Kennedy, P., Cameron, P., & Munyan, K. (2022). Advancing nursing science and practice in unison. *Journal of Doctoral Nursing Practice*. https://doi.org/10.1891/JDNP-2021-0014. JDNP-2021-0014.R1.

Kim, S. C., Ecoff, L., Brown, C. E., Gallo, A.-M., Stichler, J. F., & Davidson, J. E. (2017). Benefits of a regional evidence-based practice fellowship program: A test of the ARCC model. *Worldviews on Evidence-Based Nursing, 14*(2), 90–98. https://doi.org/10.1111/wvn.12199

McCauley, L. A., Broome, M. E., Frazier, L., Hayes, R., Kurth, A., Musil, C. M., et al. (2020). Doctor of nursing practice (DNP) degree in the United States: Reflecting, readjusting, and getting back on track. *Nursing Outlook, 68*(4), 494–503. https://doi.org/10.1016/j.outlook.2020.03.008

Melnyk, B. (2013). Distinguishing the preparation and roles of doctor of philosophy and doctor of nursing practice graduates: National implications for academic curricula and health care systems. *Journal of Nursing Education, 52*(8), 442–448.

Merriam Webster. (1999). *Merriam-Webster's collegiate dictionary* (10th ed.). Merriam-Webster Incorporated.

Moore, A., Meucci, J., & Mcgrath, J. (2019). Attributes of a successful clinical ladder program for nurses: An integrative review. *Worldviews on Evidence-Based Nursing, 16*(4), 263–270. https://doi.org/10.1111/wvn.12371

Moy, A. J., Schwartz, J. M., Chen, R., Sadri, S., Lucas, E., Cato, K. D., et al. (2021). Measurement of clinical documentation burden among physicians and nurses using electronic health records: A scoping review. *Journal of the American Medical Informatics Association, 28*(5), 998–1008. https://doi.org/10.1093/jamia/ocaa325

Murphy, M., Straffileno, B., & Carlson, E. (2015). Collaboration among DNP and PhD prepared nurses: Opportunity to drive positive change. *Journal of Professional Nursing, 31*(5), 388–394.

National Institute of Nursing Research (NINR). (n.d.). The National Institute of Nursing Research 2022–2026 strategic plan. https://www.ninr.nih.gov/aboutninr/ninr-mission-and-strategic-plan

Page, A., Halcomb, E., & Sim, J. (2021). The impact of nurse leadership education on clinical practice: An integrative review. *Journal of Nursing Management, 29*(6), 1385–1397. https://doi.org/10.1111/jonm.13393

Paton, E. A., Wicks, M., Rhodes, L. N., Key, C. T., Day, S. W., Webb, S., et al. (2022). Journey to a new era: An innovative academic-practice partnership. *Journal of Professional Nursing, 40*, 84–88. https://doi.org/10.1016/j.profnurs.2022.03.006. ISSN 8755-7223 https://www.sciencedirect.com/science/article/pii/S8755722322000400.

Powers, J. (2020). Increasing capacity for nursing research in magnet-designated organizations to promote nursing research. *Applied Nursing Research, 55*, 151286, SSN 0897-1897. https://doi.org/10.1016/j.apnr.2020.151286

Prado-Inzerillo, M. L., Rivera, R. R., & Fitzpatrick, J. J. (2023). Academic-practice partnership for doctor of nursing practice in a large medical center. *Nurse Leader, 21*(3), 366–369. ISSN 1541-4612. https://doi.org/10.1016/j.mnl.2023.02.004.

Rivaz, M., Shokrollahi, P., Setoodegan, E., & Sharif, F. (2021). Exploring the necessity of establishing a doctor of nursing practice program from experts' views: A qualitative study. *BMC Medical Education, 21*(1), 328. https://doi.org/10.1186/s12909-021-02758-w

Robertson, B., McDermott, C., Star, J., & Clevenger, C. K. (2021). The academic-practice partnership: Educating future nurses. *Nursing Administration Quarterly, 45*(4), E1–E11. https://doi.org/10.1097/NAQ.0000000000000487

Rosenfeld, P., Glassman, K., Vetter, M. J., & Smith, B. (2022). A comparative study of PhD and DNP nurses in an integrated health care system. *Nursing Outlook, 70*(1), 145–153. https://doi.org/10.1016/j.outlook.2021.07.010

Russo, C., Calo, O., Harrison, G., Mahoney, K., & Zavotsky, K. (2018). Resilience and coping after hospital mergers. *Clinical Nurse Specialist, 32*(2), 97–102. https://doi.org/10.1097/NUR.0000000000000358

Schoville, R. R., Ross, T., Szczechowski, K., Medvec, B., Pineau, M., Aebersold, M., et al. (2023). Creating the nurse executive for the future: A collaborative academic and health system partnership. *Nurse Leader, 21*(2), 268–275. https://doi.org/10.1016/j.mnl.2022.08.00

Schuelke, S., Aurit, S., Connot, N., & Denney, S. (2019). Virtual nursing: The new reality in quality care. *Nursing Administration Quarterly, 43*(4), 322–328. https://doi.org/10.1097/NAQ.0000000000000376

Shirey, M. R., Bonamer, J., Clarke, C., Hass, S., Ivory, C., Kitto, S., et al. (2021). *Multi-site research playbook: A practical guide to support multi-site research studies for greater impact.* American Nurses Credentialing Center's Research Council. American Nurses Credentialing Center.

Speroni, K. G., Mclaughlin, M. K., & Friesen, M. A. (2020). Use of evidence–based practice models and research findings in magnet–designated hospitals across the United States: National survey results. *Worldviews on Evidence-Based Nursing, 17*(2), 98–107. https://doi.org/10.1111/wvn.12428

Stevenson, J. S., & Woods, N. F. (1985). Nursing science and contemporary science: Emerging paradigms. In G. E Sorenson (Ed.), *Setting the agenda for the year 2000: Knowledge development in nursing* (pp. 6–20). American Academy of Nursing.

Strudwick, G., Jeffs, L., Kemp, J., Sequeira, L., Lo, B., Shen, N., et al. (2022). Identifying and adapting interventions to reduce documentation burden and improve nurses' efficiency in using electronic health record systems (the IDEA study): Protocol for a mixed methods study. *BMC Nursing, 21*(1), 213. https://doi.org/10.1186/s12912-022-00989-w

Wysocki, K., Underwood, P. C., & Kelly-Weeder, S. (2015). An essential piece of nursing's future: The continued development of the nurse practitioner as expert clinician and scientist. *Journal of the American Association of Nurse Practitioners, 27*(4), 178–180. https://doi.org/10.1002/2327-6924.12251

Zhang, Y., An, Y., Wang, L., Zhao, Q., Li, H., & Fan, X. (2023). Psychosocial factors associated with career success among nurses: A latent profile analysis. *Journal of Advanced Nursing, 79*, 652–663. https://doi.org/10.1111/jan.15524

23

Innovation and New Models of Evidence-Based Care

Hiyam M. Nadel, Karyn L. Boyar, and Kimberly Whalen

LEARNING OUTCOMES

After reading this chapter, you should be able to do the following:
- Define both innovation and next-level innovation.
- Describe and articulate the use of design thinking (DT) for faculty and students in prelicensure and postbaccalaureate nursing programs.
- Describe and articulate the use of DT and human-centered design for interprofessional teams in solving problems and identifying gaps and unmet needs within the clinical setting.
- Apply methods that can help turn patient-centered needs into human-centered solutions.
- Apply not only user-centered DT but humanity-centered design as we evolve to benefit society as a whole.
- Describe the benefits of diverse and inclusive teams.
- Understand DT as a model to craft meaningful, evidence-based research poster projects using the full framework of DT.
- Understand why a maker's space adds to the success of an innovation program.

KEY TERMS

Design thinking
Humanity-centered
Human-centered design
Innovation
Intellectual property
Nursing process
User-centered

For many years now, nurses have been instructed and encouraged to innovate and "think out of the box" to solve our health care challenges. Now, more than ever, we need to reimagine novel ways of working. For reimagined work to be realized, we need to think about new roles and new skills, and how to transform how we deliver care. But doing all of this future work without any training in the innovation methodology just leads to incremental changes to what is already familiar to us or becomes an exercise in a process improvement project that often lacks the input of end users. An example of this scenario is the redesign of patient education material. Without the proper training in person-centered design, a patient educational pamphlet that is not being used is redesigned by the health care system in different colors and in multiple languages, and updated with pictures to reflect the target patient population. The assumptions made here are that patients did not like the black-and-white version and that not all patients speak English, and that they wanted to see other patients that looked like them. These assumptions are made by the redesign team without seeking the input of the end user of the educational material. While the rework is still very important because it addresses important issues, it does not reflect a patient-centered innovative solution.

Innovation is defined in Boxes 23.1 and 23.2. The innovation methodology used in this chapter is design thinking (DT), which involves a framework that guides the user as they work through the five steps within the framework. The five phases are Empathy, Define, Ideate,

> **BOX 23.1 Kaya and Colleagues' Innovation Definition**
>
> Kaya and colleagues (2015) first described innovation as the application of creativity or problem solving that results in a widely adopted strategy, product, or service that meets a need in a new and different way. Innovations are about improvement in quality, cost effectiveness, or efficiency (Kaya et al., 2015).

> **BOX 23.2 Next Level of Innovation Defined**
>
> Innovation is the application of creativity or problem solving that results in a widely adopted strategy, product, technology, or service that meets a need in a new and different way. Innovations are about improvement in quality, cost effectiveness, efficiency, and cost avoidance. There is a need for innovation metrics and new business models that are different from operational models. Solutions cannot be a burden to frontline caregivers. It involves an approach that includes creativity, controlled risk taking, pivoting, and human-centered design with a trauma-informed lens.

Prototype, and Test. The process of DT is more thoroughly explained later in the chapter. Still, the above phases allow you to understand your end user (Empathy) deeply and to better Define the problem you are trying to solve. The correct problem identification then frees you up to create impactful solutions (Ideate) that move you to Prototyping and Testing your solutions. Although this seems like a linear process, it is very much an iterative one because the feedback you get from the Testing phase allows you to go back and continue enhancing your solutions while keeping your end users at the forefront.

It is vital that health care organizations listen, educate, create a pathway, and establish mentorship for nurses to innovate. Nurses are working directly with the patient to improve their health outcomes. This often involves creating new solutions to meet the specific care required by each patient. Patients' needs are varied, and the nurse often must use creative solutions to meet these needs. The problem is that nurses have always thought that is "just" what we do to meet the patient's needs and improve outcomes. Nurses need to be educated about innovation and DT to realize we need to own what we bring to improve health care outcomes that lead to decreased costs.

Some health systems are beginning to understand the need to educate and support innovation by their frontline staff; examples will be discussed later in the chapter. Innovation training should not only be implemented for staff, but equally important, training should take place for the leaders of health systems to support them and provide the resources needed to their staff.

Serious consideration should also be given to adding the innovation methodology to nursing school curricula in both baccalaureate and postbaccalaureate education, as this is the ideal place to start developing skills in innovation. However, educational competencies for educators need to be developed and implemented to accomplish this.

INNOVATION DEFINED

Because most people are unsure of what we mean when we say innovation, perhaps it is best to start by defining the word. See Box 23.1.

Innovation continues to evolve, especially in the health care setting. We propose adding the additions in Box 23.2 to Kaya and colleagues' (2015) definition to remain current.

Just as the definition of innovation continues to evolve, so does DT for healthcare. We are gradually moving from a **user-centered** approach to a **humanity-centered** approach for the collective well-being of society as a whole. What might be desirable and engaging to one end user might not be beneficial to a community or at the societal level. We propose a humanity-centered paradigm that respects human vulnerabilities and builds on values that help people thrive collectively by incorporating additional frameworks from the social sciences (see Fig. 23.1).

INNOVATION TEAMS

To bring the best and most comprehensive solutions forward, teams must be multi/intra/interdisciplinary and diverse in thought, skill set, and experience level. Because patient care is interdisciplinary, teams should also represent a variety of perspectives. Innovative solutions cannot be thought of and implemented in silos. Collaboration between interdisciplinary team members is important to the success of innovative solutions

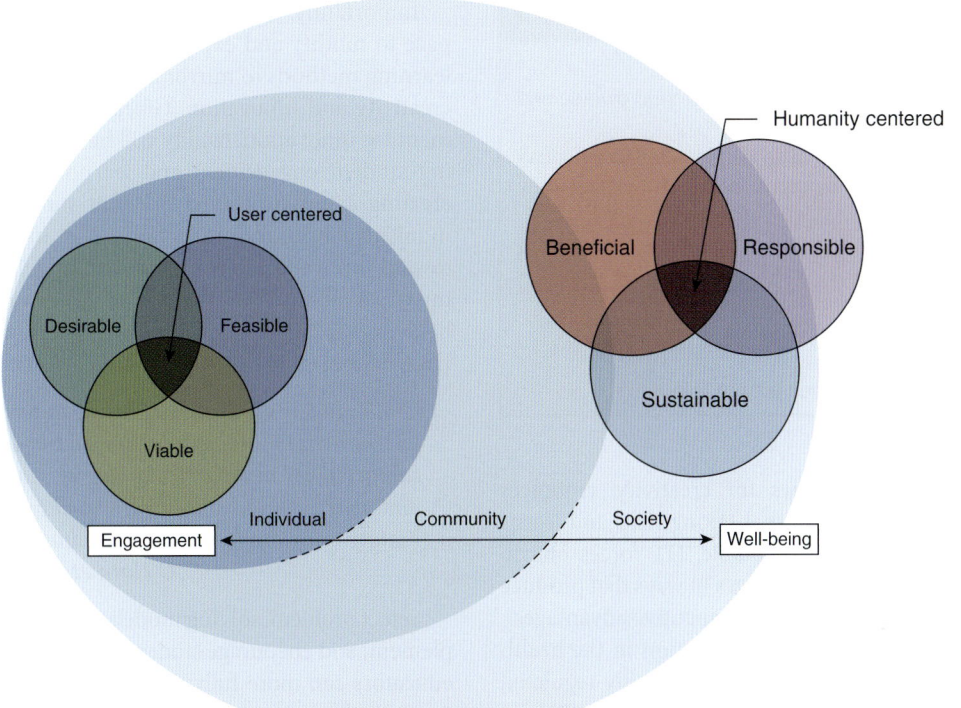

Fig. 23.1 Humanity-Centered Design Thinking. (Adapted from a figure by Rachael Acker. Human-centered AI and experience innovator. Healthero.io.https://www.healthero.io/.)

to improve patient outcomes. Atkinson and colleagues (2022) demonstrated that there is increased learning for innovation by interdisciplinary teams that benefit from a learning ecosystem, including interpersonal/interprofessional, informational, structural, and processual alignment. Examples of this might include bringing the pharmacy team to the table when working on a nurse-led solution in an oncology transfusion unit or bringing biomedical engineers to the team if the solution is a device. It is also highly recommended to bring the patients' perspectives because their experience with their healthcare adds invaluable insights.

Inclusive teams have the potential to evolve high-quality connections when diverse participants are invited to contribute. When they see the best in each other, their thinking becomes more broadened; their action repertoire expands, and they become more engaged and more open to ideas (Dutton, 2003). The end result is solutions of higher caliber.

Teams, however, need to be reminded of engagement principles as they work through the design principles. Some examples are listed in Box 23.3.

INNOVATION METHODOLOGY: DESIGN THINKING

Innovation involves DT, where the first step is the **empathy** phase. This entails digging deeper into the problem, breaking it down from the perspective of the end users, and challenging assumptions. If DT were utilized in the educational pamphlet example, as previously mentioned, one would first try to understand how the patient learns: Do they prefer reading or listening? Do they learn by words or pictures or a mixture? Which is better, paper or a digital format? Once this information has been gathered, the solution will be well investigated and thought out from the patient's perspective and may take a completely different direction from the original idea. See Fig. 23.2.

"Design thinking gets around the human biases (rootedness in the status quo) or attachments to specific behavioral norms ('That's how we do things here') that time and again block the exercise of imagination" (Liedtka, 2023, p. 2). It provides a structure that guides the work for people unfamiliar with innovation. When

> **BOX 23.3 Engagement Principles**
>
> - Incentivize collaboration.
> - Cocreate a vision, the North Star, around diverse and inclusive perspectives.
> - Entertain all ideas because all ideas are good ideas no matter where they come from or how crazy they seem.
> - Be curious. Learn from other industries. Learn from nature.
> - Learn from each other.
> - There is no failure, only lessons.
> - Learn new skills.
> - Let discomfort energize you and lean into it.

fully integrated, DT allows for creativity, embraces ambiguity, and teaches one that taking risks and learning from our failures is acceptable. DT forces one to push knowledge through the stages in ways that produce breakthrough innovations and competitive advantages.

There are many barriers to innovation in the health care setting, which is a very complex, highly regulated system that entails many policies, provides 24/7 care, involves union versus nonunion environments, and is very high stakes because of the potential of hurting a patient. New technologies, such as electronic health records, are constantly changing and often pose an additional burden to the front lines. Finally, no time is dedicated to working on innovative projects. But rather than see these as barriers, by incorporating an innovative mindset, one can instead view these as opportunities. Innovation teaches us to enjoy problems because problems can lead to innovation.

DESIGN THINKING IN THE ACADEMIC AND CLINICAL SETTING

Faculty, students, and graduates of all nursing programs should possess the knowledge and skills needed to address fast-paced technological advancements in both clinical practice and health care delivery models. In response to outsized progress, our leading nursing organizations and associations recognize the urgency of early adaptation of technology and overwhelmingly champion innovative methods that can inspire educators and students as they navigate an increasingly complex and ever-changing health care environment.

Importantly, nursing educators will need to keep pace to modify and expand their current teaching and learning methods to mirror an industry that now prizes creativity and innovation. Given this positive environment for innovation, faculty will be tasked with increasing student engagement and learning experiences by creating a unique framework that supports creativity, inquisitiveness, and reflection. The increasing push toward innovation may be summed up with the following observations from the National Innovation Summit held in 2022, and sponsored by the Royal Technical High School (KTH) Royal Institute of Technology

> *"Both students and faculty must understand and feel the need for innovation. Embedding innovation competencies into curricula, degree requirements, and metrics for advancement would promote integrating innovation into nursing education."*
>
> **O'Hara et al., 2022**, pp. 5–11

Select problem-solving models can help inspire, complement, and encourage student growth, and in this way, educators can more fully understand who our students are and where they are going. Students should graduate with the confidence that they are able to assume leadership roles that incorporate and embrace innovation, even on the graduate nurse level. Educators are critical in helping our future nurses manage the challenges created when healthcare and technology invariably converge.

One demonstrated method to foster creativity and innovation inside and outside the classroom may lie in using DT as it describes a stepwise process of applying **human-centered design** toward problem solving as an innovation tool across various disciplines. Over the last decade, we can trace the DT influence on nursing as educators strive to ensure that future nurses possess the creativity and innovation to tackle the problems facing healthcare today. The American Association of Colleges of Nursing (AACN) promotes creative thinking and empathy as critical nursing skills for both entry-level and advanced practice nursing. In fact, the AACN new *Essentials* outline domains and competencies that formally require the use of creative problem solving to understand specific populations and their focused needs (AACN, 2021). The National Council for the State Boards of Nursing seeks to create a favorable climate for innovation (Ea et al., 2022). Translating DT into clinical experiences may lead to a more creative and innovative approach to patient care.

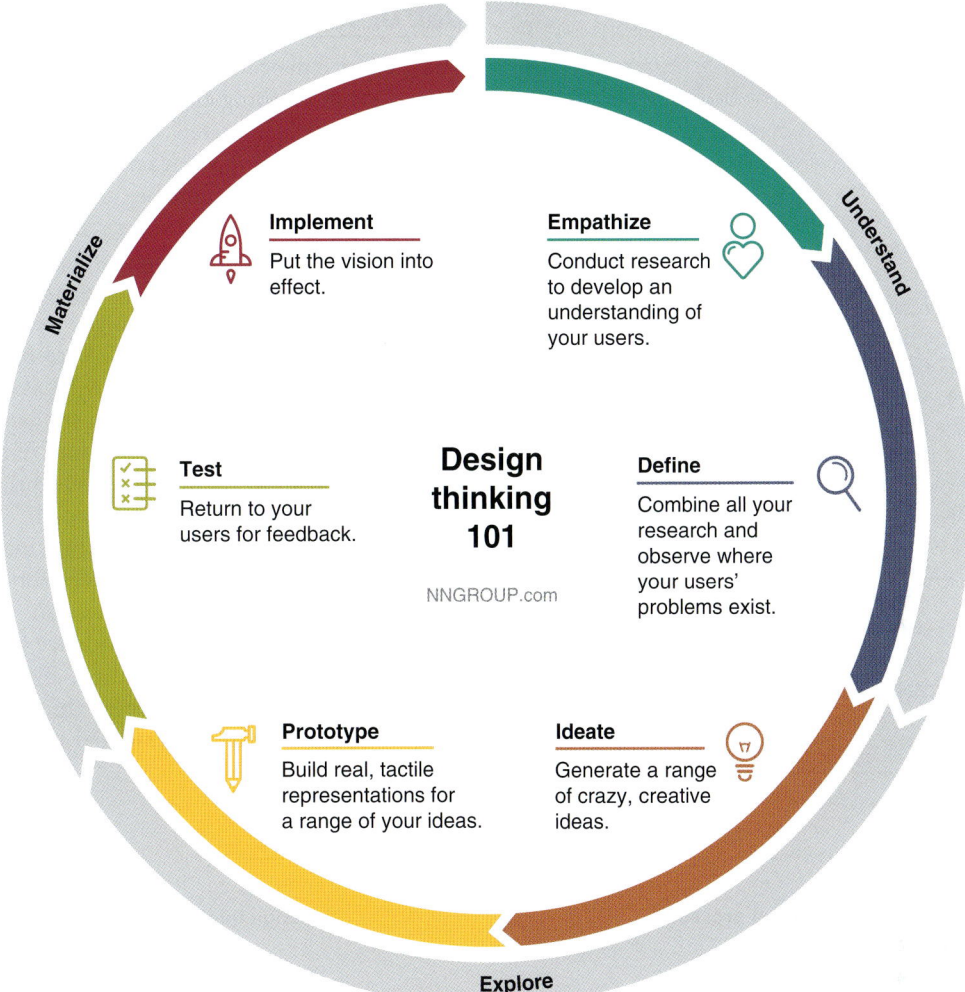

Fig. 23.2 Design Thinking 101. (Adapted from Sarah Gibbons: NN/g Nielsen Norman Group, https://www.nngroup.com/articles/design-thinking/.)

The National Academies of Sciences, Engineering, and Medicine (NASEM) specifically calls on our educators and future nurse leaders to facilitate the creation of innovative approaches by challenging the status quo, breaking down traditional barriers to change, and encouraging team members to solve problems using DT. Identifying best practices and facilitating the translation and adoption of new ideas underpins these recommendations (NASEM, 2021). See additional professional endorsements to use DT in healthcare in Box 23.4.

In many ways, the DT model of problem solving (Empathy, Define, Ideate, Prototype, Test) contrasts strikingly with the nursing process ADPIE (Assess, Diagnose, Plan, Implement, Evaluate) (Fig. 23.3).

Traditional problem solvers start thinking about the right answers to their patient issues. In contrast, design thinkers explore the right questions to ask end users of their proposed solutions. Instead of designing *for* patients, design thinkers manifest solutions with people (Table 23.1).

> **BOX 23.4 Professional Endorsements: Innovation; Design Thinking for Nurses and Healthcare**
>
> - 2008, The American Association of Colleges of Nursing promoted creative thinking and empathy as critical nursing skills
> - 2009, National Council for the State Boards of Nursing sought to create a favorable climate for innovation (NSCBN, 2009).
> - 2016, American Nurses Association's (ANA) white paper *The Innovation Road Map: A Guide for Nurse Leaders* signaled the role of educators to cultivate an innovative workforce prepared to meet the needs of the 22nd century, signifying the importance for undergraduate nursing students to develop competence with design thinking prior to entering the nursing profession
> - 2018, ANA's Quality and Innovation Conference launched their first and nursing's largest ever hackathon involving 800 participants and including the rapid prototyping method of DT
> - 2019, Society of Nurses, Scientists, Innovators, Entrepreneurs, and Leaders launched the first nursing organization solely committed to empower nurses to discover, invent, and pioneer products, processes, services, and platforms

From Ea et al., 2019.

USE OF ARTIFICIAL INTELLIGENCE

The guidance in academia regarding artificial intelligence (AI) in teaching and learning has been to integrate computer-generated information as opposed to banning it. During a hackathon that traditionally used DT to promote human creativity in health-related problem solving, course faculty integrated an AI exercise after students completed the divergent thinking phase. ChatGPT generated content that answered the same "How might we…" question. Human and computer-generated responses were compared to evaluate whether new ideas emerged or if students identified the same or similar solutions. In some groups, human ideation was reinforced by AI content; in others, additional categories of solutions were presented for continued exploration before proceeding to convergent thinking. Students critiqued the AI-generated answers for feasibility, accuracy, and fit to answer the question. They found this exercise increased their confidence that relevant potential solutions were identified. By introducing AI after they completed divergent thinking on their own, human creativity, an essential part of DT, was not impaired.

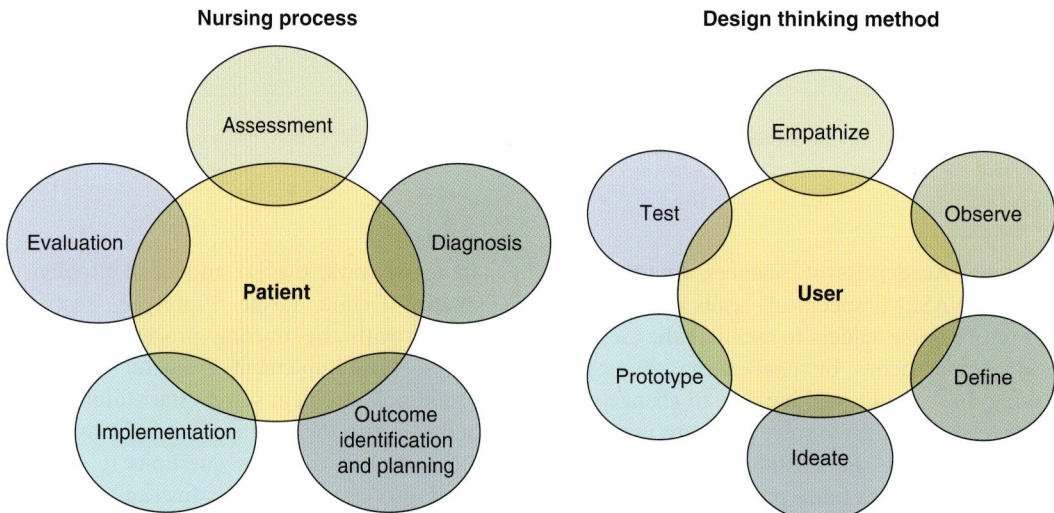

Fig. 23.3 Nursing Process versus Design Thinking Method. (Data from Ea et al., 2019.)

TABLE 23.1 Traditional Problem Solving Versus Design Thinking

How does design thinking work? How does it fit into the nursing process?

Traditional Problem Solving	Design Thinking
What is the right answer?	What is the right question?
Repeatable, proven processes	Intuitive, responsive practice
Design for	Design with
Think for insight	Built for insight
More talk	More listening
Stuck inside	Get outside
Data	Stories
Talk about likes and dislikes	Talk about experiences
Talk about facts	Talk about feelings
Silos	Collaborative
Evolutionary (boring)	Revolutionary (inspiring)

From Ea et al., 2019.

CONTINUE LEARNING

IDEO (combining form of the words "idea," as in "ideology" or "ideogram") the company is a good place to start for those seeking a more formalized way to gain practice and expertise in DT (https://www.ideou.com/products/design-thinking-certificate). The founders of DT built this online educational platform, and it offers several excellent certificate programs in both foundational and advanced DT concepts.

Additional resources around DT education should be sought out, including where to find hackathons and incubators/accelerators, as these activities help develop ideas for prototyping and then how to proceed to the next steps. Broadly defined, startup incubators/accelerators nurture new ideas assisting creative teams in obtaining necessary resources, and ancillary and other services critical to launching the prototype (Pattnaik et al., 2020). A short list of hackathons and incubators is provided (see Table 23.2) for those who would like the immersive, intense experience of a rapid exercise in DT, usually done over a weekend. As a result of attending a hackathon, a nurse's confidence has been shown to increase, allowing the nurse to take on a new venture, startup, or project (Kagan et al., 2023). Although more research is warranted in this area, these initial findings are promising, and hackathons are an excellent venue to explore.

EVIDENCE-BASED PRACTICE, INNOVATION, AND RESEARCH

In healthcare, we care for patients through evidence-based practice (EBP), but an unmet need or gap is discovered that triggers innovation, which can become evidence based. Innovation is the sweet spot before the evidence; therefore, it is important to understand the difference between innovation-based and evidence-based practices. "Innovation involves creating a solution to something when a solution or evidence does not exist (emergent) or modifying an existing solution to make an improvement (incremental or process). In both cases, the innovation brings value to the patient, clinician, health system, or all of the above" (Ackerman et al., 2018, p. 159). The relationship between EBP and innovation has been well described elsewhere (Porter et al., 2017). Innovation and EBP are the building blocks for research. Innovative ideology leads to EBP, opening the doors for original research with a nurse scientist. The authors have experienced the overlap between innovation and research in their work. Still, thought must be given as to where, within the clinical setting, a nurse scientist is available and look to academic partners if a nurse scientist is unavailable. Innovation lays the groundwork for the evidence and keeps clinical practice moving forward as we continuously question the status quo.

TABLE 23.2 Getting Involved and Resources

Innovation	Organization	Website
Accelerators	Launch Lane	https://sciencecenter.org/programs/launch-lane
	Mass Challenge	https://masschallenge.org/
	MCA Americas Nurse Innovator	https://mcamericas.org/innovation/startupsupport/entrepreneurship
	Penn Nursing Innovation Accelerator	https://www.nursing.upenn.edu/innovation/innovation-accelerator/
	Techstars	https://www.techstars.com/accelerator-hub
	Y Combinator	https://ycombinator.com/
Design Thinking (DT)	Design Thinking for Health	http://designthinkingforhealth.org
	IDEO: online learning platform offering certification courses in DT	https://www.ideou.com/products/design-thinking-certificate
Health	Health Design Thinking	https://mitpress.mit.edu/books/health-design-thinking
Entrepreneurship Education	Dreamit	https://www.dreamit.com/
	Drexel University/ Society of Nurses, Scientists, Innovators, Entrepreneurs and Leaders Nurse Innovation & Entrepreneurship Certificate Program	https://drexel.edu/close/programs/sonsiel/
Hackathons	Hack MIT	https://hackmit.org/
	Jefferson Health Hack	https://innovation.jefferson.edu/programs-events/health-hack.html
	MIT Hacking Medicine	https://hackingmedicine.mit.edu/
	NurseHack4Health	https://nursehack4health.org/
	Hacking Health Camp	https://hackinghealth.camp/en/a-propos/
	Junction Hackathon (Europe)	https://www.hackjunction.com/
	Yale Center for Biomedical Innovation & Technology Healthcare Hackathon	www.yalehackhealth.org
Incubators/Innovation	Innovation Design Excellence Awards (IDEA)	https://www.mghpcs.org/Innovations/default.shtml
	JLabs	https://jlabs.jnjinnovation.com/
	Johnson & Johnson Nurse Innovation	https://nursing.jnj.com/innovate-with-us
	Nurse Pitch	https://www.himss.org/globalconference/
	Penn Nursing Innovation	https://www.nursing.upenn.edu/innovation/

From Kagan et al., 2021.

TIP

Using Design Thinking to Create Meaningful Poster Presentations

One method to use both DT and the **nursing process** is to have teams create an evidence-based poster (Fig. 23.4) that delves creatively and deeply into the lived experiences of the population affected by the issue. As teams identify an area of concern and begin a literature search, the first phase of DT begins. Much like the nurse who assesses a new patient, this discovery process involves sensitive inquiry, data collection, and end-user preferences. The design thinker synthesizes subjective and objective findings into a cohesive picture of this patient/user. In this way, a more profound understanding of the problem helps build a relational framework that can scaffold solutions for the best person-centered care.

ADPIE (Assessment): DT (Empathy)

In the Empathy phase, design thinkers create a "persona" that encapsulates people/patients/systems. For example, if the issue is containing and curtailing drug misuse among college students, Billy (persona), fearful of social stigma (Fig. 23.4), may represent a slice of that college's population: a student vulnerable to drug misuse because of stress, environment, and academic pressures. Teams may then develop their poster project using traditional evidence-based methods to disseminate findings as seen through the lens of Billy.

ADPIE (Diagnosis): DT (Defining)

In the second step of DT, the Defining phase, design thinkers try to frame the issue by asking a "How might we..." question. "How might we increase outreach to college students by reducing stigma to seek help and treatment?" Students can benefit from a concentrated class that is designed to mimic a hackathon. Traditionally, hackathons are used to unleash the creative spirit of teamwork and to brainstorm innovative solutions to a set issue, and may last several days (Oyetade et.al., 2022). For this exercise, students work for several hours brainstorming solutions using the next three phases of DT: Ideation, Prototyping, Testing

ADPIE (Nursing Outcome/Planning): DT (Ideation)

The third phase of DT employs the Ideation phase, which uses divergent and convergent thinking to allow design thinkers to stretch their imaginative wings. Divergent thinking asks that you create as many iterations as possible of solutions to the "How might we..." question. Most design thinkers use sticky notes to keep track of these ideas. Nothing is off the table. During one mini-hackathon, this poster group (Fig. 23.5) generated 54 ideas to help Billy. When you use the divergent phase to generate ideas, removing all barriers to possible solutions is critical, so do not say no to any ideas—no "no" judgments, no sarcasm!

- Reply and build on ideas with: "Yes, and...."
- Imagine you have an unlimited budget, time, resources, and possibilities.
- There are no right or wrong ideas.
- Quantity over quality.

Once all ideas are exhausted, move on to the *convergent phase* of Ideation. This phase is about quality over quantity. Start moving your sticky notes into just a few buckets that represent recurring themes. Teams should ask:

- What themes emerged from our brainstorming?
- Are there different categories of ideas that logically organize?
- Which ideas best fit/answer our "How might we..." question?
- Which ideas serve the end user the best?
- Are there any unintended consequences of these ideas?
- Quality over quantity.

In the example provided, this team converged their ideas into three and decided to implement a celebrity ad campaign, a 24-hour anonymous hotline, and Narcan training.

ADPIE (Implementation): DT (Prototyping)

Using the materials at hand, the team designs a simple prototype of the proposed solution (Fig. 23.6). Design thinkers like to use materials found in any kindergarten classroom, modeling clay, crayons, pipe cleaners, etc. The brain works better when the hands are engaged.

- Goal is NOT to create a "perfect" prototype, but simply to create.
- You are looking for something tangible to communicate your idea.

ADPIE (Evaluation): DT: (Testing)

Share your prototype with stakeholders: patients who can identify with your persona, interested health care providers, and financial backers. Incorporate the feedback you receive from your stakeholders into your plan and redesign as needed. The Testing phase corresponds well with the nursing evaluation phase, as the nurse will adjust the plan of care based on patient preferences and provider recommendations. See Tester questions in Box 23.5.

Substance abuse, stigma and pitfalls to seeking treatment
Authors

Background/ overview of topic	Summary/ synthesis of findings	Ethical/moral nursing implications	Health policy implications	Recommendations for practice
Empathy/ persona creation	Define issue with "How might we…?"	Ideation phase	Prototyping of ideas	Testing phase - evaluate and make changes
Billy, 21 yr old college student with substance abuse feels afraid, embarrassed to ask for help	How might we reduce the stigma for substance abuse treatment?	Divergent thinking: 54 ideas generated converged to 3 categories	Social media campaign targeted to unemployed substance abusers under 30 years old - establish hotline	Add feature for caller anonymity

Application of design thinking

Fig. 23.4 Sample Evidence-Based Practice Design Thinking Poster Exercise. (From Boyar, K. (2020). NYU Meyers College of Nursing.)

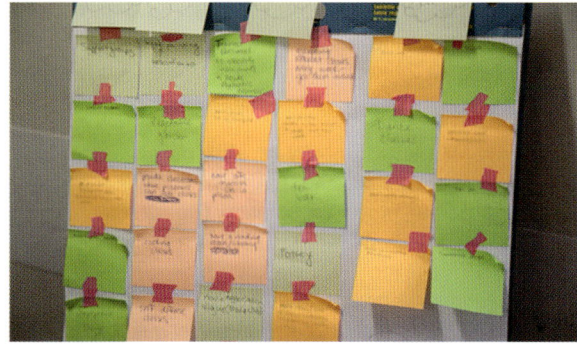

Fig. 23.5 Divergent Thinking: Quantity Over Quality. (From Boyar, K. (2020). NYU Meyers College of Nursing.)

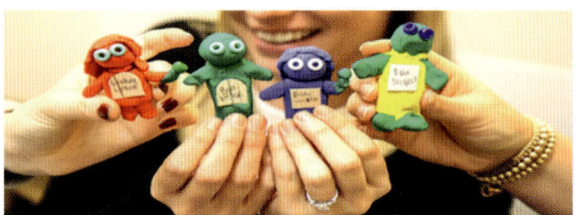

Fig. 23.6 Prototyping a Celebrity Ad Campaign. (From Boyar, K. (2020). NYU Meyers College of Nursing.)

BOX 23.5 Tester Questions

- Does the persona match the solution?
- Did the group clearly and adequately address the issue in their "How might we…?"
- Did the prototype fit the population?
- How soon could the prototype be put into action?
- How pressing is the need for the prototype to be developed and launched?
- Any barriers?
- Any unintended consequences?

NURSING INNOVATION AND TECHNOLOGY

There are many ways for nursing to innovate. Innovation can be device related, technology related, and related to improvement in patient care workflow. Using data and technology is one of the ways nursing needs to be involved in creating innovative tools to impact patient outcomes and decrease health care worker stress and burnout. *The Future of Nursing 2020–2030: Charting a Path to Achieve Health Equity* (NASEM, 2021) recommends "All public and private health care systems should incorporate nursing expertise in designing, generating, analyzing, and applying data to support initiatives focused on social determinants of health and health equity using diverse digital platforms, artificial intelligence, and other innovative technologies (pp. 366–367)."

DATA, INFORMATION, KNOWLEDGE, AND WISDOM FRAMEWORK AND ARTIFICIAL INTELLIGENCE

Nurses must be involved in creating innovative tools that incorporate data and embed nursing wisdom into all technology that comes into contact with patients. Graves and Corcoran (1989) provided the Data-Information-Knowledge-Wisdom (DIKW) Framework (Fig. 23.7) as the first widely accepted framework for nursing informatics.

Clinical decision support (CDS) provides clinicians with computer-generated clinical knowledge and patient-related information that is presented in a timely fashion to enhance patient care (Teich et al., 2005; Whalen et al., 2016; Cato et al., 2020). AI applies advanced analysis and logic-based techniques, including machine learning, to interpret events, support and automate decisions, and take action (Gartner, Inc., 2023). Carroll (2019) states, The technology is designed for decision making to provide person-centered, precision care to improve their experience and engagement, and focus on patient outcomes to affect care quality. AI will enhance CDS tools to provide nursing wisdom (Rossetti et al., 2021). Nurses must be involved in the innovation and design of AI to incorporate real-time data, nursing processes, and nursing and patient workflows. Nurse leaders must analyze practice gaps, and evaluate, design, and advocate for innovating and incorporating tools like CDS/AI to harness nursing wisdom to improve patient outcomes (Whalen et al., 2016). Including nursing input into the content and design promotes nurse autonomy and adherence to evidence-based guidelines. The DIKW Framework can be used to support nurse leaders in innovating and implementing CDS/AI (Whalen et al., 2016; Cato et al., 2020).

The CONCERN (Communicating Narrative Concerns Entered by Registered Nurses) CDS uses AI models, machine learning, and natural language processing to look at patterns of nursing documentation as an indicator of nurses' increased surveillance to predict when patients are at risk of clinical deterioration (Rossetti et al., 2021). See Box 23.6.

Box 23.7 contains some examples of health systems embracing and integrating innovation within their institutions.

MAKERSPACE

A maker's lab, also known as a makerspace or innovation lab, is a dedicated physical space equipped with tools, technologies, and resources that facilitate hands-on learning, experimentation, and the creation of prototypes and projects. These labs, commonly found in schools, libraries, and accessible community areas, encourage experimentation and rapid iteration of

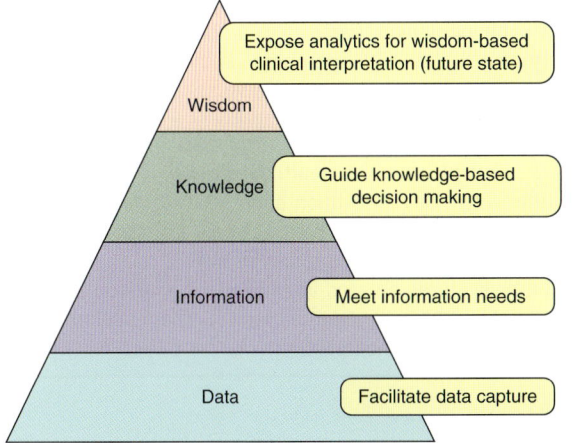

Fig. 23.7 Data-Information-Knowledge-Wisdom (DIKW) Framework. (From Whalen et al., 2016.)

> **BOX 23.6 CONCERN Study**
>
> The Communicating Narrative Concerns Entered by Registered Nurses (CONCERN) study highlights the importance of incorporating the data nurses enter to improve patient outcomes. The CONCERN clinical decision support (CDS) uses AI models, machine learning, and natural language processing to look at patterns of nursing documentation as an indicator of nurses' increased surveillance to predict when patients are at risk of clinical deterioration (Rossetti et al., 2021). The CONCERN study aims to implement and evaluate an early warning score system that provides CDS in electronic health record systems (Rossetti et al., 2021).

BOX 23.7 Examples of Health Systems Embracing Innovation

Innovation at Massachusetts General Hospital (MGH) Through the Center for Innovations in Care Delivery (CICD)

Innovation Design Excellence Awards (IDEA) was established to enhance a culture of innovation and designed to inspire further incubation with the goal to influence practice through interdisciplinary innovation. The process included sending out an email with a call for staff's pain points and their ideas for solutions. A committee was established and composed of nurse scientists, innovation partners, and patient care services leaders to review the applications. A search was done to establish if there were already existing products, ideas, or processes. The committee voted on the ideas that were unique, most needed, and feasible. A $5,000 award was awarded to the two winners. Along with the financial award, the winners worked with innovation mentors in CICD to guide the awardees through the process of innovation. This included establishing the ideas and working with engineers, patent attorneys, innovation specialists, and the industry.

Two awardees:
- Blood Transfer Shield was conceived when the national bio-threat team recognized a gap in drawing pediatric blood and transferring the fluid into another container with no protection
- PegPal was solving the problem of Amyotrophic lateral sclerosis (ALS) patients adjusting to their decline in the feeding process

Ether Dome Challenge for Patient Care Services

The pandemic allowed us to pause the IDEA program and gave us time for reflection. The IDEA program yielded only an average of 27 applications per year and we knew we could do better. We teamed up with the Health Transformation Lab to use their platform that we believed decreased barriers to entry. We called the challenge the Ether Dome Challenge (EDC) after the Ether Dome where the first anesthetic was used on a patient. We provided office hours to answer or assist with the application process. The EDC consisted of four phases. Phase 1 was the ideation phase, which allowed staff to submit their pain points and their ideas for a solution. Phase 2 was the crowd voting phase, which allowed all staff to vote for the pain or solution that resonated with them. This phase differed from the IDEA challenge in that we did not have a committee to select the winners until later in the process. We only asked for a full application if the idea was top-voted from the crowd. In Phase 3 the committee selected the winners from the top-voted ideas. The same support in terms of funding and innovation mentorship was provided to the winning teams as in the IDEA project.

Example awardees:
- A discharge medication solution to address a complex medication adherence for patients being discharged from a hematology-oncology unit
- A solution for both patients and caregivers in monitoring and documenting the intake and output for congestive heart failure patients

Ether Dome Challenge (EDC) for Patient and Family Advisory Councils (PFACs)

We engaged our patients through the same platform and process described with our staff in the previous section. At MGH, there are eight PFACs, which are organized by disease center and location (e.g., Cancer Centers, Emergency Department, Charlestown Healthcare Center). All 110 members across PFACs were invited to participate. Prior to the launch of the EDC, the planning team met with the different PFAC members to gauge their interest. The contest began only after we received buy-in from both patients and their families.

The two winning ideas proposed:
- For children with chronic conditions, a coordinated solution that communicates to patients post discharge who and when to call with the end result of avoiding unnecessary visits to the emergency department
- A resource app that answers parents' questions when their child is in the pediatric intensive care unit

These two teams will have funding and incubation help from the innovation teams. This process has been highly engaging to the PFAC members, as they are now actively involved with devising their own solutions rather than playing a more passive role.

Dartmouth-Hitchcock Health Systems:
- Ran a two-day innovation sprint that yielded two winners and generated buy-in not only from their leadership but internal accelerators as well

Other systems created innovation committees as they begin their journey in identifying how they will integrate innovation within their system.

projects without specific degree prerequisites. Integrating a maker's lab in an innovation program can bring about several benefits:

1. **Rapid Prototyping:** Access to tools like 3D printers, laser cutters, computer numerical control machines, and electronic kits as examples, allow participants to turn their ideas or solutions into tangible prototypes for testing both the concept and the feasibility. This minimally viable solution can then be iterated on in a rapid way from feedback gathered at the testing stage.
2. **Hands-On Learning:** Learning through experience is often more effective than passive methods. Maker's labs offer a practical learning environment where participants can acquire technical skills, develop a deeper understanding of materials and processes, and enhance their problem-solving abilities. Tan and colleagues (2021) showed the aforementioned to be true when they applied 3D-printed models in teaching atrial septal defect against the current passive teaching method.
3. **Risk Reduction:** Designing, prototyping, testing, and refining in a makerspace identifies potential or real issues early on. This helps with risk reduction when changes are more feasible and cost effective.
4. **Inspiration and Motivation:** The physical presence and being surrounded by tools spark motivation and encourage individuals to explore their creativity more actively.

The following are two examples:

- The Studios @ Venture Labs is a collection of workspaces and labs that house digital and analog fabrication technologies that empower the Penn community to make their ideas a reality. https://venturelab.upenn.edu/fabrication-studios.
- Maker Health, originating from the Massachusetts Institute of Technology's Little Devices Lab in 2015, aims to bring the makerspace culture into point-of-care settings with custom tools, equipment, and software. The MakerNurse community, an inventive nursing group within MakerHealth, further expands this approach to the nursing practice worldwide. The first hospital makerspace opened at the University of Texas Medical Branch's hospital makerspace in 2015 in partnership with MakerHealth and with support from the Robert Wood Johnson Foundation. This lab enabled labor and delivery nurses to craft specialized gowns for skin to skin contact, enabled a pathologist to build a remote bacteria culture plate monitoring, and assisted a hospital locksmith in designing a 3D-printed lock-setting www.makerhealth.com.

INTELLECTUAL PROPERTY

"Intellectual property" means inventions, patents, copyrights, trademarks, trade secrets, and any other intellectual or intangible property protected by law. The inventor needs a baseline understanding of the intellectual property and their relationship within the institution and the institution's right over an employee's invention. Some institutions have a **tech transfer** or **innovation office** with which the reader can connect for these policies. If the invention can be commercialized, the process is long, arduous, and complex with lots of moving parts, and professional advice is the recommended pathway.

IMPLICATIONS FOR PRACTICE SETTINGS/NEW MODELS OF CARE

It is important to look at what is happening in the health care industry today as new entrants such as Amazon, Walmart, and Apple are changing the landscape, delivering care to their employees on site and redefining the value as they bring healthcare closer to the patient.

CVS Minute Clinics, Teladoc Health, Calm, and Hospital at Home (delivers acute-level care at home), to name a few, are disrupting care models that make healthcare easier, more affordable, and more humane. These examples also contribute to redefining patient expectations.

We need to ask ourselves how we prepare staff to thrive in these new models of care. Or better yet, those of us in healthcare should be defining and driving the changes in healthcare. We cannot make these disruptive changes without upskilling staff and equipping them with the innovation methodology, including human-centered design and DT. Still, once we do, there are transformative solutions to benefit both the patient and the health system they work in.

When innovation is an expectation and permission is granted to fail and try new ideas safely, we will see the changes we need to see in healthcare.

SYNTHESIS

In conclusion, research, inquiry, curiosity, and framing/defining the problem are important to creative problem solving and designing meaningful and sustainable solutions. Given that our new generation of nurses are expected to function as patient advocates, clinical problem solvers, and innovation leaders in health care delivery models, DT offers a unique, evidence-based problem-solving tool that may help stimulate solutions to better person-/humanity-centered care. Of paramount importance is the early adoption of innovative problem solving by our nursing educators, students, and professional health care teams, and it is key to staying current and ahead of certain changes. DT requires diversity in the team makeup. It is equally important to bring together teams that are diverse in thought, skill sets, and backgrounds. Each differing perspective enriches the team process, especially the solutions. Multifunctional digital platforms, AI, and other innovative technologies, including generative AI applications such as ChatGPT, must be wisely used as we judiciously incorporate their relevance into existing frameworks.

KEY POINTS

- Nurses do not see themselves as innovators and need upskilling despite the constant innovation to provide improved patient outcomes.
- Nurses need mentorship throughout the innovation process. This is new learning for nurses because they have not been exposed to ideas of design, engineering, working with innovation teams, patent attorneys, and industry. This training should ideally begin in school.
- This is an empowering process that brings creativity to the bedside.
- Collaboration among interdisciplinary teams results in high-functioning teams and opens them to new ideas to create even better solutions.
- Innovation requires patience and remaining steadfast to the end goal. It is a long process, and there are many ups and downs through which communication must be done throughout the process.
- What leaders assume are pain points can be verified or corrected by hearing directly from the staff to better align and support their staff.
- Time needs to be given for staff to work on their solutions and not asked to do the work above and beyond their normal schedules.
- Funds must be allocated to allow the solution to mature to a phase where it can be tested and iterated. Even more, funds will be needed to reach a commercialization point.
- Just start somewhere!

REFERENCES

Ackerman, M. H., Porter-O'Grady, T., Malloch, K., & Melnyk, B. M. (2018). Innovation–based practice (IBP) versus evidence–based practice (EBP): A new perspective that assesses and differentiates evidence and innovation. *Worldviews on Evidence-Based Nursing*, *15*(3), 159–160. https://doi.org/10.1111/wvn.1229.

American Association of Colleges of Nursing (AACN). (2021). *The essentials: Core competencies for professional nursing education.* AACN. https://www.aacnnursing.org/Portals/42/AcademicNursing/pdf/Essentials-2021.pdf.

Atkinson, M. K., Benneyan, J. C., Bambury, E., Schiff, G. D., Phillips, R. S., Hunt, L. S., et al. (2022). Evaluating a patient safety learning laboratory to create an interdisciplinary ecosystem for health care innovation. *Health Care Management Review*, *47*(3), E50–E61. https://doi.org/10.1097/hmr.0000000000000330.

Carroll, W. (2019). Artificial intelligence, critical thinking, and the nursing process. *Online Journal of Nursing Informatics*, *23*(1).

Cato, K. D., McGrow, K., & Rossetti, S. C. (2020). Transforming clinical data into wisdom. *Nursing Management*, *51*(11), 24–30.

Dutton, J. E. (2003). *Energize your workplace: How to create and sustain high-quality connections at work.* Jossey-Bass.

Ea, E., Vetter, M. J., Boyar, K., & Keating, S. A. (2022). Using design thinking to thread the social determinants of health in an undergraduate curriculum. *Nurse Educator*, *48*(2), 114–115. https://doi.org/10.1097/nne.0000000000001293.

Gartner, Inc. (2023). *Gartner glossary: Augmented intelligence.* https://www.gartner.com/en/information-technology/glossary/augmented-intelligence#:~:text=Augmented%20intelligence%20is%20a%20design,decision%20making%20and%20new%20experiences.

Graves, J. R., & Corcoran, S. (1989). The study of nursing informatics. *Journal of Nursing Scholarship*, 21(4), 227–231.

Kagan, O., Nadel, H., Littlejohn, J., & Leary, M. (2021). Evolution of nurse-led hackathons, incubators and accelerators from an innovation ecosystem perspective. *Online Journal of Issues in Nursing*, 26(3).

Kagan, O., Sciasci, N. G., Koszalinski, R. S., Kagan, D. H., Leary, M., & Nadel, H. (2023). Nurses' confidence in starting a new venture, startup, or project in the context of nurse-led hackathons: Results of prehackathon survey. *Nursing Outlook*, 71(3):101961. https://doi.org/10.1016/j.outlook.2023.101961.

Kaya, N., Turan, N., & Aydın, G. Ö. (2015). A concept analysis of innovation in nursing. Procedia, Social and Behavioral Sciences. *Innovation-Based Practice (IBP) Versus Evidence-Based Practice (EBP): A New Perspective That Assesses and Differentiates Evidence and Innovation*, 195, 1674–1678. https://doi.org/10.1016/j.sbspro.2015.06.244.

Liedtka, J. (2023). *Why design thinking works Harvard Business Reveiw.* In press, 2023. https://hbr.org/2018/09/why-design-thinking-works.

National Academies of Sciences, Engineering, and Medicine (NASEM). (2021). *The future of nursing 2020–2030: Charting a path to achieve health equity.* National Academies Press. https://doi.org/10.17226/25982.

NCSBN, & The National Council of State Boards of Nursing. (2009). Unlocking the possiblities: The key to regulatory excellence. NSCBN 2009 Annual Meeting. https://www.ncsbn.org/search.page?q=Randolph&filetype=&sitefilter=&metafilter=&page=5. [Accessed 19 August 2024].

O'Hara, S., Ackerman, M. H., Raderstorf, T., Kilbridge, J. F., & Melnyk, B. M. (2022). Building and sustaining a culture of innovation in nursing: Academics, research, policy, and practice: Outcomes of the national innovation Summit. *Journal of Professional Nursing*, 43, 5–11. https://doi-org.proxy.library.nyu.edu/10.1016/j.profnurs.2022.08.001.

Oyetade, K., Zuva, T., & Harmse, A. (2022). Educational benefits of hackathon: A systematic literature review. *World Journal on Educational Technology: Current Issues*, 14, 1668–1684. https://doi.org/10.18844/wjet.v14i6.7131.

Pattnaik, N., Shukla, M., & Pandey, S. C. (2020). Design thinking and startup incubators: Towards a co-creation model for humanizing the new product development process. *Rutgers Business Review*, 5(3), 364–383. https://ssrn.com/abstract=3831676.

Porter-O'Grady, T., & Malloch, K. (2017). Evidence-based practice and the innovation paradigm: A model for the continuum of practice excellence. In S. Davidson, D. Weberg, T. Porter-O'Grady, & K. Malloch (Eds.), *Leadership for evidence-based innovation in nursing and health professions.* Jones and Bartlett Learning.

Rossetti, S. C., Dykes, P. C., Knaplund, C., Kang, M. J., Schnock, K., Garcia, J. P., Jr., et al. (2021). The Communicating Narrative Concerns Entered by Registered Nurses (CONCERN) clinical decision support early warning system: Protocol for a cluster randomized pragmatic clinical trial. *JMIR Research Protocols*, 10(12):e30238. https://doi.org/10.2196/30238. PMID: 34889766; PMCID: PMC8709914.

Tan, H. S., Huang, E., Deng, X., & Ouyang, S. (2021). Application of 3D printing technology combined with PBL teaching model in teaching clinical nursing in congenital heart surgery. *Medicine*, 100(20):e25918. https://doi.org/10.1097/md.0000000000025918.

Teich, J. M., Osheroff, J. A., Pifer, E. A., & Sittig, D. F. (2005). Clinical decision support in electronic prescribing: Recommendations and an action plan. *Journal of the American Medical Informatics Association*, 12(4), 365–376.

Whalen, K., Bavuso, K., Bouyer-Ferullo, S., Goldsmith, D., Fairbanks, A., Gesner, E., et al. (2016). Analysis of nursing clinical decision support requests and strategic plan in a large academic health system. *Applied Clinical Informatics*, 7(2), 227–237. https://doi.org/10.4338/ACI-2015-10-RA-0128. PMID: 27437036; PMCID: PMC4941835.

24

Nursing Informatics

Chin Park and Kathleen Begonia

LEARNING OUTCOMES

After reading this chapter, you should be able to do the following:
- Describe the history of nursing informatics.
- Explain the concept of the Data-Information-Knowledge-Wisdom (DIKW) framework and its application to nursing practice.
- Identify the principles of data analysis and information flow in nursing practice.
- Evaluate the use of data for making choices that affect patient care delivery.
- Describe the practical aspects of nursing support systems for decision making.
- Identify the applications of informatics solutions and technology and their potential in the future of nursing practice.
- Discuss the roles of the nurse informaticist in the health care delivery process.

KEY TERMS

Big data
Care quality
Clinical workflow
Data analytics
Decision support
DIKW (Data-Information-Knowledge-Wisdom)
Future innovation
Interprofessional collaboration
Patient safety
Technology

HISTORICAL BACKGROUND: WHY NURSING INFORMATICS?

The rise and advancement of **technology** transformed healthcare into a constantly evolving landscape. Overwhelmed by the technology, clinicians needed assistance navigating the implementation of electronic health records (EHRs) and harnessing the benefits of real-time data use implications in the delivery of quality care. The increasing need to better understand and manage health care technology gave rise to the field of health care informatics. **Informatics** is the study of how people, technology, and processes are interrelated. The field of health care informatics includes medical informatics, pharmacy informatics, public health informatics, and nursing informatics, to name a few.

Nurses are called on to develop and incorporate technical competencies into their work, which may include the use of telehealth, virtual patient observation monitors, patient portals, digital health tools, and **data analytics**. This chapter focuses on the nursing informatics specialty and its relationship to evidence-based practice (EBP) and health care quality improvement (QI). Nursing expertise is critical to the expansion of designing, generating, analyzing, and applying data to support initiatives focused on social determinants of health and health equity using diverse digital platforms, artificial intelligence, and other innovative technologies

(Wakefield et al., 2021). The goals of nursing informatics are to improve patient care and ensure safe, quality health care delivery by providing digital resources to support and enhance evidence-based nursing practice.

Nursing informatics is a specialty that integrates nursing science, information science, computer science, and cognitive science to assist in managing and communicating data, information, knowledge, and wisdom to support and enhance the quality of nursing practice (American Nurses Association [ANA], 2014; Graves & Corcoran, 1989; McGonigle & Mastrian, 2018). This discipline helps nursing achieve the recommendations of the 2020–2030 Robert Wood Johnson Foundation Future of Nursing Report to develop technical competencies and informatics thought processes to use digital health tools and data analytics appropriately and efficiently.

Domain 8 of the American Association of Colleges of Nursing (AACN) *The Essentials: Competencies for Professional Nursing Education* (2021) encompasses informatics and health care technologies. Information and communication technologies and informatics provide tools to support care, gather data, and form information to drive decision making, and support professionals as they expand knowledge and wisdom for practice. The domain focuses on using informatics to improve delivery of safe, high-quality, and efficient health care services aligned with best practice and regulatory standards (AACN, n.d.). With the increase in evolving health care technologies, all nurses have a responsibility to advocate for equitable access and assist patients with using technology to engage in their care. Patients engaged with health care technology have the potential to improve their overall health outcomes.

Table 24.1 displays the entry-level and advanced-level nursing education competencies, as well as relevant examples next to each competency. The entry-level nurse identifies the various types of technology available

TABLE 24.1 AACN Essentials Domain 8: Core Competencies for Professional Nursing Education (2021) With Examples

Entry-Level Professional Nursing Education	Example	Advanced-Level Nursing Education	Example
8.1 Describe the various information and communication technology tools used in the care of patients, communities, and populations.			
8.1a Identify the variety of information and communication technologies used in care settings.	The nurse identifies Epic as an EHR and the Zoom phone system as a method to communicate.	8.1g Identify best evidence and practices for the application of information and communication technologies to support care.	The nurse will communicate with peers, review the literature, and identify technology that has best supported clinical workflows.
8.1b Identify the basic concepts of electronic health, mobile health, and telehealth systems for enabling patient care.	The nurse defines what an EHR is and capabilities of telehealth programs.	8.1h Evaluate the unintended consequences of information and communication technologies on care processes, communications, and information flow across care settings.	The nurse understands that there are risks associated with information systems; for example, clinical staff may forget about downtime paper processes for clinical documentation if an EHR becomes unexpectedly unavailable.
8.1c Effectively use electronic communication tools.	The nurse uses Vocera devices and Zoom phones to make calls.	8.1i Propose a plan to influence the selection and implementation of new information and communication technologies.	The nurse develops or joins a steering committee to discuss new health technology introduced into the health system.

TABLE 24.1 AACN Essentials Domain 8: Core Competencies for Professional Nursing Education (2021) With Examples—cont'd

Entry-Level Professional Nursing Education	Example	Advanced-Level Nursing Education	Example
8.1d Describe the appropriate use of multimedia applications in healthcare.	The nurse understands how multimedia can be used to help improve patient health, such as by posting general information that can educate patients.	8.1j Explore the fiscal impact of information and communication technologies on healthcare.	The nurse understands the impact of regulations, such as the HIPAA Privacy Rule, on scenarios where clinicians overshare on social media.
8.1e Demonstrate best practice use of social networking applications.	The nurse keeps patient information confidential and does not overshare patient health information on social media.	8.1k Identify the impact of information and communication technologies on workflow processes and health care outcomes.	The nurse is aware of the multitude of information available to patients online and in the media and is prepared to navigate complex patient questions that may include false information.
8.1f Explain the importance of nursing engagement in the planning and selection of health care technologies.	The nurse describes how they can be engaged as super users and inspire adoption of the EHR.		
8.2 Use information and communication technology to gather data, create information, and generate knowledge.			
8.2a Enter accurate data when chronicling care.	The nurse validates accuracy of patients' vital sign data in the EHR.	8.2f Generate information and knowledge from health information technology databases.	The nurse is able to formulate appropriate plans of care for patients based on information in the EHR.
8.2b Explain how data entered on one patient impacts public and population health data.	The nurse describes how patient data entered in the EHR, if patient consents, can be used to help improve development of treatment and plans of care.	8.2g Evaluate the use of communication technology to improve consumer health information literacy.	The nurse surveys patients to determine if patient portals or emails with health information are easy to understand or helpful for patients.
8.2c Use appropriate data when planning care.	The nurse looks at relevant data in the EHR or medical devices (glucometer) to make decisions on patient care.	8.2h Use standardized data to evaluate decision making and outcomes across all systems levels.	The nurse looks at EHR reports to evaluate patient outcomes.
8.2d Demonstrate the appropriate use of health information literacy assessments and improvement strategies.	The nurse assesses health information literacy in patient populations and determines appropriate methods of teaching patients based on literacy level.	8.2i Clarify how the collection of standardized data advances the practice, understanding, and value of nursing and supports care.	The nurse questions when data are not standardized in the EHR. For example, if abdominal pain is documented as "abd pain" or "GI pain," the nurse raises awareness to the team about how the inconsistencies in documentation can impact EHR reports.

Continued

TABLE 24.1 AACN Essentials Domain 8: Core Competencies for Professional Nursing Education (2021) With Examples—cont'd

Entry-Level Professional Nursing Education	Example	Advanced-Level Nursing Education	Example
8.2e Describe the importance of standardized nursing data to reflect the unique contribution of nursing practice.	The nurse describes and uses nursing documentation standards, such as the Clinical Care Classifications terminology, to ensure clear communication of care.	8.2j Interpret primary and secondary data and other information to support care.	The nurse reviews data collected and shared by the care team to make decisions on the patient's plan of care.
8.3 Use information and communication technologies and informatics processes to deliver safe nursing care to diverse populations in a variety of settings.			
8.3a Demonstrate appropriate use of information and communication technologies.	The nurse uses the EHR in real time to document patient care and hospital-issued Zoom phones to communicate with the clinical team.	8.3g Evaluate the use of information and communication technology to address needs, gaps, and inefficiencies in care.	The nurse uses reporting tools and dashboards to determine if technology being used is helpful.
8.3b Evaluate how decision support tools impact clinical judgment and safe patient care.	The nurse assesses warning alerts when scanning patient wristbands and medications to ensure safe patient care.	8.3h Formulate a plan to influence decision-making processes for selecting, implementing, and evaluating support tools.	The nurse partners with informatics and IT to develop a technology steering committee that evaluates support tools.
8.3c Use information and communication technology in a manner that supports the nurse–patient relationship.	When using point-of-care devices with the patient, the nurse will explain the rationale behind the use of that technology, so the patient understands.	8.3i Appraise the role of information and communication technologies in engaging the patient and supporting the nurse–patient relationship.	The nurse evaluates the usefulness of technology's impact on patient engagement.
8.3d Examine how emerging technologies influence health care delivery and clinical decision making.	The nurse will participate in discussions with colleagues about how technology is impacting care.	8.3j Evaluate the potential uses and impact of emerging technologies in healthcare.	The nurse will participate in a pilot of AI health care technology and provide feedback to the hospital and vendor about the device.
8.3e Identify impact of information and communication technology on quality and safety of care.	The nurse sees the impact of publicly shared information on social media platforms on patient education.	8.3k Pose strategies to reduce inequities in digital access to data and information.	The nurse will lobby or work with government officials to develop a plan to ensure all patients have digital access to their health information.

TABLE 24.1 AACN Essentials Domain 8: Core Competencies for Professional Nursing Education (2021) With Examples—cont'd

Entry-Level Professional Nursing Education	Example	Advanced-Level Nursing Education	Example
8.3f Identify the importance of reporting system processes and functional issues (error messages, misdirections, device malfunctions, etc.) according to organizational policies and procedures.	The nurse will know the process for reporting system issues and who to contact if an error message appears on the EHR or medical device used to care for a patient.		
8.4 Use information and communication technology to support documentation of care and communication among providers, patients, and all system levels.			
8.4a Explain the role of communication technology in enhancing clinical information flows.	The nurse describes how to use Epic secure chat to communicate with the providers.	8.4e Assess best practices for the use of advanced information and communication technologies to support patient and team communications.	The nurse, along with an interdisciplinary team, utilizes a collaborative flowsheet in the EHR to determine effective plan of care.
8.4b Describe how information and communication technology tools support patient and team communications.	The nurse uses the Epic rover to receive critical alerts from the patient telemetry monitors.	8.4f Employ electronic health, mobile health, and telehealth systems to enable quality, ethical, and efficient patient care.	The nurse reviews the EHR to discuss plan of care with a patient through a telemedicine call.
8.4c Identify the basic concepts of electronic health, mobile health, and telehealth systems in enabling patient care.	The nurse differentiates among the different informatics tools when providing care to patients.	8.4g Evaluate the impact of health information exchange, interoperability, and integration to support patient-centered care.	The nurse is able to provide seamless care through the use of an integrated EHR.
8.4d Explain the impact of health information exchange, interoperability, and integration on healthcare.	The nurse explains to the patient the importance of integrated health care systems to provide efficient patient care. The nurse shows the patient that discharge instructions are available on the patient's portal.		

Continued

TABLE 24.1 AACN Essentials Domain 8: Core Competencies for Professional Nursing Education (2021) With Examples—cont'd

Entry-Level Professional Nursing Education	Example	Advanced-Level Nursing Education	Example
8.5 Use information and communication technologies in accordance with ethical, legal, professional, and regulatory standards, and workplace policies in the delivery of care.			
8.5a Identify common risks associated with using information and communication technology.	The nurse sees a coworker's computer screen left alone with patient data displayed and informs the coworker about the risks of displaying personal health information within view of bystanders.	8.5g Apply risk mitigation and security strategies to reduce misuse of information and communication technology.	The nurse uses two-factor authentication to log in to the work-issued laptop at home to document on a patient's electronic chart.
8.5b Demonstrate ethical use of social networking applications.	The nurse does not share patient interactions or photos with patients on Facebook.	8.5h Assess potential ethical and legal issues associated with the use of information and communication technology.	The nurse reviews the HIPAA Privacy Rule and implications with social media.
8.5c Comply with legal and regulatory requirements while using communication and information technologies.	The nurse does not use HIPAA noncompliant technology to communicate with providers and colleagues.	8.5i Recommend strategies to protect health information when using communication and information technology.	The nurse will collaborate with IT by recommending device time-out times to log staff out of a device that is left idle. This is to prevent bystanders from accessing patient information.
8.5d Educate patients on their rights to access, review, and correct personal data and medical records.	The nurse will educate a patient on how to use the patient portal to track and manage health information.	8.5j Promote patient engagement with their personal health data.	The nurse will talk to patients on follow-up visits about the patient portal and encourage use of the portal.
8.5e Discuss how clinical judgment and critical thinking must prevail in the presence of information and communication technologies.	The nurse will speak with colleagues about the importance of using critical thinking to determine if technology is useful for patient care and discuss ways to improve with IT.	8.5k Advocate for policies and regulations that support the appropriate use of technologies impacting healthcare.	The nurse will advocate and work with law makers to establish and enforce regulations that protect patient information.
8.5f Deliver care using remote technology.	The nurse interacts with patients through telehealth visits on Zoom (video conferencing).	8.5l Analyze the impact of federal and state policies and regulation on health data and technology in care settings.	The nurse is aware of policies enacted by Centers for Medicare and Medicaid Services on how telehealth services are provided.

AACN, American Association of Colleges of Nursing; *AI*, artificial intelligence; *EHR*, electronic health record; *HIPAA*, Health Insurance Portability and Accountability Act; *IT*, information technology.
Adapted from AACN, 2021.

to support patient care, while the advanced-level nurse understands the various technologies but critically thinks about the use-case and ways to optimize how technology is used to support care.

HISTORY OF NURSING INFORMATICS IN EDUCATION

Nursing informatics, as a field of study and practice, developed in the United States as computer technology was introduced into health care settings and the need arose to manage large amounts of patient data. The ANA recognized nursing informatics as a specialty in 1992 (Harrington, 2015), and the field has since grown to encompass a wide range of roles and responsibilities within health care organizations. Today, nursing informatics professionals work to ensure the effective use of technology and data in health care delivery, with a focus on improving patient outcomes, streamlining clinical workflows, and enhancing the overall quality and delivery of evidence-based care.

The history of nursing informatics education in the United States can be traced back to the 1970s when nurses first began to use computers for administrative purposes such as patient scheduling and record keeping. However, it was not until the 1980s and early 1990s that nursing informatics as a specialized field of study began to emerge (Ozbolt & Saba, 2008).

During this time, nursing informatics education programs were developed and offered at various universities across the country. These programs aimed to equip nurses with the necessary knowledge and skills to effectively use information technology in health care settings, improve patient outcomes, and enhance the overall quality of care provided. As technology continued to advance and EHRs became more prevalent, the demand for nursing informatics professionals grew.

Today, nursing informatics education programs continue to evolve and expand in response to the ever-changing health care landscape. Many nursing schools now offer specialized courses and degree programs in nursing informatics, ranging from undergraduate to doctoral levels. Additionally, organizations such as the American Nurses Credentialing Center (ANCC) and the Healthcare Information and Management Systems Society (HIMSS) have established competencies and certification programs to ensure that nurses have the necessary skills and knowledge to effectively navigate and leverage technology in health care settings (ANCC, n.d.; HIMSS, n.d.).

As the health care industry continues to become increasingly reliant on technology, nursing informatics education will undoubtedly continue to play a critical role in preparing nurses for the challenges and opportunities of the future. An example of nursing informatics application in nursing is the use of simulation software to educate nursing students. Simulation software allows students to practice vital nursing skills in a virtual environment, and simulated scenarios with high-fidelity manikins can replicate real-life scenarios. This provides nursing students with a safe and controlled setting to develop their skills, without the risk of harming patients.

One immersive tool for potential use in simulation education is virtual reality (VR) (Choi et al., 2022). Lifelike clinical scenarios can be recreated by VR, and nursing students can practice various interventions and procedures. The simulations can include scenarios like patient assessment, wound care, and medication administration. The students can interact with virtual patients, monitor patient vital signs, and make decisions within a safe and controlled environment.

Nursing informatics can also be applied in education using EHRs as a tool for teaching students. They can provide hands-on experience with real-world documentation practices using simulated patient data. Nursing students can review patient histories, track vital signs, and practice charting patient data and documenting patient care workflows (e.g., assessment, care planning, medication administration). In cases with simulation centers that have installed real EHR systems (e.g., Epic), students would receive relevant training on systems utilized in actual health care systems.

Other examples include the use of online learning platforms or educational apps that incorporate nursing informatics concepts, such as data management and analysis. Additionally, nursing informatics can be integrated into education through teleconferencing technologies, which allow for remote learning and virtual clinical experiences. Learning management systems (LMSs) are used in integrated health care systems to support education, training, and professional development utilizing a centralized platform. The LMS can provide a repository of continuing education, certification, and compliance courses, and tracking of earned credits can help with licensing and certification requirements. The health care organization can use the LMS to promote research literacy with training on data analysis, research methodologies, and EBPs, and clinicians can also access resources with the latest research findings. The LMS can also be used to provide performance evaluations and feedback and identify areas for improvement.

At Mount Sinai Health System, the Portal for Education and Advancement of Knowledge (PEAK) system is used for staff education (Icahn School of Medicine at Mount Sinai, n.d.). It allows all staff, clinical and nonclinical, to access and complete required training modules, such as annual mandatory education and other education required per job role. It helps track and manage training. Nurses can access EHR training on the PEAK website, and once they complete the training for their particular role, the tracking program notifies the EHR technical team to create a user ID and profile for their role. For example, emergency department nurses will complete EHR emergency department education on PEAK to understand clinical documentation associated with their new role, and once they complete the PEAK module, the EHR technical team grants access. These are similar to learning management systems, because PEAK has a collection of PowerPoint slideshow modules and quizzes.

DATA-INFORMATION-KNOWLEDGE-WISDOM

The Data-Information-Knowledge-Wisdom (DIKW) framework is the backbone of nursing practice and lays the groundwork for nursing informatics. It originated in the field of computer and information science as a subspecialty of knowledge management (Garcia-Dia, 2019; Nelson, 2020). Data are comprised of simple words and numbers; when data are labeled or defined, they become information. Nurses gather data and information when they assess their patients and draw on knowledge from their formal education and past experiences to determine a plan of care for their patients. As seen in Fig. 24.1, the DIKW framework is depicted as a battery composed of the DIKW concepts that build on each other, ultimately "charging" up to wisdom, which is the full potential (i.e., full battery/full charge).

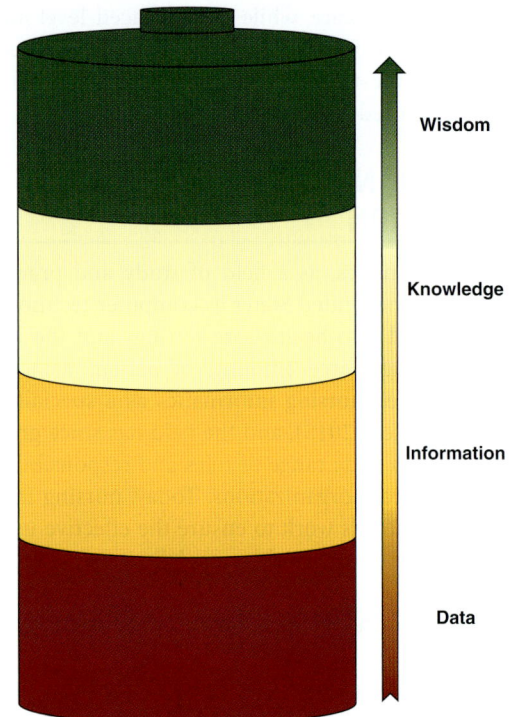

Fig. 24.1 Adapted Data-Information-Knowledge-Wisdom (DIKW) Framework Model. (Data from McGonigle et al., 2018.)

That full potential (wisdom) is the ideal position from which the nurse can make important decisions. The color gradient illustrates the constantly progressive process of building up from data to wisdom. It also represents this process as a continuum, with nurses advancing their decision-making skills in various aspects of patient care, and for any given situation, the "charge" level will move up or down based on their progression in that area.

Novice nurses start their journey through the DIKW continuum by understanding the importance of basic data and information. As they learn about the patients for whom they care with their preceptors and through continuing education, they build on their knowledge base. Wisdom is seen in experienced nurses who are able to synthesize knowledge and experience to make insightful clinical decisions. Expert nurses critically think through different scenarios to recognize symptoms of certain disease processes and anticipate patients' needs. The integration of EBP in clinical practice would be an example of wisdom on the DIKW framework (Table 24.2).

TABLE 24.2 Data-Information-Knowledge-Wisdom (DIKW)

Terms	Definition	Example	Informatics Example
DATA	Raw facts	87, blue	Raw data entered into the EHR
INFORMATION	Raw fact defined	87 beats per minute, blue lips	Organized and defined data points in patient's EHR
KNOWLEDGE	Interrelated information	Understanding that blue lips may indicate the patient is cyanotic	Clinical decision support systems developed based on EBP
WISDOM	Applying knowledge and experience to problem solve	Assessing for breathing and providing oxygen to patient with cyanosis	Using critical thinking skills to determine if a clinical decision support recommendation is appropriate for patient's situation

EBP, Evidence-based practice; *EHR*, electronic health record.

TIP

Nurse Jon considers the trends in vital sign data of his patient, as well as his knowledge of EBP from nursing school and experience in caring for patients, to determine an appropriate plan of care. The DIKW framework is at work here because data are the numerical values of the vital signs (84/52, 110, 104, 22). When these numbers are labeled, they become information (blood pressure: 84/52; heart rate: 110; temperature: 104 degrees Fahrenheit; respiratory rate: 22). He draws on his knowledge from his nursing education and past experiences caring for patients to make clinical decisions with wisdom.

PRINCIPLES OF NURSING INFORMATICS—SCOPE AND STANDARDS OF PRACTICE

Nursing informatics provides electronic decision support tools to clinicians to support documentation and enhance the care they provide. The tools allow them to make quick decisions based on the data pulled from bedside devices and applications, and within the context of EBP, they can take actions within the EHR (e.g., initiate sepsis screenings/alerts, stroke order sets, escalation pathways, etc.).

Early on, many nurses found themselves in the role of informaticist by accident or through curiosity (McGonigle & Mastrian, 2018). Competencies of nurses should include technical skills to ensure they are able to use electronic tools constantly introduced in the clinical setting. Roles of advanced practice nurses have evolved to include titles such as: project manager, consultant, educator, researcher, product developer, advocate, policy developer, clinical analyst, system specialist, entrepreneur, and business relationship manager. The combination of nursing experience and knowledge of technology is vital in providing education to staff, leading and supporting technological projects, and providing recommendations for enhancing and transforming healthcare.

Along with the evolution of technology, the role of the nursing informaticist has evolved over the years. The 1992 first edition of the standards included only *data, information, knowledge,* and in 2009, it grew to include *wisdom* (Bickford, 2009). The scope of practice statement provides answers to the "who," "what," "when," "where," "how," and "why" questions about nursing informatics. The scope and standards of practice evolved over time with the help of the ANA committee. It is critical these are constantly reviewed and updated to reflect current practice and advances in technology. The standards content presented in Table 24.3 presents each of the standards of practice and professional performance. The standards of practice reflect the incorporation of the nursing process within nursing informatics (NI) practice, while the professional performance standards address education, professional practice evaluation, quality of practice, collegiality, collaboration, ethics, research, resource utilization, advocacy, and leadership.

In 2006, the Technology Informatics Guiding Education Reform (TIGER) Initiative convened a summit of nursing stakeholders to develop, publish, and commit to an action plan to make healthcare safer, more effective, efficient, patient centered, timely, and equitable (Sensmeier et al., 2017). TIGER is focused on education reform and interprofessional community development

TABLE 24.3 ANA Scope and Standards of Practice (3rd edition)

Standards of Nursing Informatics Practice

Standard	Concept	Definition
Standard 1	Assessment	The informatics nurse collects comprehensive data and information through a variety of assessment methods, including assessment algorithms like the PIECES framework, workflow analysis, and interviews, that help define the issue or problem.
Standard 2	Diagnosis, Problems, and Issues Identification	The informatics nurse analyzes assessment data to identify problems, issues, and opportunities for improvement.
Standard 3	Outcomes Identification	The informatics nurse identifies and documents specific expected outcomes for an individualized plan to address an issue.
Standard 4	Planning	Considering clinical and business impact, the informatics nurse develops a comprehensive plan to meet expected outcomes.
Standard 5	Implementation	The informatics nurse partners with the health care team to implement a plan within budget and plan requirements.
Standard 5a	Coordination of Activities	The informatics nurse provides leadership by coordinating and documenting activities within the project plan.
Standard 5b	Health Teaching and Health Promotion	The informatics nurse introduces informatics solutions focused on education to promote health outcomes.
Standard 6	Evaluation	The informatics nurse evaluates progress toward attainment of expected outcomes.

Standards of Professional Performance for Nursing Informatics

Standard	Concept	Definition
Standard 7	Ethics	The informatics nurse practices ethically by practicing in a manner that preserves and protects health care consumer autonomy, dignity, and rights.
Standard 8	Culturally Congruent Practice	The informatics nurse considers culture and incorporates a spirit of diversity, equity, and inclusion when developing informatics solutions for healthcare.
Standard 9	Communication	The informatics nurse communicates effectively in a variety of methods (phone call, text, email), depending on consumer preferences, in all areas of practice.
Standard 10	Collaboration	The informatics nurse collaborates with others to effect change and produce positive outcomes through sharing of data, information, and knowledge.
Standard 11	Leadership	The informatics nurse demonstrates leadership by promoting the organization's strategic plan, mentoring colleagues, and influencing decision-making bodies to improve professional practice.
Standard 12	Education	The informatics nurse attains knowledge and competence that reflect current nursing and informatics practice by participating in ongoing educational opportunities, such as attending conferences and reading journals.
Standard 13	Evidence-Based Practice and Research	The informatics nurse integrates evidence and research findings into practice by using data to communicate evidence and sharing research findings with colleagues.
Standard 14	Quality of Practice	The informatics nurse collects and analyzes data to formulate recommendations to improve quality and effectiveness of nursing and informatics practice.
Standard 15	Professional Practice Evaluation	The informatics nurse engages in self-evaluation of practice regularly and participates in peer review to improve practice.
Standard 16	Resource Utilization	The informatics nurse uses appropriate resources to plan and implement informatics solutions that are safe, effective, and fiscally responsible.
Standard 17	Environmental Health	The informatics nurse assesses and advocates for appropriate use of environmentally safe products in healthcare.

ANA, American Nurses Association.

to help drive innovation and technology on a global level. The spirit of TIGER is to maximize the seamless integration of technology and informatics into nursing practice, education, and research. In order to equip every practicing nurse with informatics competencies, TIGER developed recommendations in the areas of basic computer competencies, information literacy, and information management. The TIGER International Competency Synthesis Project aims to investigate global informatics requirements in relation to core competencies to match them with national and regional needs. Informatics competencies have evolved to include project management skills, business relationship management, and administrative management skills.

In 2014, TIGER transitioned to HIMSS and shifted to a new interdisciplinary approach to managing healthcare with a broader range of health care professionals. With the incorporation of *interprofessional collaboration*, more global perspectives are included in informatics competencies.

As part of the TIGER Initiative, collaborative teams formed to accelerate the action plan within nine key topic areas. All teams worked on identifying best practices from both education and practice related to their topic, so that this knowledge can be shared with others interested in enhancing the use of information technology (IT) capabilities for nurses. Each collaborative team researched their subject with the perspective of, "What does every practicing nurse need to know about this topic?" The teams identified resources, references, gaps, and areas that need further development and provided recommendations for the industry to accelerate the adoption of IT for nursing (Table 24.4).

> **TIP**
>
> An example competency evaluation statement to assess a nurse's basic computer skills is: "I am able to work with peripheral devices (e.g., scanners and printers)." If the nurse is not comfortable with using scanners or printer hardware, this may impact their ability to use point-of-care devices, like barcode medication scanners or lab specimen label printers. They may require additional training or elbow-to-elbow support to improve their skills.

> **TIP**
>
> Another example competency evaluation statement to assess nurses' informatics knowledge is: "I am able to collect data and document information related to clinical care." Nurses need to demonstrate the ability to gather data from various clinical devices and document data in the EHR so they can create comprehensive treatment plans and improve outcomes.

DATA USE AND EVALUATION

Nursing practice involves caring for highly complex patient populations with specific disease processes. While it is important to understand the pathophysiology and treatment options available, it is also critical to understand trends in populations to enhance the overall plan of care. Informatics tools, specifically data mining concepts, provide important support to nurses' decision-making processes.

TABLE 24.4 TIGER Competencies Methodology

TIGER Component	Standard	Standard-Setting Source	Example
Basic Computer Competencies	European Computer Driving License	European Computer Driving License Foundation (www.ecdl.org)	Nurses using the computer and managing files in word processing applications
Information Literacy	Information Literacy Competency Standards	American Library Association (www.ala.org)	Nurses educating patients on where to find health information online
Information Management	(Utilizes two standards) 1. EHR Functional Model—Clinical Care Components 2. International Computer Driving License—Health	1. Health Level Seven (HL7) (www.hl7.org) 2. European Computer Driving License Foundation (www.ecdl.org)	Nurses entering vital sign documentation in the EHR

EHR, Electronic health record; *TIGER*, Technology Informatics Guiding Education Reform.

Data mining utilizes algorithms to generate actionable insights and identify patterns and relationships from large data sets, which can enhance clinical workflow and **patient safety**. Knowledge Discovery in Databases (KDD) is the very basis of most data mining concepts and involves identifying correlations or patterns within data that are hidden in large relational databases. Data are analyzed from different perspectives and categorized, and relationships among data are identified.

Developed in 2000, CRISP-DM is a more refined version of KDD and assists those interested in data mining large data sets. It is widely used today. All the data mining concepts have the common goal of identifying and eliminating problems, improving processes, and achieving better outcomes; however, the approach varies. All expect feedback at each step of the process. Table 24.5 provides an overview of some of the most common data mining concepts and relevant use cases.

When trends are identified and a quality improvement plan to change practice is developed and executed, the change in practice should be evaluated. Plan-Do-Study-Act (PDSA) is a methodology that can be used to test processes that are implemented. The four steps guide the thinking process into breaking down the task into steps and then evaluating the outcome, improving it, and testing again (Institute for Healthcare Improvement, n.d.). This is relevant for many of the informatics changes that are implemented. For example, after implementing an electronic sepsis order set, which is a clinical decision support tool that allows for the quick entry of electronic orders for an evidence-based sepsis protocol, PDSA can be used to study and refine the treatment of sepsis patients and measure their outcomes.

Though we have these popular data mining concepts in place, it is important to consider the implications of big data, artificial intelligence, and technological advancements and their effects on understanding nursing trends. These technological advancements and the accumulation of large amounts of data can impact data mining processes and how we approach data. Although these data modeling concepts exist to improve inefficiencies, without support from management and key stakeholders, process improvement would be very difficult.

TABLE 24.5 Data Mining Concepts

Data Mining Concept	Definition	Example
CRISP-DM (Cross-Industry Standard Process for Data Mining)	Designed in a cyclic iterative loop that allows movement back and forth between phases for continuous review. It provides an overview of data mining life cycle.	Project to predict hospital length of stay based on indicators that are commonly used for hospitalization (e.g., gender, age, admitting diagnosis)
Six Sigma DMAIC (Define, Measure, Analyze, Improve and Control)	Focuses on discrepancies between the data and the current process to implement successful solutions	**Define:** Improve clinic patient's waiting time to max of 15 minutes. **Measure:** Quantify the problem. What are the bottlenecks in the process? **Analyze:** Analyze the data; identify the root cause of the problem. **Improve:** Implement and verify the solution. **Control:** Maintain the solution.
SEMMA (Sample, Explore, Modify, Model, and Assess)	Explores, analyzes, and groups data to predict outcomes	**Sample:** Choose a subset of data (e.g., review only readmissions for congestive heart failure patients; subset of all cardiac patients). **Explore:** Utilize statistical analyses. **Modify:** Parse and clean the data. **Model:** Create a projected model of possible outcomes. **Assess:** Review how useful and relevant the model is for the topic; test it with the problem statement in mind.

> **TIP**
>
> Hospitals that attain ANCC Magnet status demonstrate their commitment to excellent nursing care (ANA, 2017). Magnet-designated hospitals were more likely than non-Magnet hospitals to attest to meaningful use with their EHR adoption (Lippincott et al., 2017). Hospitals can meet meaningful use criteria by ensuring that the certified EHR is used in a way that improves safety, quality, efficiency, and health care outcomes. Metrics of meaningful use are nursing sensitive or dependent on nursing documentation—for example, prioritizing meeting a meaningful use measure of continuity of care document transactions for the sharing of data, data warehousing, and continuity of data with emergency, ambulatory, and outpatient settings.

The American Recovery and Reinvestment Act of 2009 introduced the Health Information Technology for Economic and Clinical Health Act, which supported the adoption of EHRs. In 2011, the Centers for Medicare and Medicaid Services (CMS) established Medicare and Medicaid EHR incentive programs to encourage eligible professionals and health care entities to adopt, implement, upgrade, and demonstrate meaningful use of certified EHRs.

The three main components of using EHRs in the meaningful use program use certified EHRs:
- In a meaningful manner, such as e-Prescribing
- For the electronic exchange of health information to improve quality of healthcare
- To report clinical quality measures

In April 2018, CMS renamed the EHR incentive programs the Medicare and Medicaid Promoting Interoperability Programs. Promoting interoperability renewed commitment to promoting and prioritizing interoperability and exchange of health care data. The increased focus on interoperability prioritizes patient access to their health information (Anumula & Sanelli, 2012; CMS, n.d.).

> **TIP**
>
> An example of a QI project using informatics is incorporating smart order sets for sepsis protocol to increase efficiency and improve patient outcome. Clinicians do not have to spend excessive time figuring out what orders are needed.
> To learn more about how PDSA is used, the Institute for Healthcare Improvement has resources with examples of quality improvement projects (https://www.ihi.org:443/resources/Pages/Tools/PlanDoStudyActWorksheet.aspx).

> **TIP**
>
> The quality of data is very important when applying KDD to health care databases. It is important to understand and consider how data are input into EHRs, which is why standardization of data entry is a high priority for ensuring health care providers are able to obtain meaningful clinical reports and understand trends among patient populations. The Nursing Minimum Data Set (Werley et al., 1986) provided guidelines regarding the information needed about each patient, including demographic elements, nursing care elements (e.g., nursing diagnoses, nursing interventions, nursing outcomes, nursing care intensity), and service elements (e.g., admission/discharge dates, disposition). The data set needs to be continuously reviewed to ensure comprehensive socioeconomic and cultural data is gathered.

NURSING SUPPORT SYSTEMS FOR DECISION MAKING

Nursing support systems play a critical role in enhancing patient care. One aspect of nursing support systems is clinical decision support systems (CDSS), which are designed to provide clinicians with real-time information and recommendations to help facilitate accurate and efficient decision making in patient care (Ruland, 2004). These systems utilize computerized clinical knowledge bases to match the characteristics of an individual patient, which enables clinicians to make more informed decisions about their care.

CDSS are examples of technology systems that can assist critical care nurses in the surveillance process. CDSS are computer-based tools that assist nurses in making informed decisions by providing evidence-based recommendations, alerts, and reminders at the point of care (Nibbelink et al., 2018). Practical aspects of nursing support systems using CDSS include the following:

1. Data integration: CDSS integrates the data from various sources, such as EHRs, laboratory results, medication databases, and patient medical histories. The system consolidates and analyzes this information to generate relevant recommendations.

2. Evidence-based guidelines: CDSS incorporates evidence-based guidelines and best practices. These guidelines are derived from reputable sources, such as clinical practice guidelines and research studies. By following these guidelines, nurses can provide standardized and high-quality care.
3. Decision support tools: CDSS provides nurses with decision support tools that aid in the assessment, diagnosis, and treatment of patients. These can include screening tools, risk calculators, symptom checkers, diagnostic algorithms, and treatment protocols. Nurses can input patient data into these tools to receive personalized recommendations.
4. Alerts and reminders: CDSS can generate real-time alerts and reminders to notify nurses of critical information or potential issues related to patient care. For example, if a patient has a drug allergy or a potentially harmful drug interaction, the system will alert the nurse to take appropriate action (e.g., Sepsis Alerts, PEWS [Pediatric Early Warning Signs], MEWS [Modified Early Warning System]).
5. Clinical documentation: CDSS can assist nurses in documenting patient information accurately and efficiently. It can automatically populate certain fields in the EHR based on the data input and provide templates for documentation. This feature helps in reducing documentation errors and saves time for nurses.
6. Education and training: CDSS can serve as an educational tool for nurses by providing access to up-to-date medical knowledge, clinical guidelines, and educational resources. It can help nurses stay updated with the latest developments in their field and enhance their clinical decision-making skills.
7. Monitoring and surveillance: CDSS can support nurses in monitoring patient conditions and identifying potential complications. It can analyze data trends and notify nurses if any abnormal values or patterns are detected, allowing for early intervention and proactive management.

Overall, nursing support systems using CDSS empower nurses by providing them with evidence-based recommendations, clinical tools, alerts, and educational resources. By leveraging these systems, nurses can make more informed decisions, deliver safer care, and improve patient outcomes.

> **TIP**
>
> Nurses are encouraged to stay updated with the latest evidence-based guidelines and follow them when making clinical decisions. These guidelines are developed based on rigorous research and provide recommendations for optimal patient care. By adhering to evidence-based guidelines, nurses can ensure that their decisions are supported by the best available evidence, leading to improved patient outcomes.

> **TIP**
>
> It is important for nurses to pay attention to the real-time alerts or reminders and act on them promptly, despite the risk of the "alert fatigue" phenomenon. These alerts can warn about drug allergies, potential medication interactions, or other important safety considerations. By responding in a timely manner, nurses can prevent or mitigate adverse events and work to ensure patient safety.

FUTURE OF NURSING INFORMATICS

Looking ahead, the field of nursing informatics is poised for continued growth and development, driven by advances in technology and future innovations. The progression of technological development can potentially harness the vast potential of existing informatics solutions. Some examples include the following:
- Patient decision support (PDS)
- Personal health records (PHRs)
- Regional health information exchange (HIE)
- Clinical data registries
- Mobile health (mHealth)
- Big data analytics
- Artificial intelligence (AI)
- Internet of Things (IoT)

PDS systems can help patients actively participate in care and treatment planning to promote shared decision making. They provide patients with access to evidence-based information that can often be periodically updated on the PDS systems. It encourages a patient-centered approach that respects individual preferences and values while promoting evidence-based treatment plans.

PHR is a digital tool that allows patients to access and manage their own health information in a secure, convenient manner (Lester et al., 2016). Patients can share their data with health care providers, and PHRs often include educational resources based on evidence-based guidelines. Lack of interoperability is a technical challenge facing the utilization of PHRs, as they struggle in the integration to the EHRs of health care systems. Data privacy can also be a concern with PHRs when considering vulnerable populations (e.g., adolescents, patients with HIV).

Regional HIEs are electronic networks that facilitate the secure exchange of health data and information among health care organizations (Holmgren & Adler-Milstein, 2017). They can support EBP by improving access to comprehensive patient data and promoting care coordination. Regional HIEs can help prevent unnecessary duplication of services and medical tests, and with a complete medical history, a provider can make more informed decisions. This can help reduce health care costs and minimize the potential harm to patients.

Clinical data registries are structured databases that house clinical data about patients and the care they have received. Integrated CDSS tools can provide health care providers with real-time alerts and evidence-based recommendations based on registry data. This assists in clinical decision making and adherence to evidence-based guidelines.

mHealth refers to the use of mobile devices (e.g., smartphones, tablets, wearables, and other wireless technologies) to support patient health management, health care delivery, and patient engagement. mHealth apps can provide access to evidence-based clinical guidelines and treatment recommendations for providers. They can also empower patients with evidence-based health information and educational materials.

The use of big data in nursing informatics is becoming increasingly common as health care delivery becomes more driven by data. **Big data** can help identify opportunities for streamlining health care delivery, identifying areas of clinical excellence, and providing insights into population health trends (Gephart et al., 2018). However, the use of big data also presents several challenges, including data security and privacy concerns, as well as the need for specialized data analytics skills and tools to effectively manage and analyze the large amounts of data generated by health care organizations.

The use of AI in nursing informatics has the potential to revolutionize patient care by leveraging machine learning algorithms and predictive analytics to support clinical decision making (Robert, 2019). By analyzing vast amounts of patient data, AI can help identify patterns and trends that may be missed by human clinicians, providing more accurate diagnoses and treatment plans, and ultimately improving patient outcomes. For example, AI algorithms can analyze medical images to detect tumors or lesions (Olveres et al., 2021).

AI technologies can optimize nursing workflows and improve efficiency. AI algorithms can automate routine tasks, such as data entry, documentation, and scheduling, reducing the administrative burden on nurses. Natural language processing enables AI systems to interpret and extract relevant information from unstructured data sources like clinical notes, enabling faster and more accurate data analysis.

However, the integration of AI in nursing informatics also presents several ethical and legal considerations, including privacy concerns and potential biases in algorithm development. Therefore, AI systems must be designed and implemented in a manner that ensures patient safety and privacy while also minimizing biases and errors. In addition, nursing informatics professionals must ensure that AI systems are regularly monitored and evaluated to ensure their ongoing effectiveness and safety.

IoT is another technology that has significant potential to transform patient care. IoT is a system of interconnected devices and sensors that can collect and transmit data in real time (Ghosh et al., 2018). In healthcare, IoT can help in monitoring patients remotely, capturing patient data continuously, and detecting changes in patient conditions to facilitate early intervention.

IoT can be used to track patient vital signs and activity levels in real time, providing clinicians with up-to-date information that can inform clinical decision making. Additionally, IoT in nursing informatics can help automate certain processes such as medication dispensing and tracking, thus helping to reduce errors and improve efficiency. IoT devices enable virtual nursing teams to set up alerts and notifications for abnormal readings or notable changes in the patient data, and this would allow for timely interventions and potentially reduce hospital admissions.

IoT devices empower patients to actively participate in their own care and self-management. This promotes patient engagement and self-care, and facilitates shared decision making between patients and nurses.

Nonetheless, the use of IoT in nursing informatics also presents several challenges, including data management and interoperability issues. For example, the vast amounts of data generated by IoT devices require robust data management strategies to ensure that the data is accurate and accessible when needed. The security and privacy of the IoT-generated data are also essential priorities.

The COVID-19 pandemic highlighted the critical importance of nursing informatics in supporting remote patient monitoring and telehealth initiatives (Kaminski, 2020). During the height of the pandemic, nurses were able to utilize telehealth technologies to provide care to patients with COVID-19 and other illnesses, while minimizing the risk of person-to-person transmission. Nurses were also able to help patients stay in contact with their families with communication technologies, such as video conferencing and messaging apps. Other telehealth applications include remote nursing consultations or medication adherence tracking through IoT-connected medication dispensers, which dispense the correct medications at the correct time and send alerts/reminders to the patients and caregivers (Pal et al., 2022).

These all have the potential to revolutionize health care delivery and improve patient outcomes.

ROLES OF THE NURSE INFORMATICIST

Nursing informatics has become an essential component of modern health care delivery, with a focus on leveraging technology and data to improve patient outcomes and enhance the overall quality of care (ANA, 2022). There are various roles within nursing informatics, each with its own set of duties and responsibilities. These positions may differ depending on the health care organization or regional setting, but common roles include the following:

- Clinical analyst/nurse informaticist: Registered nurses with specialized training in informatics. They are responsible for collecting, analyzing, and interpreting health care data. They work with various data sources, including EHRs, to identify trends, monitor patient outcomes, and assist in research projects. They design, implement, and maintain health care information systems, ensuring that they meet the needs of nurses and other health care professionals. They also provide training and support to health care staff on using these systems effectively.
- Nursing informatics project manager: Oversee the planning, execution, and completion of informatics projects. They assemble and lead interdisciplinary teams and manage resources to ensure project success. They coordinate with various stakeholders, ensure that projects are on schedule and within budget, and communicate progress to leadership.
- Chief nursing informatics officer (CNIO): Crucial member of a system's senior-level executive team, and their role is to provide strategic guidance and strong leadership in the implementation and integration of information systems in health care organizations using DIKW (Ventura, 2018). They collaborate with other members of the executive team to align nursing informatics initiatives with the organization's goals. CNIOs often oversee informatics teams and ensure that nursing standards and best practices are integrated into technology solutions.

The field of nursing informatics will continue to be a dynamic and rapidly evolving specialty, with the potential to make a significant impact on the future of health care delivery and patient care. As such, health care organizations can continue to invest in the development and implementation of nursing informatics initiatives, to ensure that they remain at the forefront of health care innovation and can provide the highest quality care to patients in an increasingly complex and rapidly changing health care landscape. This will require ongoing education and training for nursing informatics professionals, as well as collaboration between health care organizations, technology companies, and regulatory bodies, to ensure that nursing informatics initiatives are developed in a manner that is safe, effective, and aligned with best practices in patient care (Farzandipour et al., 2020).

As healthcare continues to evolve, nursing informatics will undoubtedly play a crucial role in shaping the future of patient care and advancing the field of nursing. It is exciting to consider the possibilities that lie ahead for nursing informatics as new technologies continue to emerge and health care delivery models evolve.

> **TIP**
>
> Workflow analysis and design are key tools used by nursing informaticists to better understand and enhance day-to-day processes. For example, when planning to change from one EHR system to another, it is important to understand the current state in order to map out a more efficient future state.

> **TIP**
> Social media is a frequently used platform to communicate and share photos and information. The National Council of State Boards of Nursing (NCSBN) created a guide for nurses on best practices for using social media and how to avoid associated risks (https://www.ncsbn.org/brochures-and-posters/nurses-guide-to-the-use-of-social-media).

> **TIP**
> To decrease the wait time for patients to see medical specialists in the hospital, the hospital can incorporate telehealth visits from specialists. For example, if a patient is admitted for stroke and is experiencing a rash, a dermatologist may need to be consulted. Instead of waiting days for a visit from a dermatologist, a telehealth visit can be scheduled, and a clinician at the bedside can help facilitate the visit over a hospital-provided telehealth device.

> **TIP**
> During the pandemic, Zoom was used on computers/smart devices to help patients communicate with their remote family members. Zoom for video calls can be used for infectious patient isolation to reduce usage of personal protective equipment, for group video visits, and to allow patients to stay connected to family and friends from inpatient rooms. Nursing informaticists helped implement the Zoom technology to ensure it met the needs of patients and clinicians.

> **BOX 24.1 Reflections on Knowledge Application of Nursing Informatics**
>
> - Think about a time when you used technology to provide care to your patient. What informatics competencies did you use?
> - What nursing informatics (NI) competencies are required to implement telehealth?
> - How is the DIKW continuum utilized in your nursing practice?
> - How can we bring care to underserved or underrepresented populations using technology?
> - Take time to interview a nursing informatics specialist to learn more about nursing informatics.

SYNTHESIS

Since being recognized in 1992, the field of nursing informatics has significantly evolved, and it continues to keep pace with the innovations of technology and nursing science. And as the landscape of nursing informatics continues to develop, the core principles of this field will always be the safety of the patient, the quality of patient care, and the optimization of the nurse's role and efforts. The DIKW framework can continue to guide care delivery and improve patient outcomes, because healthcare processes depend on data use and information sharing. The nurse informaticist will continue to partner with interdisciplinary team members to provide crucial improvement in nursing practice. Reflections to consider in the application of the nursing informatics process can be found in Box 24.1.

KEY POINTS

- Nursing informatics integrates nursing science, information science, computer science, and cognitive science to manage and communicate data, information, knowledge, and wisdom.
- Nurses gather data and information, draw on their knowledge, and apply wisdom to determine an optimized plan of care for patients.
- Nursing informatics applications seek to improve patient care and ensure safe, quality health care delivery with digital resources to support and enhance nursing practice.
- The ANA created the Scope and Standards of Practice for nursing informatics, which helped guide the development of this field.
- The TIGER Initiative is focused on education reform and interprofessional community development to maximize seamless integration of technology and informatics into nursing practice, education, and research.
- Nurses can use data mining concepts to observe trends in their patient populations and develop uniquely relevant care plans.

- CDSS provide real-time information and recommendations to help facilitate accurate and efficient decision making for clinicians.
- The future of nursing informatics will embrace technological advancements to revolutionize the delivery of evidence-based healthcare and improve patient outcomes.
- Ongoing education and training for nursing informaticists can ensure that initiatives are developed to be aligned with best practices in patient care.

REFERENCES

American Association of Colleges of Nursing (AACN). (n.d.). *Domain 8: Informatics and healthcare technologies*. https://www.aacnnursing.org/essentials/tool-kit/domains-concepts/informatics-and-healthcare-technologies.

American Association of Colleges of Nursing (AACN). (2021). *The Essentials: Core competencies for professional nursing education*. https://www.aacnnursing.org/Portals/42/AcademicNursing/pdf/Essentials-2021.pdf.

American Nurses Association (ANA). (2014). *Nursing informatics: Scope and standards of practice* (2nd ed.). American Nurses Association.

American Nurses Association (ANA). (2017). *Magnet recognition program | ANCC*. https://www.nursingworld.org/organizational-programs/magnet/.

American Nurses Association (ANA). (2022). *Nursing informatics: Scope and standards of practice* (3rd ed.). American Nurses Association.

American Nurses Credentialing Center (ANCC). (n.d.). *Informatics nursing certification*. https://www.nursingworld.org/our-certifications/informatics-nurse/.

Anumula, N., & Sanelli, P. C. (2012). Meaningful use. *AJNR: American Journal of Neuroradiology*, 33(8), 1455–1457. https://doi.org/10.3174/ajnr.A3247.

Bickford, C. (2009). Nursing informatics: Scope and standards of practice. *Studies in Health Technology and Informatics*, 146, 855.

Centers for Medicare and Medicaid Services (CMS). (n.d.). *Promoting interoperability programs*. https://www.cms.gov/medicare/regulations-guidance/promoting-interoperability-programs.

Choi, J., Thompson, C. E., Choi, J., Waddill, C. B., & Choi, S. (2022). Effectiveness of immersive virtual reality in nursing education: Systematic review. *Nurse Educator*, 47(3), E57–E61. https://doi.org/10.1097/NNE.0000000000001117.

Farzandipour, M., Mohamadian, H., Akbari, H., Safari, S., & Sadeqi, M. (2020). *HIMSS self-assessment of nursing informatics competencies in hospitals*. https://www.himss.org/resources/self-assessment-nursing-informatics-competencies-hospitals.

Garcia-Dia, M. (2019). *Project management in nursing informatics*. Springer Publishing Company.

Gephart, S. M., Davis, M., & Shea, K. (2018). Perspectives on policy and the value of nursing science in a big data era. *Nursing Science Quarterly*, 31(1), 78–81. https://doi.org/10.1177/0894318417741122.

Ghosh, A., Chakraborty, D., & Law, A. (2018). Artificial intelligence in Internet of things. *CAAI Transactions on Intelligence Technology*, 3(4), 208–218. https://doi.org/10.1049/trit.2018.1008.

Graves, J. R., & Corcoran, S. (1989). The study of nursing informatics. *Journal of Nursing Scholarship*, 21, 227–231.

Harrington, L. (2015). American Nurses Association releases new scope and standards of nursing informatics practice. *AACN Advanced Critical Care*, 26(2), 93–96. https://doi.org/10.1097/NCI.0000000000000065.

Healthcare Information and Management Systems Society (HIMSS). (n.d.). *Certification*. https://www.himss.org/resources-certification/overview.

Holmgren, A. J., & Adler–Milstein, J. (2017). Health information exchange in US hospitals: The current landscape and a path to improved information sharing. *Journal of Hospital Medicine*, 12(3), 193–198.

Icahn School of Medicine at Mount Sinai. (n.d.). *PEAK (portal for education and advancement of knowledge)*. https://researchroadmap.mssm.edu/reference/systems/peak/.

Institute for Healthcare Improvement. (n.d.) *Plan-Do-Study-Act (PDSA) worksheet*. https://www.ihi.org:443/resources/Pages/Tools/PlanDoStudyActWorksheet.aspx.

Kaminski, J. (2020). Informatics in the time of COVID-19. *Canadian Journal of Nursing Informatics*, 15(1), 1. https://cjni.net/journal/?p=6820.

Lester, M., Boateng, S., Studeny, J., & Coustasse, A. (2016). Personal health records: Beneficial or burdensome for patients and healthcare providers? *Perspectives in Health Information Management*, 13(Spring) 1h.

Lippincott, C., Foronda, C., Zdanowicz, M., McCabe, B. E., & Ambrosia, T. (2017). The relationship between magnet designation, electronic health record adoption, and Medicare meaningful use payments. *Computers, Informatics, Nursing*, 35(8), 385–391. https://doi.org/10.1097/CIN.0000000000000336.

McGonigle, D., & Mastrian, K. (2018). *Nursing informatics and the foundation of knowledge* (4th ed.). Jones & Bartlett Learning.

Nelson, R. (2020). Informatics: Evolution of the Nelson data, information, knowledge and wisdom model: Part 2. *The Online Journal of Issues in Nursing, 25*(3).

Nibbelink, C. W., Young, J. R., Carrington, J. M., & Brewer, B. B. (2018). Informatics solutions for application of decision-making skills. *Critical Care Nursing Clinics of North America, 30*(2), 237–246. https://doi.org/10.1016/j.cnc.2018.02.006.

Olveres, J., González, G., Torres, F., Moreno-Tagle, J. C., Carbajal-Degante, E., Valencia-Rodríguez, A., et al. (2021). What is new in computer vision and artificial intelligence in medical image analysis applications. *Quantitative Imaging in Medicine and Surgery, 11*(8), 3830–3853. https://doi.org/10.21037/qims-20-1151.

Ozbolt, J. G., & Saba, V. K. (2008). A brief history of nursing informatics in the United States of America. *Nursing Outlook, 56*(5), 199–205.e2. https://doi.org/10.1016/j.outlook.2008.06.008.

Pal, K., Ari, S., Bit, A., & Bhattacharyya, S. (Eds.). (2022). *Advanced methods in biomedical signal processing and analysis*. Academic Press.

Robert, N. (2019). How artificial intelligence is changing nursing. *Nursing Management, 50*(9), 30–39. https://doi.org/10.1097/01.NUMA.0000578988.56622.21.

Ruland, C. M. (2004). Improving patient safety through informatics tools for shared decision making and risk communication. *International Journal of Medical Informatics, 73*(7–8), 551–557. https://doi.org/10.1016/j.ijmedinf.2004.05.003.

Sensmeier, J., Anderson, C., & Shaw, T. (2017). International evolution of TIGER informatics competencies. *Studies in Health Technology and Informatics, 232*, 69–76.

Ventura, R. (2018). The role of the chief nursing informatics officer. *American Nursing Informatics Association*. https://www.ania.org/assets/documents/position/cnioPosition.pdf.

Wakefield, M. K., Williams, D., Le Menestrel, S., & Flaubert, J. (2021). *The future of nursing 2020-2030: Charting a path to achieve health equity*. National Academies Press.

Werley, H. H., Lang, N. M., & Westlake, S. K. (1986). The nursing minimum data set conference: Executive summary. *Journal of Professional Nursing, 2*(4), 217–224. https://doi.org/10.1016/s8755-7223(86)80043-6.

25

Population and Public Health

Jenna Blind, Stacen A. Keating, Robin Toft Klar, and Jeanmarie Moorehead

LEARNING OUTCOMES

After reading this chapter, you should be able to do the following:
- Define population health.
- Recognize principles of population health across the continuum of care.
- Discuss the role of clinical leaders in population health.
- Describe the impact of health equity across populations.
- Identify strategies to promote population health and evidence-based disease management across the care spectrum.
- Analyze the nurse's participation in the collection of data used in population health.
- Analyze process and outcome measures to use in evaluation of population health data.
- Determine the role of the nurse in public health emergencies.
- Differentiate between epidemic, endemic, and pandemic.

KEY TERMS

Community
Epidemiology
Health equity
Population health
Public health
Social determinants of health
Syndromic surveillance

Population health as a concept and science has evolved from the earlier sciences of epidemiology, the study of disease, and public health. The Centers for Disease Control and Prevention (CDC) defines **public health** as a science whose primary focus is to protect and improve the overall health and well-being of people and their respective communities (CDC, 2023). The necessity of understanding population health came from decades of realizing the intersection of epidemiology and the medical focus of health care delivery. The health care system alone was not enough to understand why overall health of individuals was declining. As part of the National Academies of Sciences, Engineering, and Medicine's (NASEM) Roundtable on Population Health Improvement (2016), proceedings were published that examined how to advance the science of population health. Key takeaways included the discussion of the term embodiment. An individual's health does not add up to 100%, as there are intertwined and multilevel actions occurring over a lifetime that create the human and their human condition, which are presented in every encounter with a health care provider.

HISTORY OF POPULATION HEALTH

Conveners at the 2017 NASEM meetings highlighted the importance in identifying the cross-tabulation of the state of evidence and *consensus* and the state of evidence-based *action* around population-focused policies. This is an important and critical analysis as many of the weak actions are a result of their politicized nature. As the COVID-19 pandemic has illustrated, the politicization of health direction and advice can lead to misinformation. Communication from trusted health care providers and their partners can assuage mistrust and hesitancy to make evidence-based changes in everyday health care behaviors.

An evidence-based understanding of the impact of programs, policies, and projects that support the health of populations is imperative. Many programs and projects are implemented as the activity of funded research or practice initiatives. The peer-reviewed literature describing the outcomes of the program often do not relay the critical analysis of how the actions of the initiative allowed for participant buy-in or if the program or project was funded after the study. Conducting a health impact assessment of the program, policy, or project within specific populations of interest can bring to the forefront where the positive and negative impacts are and if some aspects of deimplementation are the next steps to address all six A's of access: availability, accessibility, affordability, appropriateness, adequacy, and acceptability (U.S. Department of Health and Human Services, 1995).

A follow-up meeting of NASEM's Roundtable on Population Health Improvement met in 2022, and the resultant report delineated trends, evidence, and policy implications (NASEM, 2023) highlighting the importance of collecting and analyzing population-level data from all geographies and demographics. The United Nations Sustainable Development Goals (Fig. 25.1), 17 in total, are global goals directed to support social and physical determinants of health along with regular and reliable measurement of goals met. The Sustainable Development Goals (SDGs) and NASEM's Roundtable emphasize equitable distribution of resources. The impact of these resources plays a more significant role in the health of populations than most policies. Globally, the SDGs were identified in 2015 by a United Nations task force that ultimately described 17 areas of impact that all nations should work toward to improve the lives of populations around the world (United Nations, 2015). Specifically, Goal 3 relates to world health priorities and notes that all countries should strive to care for their people in a way that would enable them to live healthy

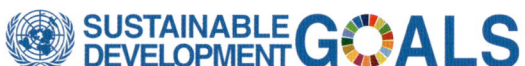

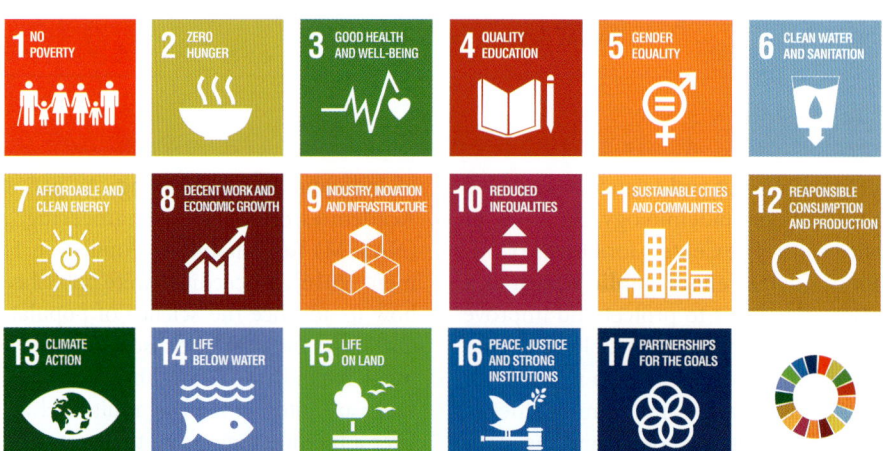

Fig. 25.1 United Nations Sustainable Development Goals. (From United Nations. UN Office for Sustainable Development. Sustainable Development Goals (SDGs). https://unosd.un.org/content/sustainable-development-goals-sdgs. Copyright © United Nations. All rights reserved.)

lives and experience well-being at all ages. Sachs and colleagues (2021) have noted that overall sustainable development efforts notably declined due to the COVID-19 pandemic and that preparation, resources, and prompt intervention are needed going forward when population health issues of this magnitude occur around the world.

EPIDEMIOLOGY

Identifying major health issues and improving care for populations requires a unique set of evidence-based competencies for clinical leaders and others. The American Association of Colleges of Nursing (AACN) *The Essentials: Core Competencies for Professional Nursing Education* define advanced-level nursing competencies in Domain 3 and encompass the management of population health needs, including the ability to study and evaluate population health data in order to address pressing concerns (AACN, 2021). **Epidemiology** is the science of population health and is considered both a methodology and a body of scientific knowledge (Khaliq, 2020). A sound understanding of epidemiology is foundational to identifying health issues, intervening to improve health outcomes, and evaluating interventional effectiveness for target populations. For advanced practice-level nurses and nursing leaders, it is important to know that epidemiological principles provide essential knowledge needed to improve population health. According to the CDC, epidemiology is succinctly described as follows:

> By definition, **epidemiology** is the study (scientific, systematic, and data-driven) of the distribution (frequency, pattern) and determinants (causes, risk factors) of health-related states and events (not just diseases) in specified populations (neighborhood, school, city, state, country, global).

Gaining a broader understanding of epidemiology means understanding what happens when disease outbreaks occur, including those that stem from infectious agents or perhaps foodborne illness, and many other conditions and disease states. At the height of the COVID-19 pandemic epidemiologists were key to investigating the infectious nature of the virus as it related to various populations, including those of varying age groups, those with underlying chronic illness, and variables related to the **social determinants of health** (SDOH). Nurses in public health roles were also actively working to understand the nature of this global pandemic and the populations most at risk in order to provide evidence-based care.

It is important to note the difference in disease outbreak magnitude by understanding the concepts of epidemic, endemic, and pandemic (Khaliq, 2020). An **epidemic** relates to a public health issue or disease that is impacting a significant number of people within a **community**, population, or set geographic area. For example, gun violence is an epidemic problem within the United States when compared to other global regions. A public health issue or disease that is **endemic** occurs within a particular group of people or country. Malaria is endemic to a number of countries around the globe but is not problematic, currently, in the United States. A **pandemic** concerns an issue that affects populations from multiple countries or continents around the world. COVID-19 is the most recent example of an infectious disease that started in China and spread quickly and with virulence across Europe, the United States, and the majority of the world in 2020 (World Health Organization, 2020).

Epidemiology is focused on understanding and investigating issues of concern to specific populations. At its core, epidemiology seeks to look at the magnitude of a health issue or disease occurrence in a population and determine why this is happening so that action can be taken to improve outcomes for those most at risk. Key areas of investigation include environmental exposures (lead in water sources), infectious disease (SARS, giardia, tuberculosis, etc.), injuries (gun violence, falls, etc), noninfectious disease (chronic illnesses), natural disasters (hurricanes, floods, etc.), and terrorism. Concerns around climate health and the effects of global warming are more recently being researched in terms of the magnitude these climate changes will have for large populations around the globe. Within the U.S. Office of Disease Prevention and Health Promotion, the Healthy People 2030 (HP2030) framework provides clinical nurses and nurse leaders with an outline of the key population health issues facing our nation (U.S. Office of Disease Prevention and Health Promotion, n.d.). Currently, HP2030 data-driven national objectives include 358 core measurable topics that help guide the work of nurses leading quality improvement efforts for their target populations.

As a methodology, epidemiology uses several techniques of investigation. Most commonly, observational

TABLE 25.1 Ongoing Longitudinal Studies in Population Health

Name of Study	Study Description	Link to Study
Framingham Heart Study	• Directed by the National Institute of Health • Cohort study, longitudinal • Began in 1948 • Participants are men and women between the ages of 30 and 62 from Framingham, Massachusetts • Focusing on cardiovascular health	https://www.framinghamheartstudy.org/fhs-about/
Grant Study	• Directed by 268 Harvard University graduates • Cohort study, longitudinal • Began in 1938 • Participants are graduates from Harvard University • Focusing on the psychological predictor of healthy aging	https://www.adultdevelopmentstudy.org/grantandglueckstudy
Nurses' Health Study	• Directed by Brigham and Women's Hospital and the Harvard Medical School and Harvard T. H. Chan School of Public Health • Prospective investigation, longitudinal • Began in 1976 • The participants are male and female nurses • Focusing on risk factors for major chronic diseases in women	https://nurseshealthstudy.org/about-nhs

studies are done (see Chapter 9). These are nonexperimental in nature and involve the following types of studies: cross-sectional, case-control, and cohort. Observational methods then are key to this area of population health science and are concerned with variables related to time, place, and person.

Cross-sectional studies allow the investigator to study exposures and outcomes for a number of individuals and multiple variables at a given point in time. As a result, these studies do not require follow-up and are less costly to perform. This method is analogous to taking a snapshot of the problem at hand and describing the prevalence of desired characteristics in a population. For this reason, cross-sectional studies may also be termed prevalence studies as they can readily describe the prevalence of multiple characteristics or variables at a given point in time. Often surveys are used with participants to collect the desired data. Of note is the fact that these studies do not provide insight into any type of cause-and-effect relationship of the variables of interest.

Case-control studies are another means of conducting epidemiological research. In this method of study, *cases* are chosen because they have the disease and *controls* are chosen because they do not have the disease. Then the two groups can be compared to see how they differ in terms of exposures and outcomes. An example is the use of a case-control study to look at the association of a drug exposure and a health outcome. Investigators need to pay great attention to how controls are chosen to reduce selection bias in the study.

Cohort studies are most often prospective in nature, although they can be done retrospectively too, but they contain a level of increased risk of bias when done this way. The goal of a cohort study is to follow a group of people over time to observe for disease occurrence. There are a variety of examples of valuable ongoing longitudinal studies in population health that provide insight into patterns of health and illness (Table 25.1). A benefit of cohort studies is the ability to look at cause and effect when drawing conclusions from the data. For example, at the outset of the study, participants likely do not have significant disease but may develop the disease over time due to certain exposures or behaviors that can be tracked. Following numerous people over long periods of time (many years for some of the large well-known cohort studies) has challenges related to being time and labor-intensive as well as costly. Participants may drop out of these studies, causing bias in terms of the analysis and conclusions.

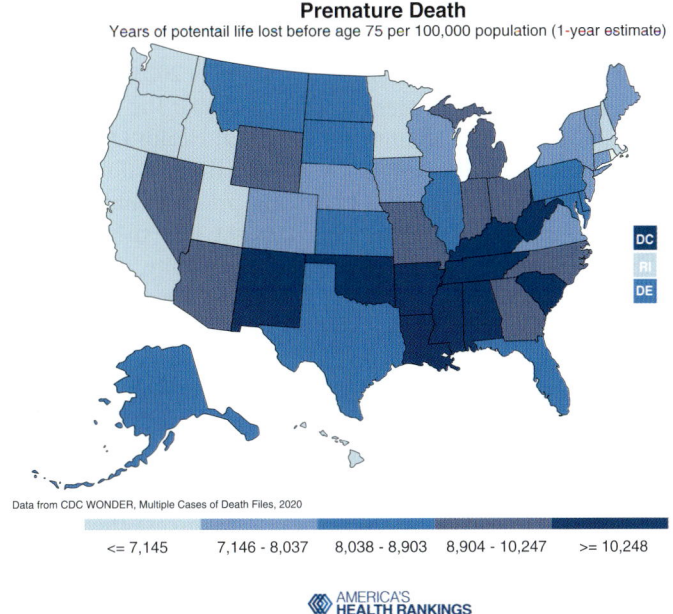

Fig. 25.2 Premature Death in the United States. Health outcomes in the United States by state. (From America's Health Rankings: United Health Foundation. Premature Death in United States. https://www.americashealthrankings.org/explore/measures/YPLL. © Copyright United Health Foundation. All Rights Reserved.)

Overall, principles of epidemiology provide clinical nurses and leaders with the competencies and tools needed to identify population health issues for diverse populations. Understanding how epidemiology is core to population health enables advanced-level nurses and leaders to then employ the best study design, data collection, and evaluation techniques for the population health issue at hand. Analyzing the data allows for unearthing clues as to the potential causes and the identification of potential interventions to address the issues in ways that are hopefully beneficial to the target population. A solid plan of identification of at-risk populations, intervention planning, implementation, and evaluation of any quality improvement initiative is key to success in improving population health across the United States and globally. A heat map is a data visualization tool to graphically illustrate trends and impact in particular geographic areas. See Fig. 25.2 for the premature death heat map in the United States. Advanced practice nurses can utilize national and state-level health rankings to evaluate premature death in their communities and implement evidence-based strategies to address disparities.

INFORMATICS AND POPULATION HEALTH

Robust data collection and analysis procedures are a critical component of epidemiology and public health principles. These procedures (i.e., collection, surveillance, investigation) are used to guide nurses and other health care providers' understanding of the health of populations to improve public health decision making on a micro, meso, and macro level. With the inception of the electronic health record (EHR) and other health information systems, the use of this data for public health surveillance has become more prominent. The American Recovery and Reinvestment Act of 2009, also known as the Recovery Act, was a program implemented by the Centers for Medicare and Medicaid Services to incentivize health care organizations to successfully demonstrate meaningful use of EHR data. To achieve meaningful use, one requirement is to collect public health data and conduct **syndromic surveillance**, defined as early alerts that track symptoms that are publicly reported within hours, thereby arming organizations with the ability to prevent and manage disease. As a result, communication regarding diagnosis and treatment can be facilitated across the health care spectrum and continuum of care.

Health care organizations that achieve the coveted Magnet designation from the American Nurses Credentialing Center (ANCC) are recognized for their abilities to promote excellence in nursing practice, intraprofessional collaboration, innovation, and outcomes. This model emphasizes health care organizations' abilities to promote population health through the collection of community-level data such as the Community Health Rankings data set. This data set relies on county-level data at the population level, reporting on SDOH that align with Healthy People decennial targets and SDGs.

DATA COLLECTION AND DATA SETS FOR POPULATION HEALTH

General public health data are provided to CDC databases and other public health data sets to improve access to this information. These data sets are typically organized in categories such as chronic conditions, communicable diseases, environmental health, health practice and prevention, injury prevention, and occupational health. Examples of data that are available at the local, regional, national, or international level include:

Local: In March 2020, the New York City (NYC) Health Department implemented the COVID-19 Population Health Survey. This is a representative population-based survey aimed at understanding past COVID-19 infection in association with demographics, housing, employment, and other characteristics. As the pandemic progressed, there was increased attention to the systemic effects of the virus on the overall health of NYC residents. (NYC COVID-19 Population Health and Serologic Surveys, 2023, https://www.nyc.gov/site/doh/data/data-sets/covid-19-serologic-surveys.page)

Regional: The New York State Department of Health (NYSDOH) published data regarding the COVID-19 pandemic, including testing, vaccinations, hospitalizations, and mortality. This information is accessible to the public and can be accessed via the NYSDOH website. (COVID-19 Data in New York: Monitoring the Key Aspects of the Epidemic, 2023, https://coronavirus.health.ny.gov/covid-19-data-new-york)

National: The U.S. Department of Health and Human Services has a research database maintained by the National Institutes of Health. This database contains population health data and focuses on the intersection of biology, environment, and lifestyle. (National Institutes of Health: All of Us Research Program, 2023, https://allofus.nih.gov/)

International: The World Health Organization's (WHO) Global Health Observatory is a robust global health database including over 1,000 indicators representing priority public health data topics that provide insight into the burden of disease, environmental health, equity, and mortality worldwide. (The Global Health Observatory: Explore a World of Health Data, 2023, https://www.who.int/data/gho)

COVID-19 magnified the importance of a reliable and resilient emergency preparedness plan for **public health emergencies**. These events require constant preparedness simulations and participation of personnel from organized health care systems and community health resources. The increase in occurrence of public health emergencies, such as wildfires, floods, earthquakes, and extreme heat events, demand a continuous update in training for the aforementioned resources. The knowledge, skills, and abilities of those involved in said emergencies, including first responders, health care personnel, and government officials, must take priority to mitigate financial and human impact. This planning and preparation ultimately impacts and protects the health and wellness of populations.

The Gravity Project, which was developed in 2017, brought together stakeholders to develop a collaborative focused on the importance of data sharing as it relates to SDOH (Health Level Seven International, n.d.). This pivotal project focused on the criticality of **interoperability** of this standardized data set to support patient care. Interoperability is defined as the ability of different information systems to communicate data in a coordinated manor. The Gravity Project has since defined 830 data elements across the population and public health spectrum that can be exchanged across disparate digital health platforms. These data elements can be categorized into value sets including, but not limited to, food insecurity, housing instability, homelessness, educational attainment, and social connection, etc.

The quality of individuals' or a population's life is affected by their SDOH. As defined by the AACN *Essentials* (2021), advanced practice nurses are equipped with the knowledge, skills, and abilities to assess population health data across the continuum of care. These competencies imply a shared responsibility of health care providers to strive for improved healthcare for all, regardless of their SDOH.

WHERE YOU LIVE MATTERS TO YOUR HEALTH

Social Determinants of Health and Health Equity by U.S. Rankings

In the United States, a person's zip code is a SDOH outcome, including premature mortality of infants, children, and adults, and health behaviors such as the likelihood of smoking, suffering from obesity, and poor access to healthy foods. According to the Robert Wood Johnson Foundation, health disparities exist by race, ethnicity, and place. Birthweight is an essential quality indicator of life for babies and mothers—babies born to Black mothers in the United States are likelier to be low birthweight and twice as likely to die under the age of 1 than White babies (Fig. 25.3). Clinical, educational, and administrative leaders must understand the social determinants of their community's health outcomes, which is essential knowledge in caring for a population.

Digital Redlining Checkpoint

As a result of broadband (high-speed internet) being unavailable to communities experiencing poverty, unemployment, and profoundly low educational levels, the health and wellness of individuals is disproportionately being impacted. Broadband is essential in that it promotes healthy communities by removing barriers to healthy outcomes and promoting access to healthcare (i.e., telemedicine), education (i.e., remote schooling), and employment (i.e., job postings). Digital redlining is a prime example of how SDOH influence a population's ability and opportunity to adequately manage their health in the same way that populations with access to broadband are able to do so (County Health Rankings and Roadmaps, n.d.).

ESSENTIAL SKILLS IN POPULATION HEALTH

Population Health Competencies: Essential Skills for Clinical, Educational, and Administrative Leaders for Population Health

The Council on Linkages Between Academia and Public Health Practice (Council on Linkages) is a joint venture between 24 U.S.-based public health organizations, including the CDC, AACN, and the American Public Health Association. See Box 25.1 for the complete list of the Council on Linkages partners. The Council on Linkages collaborates to establish core competency skills for public health professionals in academia and practice. The eight domains of the competencies are (1) Data Analytics and Assessment, (2) Policy Development and Program Planning, (3) Communication, (4) **Health Equity**, (5) Community Partnership, (6) Public Health Sciences, (7) Management and Finance, and (8) Leadership and Systems Thinking. This section will explore the essential skills of communication, community partnerships, and leadership and systems thinking skills related to population health.

Communication Skills and Community Partnerships

It is essential to develop relationships in the community to build partnerships. To achieve meaningful community connections, you need to appreciate the partner's culture with an awareness of any biases you may have. Effective communication with local, regional, national, and global health stakeholders is a skill that clinical, educational, and administrative leaders must possess. In a time of vast health information, nurse leaders are responsible for controlling the spread of health misinformation. Knowing the stakeholders in the population you serve is a crucial element in disseminating

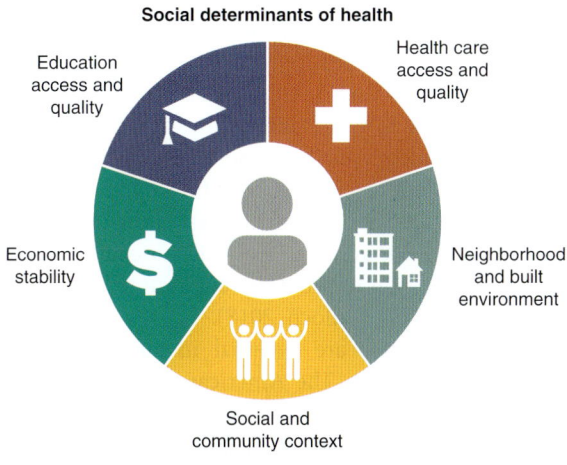

Fig. 25.3 Social Determinants of Health. (From Healthy Lakewood Foundation. Social Determinants of Health. https://healthylakewoodfoundation.org/social-determinants-of-health/. © Healthy Lakewood Foundation.)

> **BOX 25.1 The Council on Linkage Between Academia and Public Health Practice**
>
> 1. American Public Health Association
> 2. American Association of Colleges of Nursing
> 3. American College of Preventive Medicine
> 4. Association for Prevention Teaching and Research
> 5. Association of Accredited Public Health Programs
> 6. Association of Public Health Laboratories
> 7. Association of Schools and Programs of Public Health
> 8. Association of State and Territorial Health Officials
> 9. Association of University Programs in Health Administration
> 10. Centers for Disease Control and Prevention
> 11. Community-Campus Partnerships for Health
> 12. Council of Public Health Nursing Organizations
> 13. Council of State and Territorial Epidemiologists
> 14. Council on Education for Public Health
> 15. Health Resources and Services Administration
> 16. National Association of County and City Health Officials
> 17. National Association of Local Boards of Health
> 18. National Board of Public Health Examiners
> 19. National Environmental Health Association
> 20. National Library of Medicine
> 21. National Network of Public Health Institutes
> 22. Public Health Accreditation Board
> 23. Society for Public Health Education
> 24. Veteran's Health Administration (VHA)

From Public Health Foundation. (2023). *Advancing the public health workforce to achieve organizational excellence.* Public Health Foundation.

evidence-based health information. As health care leaders, conducting a critical appraisal of the evidence, summarizing evidence-based practice recommendations, and disseminating this information to individuals and the community in your health service area is crucial.

The AACN *Essentials* (2021) Domain 3 is devoted to population health competencies for nursing education. The advanced-level population health competencies include (1) managing population health, (2) engaging in effective partnerships, (3) considering the socioeconomic impact of the delivery of healthcare, (4) advancing equitable population health policy, (5) demonstrating advocacy strategies, and (6) advancing preparedness to protect population health during disasters and public health emergencies.

Partnering with local and regional elected and appointed government officials and policy makers, schools, clergy, business owners, community centers such as local Boys and Girls Clubs, and the media is essential in circulating evidence-based population health information. Engaging with other health professionals to address population health, demonstrating effective collaboration and mutual accountability with appropriate stakeholders, and using cultural and linguistic-appropriate communication strategies are entry-level competencies for nurses to possess (AACN, 2021).

> **TIP**
>
> Interprofessional collaboration between nurses, physicians, and community health workers can be an effective strategy for disseminating public health information to local officials, community partners, and the media.

Leadership and Systems Thinking in Population Health

The interconnectedness of systems plays a role in the health of populations. The world learned quickly from the COVID-19 pandemic just how interconnected and dependent the population of the world's health is on systems. Global, national, and local health care systems depend on a chain of industries from banking and capital markets, basic science, including research and development of vaccines, the supply chain, policy makers, and the media (Tooley, 2021). Although it is well known that attention to the SDOH is lacking in the United States, the recent pandemic further exposed the inequities vulnerable populations experience within our health care system. The survival of a system is less about competing and more about shared survival skills, including adaptation and the skill to build the community's response (Porter-O'Grady & Malloch, 2018).

Leadership skills are essential in affecting health policy and outcomes. The American Organization for Nursing Leaders (AONL) issued *Nurse Executive Competencies: Population Health* in 2015, recognizing that nurse leaders, as community advocates, need a skill set related to improving the health of the communities served (Association of Nurse Executives [AONE] & AONL, 2015). The AONL competencies are comprised of five domains: communication and relationship building, health care environment knowledge, leadership, professionalism, and business skills. The domains contain subdomains that expand on the knowledge and skills necessary for nurses in practice and academic leadership. Population health skills for nurse leaders include foundational thinking, such as a critical analysis of research-based evidence; systems thinking to consider nursing decisions' impact on the health of populations; personal journey disciplines, including seeking and providing mentorship; forging professional relationships; and succession planning (AONL, 2023).

THE MOST COVETED HEALTH OUTCOME: HAPPINESS

Happiness has been linked with improved mental health, reduced inflammation, improved cardiovascular health, lower risk of heart disease and stroke, and increased survival and longevity (Helliwell et al., 2013). Did you know the happiness of a country can be measured? The World Happiness Report (WHR) ranks a countries' happiness on a scale of 0 to 10 (Helliwell et al., 2023). The 2023 WHR found that (1) social support, (2) gross domestic product per capita, (3) healthy life expectancy, (4) freedom to make life choices, (5) generosity, and (6) absence of corruption are among the most essential factors in happiness. In the 2023 WHR, Finland, with an overall score of 7.8, leads the world in happiness and has been at the top of the happiness scale for the past six years, along with other Nordic countries. The United States ranked 15th out of 130 participating countries in the 2023 WHR with a world happiness score of 5.5. Focusing on happiness may be a key element in the population's health. Happiness has caught the interest of gerontologists because of emerging studies that link happiness with overall health and longevity over a lifetime. Among the questions researchers are asking are, if there is a *protective factor* for morbidity and mortality and overall survival predictions in older adults as an independent variable (Miething et al., 2020; Steptoe, 2019).

IMPLICATIONS FOR PRACTICE

Population health requires the acknowledgment of how embodiment, intertwined and multilevel lifetime actions, sets the context for both members of populations and subpopulations and their care providers. Members of the health care team should evaluate how evidence informs causes and actions to put forward a consistent message to populations. Small changes at the local level and of a socially determined nature have a larger impact on the health of populations than individual actions. A regular and systematically scheduled evaluation of population data may identify an incremental or larger change that may not be detected during the daily, busy practice of care. Knowing the stakeholders of your practice setting and population is imperative. Updating contacts at least annually is recommended, as people and their programs are dynamic.

Ongoing discussions about the business of healthcare, from the bedside to the boardroom, are foundational to the success of the provision of healthcare for populations. Improving business acumen to support skills such as inventory management, short- and long-term budgeting appropriations around services provided, and deimplementation analysis are critical to ensuring that high-quality care is maintained for a variety of populations. For example, during the first wave of the COVID-19 pandemic, a gap was quickly identified regarding the responsibility of nurses in ensuring proper inventory of personal protective equipment (PPE) including type of PPE, location of storage, and quantity needed to safely protect patients and their providers.

SYNTHESIS

An understanding of population health is critical to enable health care professionals to identify and respond to the needs of an increasingly complex health care landscape. Having the knowledge, skills, and competencies to view healthcare in terms of the most pressing needs impacting larger and larger segments of the population is crucial for meeting the diverse needs of people across the life span. Going forward, an understanding of population health will be required of all practitioners to improve health through education, interventions, more effective use of limited resources, and better policies from governing bodies. As a long-studied concept among the public and community health professionals, population health may be a newer term to some in the health care field. It is certainly receiving more attention in the form of research priorities and funding mechanisms. This is the result of current and emerging evidence that supports the impact of a population focus on the health of all people.

The collection, analysis, and synthesis of data help identify patterns and prevalence of all aspects of health. Advanced health practitioners use these data to support care and as evidence for practice changes. Critical to population health is the development of and maintenance of relationships across the entire spectrum within the community of care. There is more to a population's health than individual physiologies. There are collectives and subcollectives of human and societal interactions that create a climate of health that leads to happiness and long, productive lives. As nurses, we take an oath upon completing our academic studies cited at our graduation ceremony. This oath notes that *"In the full knowledge of responsibilities I am undertaking, I promise to care for my patients with all the knowledge, skills and understanding I possess, without regard to race, color, creed, politics or social status, sparing no effort to conserve meaningful life, to alleviate suffering, and to promote health."* In order to promote health effectively for all segments of society, practitioners need to be grounded in the science surrounding population health.

KEY POINTS

- Data are critical in identifying opportunities and strategies to promote population health and disease management across the continuum of care as well as epidemics, endemics, and pandemics.
- Nurses are responsible for analyzing and developing interventions to support all aspects of a population's health including, but not limited to, SDOH, physiology, and pharmacology.
- Nurses should lead the health care team in continuous, evidence-based quality improvement that addresses the impact of health equity across populations.
- Nurses are essential in informing policy makers on decisions and policies that impact the health of populations.
- In public health emergencies, nurses are key stakeholders in all phases of planning and preparedness to protect the health and wellness of populations.

REFERENCES

American Association of Colleges of Nursing (AACN). (2021). *The essentials: Core competencies for professional nursing education.* AACN. https://www.aacnnursing.org/Portals/42/AcademicNursing/pdf/Essentials-2021.pdf.

Association of Nurse Executives (AONE), & Association of Nurse Leaders (AONL). (2015). AONL nurse manager competencies. *AONE, AONL.* www.aonl.org/competiences.

Association of Nurse Leaders (AONL). (2023). *AONL nurse leader core competencies.* AONL.

Centers for Disease Control and Prevention (CDC). (2023). *What is public health?.* https://www.cdcfoundation.org/what-public-health.

County Health Rankings and Roadmaps. (n.d.). *Digital redlining: A digital disadvantage: Low broadband rates in urban, segregated pockets compound inequities.* County Health Rankings and Roadmaps. https://www.countyhealthrankings.org/reports/digital-redlining

Health Level Seven International. (n.d.). The Gravity Project. https://confluence.hl7.org/display/GRAV/The+Gravity+Project.

Helliwell, J. F., Huang, H., Norton, M., Goff, L., & Wang, S. (2023). World happiness, trust and social connections in times of crisis. In *World happiness report 2023* (11th ed., Chapter 2). UN Sustainable Development Solutions Network.

Helliwell, R., Layard, R., & Sachs, J. (2013). World happiness report. *UN Sustainable Development Solutions Network.*

Khaliq, A. A. (2020). *Managerial epidemiology: Principles & applications.* Jones & Bartlett Learning.

NASEM. (2023). *2022 annual report of the National Academies: Roundtable on Population Health Improvement.* Retrieved from https://nap.nationalacademies.org/catalog/27077/roundtable-on-population-health-improvement-annual-report-2022.

Miething, A., Mewes, J., & Giordano, G. N. (2020). Trust, happiness and mortality: Findings from a prospective US population-basted survey. *Social Science & Medicine, 252.* https://doi.org/10.1016/j.socscimed.2020.112809.

National Academies of Sciences, Engineering, and Medicine; Health and Medicine Division; Board on Population

Health and Public Health Practice; Roundtable on Population Health Improvement. (2016). *Advancing the science to improve population health: Proceedings of a workshop*. Washington (DC): National Academies Press (US). Roundtable on Population Health Improvement. Available from https://www.ncbi.nlm.nih.gov/books/NBK447172/.

Porter-O'Grady, & Malloch, K. T. (2018). *Quantum leadership: Creating sustainable value in health care* (5th ed.). Harper Collins.

Sachs, J., Kroll, C., Lafortune, G., Fuller, G., & Woelm, F. (2021). *The decade of action for the Sustainable Development Goals: Sustainable development report 2021*. Cambridge University Press.

Steptoe, A. (2019). Investing in happiness: The gerontological perspective. *Gerontology*, 65(6), 634–639. https://doi.org/10.1159/000501124.

Tooley, C. (2021). What "systems thinking" actually means—and why it matters for innovation today. https://www.weforum.org.

United Nations. (2015). Sustainable development. *The 17 Goals*. https://sdgs.un.org/goals.

U.S. Department of Health and Human Services. (1995). *Community-based health care: Nursing strategies—a report of an NINR priority expert panel. National nursing research agenda. Developing knowledge for practice: Challenges and opportunities*. U.S. Department of Health and Human Services.

U.S. Office of Disease Prevention and Health Promotion. (n.d.). Healthy people 2030. U.S. Department of Health and Human Services. https://health.gov/healthypeople.

World Health Organization (WHO). (2020). *A year without precedent: WHO's COVID-19 response*. https://www.who.int/news-room/spotlight/a-year-without-precedent-who-s-covid-19-response.

26

Health Policy

Kimberly S. Glassman and Dewi Brown-Deveaux

LEARNING OUTCOMES

After reading this chapter, you should be able to do the following:
- Describe the difference between policy and health policy.
- Identify levels of health policy within the policy process.
- Integrate evidence to develop and influence health polices at multiple levels (federal, state, local).
- Implement a policy change at the organizational level.
- Engage with professional organizations to influence policies to improve health and health equity.

KEY TERMS

Health equity   Health policy   Nursing and health policy

OVERVIEW OF POLICY AND HEALTH POLICY

This chapter describes the ways that the nursing profession participates in the development of health policy, including identifying a policy problem, engaging stakeholders, moving a policy agenda through the legislative process, and implementing the final policy. The historical context of nursing's role in policy development through the contemporary issues faced by the profession, including pandemics, well-being, and workforce issues, are explained. The role of advanced practice nurses in shaping health policy and the importance of research in developing health policy are discussed, in addition to the landscape of professional nursing and nursing organizations' contributions to health and health policy development and implementation. Nurses' obligation to address organizational and local, state, and federal policies is noted.

Nurses, as one of the most trusted professions, have many opportunities to influence the care of people in their communities and beyond. One of nursing's greatest advantages is that people listen to what they have to say about most topics. However, nursing's power cannot be leveraged to help the community at large if they do not know how to influence policy.

Policy is defined as a set of standards, law, regulation, procedure, administrative action, and/or incentive, established by the governments, whereas institutional policies are developed by organizations to guide internal practices and actions (Pollack Porter et al., 2018). Policy decisions are often reflected in resource allocations by legislative bodies or the individual organization through well-formed and data-driven presentations to organizational leaders.

Health policy refers to the decisions, plans, and actions that are assumed by governments, organizations, and stakeholders to achieve population health, and safeguard access to quality health care services (World Health Organization [WHO], 2020). This broad definition covers all aspects of how health policy shapes our lives, but the actual "doing policy" is more complex (Keller & Ridenour,

2021). Our own health is influenced by policies in different sectors, such as transportation policies that encourage physical activity by creating bicycle-friendly community design or schools' policies used to improve nutritional content of school meals (Centers for Disease Control and Prevention [CDC], 2024; https://www.cdc.gov/active-people-healthy-nation/php/get-started/index.html).

Health policy has been shaped over time by a range of factors, including scientific advancements, societal changes, political ideologies, and evolving health care systems (Annesley, 2019). Health policy has further developed by advancement in technology, increased health care costs, and the unending quest for Sustainable Development Goals (Buzeti et al., 2020). The COVID-19 pandemic also highlighted the importance of how increased awareness of the need for international partnerships have shaped global health policy (Chelak & Chakole, 2023).

Health policy seeks to improve population health, access to quality care, and impact the challenges of an ever-shifting health care landscape (National Academies of Sciences, Engineering, and Medicine [NASEM], 2021). Nurses play an important role in advocating for policy that impacts patients and the profession, especially when working together on issues that affect nursing practice and health outcomes. Nurses can have an insightful influence on health policy by becoming engaged in the policy process on many levels. This engagement includes identifying those policies to impact, as well as evaluating the evidence for or against the policy and leading policy change (American Association of Colleges of Nursing, 2021).

HISTORICAL CONTEXT OF NURSING'S CONTRIBUTION IN HEALTH POLICY

Nursing's role in shaping health policy has evolved significantly over time, informed by various sociopolitical factors, advancements in healthcare, and nurses' changing roles and responsibilities. Nursing's transition to a "formal" profession in the 19th century was informed by the pioneering work of figures like Florence Nightingale (Harper et al., 2014) and Mary Seacole (Mary Seacole Trust, 2023) working to improve care to soldiers in the Crimean War. During this period, nursing health policy was focused on creating nursing care standards and professionalizing nursing practice. In the early 20th century, nursing policy work expanded toward regulation and licensure (Chiu et al., 2021). The scope of and legal recognition of nursing practice was defined by the establishment of state nursing boards and legislation of state nurse practice acts (Keeling, 2015). These policies regulated the practice of nursing to protect the public and ensure skilled nursing care.

The World Health Organization's Alma-Ata Declaration in 1978 underscored the significance of primary healthcare and nurse's involvement in achieving equitable access to health services worldwide (Hajizadeh et al., 2021). The declaration prompted the development of policies to achieve health for all, with nurses in a pivotal role to promote primary health care and creating preventative health measures (WHO, 2018).

The late 20th century brought a significant emphasis on patient safety, quality improvement, and evidence-based practice with the dramatic shift to care for people in hospitals rather than in their homes—the predominant model of the early 1900s (Keeling, 2015). National, state, and organizational policies were implemented to reduce patient harm such as health care-associated infections, medication errors, and hospital-acquired conditions (Bates & Singh, 2018). In addition, the rapid inception of health care technology prompted the development of federal policies such as the Health Insurance Portability and Accountability Act of 1996 (HIPAA) to protect patients' personal and health-related information in all forms of health records. Additional regulation followed with the Health Information Technology for Economic and Clinical Health Act of 2009, which strengthened the HIPAA Privacy and Security Rules protections by including business associates, while also incentivizing the adoption of electronic health records. Telehealth and additional digital health innovations soon followed and continue to expand at exponential rates. Many of these federal policies come with financial rewards and penalties to health care organizations, such as withholding Medicare payment for high infection or injury rates and subsidies for hospitals and practices to implement electronic health records (Bates & Singh, 2018).

In 2019, the COVID-19 pandemic prompted the National Academy of Medicine (NAM) to convene a group of experts across the health, payer, and government sectors to identify strengths and areas of opportunity that arose out of caring for people and communities during the pandemic (NAM, 2023). This publication identifies several strategies and implications for changing and developing new policies to guide future pandemic care. The pandemic has further highlighted the critical role of nurses in health care systems worldwide. It prompted policy responses to address the challenges nurses face and ensure their safety, well-being, and support during times of crisis (Anders, 2021).

There is a growing recognition of the importance of nursing leadership in policy. Nurses are increasingly involved in shaping health policy at local, national, and international levels, advocating for the needs of patients and the profession (Anders, 2021). The American Academy of Nursing serves as the policy voice for the nursing profession. This membership organization, made up of expert nurses who have made significant contributions to the profession, healthcare, and health policy, shapes health policy at the national level (aannet.org).

Nursing policy has evolved from focusing on professionalism and regulation to encompass broader issues of access, quality, safety, and leadership (Limoges et al., 2022). Nurses shape policies that improve health care delivery, promote health equity, and address emerging health challenges (Chiu et al, 2021).

ADVANCING HEALTH POLICY INTO PRACTICE

Moving policy into practice is an iterative process that involves the transition and implementation of policies into tangible actions and changes in health care delivery. The development of policies frames direction, but policies impact health care practices through effective and robust implementation.

A useful tool for understanding the policy process is illustrated in Fig. 26.1.

The following steps outline how policy moves into practice (CDC, 2024). For nurses interested in developing, changing, or evaluating policies, it is important to understand where the policy sits in the policy process. For example, if a problem has been identified, but not yet shaped into a policy, the issue is at the *problem identification* stage. It is important to note that the lack of an existing policy is not a "policy problem."

1. **Problem Identification**: Policies are developed by collecting, summarizing, and interpreting data related to a problem identified. The data are then assessed for potential gaps to frame the problem, which then lends itself to a potential policy solution. This stage defines the goals and objectives, targeted

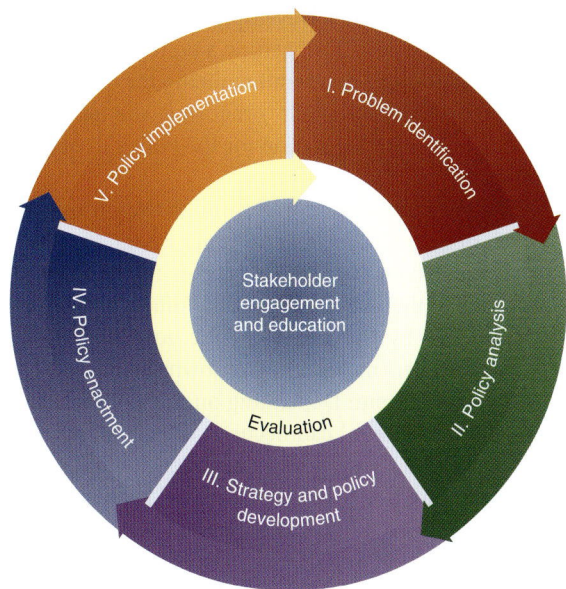

Fig. 26.1 The Policy Process. (From Centers for Disease Control and Prevention (CDC), Office of Policy, Performance, and Evaluation. (n.d.). The CDC policy process. https://www.cdc.gov/policy/polaris/policyprocess/index.html.)

population, health care issues, strategies, and interventions.

A policy may have been identified and proposed but is not moving forward. This is an opportunity to explore who is sponsoring the policy (regulation) and why this person or organization is involved. Perhaps the issue or problem has not been well defined, and the nurse has the knowledge and expertise to offer different wording or additional examples, or to clarify the issue from the perspective of the people served. There may be a need for more compelling research to reassure the legislators that this is the best action to solve the problem.

2. **Policy Analysis**: Recognition of varied policy to address the problem by utilizing research studies to assess the greatest efficiency.

This phase of the policy process requires knowledge of the legislative process. The nurse needs to know which legislator is supporting the policy, and where the proposed policy sits in the legislative process—which committee is it in, where is it stuck, and which legislators need to be contacted are all spaces that nurses can work in to move a policy forward.

3. **Strategy and Policy Development:** Recognize and strategize the process of getting a policy adopted and the methodology of operationalizing the policy. The adoption process entails procuring the necessary endorsements or legislation for the policy to become official (CDC, 2024).

   When the policy has moved through the various levels of federal, state, or local government, the policy is then voted on, and if passed, is finalized by the head of the relevant legislative office, and signed into law by the president, the governor, or the local leader (mayor, chair of town council, etc.).

4. **Policy Enactment:** Depending on the jurisdiction of the policy, espousal can occur at the organizational, regional, or national level. Enactment or passing of the policy follows internal or external procedures.

   Finally, the policy that is now the law needs to be implemented, and that is done by various branches of government. At the federal level, laws are implemented by the executive branch—the Office of the President. The relevant sector will need to write the rules on how to implement the law. There is a similar process at the state and local level—there is another legislative body responsible for writing the implementation plan.

5. **Policy Implementation:** Implementation of the policy involves translating the enacted policy into practical steps and activities. Implementation requires clear communication and resource allocation to build the capacity of the personnel implementing the policy (CDC, 2024).

   Policy moving into practice is an iterative and multifaceted process, involving effective implementation, evaluation, and monitoring to measure impact and identify barriers, gaps, or progress to track its process. The policy, however, can be adapted or adjusted by policy makers and stakeholders during monitoring. This might include revising of guidelines, reallocating resources or implementing new strategies. Once the policy has been deemed successful, it is then integrated into routine health care practices, regulations, and organizational structures.

Identifying an issue or problem requires an understanding of where the issue is in the policy process. Some issues, such as nurse staffing ratios, may be discussed in policy circles (stakeholders, etc.) and never get traction as a bill. Sometimes, these bills languish in legislative committees and never move forward, and others speed through the process. Nurses must be able to identify where the issue fits in the policy process so that an action can be developed and implemented. Perhaps a regulation exists but is no longer relevant to the current issues faced today and require revision. Those actions would be different from the action necessary to move a bill out of a committee to the next step in the legislative process. Nursing's effectiveness as a profession is only as good as our knowledge of the process.

THE ROLE OF GOVERNMENT AND LEGISLATIVE BODIES IN HEALTH POLICY

Health policies are shaped and influenced by the three layers of government, federal, state/provincial, and local. At the national level, the federal government frames overarching health policies, enacts legislation, and allots health care funding and resources (Pollack Porter et al., 2018). The federal government develops regulations and promotes intersectoral collaboration to enhance health by addressing social determinants of health (SDOH). Regional governments implement federal health policies, allocate resources, and engage in health planning that address local needs and have jurisdictional authority to mitigate health disparities by modifying policies to address specific contexts (Pollack Porter et al., 2018). Local government implements public health initiatives to facilitate access to health care services and address local affairs (Pollack Porter et al., 2018). Each level of government—federal, state, and local—is collectively essential for the improvement of population health outcomes.

NURSES IMPACT HEALTH POLICY AT THE THREE LEVELS OF GOVERNMENT

Nurses wield considerable influence on policy at every level of government. The commitment to advance patient care and being the largest group of health professionals positions nurses as valuable partners in shaping health care policies. Professional organizations are an important partner in providing a unified voice and advocacy strategies to drive policy at both the state and national level. The American Academy of Nursing (aannet.org) serves as the policy arm of the American Nurses Association (www.nursingworld.org) and demonstrates an unwavering commitment to policy advocacy. Through the filing of several amicus briefs and publishing policy briefs, they take definitive stances on critical issues, contributing to policy formulation and implementation. Equally vital is the contribution of the American Association of Colleges of Nursing (aacnnursing.org), which represents higher education and lobbies for increased funding for nursing education to ensure a robust and skilled pipeline for nurses. The Health Resources and Services Administration-sponsored Nurse Faculty Loan Program (https://bhw.hrsa.gov/funding/apply-loan-repayment#faculty-lrp) provides low-interest loans to nurses seeking master's and doctoral degrees who commit to a teaching career. Designed to bolster the nursing faculty shortage, these federal policies are an important method for developing nursing education as a career option. In addition to these pivotal efforts, nursing specialty organizations, such as the National Black Nurses Association, the National Hispanic Organization, the Oncology Nursing Society, the American Association of Critical-Care Nurses, and many others provide lobbying support for their members on issues relevant to that organization.

At the national level, nurses influence health policy through:

a. Advocacy: Nurses are positioned to collaborate with professional and nursing associations to increase awareness of key health care issues and advocate for evidence-based policies (Chiu et al., 2021; American Nurses Association, 2023).
b. Expertise and Research: By conducting research, publishing studies, and participating in advisory committees, nurses provide valued insights and evidence to help shape effective health policies (Hajizadeh et al., 2021).
c. Professional Nursing Associations: Nurses influence health care legislation and policy decisions by collaborating with professional organizations that have dedicated policy committees and lobbying efforts (Hajizadeh et al., 2021).

At the regional or state level, nurses can impact policy by:

a. Grassroots Advocacy: Nurses can attend public health hearings, contact policy makers, and share experiences related to health care issues in grassroots advocacy (Gerber, 2018; NASEM, 2021).
b. Coalition Building: Nurses are situated to amplify their voices and advocate for policy change by joining or forming coalitions with community organizations, health care professionals, and advocacy groups (Chiu et al., 2021).
c. Policy Analysis and Development: Nurses can provide expertise to health care task forces, communities, and advisory boards to shape polices and regulations by actively participating in policy analysis and developmental processes (Anders, 2021).

At the local level, nurses can influence policy by:

a. Community Engagement: Nurses are essential partners to enhance the community by listening to community needs and concerns by attending community public meetings, and joining community health boards to advocate for policies that address health issues and community well-being locally (Chiu et al., 2021). Community organizations can collaborate to improve the health of communities and support legislation to accomplish changes. Community boards, businesses, schools, etc. are all important partners in achieving better health for communities. Because most of these people are not health care providers, nurses become key partners and advisers to these local committees.
b. Partnerships With Local Leaders: Nurses can foster partnerships with local leaders, such as council members, mayors, and community influencers, to influence policy decisions and drive attention to health care issues affecting the local population (Chiu et al., 2021).

Leveraging expertise, experiences, and strong advocacy skills, nurses impact policy at all levels of government. Nurses' involvement help ensure that policies are patient centered and evidence based, and address the needs of the communities they serve.

IMPACT OF HEALTH POLICY ON NURSING PRACTICE

Health policy and nursing practice share corresponding roles and interrelationships within the health care system. Health policies are geared toward improving health outcomes, health care equity, and the allocation of resources to address individual and community health care needs (Hajizadeh et al., 2021). Pope et al. (1995) defines nursing practice as a caring-based practice in which processes of diagnosis and treatment are applied to human experiences of health and illness. Nursing practice incorporates a wide range of responsibilities, inclusive of health assessment, direct patient care, health education, medication administration, coordination of care, and advocacy for patients' rights and well-being (Pope et al., 1995). Additionally, nursing practice is grounded in evidence-based guidelines, ethical principles, and professional standards (Pope et al., 1995). Health policy and nursing practice are closely intertwined as health policies influence nursing practice resources and regulations, impact the environment where nurses deliver care, shape the frameworks of nursing practice, and provide health care financing for accessibility of health care services (Anders, 2021).

The scope of nursing practice, professional standards, and patient safety are guided by regulations and licensing policies (Annesley, 2019). As frontline health care providers, nurses are uniquely positioned to recognize health care gaps, advocate for patient needs, and contribute to policy development (Anders, 2021; Limoges et al., 2022). Nurses have myriad roles within the health care system, and through these roles—patient care, education, research, leadership—they offer a firsthand perspective into the effectiveness, or lack thereof, of health policies within organizations and in the communities they serve.

HARNESSING EVIDENCE AND RESEARCH TO INFORM POLICY

Evidence and research inform policy through the process of using the extant evidence and new research findings to outline and guide the advancement of effective policies in the field of healthcare (White, 2021). Utilizing evidence ensures that policy decisions are substantiated by reliable and valid evidence for desired outcomes that optimizes the distribution of resources (Pollack Porter et al., 2018).

Policy makers hope to make informed decisions through scientific knowledge to minimize ideological preferences, biases, and independent opinions that could influence policy decisions (White, 2021). Evidence-based policy making underscores the use of empirical data and research to assess the probable impacts and outcomes of varied policy options such as safety, effectiveness, interventions, and cost effectiveness (McKee, 2019). Evidence-based policy also promotes transparency and accountability, which increases the legitimacy and reliability of polices to achieve the desired outcomes. This allows policy makers to prioritize efficient, effective, and reasonable interventions. Evidence alone, however, cannot dictate policy decisions. The development of policy is a multifaceted interplay of values, political considerations, evidence, and stakeholders' agreement. Evidence is utilized to inform and support policy choices by balancing the best available evidence in conjunction with all applicable considerations (Pollack Porter et al., 2018).

The National Institute of Nursing Research (NINR) recently communicated their 2022–2026 strategic plan and highlighted five research areas for nurses to focus their science: health equity, SDOH, population and community health, prevention and health promotion, and systems and models of care (NINR, 2022). Through these research lenses, the NINR recognizes the need for innovative systems and models of care that are comprised of partnerships and coalitions that span clinical and community settings and address social factors and needs for populations and individuals. NINR strongly encourages nurse-led systems and models of care that consider how to leverage the public's trust in and the expertise of the nursing workforce; employ policy and organizational solutions informed by on-the-ground experiences of nurses; and focus on health-promoting care that encompasses the whole person in the context of their lives and living conditions, before, during, and after their points of care.

ROLES FOR CLINICAL LEADERS IN POLICY

Clinical leaders are an essential part of the health care system. Prepared at the master's and doctoral levels, they hold a unique position to effect positive change in policies both within their organization and on a broader scale. Clinical leaders possess the knowledge and proficiency to recognize areas where policies may enhance efficient and evidence-based care because of their advanced education and specialized training. By closely evaluating patients' data and benchmarking against best practices and guidelines, clinical leaders can lead initiatives to close the gap between patient care and patient outcomes by recommending new organizational policies and evidence-based changes. Furthermore, clinical leaders are proficient at finding and leveraging data to support their recommendations for enhancing care. Whether it entails wellness measures such as cancer screenings or vaccinations, or adopting a practice guideline with proven improvements to care, the clinical leader can use the best available evidence with organization data to demonstrate the need to change a practice. The clinical leader is skilled at presenting data reflecting the best practice to organizational leaders, and in designing the improvement methodologies to implement the new practice. By leading the identified care team through iterative, small tests of change, using an established methodology, clinical leaders can drive the effort to improve care outcomes.

In addition to influencing policies within an organization, clinical leaders can take advocacy to the next level by engaging with local legislators at the municipal and state level. Armed with data and evidence, clinical leaders can effectively present the need for change in regulations that impact health care delivery. Clinical leaders successfully lobbied and advocated for the elimination of practice restrictions in several states supporting the move toward greater autonomy and independent practice (NASEM, 2021). As champions of evidence-based care and advocates for policy change, clinical leaders not only serve as leaders but are positioned to serve as partners in improving health outcomes and ensuring that policies align with evidence for the future.

ADDRESSING HEALTH DISPARITIES THROUGH POLICY INTERVENTIONS

Policies impact SDOH, the conditions in which people are born, grow, live, work, and age, and the environment that shape their health outcomes (Saunders et al., 2017). Evidence suggests that policies that address SODH aid in reducing health disparities and improve overall population health (NASEM, 2021). The impact of policy on SDOH can be seen in the following ways:

1. **Education**: Policies that support access to equitable education help reduce educational disparities and improve health literacy, which positively influences health outcomes and creates opportunities for socioeconomic advancement (Ramirez-Rubio et al., 2019; Buzeti et al., 2020).
2. **Income and Employment**: Minimum wage, income support programs, and employment opportunities policies influence individuals' and families' financial resources and stability (Buzeti et al., 2020). Sufficient income and employment opportunities influence access to healthcare, safe housing, nutritious food, and essential resources for health and well-being (Ramirez-Rubio et al., 2019).
3. **Housing**: Access to safe, affordable, and stable housing policies have a direct impact on health (Chelak & Chakole, 2023). Appropriate housing conditions impact physical and mental health. They safeguard environmental hazards and reduce risk of infectious diseases (Buzeti et al., 2020).
4. **Health Care Access**: Expansive access to affordable, comprehensive, and quality health care services policies addresses health inequities. It ensures access to healthcare for all individuals, irrespective of social determinants or socioeconomic status, thus reducing health care disparities and negative health outcomes (Chelak & Chakole, 2023).
5. **Environmental Factors**: Policies connected to pollution control, environmental protection, and sustainable development impact the physical environment in which people live (Chelak & Chakole, 2023). A healthy environment and clean water help avert illness by decreasing exposure to environmental hazards and encourage healthy lifestyle and activities (Ramirez-Rubio et al., 2019).
6. **Social and Racial Equity**: Policies that unambiguously address social and racial injustices can profoundly impact health outcomes (Buzeti et al., 2020). Policies can promote social justice and health equity by addressing systemic discrimination, bias, and unequal distribution of resources (Chelak & Chakole, 2023).

The Future of Nursing 2020–2030 (NASEM, 2021) report calls for the nursing profession to leverage their expertise in patient care, quality, and safety, to focus efforts on achieving health equity for all people. Nurses recognize that poorly informed public policy, like poor healthcare and compromised SDOH, can undermine the health of patients, families, and communities. Actions to address SDOH are often rooted in long-standing policies that contribute to inequity in housing, employment, education, and other key precursors to health. The authors of the report see a major role for the nursing profession in engaging in the complex work of aligning public health, healthcare, social services, and public policies to eliminate health disparities and achieve health equity. The recommendations address how nursing, in partnership with others, can address important system changes, including preparing nurses to act individually, in teams, and across sectors to find solutions to address the needs of an aging population, improve access to primary care, mental and behavioral health, structural racism, high maternal mortality and morbidity, and eliminate the disease burden carried by specific segments of the U.S. population (NASEM, 2021). The recommendations include:

1. All national nursing organizations working together to develop a shared agenda for addressing SDOH and achieving health equity with explicit priorities across nursing practice, education, leadership, and health policy.
2. Developing coalitions of key stakeholders in state and federal government, healthcare, and public health organizations, payers, and foundations—to develop actions that enable the nursing workforce to address the SDOH and health equity in all practice settings.
3. Promotion of nurses' health and well-being needs to be supported by nursing education, employers, nursing leaders, licensing boards, and nursing organizations as nurses assume new roles to advance health equity.
4. All organizations, including state and federal, need to remove barriers to enable all nurses to practice to their full scope to advance health equity. The barriers include regulatory, public, and private payment limitations; restrictive policies and practices; and other legal, professional and commercial impediments.
5. All payers (federal, tribal, state, local, private, and public health agencies) should establish sustainable and flexible payment mechanisms to support nurses in both healthcare and public health, including school nurses, to address social needs, SDOH, and health equity.
6. All private and public health care systems should incorporate nursing expertise in designing, generating, analyzing, and applying data to support initiatives directed toward SDOH and health equity using digital platforms, artificial intelligence, and other innovative technologies.
7. Nursing education programs, including continuing education, and accreditors and the National Council of State Boards of Nursing should ensure that nurses are prepared to address SDOH and health equity.
8. To enable nurses to address inequities within communities, federal agencies, and other stakeholders within and outside of the profession, nursing should strengthen and protect the nursing workforce during the response to such public health emergencies as the COVID-19 pandemic, and natural disasters, including those related to climate change.
9. Federal agencies that fund research, together with private organizations and foundations, should convene representatives from nursing, public health, and healthcare to develop and support a research agenda and evidence base describing the impact of nursing interventions on SDOH, environmental health, health equity, and nurses' health and well-being (NASEM, 2021, pp. 355–376).

Policies alone, however, cannot fully address all SDOH. Incorporating well-designed and all-inclusive policies that prioritize health equity and social justice can enable an environment that supports individuals and communities in achieving optimal health and well-being. Addressing social determinants of health through health policy interventions makes it possible to make significant strides in reducing health inequities and improving overall population health.

SYNTHESIS

The policies that shape our health, and our lives, are important for nurses to identify, review, and determine if such policies are supporting the health of individuals and populations or if those policies no longer serve the public need to be changed. Nurses are in a pivotal role to influence where the world moves to create policies that support people where they live, work and play, and to ensure that all people can lead a full and productive life. Enhancing one's understanding of the policy process and the legislative process is essential for nurses to advocate for better health and health equity for all people. Using evidence to inform care, evaluating the outcomes of that evidence-based care, and making changes to care with those evaluative data are important steps to bringing polices in alignment with public interests.

KEY POINTS

- Nurses play an important role in shaping health policy to improve the lives of people and their communities.
- Nurses' role in shaping health policy has evolved from focusing on regulation and standardization of practice to advancing health equity.
- Health policy is shaped by evidence-based practice and research to inform regulations at all levels of government—local, state, and federal.
- Clinical leaders have an important role in advancing health policy for population health to benefit people and the communities we serve.

REFERENCES

American Association of Colleges of Nursing. (2021). *The essentials: Core competencies for professional nursing education*. American Association of Colleges of Nursing.

American Nurses Association. (2023). *Health policy*. https://www.nursingworld.org/practice-policy/health-policy/.

Anders, R. L. (2021). Engaging nurses in health policy in the era of COVID-19. *Nursing Forum, 56*(1), 89–94. https://doi.org/10.1111/nuf.12514.

Annesley, S. H. (2019). The implications of health policy for nursing. *British Journal of Nursing (Mark Allen Publishing), 28*(8), 496–502. https://doi.org/10.12968/bjon.2019.28.8.496.

Bates, D. W., & Singh, H. (2018). Two decades since *to Err Is Human*: An assessment of progress and emerging priorities in patient safety. *Health Affairs, 37*, 1736–1743.

Buzeti, T., Madureira Lima, J., Yang, L., & Brown, C. (2020). Leaving no one behind: Health equity as a catalyst for the sustainable development goals. *European Journal of Public Health, 30*(Suppl. 1), i24–i27. https://doi.org/10.1093/eurpub/ckaa033.

Centers for Disease Control and Prevention. (2024). Active people, healthy nation. https://www.cdc.gov/active-people-healthy-nation/php/about/index.htmlaccessed 12082024.

Chelak, K., & Chakole, S. (2023). The role of social determinants of health in promoting health equality: A narrative review. *Cureus, 15*(1), e33425. https://doi.org/10.7759/cureus.33425.

Chiu, P., Cummings, G. G., Thorne, S., & Schick-Makaroff, K. (2021). Policy advocacy and nursing organizations: A scoping review. *Policy, Politics & Nursing Practice, 22*(4), 271–291. https://doi.org/10.1177/15271544211050611.

Gerber, L. (2018). Understanding the nurse's role as a patient advocate. *Nursing, 48*(4), 55–58. https://doi.org/10.1097/01.NURSE.0000531007.02224.65.

Hajizadeh, A., Zamanzadeh, V., Kakemam, E., Bahreni, R., & Khodayari-Zarnaq, R. (2021). Factors influencing nurses' participation in the health policymaking process: A systematic review. *BMC Nursing, 20*, 128. https://doi.org/10.1186/s12912-021-00648-6.

Harper, D. C., Davey, K. S., & Fordham, P. N. (2014). Leadership lessons in global nursing from Nightingale from Nightingale letter collection at the University of Alabama at Birmingham. *Journal of Holistic Nursing, 32*, 44–53. https://doi.org/10.1177/0898010113497835.

Keeling, A. W. (2015). Historical perspectives on an expanded role for nursing. *Online Journal of Issues in Nursing, 20*(2), 2.

Keller, T., & Ridenour, N. (2021). Ethics. In J. Giddens (Ed.), *Concepts for nursing practice*. Elsevier.

Limoges, J., Mclean, J., Anzola, D., & Kolla, N. J. (2022). Effects of the COVID-19 pandemic on healthcare providers: Policy implications for pandemic recovery. *Healthcare policy = Politiques de sante, 17*(3), 49–64. https://doi.org/10.12927/hcpol.2022.26728.

Mary Seacole Trust. (2023). *Mary Seacole trust*. https://www.maryseacoletrust.org.uk/.

McKee, M. (2019). Bridging the gap between research and policy and practice: Comment on "CIHR health system impact fellows: Reflections on 'driving change' within the health system." *International Journal Health Policy Management, 8*(9), 557–559. https://doi.org/10.15171/ijhpm.2019.46.

National Academies of Sciences, Engineering, and Medicine (NASEM). (2021). *The future of nursing 2020–2030: Charting a path to achieve health equity*. National Academies Press. https://doi.org/10.17226/25982.

National Academy of Medicine (NAM). (2023). *Emerging stronger from COVID-19: Priorities for health system transformation*. National Academies Press. https://doi.org/10.17226/26657.

National Institute for Nursing Research (NINR). (2022). Mission and strategic plan. https://www.ninr.nih.gov/aboutninr/ninr-mission-and-strategic-plan/research-framework.

Pollack Porter, K. M., Rutkow, L., & McGinty, E. E. (2018). The importance of policy change for addressing public health problems. *Public Health Reports, 133*(1_Suppl.), 9S–14S. https://doi.org/10.1177/0033354918788880.

Pope, A. M., Snyder, M. A., & Mood, L. H. (Eds.); Institute of Medicine (US) Committee on Enhancing Environmental Health Content in Nursing Practice. (1995). Chapter 3, Nursing practice. In *Nursing health, & environment: Strengthening the relationship to improve the public's health*. Washington (DC): National Academies Press (US). Available from: https://www.ncbi.nlm.nih.gov/books/NBK232401/.

Ramirez-Rubio, O., Daher, C., Fanjul, G., Gascon, M., Mueller, N., Pajín, L., et al. (2019). Urban health: An example of a "health in all policies" approach in the context of SDGs implementation. *Globalization and Health, 15*(1), 87. https://doi.org/10.1186/s12992-019-0529-z.

Saunders, M., Barr, B., McHale, P., & Hamelmann, C. (2017). *Key policies for addressing the social determinants of health and health inequities (Health Evidence Network Synthesis Report, No. 52)*. WHO Regional Office for Europe. https://www.ncbi.nlm.nih.gov/books/NBK453566/.

White, K. M. (2021). Translation of evidence in health policy. In K. M. White, S. Dudley-Brown, & M. F. Terharr (Eds.), *Translation of evidence into nursing and healthcare* (pp. 144–164). New York: Springer Publishing.

World Health Organization (WHO). (2020). *Health policy*. http://www.who.int/topics/health_policy/en/.

World Health Organization (WHO). (2018). WHO called to return to the Declaration of Alma-Ata. http://www.who.int/social_determinants/tools/multimedia/alma_ata/en/.

27

Nurse Wellness: An Evolving Concept and Its Connection to Health Care System Outcomes

Kathleen DeMarco and Sean Clarke

LEARNING OUTCOMES

After reading this chapter, you should be able to do the following:
- Explain the high interest in nurse wellness and the significance of nurse wellness for workforce stability.
- Identify the similarities and differences in various definitions of health, wellness, and well-being as applied to nurses.
- Describe various ways of assessing nurse wellness.
- Describe strategies that can be used to promote nurse wellness at various levels within health care organizations.
- List strategies and pitfalls in research and quality improvement directed at improving nurse wellness.

KEY TERMS

Avocational interest
Burnout
Code Lavender
Compassion fatigue
Compassion satisfaction
Employee assistance program
Engagement
Health
Just culture
Meditation
Mindfulness
Peer-to-peer support
Psychological safety
Resilience
Schwartz Center Rounds
Well-being
Wellness
Work–life integration

Health, wellness, and well-being are overlapping ideas. The World Health Organization (2020) defines **health** as "a state of complete physical, mental and social well-being and not merely the absence of disease or infirmity." Such a definition, common to many areas in nursing and health science, is not only broader than lay definitions of being "healthy" or not (i.e., "ill" versus "not ill") emphasizing physical ailments, but it also pulls in the idea of contentment. **Wellness** implies living optimally in various dimensions and in a manner intended to maintain this positive state (i.e., engaging in self-care). **Well-being** is a state of happiness or harmony with one's life and environment in addition to living well (Holdsworth, 2019). Well-being is perhaps the most comprehensive of these concepts and can be thought of as an ideal or aspirational state.

The concept of a healthy workforce has existed since the 1960s and employers have long noted that worker wellness and engagement are critical to the productivity and reputation of an organization. Workforce health was an extension of emerging ideas regarding healthy communities. That special attention might need to be paid to the health of nurses and other health care workers, not only because of the stresses of their work but also because of the consequences of their health for workforce stability and service delivery, is a relatively new idea. Put otherwise, despite shortages being a recurrent problem for nursing for well over a century, it is

401

only over the last two to three decades that researchers and leaders have systematically worked to "connect the dots" between wellness, the supply of health care workers, and the quality of healthcare. The COVID-19 pandemic raised the profile of health care worker wellness. In addition to the stresses of daily life experienced by everyone in communities worldwide, nurses and other health workers bore witness to the suffering of patients and loved ones through the waves of the pandemic and endured special personal risks in delivering patient care (Gee et al., 2022). We are still watching the effects of the crisis unfold. It is important to remember that while COVID-19 may have jump-started interest in well-being, work in this area began several decades earlier—perhaps in line with a culture change in healthcare and new focus on the many factors affecting patient safety. There is still much to be done in terms of promoting wellness in health care workplaces, both in terms of local, national, and international approaches, as well as research that remains to be conducted.

Noting stress among students as well as concerns about the well-being of the workforce, the national association for baccalaureate and higher nursing education in the United States, the American Association of Colleges of Nursing (AACN), gave priority to wellness and resilience in Domain 10 of the new *Essentials* and adopted a resolution to encourage the development of curriculum and other resources to promote mental health, physical health, healthy lifestyle behaviors, and well-being in students, faculty, and staff (AACN, 2020, 2021). The American Organization of Nurse Leaders (AONL) recently incorporated well-being into their nursing leadership competencies for nurse managers and chief nurse executives (AONL, 2022).

It is not surprising that nurse wellness is a topic that frequently emerges as a theme for literature searches and sometimes even research by clinical nurses and nursing students as well as managers. As a clinical leader you will see the impact that nurse wellness has on your practice, and will have opportunities to directly influence aspects of nurse wellness as well as find creative strategies to cover vacancies, manage overtime, advocate for appropriate staffing practices, and create orientation processes within the constraints of tight budgets (which all indirectly affect nurse wellness), all the while ensuring that high-quality care is being delivered.

This chapter will review concepts related to nurse wellness and resilience and evidence related to leadership strategies that you can incorporate into your practice to promote a healthy work environment for you and your staff and enhance the quality of the healthcare you deliver.

THE CONTEXT FOR HEIGHTENED ATTENTION TO NURSE WELLNESS

The nursing profession's pivotal role in health care systems' ability to achieve optimal patient outcomes hinges on the adequacy and the well-being of the workforce. The National Academies of Sciences, Engineering, and Medicine (NASEM) Future of Nursing 2020–2030 report (NASEM, 2021) stated that well-being affects individual nurses' physical and mental health and joy and meaning in their work, professional satisfaction, and job engagement, as well as patient care quality and patient perceptions of the care they receive. The interconnection of health care worker wellness and quality of care is reflected in the Institute for Healthcare Improvement's recommendation that quality improvement efforts move from prioritizing a Triple Aim (that is, targeting enhanced population health outcomes and patient experience, as well as reductions in per capita costs of care) to a Quadruple Aim by adding improved work–life of clinicians and staff (Bodenheimer & Sinsky, 2014).

The health care sector faces challenges in delivering high-quality services, ensuring ready access to services, and delivering care at reasonable costs; turbulent conditions in society continue to place strains on both nurses and their patients. Turnover of nurses in specific positions and attrition of nurses from specific workplaces and from the profession at large can have serious impacts on working conditions. This is especially true when departing nurses cannot be replaced with new hires and recruits to the profession, but is seen even in situations where nurse supply can be replenished. The stress created by working with fewer nurses than optimal or without an adequate mix of experienced colleagues can make it difficult to provide excellent nursing care and can increase the risks of compassion fatigue and burnout (among other problems) in the staff who remain (Stephenson, 2022). A vicious cycle may be created whereby nurses who stay are at increased risk for attrition and then safety and quality of patient care increasingly suffers. The costs associated with nurse turnover are high. According to the most recent annual national health care retention and registered nurse (RN) staffing statistics, the average cost associated with the replacement of a direct-care hospital RN is $52,350. These expenses are growing and the average hospital is estimated to lose between $6.6 million and $10.5 million annually. It has been estimated that a 1% change in turnover can generate annual costs (or savings) of approximately $380,600 for the average hospital (Colosi, 2023).

With more than 1 million nurses projected to retire between 2020 and 2030, retaining established nurses and supporting newly educated nurses is vital to the growth and sustainability of the workforce (NASEM, 2019). Newly licensed nurses are a particularly vulnerable segment of the nurse workforce, because they may not have the support, resources, and strategies to cope with the transition to clinical practice. They can develop potentially unhealthy patterns early in their careers, such as neglecting self-care, which may lead to shorter or less-productive careers. Promoting wellness and self-care and providing appropriate resources to help mitigate newly hired nurses' stress levels during their transition to practice will have impacts not only on their overall health and wellness but also their patients' outcomes (Windey et al., 2019).

It is impossible to consider nurse wellness without again mentioning the impact of the COVID-19 crisis. The toll of the COVID-19 pandemic on health care workers has yet to be fully understood, from the stresses faced by direct care providers during the surges in cases and high patient mortality rates before vaccines became available (Shechter et al., 2020), to the lasting impacts of the crisis that continue today (American Nurses Foundation, 2022; Gee et al., 2022). Even in hospitals known for having superior work environments in managing their workforces, half or more of the nurses and physicians surveyed in 2021 reported heightened job-related stress, high sleep disturbance, and low confidence that their patients were able to manage post discharge care (Aiken et al., 2023).

Many aspects of the work of nurses and other health care professionals were identified as stressful long before the pandemic (ANA, 2017). These include risks to physical safety (including violence), musculoskeletal wear and tear, infectious disease risks, stresses introduced by cumbersome IT (information technology) systems like electronic health records, ethical distress related to constraints on health workers' ability to act on a patient's wishes and/or their best interests, challenging relationships with coworkers and managers, and scheduling concerns. Furthermore, suboptimal engagement in self-care and health promotion activities (ANA, 2017) has long been noted among nurses.

Clearly, many aspects of health care work can undermine well-being; these areas deserve study and intervention. A practical problem for the leader attempting to make change at the local level is getting a sense of what specific aspect of well-being can be addressed in a specific setting at a particular moment in time. That requires clarifying stakeholders' understandings of well-being and choosing relevant indicators of well-being.

WELLNESS FRAMEWORKS AND LINKS OF WELLNESS TO OTHER OUTCOMES

As mentioned at the outset, promoting wellness may include, but may also go beyond prevention, early identification, and treatment of physical health problems that employees may be vulnerable to because of (and may be affected by) their work. It may also include establishing or reestablishing safe and supportive work environments and promoting psychological and social health and contentment. It is widely assumed that healthy workers deliver higher quality care and, indeed, it is difficult to imagine that the opposite could be true. However, perhaps because of the complexity of the connections and paths that link worker wellness with patient outcomes, the associations are not always seen, and when they are, they may be relatively small.

The Mayo Clinic framework involves an interrelationship of the three dimensions posited to optimize the functioning of a workforce and is summarized below (Swensen & Shanafelt, 2020). *Wellness* refers to being in good physical and mental health. Wellness also includes sleep, exercise, fitness, nutrition, rest, and preventative services, as well as whatever care is indicated to treat health problems that may have emerged. Resilience is the flexibility and capacity to recover rapidly from stressful encounters. *Resilience* gives humans the ability to adapt to and recover from the challenges and disruptions that are a part of life. For some components of resilience, individuals have limited or no control. However, many aspects of resilience can be intentionally strengthened and developed, such as self-compassion, cognitive flexibility, moral code growth, mindset, forgiveness, religion, spirituality, mindfulness, and gratitude. *Contentment* requires an understanding of one's values and having a sense of peace of mind and fulfillment. Contentment involves good spiritual, emotional, and intellectual health, as well as work–life integration where nurturing relationships, hobbies, and educational activities. *Cultivating growth* beyond contentment is a broad concept that relates to building healthy levels of social, physical, and mental resources that can be replenished. In contrast, burnout is characterized by a depletion of social, physical, and mental resources caused by unrealistic professional demands. A person's energy engagement and enthusiasm are determined by the difference between their "burn rate" and their "replenishment rate." Of course, certain aspects of health and potential targets for intervention influence multiple areas of both physical and psychological health, for instance, the sleep disruption that is common in nursing given the need for many staff members to work evening and night hours on rotating schedules.

Workplace well-being interventions can address areas well beyond specific physical and psychological health risk factors, behaviors, and habits to target contentment with one's work, including having a sense of community with fellow team members and having opportunities to offer meaningful input into the work of their teams and running of their organizations. Intervening to improve well-being requires defining it, thinking about what factors might affect it in terms of risk factors for poor outcomes, and considering the types of interventions that might be successful. Zeroing in on which among many health issues or concerns will be the target of interventions is an important first step, in addition to clarifying which aspect or aspects of well-being (and which indicators of well-being) are expected to show change.

A critical mass of evidence ties well-being and work engagement in nurses and other health care workers to quality of care outcomes for patients (Cho & Steege, 2021; Hall et al., 2016; Wee & Lai, 2022; Welp & Manser, 2016). While such findings justify continued attention to nurse wellness, they suggest that it might be unrealistic to expect patient outcomes to consistently shift in response to nurse wellness interventions.

MEASURES/INDICATORS OF WELLNESS

Health, wellness, and well-being can be measured in a variety of ways. We can consider physical health in the form of specific diseases or physical health issues and ask about symptoms and/or diagnoses. We can consider markers and risk factors for developing physical health problems (which are affected by a range of health behaviors such as eating patterns and exercise) such as obesity and operationalize them in terms of body mass index (BMI), stress hormones, or lipid levels. It is notable that research suggests nurses as a group may have higher BMIs than some other populations and that work-related factors may be partly responsible (Chin et al., 2016). We can consider nurses' health behaviors, such as eating (quantity and quality of food intake), exercise, and alcohol and tobacco use that may reflect multiple aspects of their personal and work lives.

Psychological health can be measured broadly, for instance, by asking about the frequency and/or severity of negative emotions like anxiety and depression or invasive thoughts about difficult or traumatic experiences. Some measures and scales identify levels of symptoms and negative emotions that make it likely that an individual is suffering from a diagnosable mental health condition. We can also examine the psychological experience of work in terms of concepts like **burnout**, which is a sense of emptiness and loss of meaning accompanying high-stress work, especially in the helping professions (Woo et al., 2020). **Compassion fatigue**, a phenomenon related to but distinct from burnout, relates to a diminished reserve for feeling resulting from excessive exposures to suffering and trauma without adequate supports (Sinclair et al., 2017). It is important to note that there are also measures of positive emotions and positive psychological experiences of work. For instance, work **engagement**, a full energetic connection with one's work on physical, emotional, and cognitive levels, has been contrasted with burnout (Bakker et al., 2014). Another example would be **compassion satisfaction**, the purpose and gratification in one's contacts working with patients and families, which could be considered the flip side of compassion fatigue (Sacco & Copel, 2018). There is also a positive psychology concept known as **resilience**, which refers to an ability to bounce back (recover and/or adjust) from potentially challenging and difficult experiences and situations and to persevere and remain future-oriented (Winkel et al., 2018). Tools exist to measure all of these concepts.

Nurses can be asked to provide an overall rating of their health taking all dimensions of their health into account together. Similar questions can be asked about their satisfaction with various elements of their health and whether health issues limit their ability to work or to function in and enjoy other areas of their lives. We can also expand into explorations of nurses' perceptions and experiences of the workplace—which edges into the territory of well-being.

Many of these aspects of wellness or well-being can be assessed together using carefully designed series of questions and tools strung together that provide a wide-ranging look at the health of a workplace. Such questionnaires are usually part of a "deep dive" into a health care work community, because the demands they create for those answering them are heavy and the data they produce are typically not specific enough to form a clear focus for a research project or a quality improvement initiative. Recently, the occupational health arm of the Centers for Disease Control and Prevention (CDC), the National Institute for Occupational Safety and Health (NIOSH), developed the Worker Well-Being Questionnaire (NIOSH WellBQ), which has been described as "an integrated assessment of worker well-being across multiple spheres, including individuals' quality of working life, circumstances outside of work, and physical and mental health status "(CDC, 2021). This comprehensive tool is composed of validated questions and its use is generally free. However, at over 80 questions, it is somewhat long (even though it reportedly takes an average of 15 minutes for most to answer the questions) and not all workers will have the time or inclination to complete it. Other researchers and health care organizations, such as the Mayo Clinic, have developed tools like Mayo's Wellbeing Index (mywellbeingindex.org) to assist organizations to benchmark the health of their workers and select targeted interventions.

WELLNESS/WELL-BEING INTERVENTIONS

Interventions to maintain and strengthen wellness and well-being can take many forms: they can be educational programs, support services and programs, and/or decisions by managers to change policies and leadership gestures intended to shape work environments. Existing workplace wellness programs can play a more significant role than they currently do by including protective and preventive offerings against stress and burnout (Belton, 2018). Given the increasing workload stressors in today's health care environment, it is essential to equip health care workers with knowledge and skills to thrive despite adversity (i.e., to become resilient).

The literature is filled with potential strategies, many of them scalable to settings of varying sizes, that are ripe for replication.

A purposeful approach to identifying targets for improvement and then selecting interventions has been recommended. In 2017, the Institute for Healthcare Improvement (IHI) published a framework for creating and enhancing joy in work, especially for health care employers (Perlo et al., 2017). This framework draws on evidence regarding the workplace and organizational elements that contribute to better staff engagement and experience. The Joy in Work Framework proposes programming aimed at individual workers to promote well-being and resilience, a further set of interventions at the team level to promote camaraderie, teamwork and participative management, and finally, actions at the senior level to promote physical and psychological safety, reward and recognition, choice and autonomy, and connection to meaning and purpose. This framework proposes a systematic quality improvement approach for teams to take ownership of the process of change through developing ideas, testing changes, and measuring impact.

The discussion that follows identifies selected work wellness interventions or programs that have been widely discussed or researched, or are notable for one or more reasons. We group together approaches by level of intervention—individuals, teams, and organizations.

Interventions Targeting Individuals

Training focused on building individual resilience is often offered to assist nurses to offset fatigue, stress, workload, and burnout. Workplace wellness programs include mindfulness-based interventions targeted at reducing stress, burnout, emotional reactivity, and anxiety while improving personal resiliency and coping. Formats vary and there are indications that programs that are either web based (Henshall et al., 2022) or are very short (Heppner & Shirk, 2018) can be effective. Sleep-related behaviors and skills have also been addressed in a number of interventions.

Mindfulness training involves helping individuals from a variety of walks of life become more attentive to their emotional and physical states to enable them to purposefully choose thought patterns or actions that can improve performance or reduce stress. Mindfulness involves using a family of techniques or approaches that include yoga and tai chi. These strategies are increasingly popular: in national surveys in 2007 and 2012, approximately 14% of American workers reporting using at least one of these techniques in the prior year (Kachan et al., 2017). Much published evidence suggest that these interventions are useful in improving short- and longer-term outcomes. For instance, a meta-analysis of 19 intervention studies in working adults found that mindfulness-based interventions appear to reduce psychological distress (Virgili, 2013). Another review and meta-analysis on intervention to reduce stress in university students found that cognitive, behavioral, and mindfulness interventions were associated with decreased symptoms of anxiety. Secondary benefits included lower levels of depression and cortisol (Regehr et al., 2013). Research into the value of mindfulness and mindfulness training continues to grow, and evidence from neurophysiological, neuropsychological, psychological, and applied clinical approaches all suggest that the mindfulness is beneficial (Heppner & Shirk, 2018).

Meditation is a type of mindfulness strategy where individuals work on focusing mental energy. Many studies have supported the effectiveness of meditation on multiple outcomes, including mental health. As little as five minutes of mindfulness can have momentary cardiovascular benefits, supporting the use of mindfulness meditation to proactively deal with stress (Johnson et al., 2019). Current literature largely links brief meditation (20 minutes or less) to a number of cognitive, emotional, social, and health benefits (Heppner & Shirk, 2018).

Adequate sleep is fundamental to wellness. However, health care jobs frequently require evening and/or night work and rotating shifts. Not surprisingly, sleep disturbance is very common in nurses, with prevalence estimates of around 61% (Zeng et al., 2020). Sleep deprivation has important consequences for both physical and psychological health. The amount of sleep received impacts metabolic function, which has ramifications for weight gain and risk of diabetes. Inadequate sleep may also negatively impact the immune system, as well as increase the risk of serious illness such as heart disease, cancer, and depression. Nurse fatigue has also been associated with poor patient and worker safety and worse organizational outcomes (Cho & Steege, 2021). One analysis of interventions to improve sleep duration and quality in worker populations found that educational interventions addressing principles of sleep hygiene and how to deal with fatigue (the single most common type of intervention), as well as other interventions including recommendations for napping and activity, screening, and referral for sleep disorders treatment, generally had positive influences on sleep, but the heterogeneity and weaknesses in study designs precluded drawing firmer conclusions (Redeker et al., 2019).

Group/Team Interventions

Much healthcare is delivered in specialized settings and by fairly stable and often interdisciplinary teams. The clinical microsystems movement sets forth the idea of focusing attention of specific teams on what works and what could be improved as key to quality improvement on a larger scale (Nelson et al., 2008). Shanafelt and colleagues (2023) describe in detail how a team-based focus on quality can be applied to wellness promotion.

Smooth teamwork in and of itself and interventions to promote optimal clinical care by improving communication and coordination have often been linked to worker health outcomes (Turcotte et al., 2022; Welp & Manser, 2016). However, in addition to initiatives attempting to foster effective collaboration to optimize clinical care, there have been a number of wellness interventions aimed at team member well-being. Two examples of such programs are peer-to-peer support programs and Code Lavender response teams. Helpers, facilitators, and recipients of the teams in these interventions can include individuals who work with each other in close collaboration (perhaps in the same physical unit or clinic) or they can be members of the same discipline who provide similar services across an institution. Supportive teams can mitigate the negative effects of occupational stress and create a refuge for health care professionals involved in adverse patient care events (DeMarco & Resnicoff, 2024).

Linking peers can be a useful way of supporting health professionals dealing with adverse events, distress, and other personal or professional challenges in a way that minimizes practical barriers and potential stigma (Carbone et al., 2022; Crandall et al., 2022). Peer-to-peer support programs may reach some health care professionals who would not otherwise directly pursue a mental health consultation. Peer support using a coaching framework is an established approach that can provide support for diverse challenges and be a bridge to connect those dealing with issues to mental health professionals if needed. The Center for Professionalism and Peer Support at Brigham and Women's Hospital redesigned their peer support program in 2009 to provide one-on-one peer support; it was one of the first of its kind and over 25 national and international programs have been based on it. Important components of peer support conversations include the outreach call, invitation/opening, listening, reflecting, reframing, sense-making, coping, closing, and resources/referrals. The authors argue that creating a peer support program shifts an organization away from a culture of invulnerability, isolation, and shame, and toward a culture of shared organizational responsibility for clinician well-being and patient safety (Shapiro & Galowitz, 2016). Several other group-based approaches to peer support are worthwhile to briefly reference. **Balint groups**—originally developed for medical students and primary care physicians—involve stable groups of clinicians and leaders debriefing about difficult psychosocial situations in a protected setting. A recent review was guarded in the conclusions it reached but asserted that there was sufficient promise in Balint groups to continue to study them (Van Roy et al., 2015). Schwartz Center Rounds, a related but separate type of program, offer opportunities of teams of professionals and other health care workers to engage in structured discussions to explore the psychological, spiritual, and moral aspects of specific care situations they have experienced together. Appeal of these groups is strong, and while evidence of the effect of these Rounds on health care worker wellness and team functioning have been mixed, they are thought worthy of continued evaluation (Maben et al., 2021).

A second example of a type of intervention having a team as the target for intervention is the Code Lavender model, developed at North Hawaii Community Hospital in 2004 and brought to the Cleveland Clinic in 2008 by its first chief experience officer. The term "Code Lavender" was coined to suggest an emergency call to mobilize a planned response for emotional or spiritual distress, with a reference to lavender oil's reputation for calming the anxious. Over time, other hospital systems incorporated Code Lavender as a support for employees, each one tailoring the concept and program to their specific organization's culture and circumstances. In a model from the Cleveland Clinic, a chaplain, a holistic nurse, and volunteers respond and upon request offer not only emotional support but certain complementary and alternative medicine therapies within their scope of training (Johnson, 2014; Stone, 2018). At a medical center in San Diego, another version of Code Lavender was structured as an "act of kindness" toward a colleague. Special bags (with aromatherapy, chocolate, a written message offering kind words, and referral information for employee assistance) are prepared by staff, faculty, and administrators in the hospital and then given by peers to each other when someone was having a particularly tough day (Davidson et al., 2017). This program was then expanded by adding a Caregiver Support Team where designated unit staff members offer first-level reachouts to coworkers in distress (Graham et al., 2019).

Despite the clear appeal of strategies like Code Lavender programs and overwhelmingly positive feedback from participants about their usefulness, there has been very little research to evaluate their effects and data do not suggest measurable differences in psychological well-being of unit staff following their implementation (Davidson et al., 2017; Graham et al., 2019). Overall, Code Lavender-related initiatives are low-cost, relatively easily implemented strategies that can be rolled out across complex health systems to build a culture where staff care for each other through the stresses of their jobs (DeMarco & Resnicoff, 2024).

Organizational Interventions

A number of organization-level policies may also improve nurse wellness. It has been noted that an integrated and systematic approach to wellness requires the involvement of a broad range of stakeholders, including nurse leaders, educational institutions, health care organizations, and other employers of nurses, policy makers, and professional associations. Inclusion of program outcomes focused on well-being and ethical competencies highlight developing and sustaining wellness. The latest AACN *Essentials for Nursing Education* (2021) highlights their foundational role for the profession. Nurse leaders have a duty to create a safe work environment with a culture of inclusivity and respect, must implement and enforce strong policies to protect nurses, and must recognize and respond strategically to toxic conditions.

Individual nurses' commitment to their personal well-being is affected by the support of their employers, their leaders, and the organizational cultures in their workplaces. Enhancing well-being and a feeling of psychological safety within teams is enabled by a culture of safety, norms of professional responsibility and organizational expectations to speak up, support from peers and leaders, and familiarity with team members who value inclusion.

Leaders at all levels in organizations, including senior staff in nonmanagerial roles, play a critical role in shaping cultures and expectations. They do this not only through the messages they send in formal settings but also in their daily work, through the things said in a range of forums, their investments of time and other scarce resources, and their handling of problems that arise.

Psychological Safety and Fair and Accountable Systems

Several types of work-related stress are especially notable in healthcare. Leader initiatives to create positive cultures around these issues can make big differences in nurses' experiences of the workplace. The first, the stress associated with not feeling able to speak up for fear of negative consequences, can be countered by infusing a culture with **psychological safety** (Newman et al., 2017). This term, which originated in the research literature, has been increasingly embraced by managers and others and refers to the norms in a group of workers regarding the acceptability of raising concerns, voicing alternative opinions, and proposing different courses of action. Psychological safety is considered vital to worker self-esteem and essential to ensuring strong performance in situations where creative solutions, teamwork, and sharing of expertise are needed on an ongoing basis.

Another challenging aspect of health care work is coping with high-pressure, complicated systems where errors must be kept to a minimum. Health care professionals need to work in an environment free of hostility and in one where they trust in the integrity of the leaders. They must believe that overall, systems are designed to improve care. Generally speaking, unless errors have occurred because of expressly bad intent, unauthorized substance use, or willful and reckless disregard for policies and procedures, nonpunitive corrective responses are appropriate. Fair and just accountability systems reflect an understanding that process deficiencies rather than individual failings cause most adverse events and serious safety events (Catino, 2008). Individuals involved in an adverse event and their coworkers pay close attention to the treatment of the workers involved. If the principles of fair and just accountability are followed (i.e., **just culture**) health care professionals feel an appropriate level of concern for ensuring safety and are comfortable reporting all near-misses and adverse events (Dekker, 2007). Just culture enhances health care worker peace of mind (Swensen & Shanafelt, 2020). However, if a culture of fairness around errors does not exist, health care workers live with unnecessary ongoing fear, may feel compelled to stay silent or even to actively hide errors, and may endure more stress than warranted when adverse events and errors occur.

Work–Life Integration

Work–life integration, or perceptions of the harmony or disharmony between work and nonwork activities in one's life, is a rethinking of the popular concept of work–life balance (Brough et al., 2020; Sirgy & Lee, 2018). Achieving a degree of satisfaction about the blend between work and life outside work requires attention to hard lines in one's personal life as well as boundaries and choices about workload in addition to social support, self-care, and cultivation of **avocational interests** (i.e., enjoyable hobbies and pastimes or projects outside of work). Excessive workload and job demands are consistent drivers of burnout. Improving work–life integration is a shared responsibility between employees and employers. Many, if not all, health care professionals have some control over how much they work, and in some circumstances working fewer hours (especially in the face of competing life demands) can be the best even when financial implications are considered. At the very least, caution should be exercised whenever it is possible so that nurses do not interpret overwork or working sick (presenteeism) as an expectation or even a valued form of contributing to the organization.

It has long been recognized that competing home and work responsibilities are heavily shouldered by women in the workforce, and the disruptions created by the COVID-19 crisis brought further attention to this. Many elements of work across sectors of the economy are being rethought in the wake of pandemic. It would be a mistake for health care organizations to close off discussions about new models of on-site versus off-site work and work hours on the basis of in-person direct care being the historic norm in organizations. Changing patient needs and preferences and technological solutions continue to stimulate new approaches to delivering patient care that offer unprecedented levels of flexibility. Cautious optimism about the potential for matching nurses' work-related needs and preferences with service needs is warranted. However, it should be remembered that teleworking can have unforeseen consequences such as the blurring of personal and work involvements and the risks and dangers of multitasking.

Leaders throughout an organization are essential role models for work–life integration. Leaders demonstrating attention to maintaining their work–life personal boundaries can be a powerful inducement for all to adopt the same stance. Furthermore, leaders can demonstrate that stepping away from work as needed and allowing others to shoulder burdens temporarily is both appropriate and encouraged, and that the organization supports spending time with loved ones as not just a legitimate choice but fundamental to a full and meaningful life. Not surprisingly, healthy work–life integration promotes mental health, appears to show other benefits, and can raises effectiveness for those in all roles in organizations (Brough et al., 2020).

Entry to Practice and Early Career Interventions

Many professionals find the end of their formal, mostly theoretical training and the beginning of their full-time real-world experience to be a stressful and vulnerable time, especially those working in close contact with both service recipients/clients in time-constrained settings and with fellow professionals and other workers. Nurses are no exception: the year after obtaining initial licensure is an especially critical time, where turnover rates can be quite high. Across societies, researchers have documented that newly licensed nurses face common challenges adapting to their workplace and adopting a professional persona, while gaining clinical skills and learning to manage patient loads. It is also clear that adapting to real-world practice can be isolating and create strains on mental health (Hirani et al., 2022; Hallaran et al., 2023; Mellor et al., 2022).

Initiatives to smooth the transition to practice fall into six categories: preceptorship/mentoring programs, residency programs, internships, externships, transition or orientation to practice programs, and clinical ladder programs (McDonald & Ward-Smith, 2012). In reality, there is substantial overlap between different types of interventions to support the transition from student nurse to practitioner and encourage the retention of nurses. Offering a transition to practice program of any type signals to a newly qualified nurse that their challenges are recognized and an organizational investment is being made to help them succeed. This alone can be enough to positively influence recruitment and retention, especially if recruits and orientees perceive that early-career nurses in a particular organization are valued as strongly if not more so as they are competing employers. There is a growing body of literature that explores the effectiveness of early-career retention strategies. Effectiveness may be measured in terms of job satisfaction, confidence, or competence, and alternatively, a decrease in voluntary turnover. While these interventions are widely accepted across the profession and standards and accreditation for residency programs are increasingly common, there is limited evidence about the most important features of the programs for optimizing workplace outcomes. Thus, leaders are forced to rely on tradition and instincts to guide their choices in terms of programming; however, the stakes in terms of excessive turnover have led nearly all health care organizations to adopt at least one type of strategy in onboarding and guiding early-career nurses.

Policies, Procedure, and Culture Around Mental Health Issues in Health Care Workers

Organizational culture refers to ways of being, thinking, and doing that are unknown to outsiders, are learned mostly by observation by newcomers, and become so familiar to insiders that they become almost invisible (Schein, 2004). Specific organizations and workplaces have cultures, as do professions and sectors. As just noted, the patient safety movement that began several decades ago has attempted to dismantle a cultural belief in healthcare that human inadequacies and character deficits are the main cause of errors, and that blame and punishment are the correct responses to adverse events. As mentioned earlier, "just culture" is an attempt to undo these notions. Another damaging element of health care culture has been the idea that only patients and families have psychosocial needs tending to and that competent professionals manage any psychosocial needs on their own. Holding such beliefs, health care workers can come to accept that they must always maintain a veneer or cloak of invulnerability and infallibility. Extending this idea, they may believe that admitting to mental health issues and seeking help for them can expose them and others to reputational damage and threats to their jobs and their licensure status and may even open them to legal liability. Carrying these beliefs can further lead workers to blame themselves for their reactions to the stresses in their work and personal lives and drive them to hide their vulnerabilities from others. Taken to an extreme, workers may avoid seeking help for mental health problems, including substance use disorders, until it is perhaps too late (such as when either their safety or that of their patients has been endangered).

Even before the onset of the COVID-19 pandemic, the NASEM published *Taking Action Against Clinician Burnout* (NASEM, 2019), a systems approach to professional well-being. One of the six recommended approaches was to provide support to clinicians and learners by reducing the stigma and eliminating the barriers associated with obtaining support and services needed to prevent and alleviate burnout and other mental health challenges. Specifically, the report recommended that state licensing boards, health systems, credentialing bodies, disability insurance carriers, and malpractice insurance carriers should choose between not collecting clinician personal health information at all or limiting their queries to clinicians' current impairments and health conditions more broadly. Rather than bringing current and past diagnoses or treatment for mental health conditions into decision making indiscriminately, organizations should be transparent about how they use clinicians' health data and be supportive of clinicians who seek help. The report further recommended that state laws be enacted to bar participation of employee assistance programs, peer support programs, and mental health providers from consideration as evidence in malpractice litigation. Furthermore, health professions organizations, educational institutions, health care organizations, and affiliated training sites were urged to identify and address those aspects of the learning environment, institutional culture, infrastructure, and resources and policies that prevent or discourage access to professional and personal support programs for individual learners and clinicians.

The American Nurses Association (ANA) also has recognized the need to address stigma and regulatory issues that can become barriers to nurses addressing their mental health needs. During the first year of the COVID-19 pandemic, the ANA Board of Directors (2020) issued a position statement that accessible, affordable (or free), and confidential mental health services should be available to all nurses. Most recently, the NASEM Future of Nursing report (NASEM, 2021) recommended that nurse leaders evaluate and strengthen policies, programs, and structures within employee organizations and licensing boards to reduce stigma associated with mental and behavioral health treatment for nurses.

Moving forward, nurse leaders must address and eliminate systematic barriers to optimizing mental health in the nurse workforce. While other issues like staffing must be considered and addressed to bring about more systematic change, a shift to a culture to normalize self-care and fully use available supports is needed. Messaging from leaders should emphasize that the pandemic created extraordinary stress for all in the health care system and reaching out for help is both normal and necessary (Weston & Nordberg, 2022). Nurse leaders can normalize self-care by both role modeling appropriate attention to their own mental health and by sharing their experiences addressing their emotional and mental health needs.

Employee and Student Assistance Programs

Students and working professionals can find it difficult to access mental health counseling and related services for any number of financial or practical reasons. It can be very helpful to have a path to assistance through one's workplace or educational institution. Understandably, concerns about stigma, as just mentioned, and also confidentiality can make participants reluctant to seek care. An **employee assistance program** (EAP) that provides access to counselors and therapists available at no cost can be an important resource for health care professionals experiencing personal and emotional difficulties related to work stressors associated with clinical care or challenges in reconciling personal and work-related responsibilities. Services must be strictly confidential and all records regarding who receives them and the content of the discussions and assistance must be protected to the greatest extent possible. Considerations can be similar but slightly different for nursing students. Building a combination of academic advising and college/university health service involvement to identify students in need and deliver services to them, with possibilities for self-referral and referrals by others, is the most common approach. Students will often have the same concerns about confidentiality and stigma. However, the opportunity to intervene during nurses' educations to foster self-care (Slemon et al., 2021) or deal with crises can help build resilience for the life of their careers.

Researchers have studied EAPs, both in terms of what they do (who presents for care, what is done for them) and outcomes they achieve. The body of published evaluation research, varied as it is, suggests measurable benefits (Csiernik et al., 2021). It is possible and perhaps even desirable for employee and student assistance and health programming to go beyond responding to immediate crises and extend to health promotion activities. Adequate sleep breaks, rest, exercise and nutrition, or replenishing reserves leads to optimal well-being. Individual wellness can be improved in several ways. Organizations should respond to accessible wellness programs and encourage health professionals to take advantage of them. Five important wellness factors that are relatively straightforward to promote are adequate sleep, sunlight, movement, laughter, and midday breaks. However, all such programming requires investments of time and personnel and is best shaped by stakeholder (i.e., worker and management) engagement in identifying subjects and selecting approaches that are most likely to be effective.

IMPLICATIONS FOR PRACTICE SETTINGS

For many reasons, nurse wellness is a popular topic both for nurse leaders and for nurses across the profession dipping their toes into research, research utilization, or evidence-based practice (EBP). Concepts and ideas around wellness tend to have resonance (they "make sense" or "ring true") and are widely discussed in the professional and even the lay press, and nurses from all corners of the profession tend to have personal experiences and reference points for them. The language of psychology and wellness has infused the way nurses and others talk about work in using terms like burnout, compassion fatigue, and self-care. Some, but not all, writing dealing with wellness is grounded in theory and research, uses clear operational definitions, and meticulously distinguishes what can and cannot be concluded from data on hand. We offer a number of suggestions for new and experienced travelers in EBP, quality improvement, and research in the nurse wellness space.

Research and scholarship dealing with nurse wellness tends to either be extremely rigorously reported or to be very loose in the use of terms. Some writers use terminology and methods in a highly specific and technical sense that may be at odds with the way nonspecialists think and speak. For instance, people speak of burnout relatively casually to mean exhaustion from sustained high-intensity work, without referencing Maslach and Jackson's definition of burnout as emotional depletion in the face of human services work accompanied by depersonalization of clients and a feeling that one's work may be pointless (Maslach & Jackson, 1981) or other established definitions. It is natural to skim for what appears worthwhile and appealing when new to the literature, but it is important to recognize that the social or behavioral science or administrative/management science of foundations behind these ideas, tools, and programs may be quite different from the biomedical and clinical paradigm that many nurses are familiar with. Studying wellness and interpersonal aspects of healthcare may require time and effort to learn a new vocabulary and approach to research.

Popular and folk psychology are terms that refer to commonly held wisdom about human behavior based on mass media reports, other less formal presentations, or "received wisdom" passed down from person to person. Some of what falls in this category is referred to as "common sense," including appealing and widely accepted ideas based on unstated and unverified assumptions. The wellness field contains a great number of such assumptions. For instance, it might be assumed that dealing with challenging situations (for instance, working with patients and families facing severe illnesses and/or threats to life) is uniformly experienced as stressful by nurses, when in reality there is a very wide range of nurse experiences in dealing with critical and life-threatening illnesses. This is true even when we acknowledge that seismic events like a global pandemic can affect many health care providers deeply. Another assumption is that workers have common and/or uniform responses to interventions and programs to reduce or deal with stress or promote wellness. Clinical practice and quality improvement teach us that there is much variation in how different clinicians and settings think and function—it behooves us to pay attention to this variation and to ask critical questions about hoped-for and unintended consequences of various interventions. For instance, the initially high enthusiasm for Critical Incident Stress Debriefing (CISD) among some clinicians and leaders, a technique involving facilitated group discussions for health professionals dealing with sudden and unexpected trauma clinical events, later faded after research data accumulated. CISD provides an excellent cautionary tale about the dangers of failing to evaluate before wide diffusion of wellness interventions (Burchill, 2019). However, it is important to be sensitive to nuance even here because there are indications that some forms of debriefing may be useful for health care workers, even if many questions in this area remain unanswered (Evans et al., 2023).

Change theory teaches that interest in altering or learning behaviors is linked to the sense of urgency around accomplishing a goal and/or improving specific outcomes: the intensity of effort people in a particular setting are willing to expend on adopting new practices is linked closely with the severity of the underlying problem as they understand it. The scale of undertakings needs to reflect local resources and shared stakeholder understandings of the urgency of the situation. Wellness and wellness interventions are no exception, and it is best to check out assumptions about buy-in before embarking too far.

A literature search on nurse wellness and related topics will quickly reveal survey instruments and/or interventions that might seem to be good fits for direct application to a new project. However, it is vital to take a close look at the actual article or articles, and then consider local context and the relevance of the measure or approach for the fundamental area or problem of interest in addition to practicalities, resources, and preferences of various stakeholders in a particular workplace. Choosing measurements or interventions based on appeal rather than information about their suitability for a particular setting or situation or the quality of evidence is a form of committing to a solution before fully understanding the problem or question that hampers many quality improvement efforts. It is vital to critically examine the intervention or the measurement tool and the evidence supporting it, as well as the distance between what is feasible in a particular setting (often trimming from a larger tool or program) and your own setting, as well as what has been shown in earlier research or writing to be valid or effective. Aiming for smaller-scale early wins is often best when starting out.

Surveys are very popular as a way of collecting data but always impose a burden on respondents, and, in almost all cases, the interpretation of results is seriously limited by not knowing much about the individuals who have chosen not to complete them. In the case of wellness surveys, it could be those at the extremes of high and low levels of health or happiness who may be most likely to take up an opportunity to answer questions, but it is difficult to know with certainty. Furthermore, in a worst-case scenario, carrying out surveys dealing with perceived needs and hoped-for programming can raise unrealistic expectations about the speed and scale of planned changes. Smaller-scale questionnaires are almost always better than larger tools unless the goal is a broad needs assessment; however, either way, a clear explanation of how results will be used should always be provided to the nurses being approached.

The interests of clinicians and clinician understandings of what might be most helpful to them might be at odds with some of the resources leaders and researchers may be most likely to offer them. In 2021 surveys, distinct minorities of nurses and even smaller numbers of physicians believed that resilience training, wellness surveys, committees, and champions or times and spaces for meditation would be very important to their well-being, relative to improved staffing, uninterrupted breaks, electronic health record improvements, and reductions in documentation burden (Aiken et al., 2023). The wellness interventions we might foresee providing may not align particularly well with expectations; it may be necessary to emphasize that wellness programs are intended to complement rather than replace attention to staffing and other work environment features.

It is also important to realize that the interventions we provide may not produce quantifiable impacts on health outcomes or certainly on patient outcomes, either right away or in the long term. Being realistic about the impacts of wellness interventions is very important. If nurses and other health care workers find programs to be appealing and users are pleased, continuing to make them available may be justified. In research as well as in practice and quality improvement dealing with wellness, the optimal stance may be to always include qualitative feedback from various stakeholders and to be realistic in designing quantitative evaluations (i.e., not to expect large statistically significant improvements across all measures). As important as it is to continue to shine a light on work-related stress and health concerns in nurses and to evaluate efforts to support wellness, belonging, and joy, it is also important to remember that it will not be possible to eliminate turnover, nor may it be possible to quantify or manage the degree to which we celebrate accomplishments and help each other handle sadness, disappointments, and loss. Likewise, we may need to be content to know that we are strengthening our workforces through our efforts, without expecting to see direct impacts on organizational and patient clinical outcomes all that frequently. A combination of sound theory and science when they are available, careful local needs assessments, and thoughtful program evaluations, along with tolerance for the limitations of research data to guide complex decisions would seem to be the best strategy for quality improvement addressing nurse wellness, as is the case for all EBP and quality improvement work.

Finally, research and improvement projects on nurse wellness are potentially ripe territory for academic–practice partnerships. Many schools and colleges of nursing have faculty experts on topics related to wellness and all have faculty members who are proficient in various modes of research and EBP. Furthermore, as mentioned elsewhere in this chapter, building self-care competencies and priming nurses for resilience begins in nursing education programs. Practice-site initiatives can benefit from bringing in academic partners early and often to review evidence and data about setting-specific needs, and to plan next steps including interventions and when appropriate, formal research and/or evaluation. Academics and educators, practice leaders, and clinicians share responsibility for the stability of the workforce and thus the promotion of nurse wellness ought to joint goal for schools of nursing and their larger communities.

SYNTHESIS

Nurse wellness has physical, mental, moral, and social components, is affected by a wide range of factors, and has important consequences for workforce stability. Improving nurse wellness requires leadership decisions at multiple levels in organizations. Much research and writing outlines the interrelationship of various aspects of well-being and the potential consequences of health care operations failing to attend to nurse health. Not all commonly accepted approaches for promoting nurse wellness are necessarily supported by strong research evidence, but benefits appear to outweigh costs and risks for many. There is still much potential for research and quality improvement dealing with well-documented needs and understandings to improve outcomes for individual nurses, the workforce, and health care systems more broadly.

KEY POINTS

- Wellness and well-being are expansions of broad definitions of health that encompass psychological and physical well-being, as well as contentment with various aspects of work and one's personal life.
- The COVID-19 pandemic produced a great deal of stress for health care workers and heightened concerns that inattention to nurse wellness, especially in younger nurses, might endanger the adequacy of the health workforce.
- There are multiple measures of nurse health and wellness available that examine each dimension of health and well-being, as well as responses to health care work and its stressors such as burnout and compassion fatigue. Sometimes broad surveys of health status among nurses in a setting can be a helpful part of a needs assessment.
- Interventions to address nurse well-being include training in skills to reduce psychological distress and improve health behaviors like sleep, and engaging peers in providing social and emotional support for each other. They may also include leader interventions across organizations to show concern for nurse psychological safety and increase nurses' confidence that they will be treated fairly when errors and adverse events occur, demonstrate commitment to helping nurses integrate their work and personal lives and assisting new graduates with the stresses of entering practice, and ensure access to and reduce stigma around mental health service use by nurses and other health care workers.
- Research and EBP addressing nurse wellness are both rewarding and challenging; a number of caveats are warranted when planning projects in this territory.
- Fostering nurse wellness is a shared responsibility between educators, researchers, clinicians, and health care leaders, and is fruitful territory for academic–practice partnership initiatives.

REFERENCES

Aiken, L. H., Lasater, K. B., Sloane, D. M., & U.S. Clinician Wellbeing Study Consortium., et al. (2023). Physician and nurse well-being and preferred interventions to address burnout in hospital practice: Factors associated with turnover, outcomes, and patient safety. *JAMA Health Forum*, *4*(7): Article e231809. https://doi.org/10.1001/jamahealthforum.2023.1809

American Association of Colleges of Nursing (AACN). (2020). A call to action for academic nurse leaders to promote practices to enhance optimal well-being, resilience and suicide prevention in schools of nursing across the U.S. https://www.aacnnursing.org/portals/0/pdfs/position-statements/7-2020-Resolution-For-AACN-Nurse-Wellness-Suicide-Prevention.pdf

American Association of Colleges of Nursing (AACN). (2021). *The essentials: Core competencies for professional nursing education*. AACN. https://www.aacnnursing.org/Portals/0/PDFs/Publications/Essentials-2021.pdf

American Nurses Association (ANA). (2017). Executive summary: American nurses association health risk appraisal (key findings: October 2013–October 2016). *American Nurses Association*. https://www.nursingworld.org/~4aeeeb/globalassets/practiceandpolicy/work-environment/health--safety/ana-healthriskappraisalsummary_2013-2016.pdf

American Nurses Association (ANA), Board of Directors. (2020). Promoting nurses' mental health [Position statement]. *American Nurses Association*. https://www.nursingworld.org/globalassets/practiceandpolicy/nursing-excellence/ana-position-statements-secure/workplace-advocacy/ana-mental-health-position-statement.pdf

American Nurses Foundation. (2022). *Pulse on the nation's nurses survey series: COVID-19 two-year impact assessment survey*. https://www.nursingworld.org/~492857/contentassets/872ebb13c63f44f6b11a1bd0c74907c9/covid-19-two-year-impact-assessment-written-report-final.pdf

American Organization of Nurse Leaders (AONL). (2022). AONL nurse leader core competencies. *AONL*. https://www.aonl.org/system/files/media/file/2023/08/AONL%20Core%20Competencies.pdf

Bakker, A. B., Demerouti, E., & Sanz-Vergel, A. I. (2014). Burnout and work engagement: The JD–R approach. *Annual Review of Organizational Psychology and Organizational Behavior*, *1*, 389–411. https://doi.org/10.1146/annurev-orgpsych-031413-091235

Belton, S. (2018). Caring for the caregivers: Making the case for mindfulness-based wellness programming to support nurses and prevent staff turnover. *Nursing Economics*, *36*(4), 191–195.

Bodenheimer, T., & Sinsky, C. (2014). From triple to quadruple aim: Care of the patient requires care of the provider. *Annals of Family Medicine*, *12*(6), 573–576. https://doi.org/10.1370/afm.1713

Brough, P., Timms, C., Chen, X. W., Hawkes, A., & Rasmussen, L. (2020). Work–life balance: Definitions, causes, and consequences. In T. Theorell (Ed.), *Handbook of socioeconomic determinants of occupational health [Handbook series in occupational health sciences]* (pp. 473–488). Springer Nature. https://doi.org/10.1007/978-3-030-31438-5_20

Burchill, C. N. (2019). Critical incident stress debriefing: Helpful, harmful, or neither? [Letter to the editor]. *Journal of Emergency Nursing*, *45*(6), 611–612. https://doi.org/10.1016/j.jen.2019.08.006

Carbone, R., Ferrari, S., Callegarin, S., et al. (2022). Peer support between healthcare workers in hospital and out-of-hospital settings: A scoping review. *Acta Biomedica*, *93*(5): Article e2022308. https://doi.org/10.23750/abm.v93i5.13729

Catino, M. (2008). A review of literature: Individual blame vs. organizational function logics in accident analysis. *Journal of Contingencies and Crisis Management*, *16*, 53–62. https://doi.org/10.1111/j.1468-5973.2008.00533.x

Centers for Disease Control and Prevention (CDC), National Institute of Occupational Health and Safety (NIOSH). (2021). *NIOSH Worker Well-Being Questionnaire (WellBQ)*. https://www.cdc.gov/niosh/twh/wellbq/default.html#:~:text=The%20NIOSH%20Worker%20Well%2DBeing,physical%20and%20mental%20health%20status

Chin, D. L., Nam, S., & Lee, S. J. (2016). Occupational factors associated with obesity and leisure-time physical activity among nurses: A cross sectional study. *International Journal of Nursing Studies*, *57*, 60–69. https://doi.org/10.1016/j.ijnurstu.2016.01.009

Cho, H., & Steege, L. M. (2021). Nurse fatigue and nurse, patient safety, and organizational outcomes: A systematic review. *Western Journal of Nursing Research*, *43*(12), 1157–1168. https://doi.org/10.1177/0193945921990892

Colosi, B. (2023). *NSI national health care retention & RN staffing report*. NSI Nursing Solutions, Inc. https://www.nsinursingsolutions.com/Documents/Library/NSI_National_Health_Care_Retention_Report.pdf

Crandall, C. J., Danz, M., Huynh, D., et al. (2022). *Peer-to-peer support interventions for health care providers: A series of literature reviews*. RAND Corporation. https://www.rand.org/pubs/research_reports/RRA428-2.html

Csiernik, R., Cavell, M., & Csiernik, B. (2021). EAP evaluation 2010–2019: What do we now know? *Journal of Workplace Behavioral Health*, *36*(2), 105–124. https://doi.org/10.1080/15555240.2021.1902336

Davidson, J. E., Graham, P., Montross-Thomas, L., Norcross, W., & Zerbi, G. (2017). Code lavender: Cultivating intentional acts of kindness in response to stressful work situations. *EXPLORE*, 13(3), 181–185. https://doi.org/10.1016/j.explore.2017.02.005

Dekker, S. (2007). *Just culture: Balancing safety and accountability*. Ashgate.

DeMarco, K. A., & Resnicoff, M. (2024). Launching lavender response teams across a health care system. *Nurse Leader*, 22(2), 182–186. https://doi.org/10.1016/j.mnl.2023.09.008

Evans, T. R., Burns, C., Essex, R., et al. (2023). A systematic scoping review on the evidence behind debriefing practices for the wellbeing/emotional outcomes of healthcare workers. *Frontiers in Psychiatry*, 14. Article 1078797. https://doi.org/10.3389/fpsyt.2023.1078797

Gee, P. M., Weston, M. J., Harshman, T., & Kelly, L. A. (2022a). Beyond burnout and resilience: The disillusionment phase of COVID-19. *AACN Advanced Critical Care*, 33(2), 134–142. https://doi.org/10.4037/aacnacc2022248

Graham, P., Zerbi, G., Norcross, W., et al. (2019). Testing of a caregiver support team. *EXPLORE*, 15(1), 19–26. https://doi.org/10.1016/j.explore.2018.07.004

Hall, L. H., Johnson, J., Watt, I., Tsipa, A., & O'Connor, D. B. (2016). Healthcare staff wellbeing, burnout, and patient safety: A systematic review. *PloS One*, 11(7): Article e0159015. https://doi.org/10.1371/journal.pone.0159015

Hallaran, A. J., Edge, D. S., Almost, J., & Tregunno, D. (2023). New nurses' perceptions on transition to practice: A thematic analysis. *The Canadian Journal of Nursing Research*, 55(1), 126–136. https://doi.org/10.1177/08445621221074872

Henshall, C., Ostinelli, E., Harvey, J., et al. (2022). Examining the effectiveness of web-based interventions to enhance resilience in health care professionals: Systematic review. *JMIR Medical Education*, 8(3): Article e34230. https://doi.org/10.2196/34230

Heppner, W. L., & Shirk, S. D. (2018). Mindful moments: A review of brief, low-intensity mindfulness meditation and induced mindful states. *Social and Personality Psychology Compass*, 12(12): Article e12424. https://doi.org/10.1111/spc3.12424

Hirani, S., Tharani, A., Jetha, Z., & Khan, S. (2022). Insights from nursing students about factors affecting and strategies supporting their mental health. *Journal of Wellness*, 4(1), 10. https://doi.org/10.55504/2578-9333.1101

Holdsworth, M. A. (2019). Health, wellness and wellbeing. *Revue Interventions Économiques/Papers in Political Economy*. https://doi.org/10.4000/interventionseconomiques.6322

Johnson, B. (2014). Code lavender: Initiating holistic rapid response at the Cleveland clinic. *Beginnings: (American Holistic Nurses' Association)*, 34(2), 10–11.

Johnson, K. T., Merritt, M. M., Zawadzki, M. J., Di Paolo, M. R., & Ayazi, M. (2019). Cardiovascular and affective responses to speech and anger: Proactive benefits of a single brief session of mindfulness meditation. *Journal of Applied Biobehavioral Research*, 24(3). https://doi.org/10.1111/jabr.12167

Kachan, D., Olano, H., Tannenbaum, S. L., et al. (2017). Prevalence of mindfulness practices in the US workforce: National health interview survey. *Preventing Chronic Disease*, 14. https://doi.org/10.5888/pcd14.160034

Maben, J., Taylor, C., Reynolds, E., McCarthy, I., & Leamy, M. (2021). Realist evaluation of Schwartz rounds for enhancing the delivery of compassionate healthcare: Understanding how they work, for whom, and in what contexts. *BMC Health Services Research*, 21(1), 709. https://doi.org/10.1186/s12913-021-06483-4

Maslach, C., & Jackson, S. E. (1981). The measurement of experienced burnout. *Journal of Occupational Behavior*, 2(2), 99–113. https://doi.org/10.1002/job.4030020205

McDonald, A. W., & Ward-Smith, P. (2012). A review of evidence-based strategies to retain graduate nurses in the profession. *Journal for Nurses in Staff Development*, 28(1), E16–E20. https://doi.org/10.1097/NND.0b013e318240a740

Mellor, P. D., De Bellis, A., & Muller, A. (2022). Psychosocial factors impacting new graduate registered nurses and their passage to becoming competent professional nurses: An integrative review. *Journal of Nursing Regulation*, 13(3), 24–51. https://doi.org/10.1016/S2155-8256(22)00081-3

National Academies of Sciences, Engineering, and Medicine (NASEM). (2019). *Taking action against clinician burnout: A systems approach to professional well-being*. National Academies Press. https://doi.org/10.17226/25521.

National Academies of Sciences, Engineering, and Medicine (NASEM). (2021). *The future of nursing 2020–2030: Charting a path to achieve health equity*. National Academies Press. https://doi.org/10.17226/25982.

Nelson, E. C., Godfrey, M. M., Batalden, P. B., et al. (2008). Clinical microsystems, Part 1: The building blocks of health systems. *Joint Commission Journal on Quality and Patient Safety*, 34(7), 367–378. https://doi.org/10.1016/s1553-7250(08)34047-1

Newman, A., Donohue, R., & Eva, N. (2017). Psychological safety: A systematic review of the literature. *Human Resource Management Review*, 27(3), 521–535. https://doi.org/10.1016/j.hrmr.2017.01.001

Perlo, J., Balik, B., Swensen, S., Kabcenell, S., Landsman, A., & Feeley, D. (2017). IHI framework for improving joy in work. http://www.ihi.org/resources/Pages/IHIWhitePapers/Framework-Improving-Joy-in-Work.aspx.

Redeker, N. S., Caruso, C. C., Hashmi, S. D., Mullington, J. M., Grandner, M., & Morgenthaler, T. I. (2019). Workplace interventions to promote sleep health and an alert, healthy workforce. *Journal of Clinical Sleep Medicine*, 15(4), 649–657. https://doi.org/10.5664/jcsm.7734

Regehr, C., Glancy, D., & Pitts, A. (2013). Interventions to reduce stress in university students: A review and meta-analysis. *Journal of Affective Disorders*, 148(1), 1–11. https://doi.org/10.1016/j.jad.2012.11.026

Sacco, T. L., & Copel, L. C. (2018). Compassion satisfaction: A concept analysis in nursing. *Nursing Forum*, 53, 76–83. https://doi.org/10.1111/nuf.12213

Schein, E. (2004). *Organizational culture and leadership* (3rd ed.). Jossey-Bass.

Shanafelt, T. D., Larson, D., Bohman, B., et al. (2023). Organization-wide approaches to foster effective unit-level efforts to improve clinician well-being. *Mayo Clinic Proceedings*, 98(1), 163–180. https://doi.org/10.1016/j.mayocp.2022.10.031

Shapiro, J., & Galowitz, P. (2016). Peer support for clinicians. *Academic Medicine*, 91(9), 1200–1204. https://doi.org/10.1097/acm.0000000000001297

Shechter, A., Diaz, F., Moise, N., et al. (2020). Psychological distress, coping behaviors, and preferences for support among New York healthcare workers during the COVID-19 pandemic. *General Hospital Psychiatry*, 66, 1–8. https://doi.org/10.1016/j.genhosppsych.2020.06.007

Sinclair, S., Raffin-Bouchal, S., Venturato, L., Mijovic-Kondejewski, J., & Smith-MacDonald, L. (2017). Compassion fatigue: A meta-narrative review of the healthcare literature. *International Journal of Nursing Studies*, 69, 9–24. https://doi.org/10.1016/j.ijnurstu.2017.01.003

Sirgy, M. J., & Lee, D. J. (2018). Work–life balance: An integrative review. *Applied Research in Quality of Life*, 13(1), 229–254. https://doi.org/10.1007/s11482-017-9509-8

Slemon, A., Jenkins, E. K., & Bailey, E. (2021). Enhancing conceptual clarity of self-care for nursing students: A scoping review. *Nurse Education in Practice*, 55. : Article 103178. https://doi.org/10.1016/j.nepr.2021.103178

Stephenson, J. (2022). US Surgeon General sounds alarm on health worker burnout. *JAMA Health Forum*, 3(6): Article e222299. https://doi.org/10.1001/jamahealthforum.2022.2299

Stone, R. B. (2018). Code lavender. *Nursing*, 48(4), 15–17. https://doi.org/10.1097/01.nurse.0000531022.93707.08

Swensen, S., & Shanafelt, T. (2020). *Mayo Clinic strategies to reduce burnout*. Oxford University Press. https://doi.org/10.1093/med/9780190848965.001.0001

Turcotte, M., Etherington, C., Rowe, J., et al. (2022). Effectiveness of interprofessional teamwork interventions for improving occupational well-being among perioperative healthcare providers: A systematic review. *Journal of Interprofessional Care*, 1–18. https://doi.org/10.1080/13561820.2022.2137116

Van Roy, K., Vanheule, S., & Inslegers, R. (2015). Research on Balint groups: A literature review. *Patient Education and Counseling*, 98, 685–694. https://doi.org/10.1016/j.pec.2015.01.014

Virgili, M. (2013). Mindfulness-based interventions reduce psychological distress in working adults: A meta-analysis of intervention studies. *Mindfulness*, 6(2), 326–337. https://doi.org/10.1007/s12671-013-0264-0

Wee, K. Z., & Lai, A. Y. (2021). Work engagement and patient quality of care: A meta-analysis and systematic review. *Medical Care Research and Review*, 79(3), 345–358. https://doi.org/10.1177/10775587211030388

Welp, A., & Manser, T. (2016). Integrating teamwork, clinician occupational well-being and patient safety—development of a conceptual framework based on a systematic review. *BMC Health Services Research*, 16, 281. https://doi.org/10.1186/s12913-016-1535-y

Weston, M. J., & Nordberg, A. (2022). Stigma: A barrier in supporting nurse well-being during the pandemic. *Nurse Leader*, 20(2), 174–178. https://doi.org/10.1016/j.mnl.2021.10.008

Windey, M., Craft, J., & Mitchell, S. L. (2019). Incorporating a wellness program for transitioning nurses. *Journal for Nurses in Professional Development*, 35(1), 41–43. https://doi.org/10.1097/nnd.0000000000000498

Winkel, A. F., Robinson, A., Jones, A.-A., & Squires, A. P. (2018). Physician resilience: A grounded theory study of obstetrics and gynaecology residents. *Medical Education*, 53(2), 184–194. https://doi.org/10.1111/medu.13737

Woo, T., Ho, R., Tang, A., & Tam, W. (2020). Global prevalence of burnout symptoms among nurses: A systematic review and meta-analysis. *Journal of Psychiatric Research*, 123, 9–20. https://doi.org/10.1016/j.jpsychires.2019.12.015

World Health Organization. (2020). *Basic documents* (49th ed.). World Health Organization. https://apps.who.int/gb/bd/pdf_files/BD_49th-en.pdf.

Zeng, L. N., Yang, Y., Wang, C., et al. (2020). Prevalence of poor sleep quality in nursing staff: A meta-analysis of observational studies. *Behavioral Sleep Medicine*, 18(6), 746–759. https://doi.org/10.1080/15402002.2019.1677233

28

Harnessing the Power of Diversity, Equity, Inclusion, and Belonging to Advancing Health Care Systems Outcomes

Emerson E. Ea, Kathryn Lang, Peter Rodney, and Kathleen Evanovich Zavotsky

LEARNING OUTCOMES

After reading this chapter, you should be able to do the following:
- Discuss the principles of diversity, equity, inclusion, and belonging (DEIB).
- Describe the importance and need to integrate DEIB in the health care systems.
- Review the influence that DEIB has on health care outcomes.
- Describe the role of health care systems and nursing administrators and leaders in designing, implementing, evaluating, and sustaining DEIB in the workplace.
- Outline evidence-based strategies and examples in practice that promote and champion DEIB.

KEY TERMS

Belonging
Diversity
Equity
Harassment
Implicit bias
Inclusion
Microaggressions
Social determinants of health
Stereotyping
Systemic discrimination

Incorporating the principles of diversity, equity, inclusion, and belonging (DEIB) into the workplace is crucial for health care systems to deliver high-quality care and achieve positive outcomes. By embracing DEIB initiatives, health care systems cultivate a workforce that values diversity and possesses cultural competence, enabling them to meet the health care needs of the population they serve. In addition, these principles encourage and enhance collaboration with academic partners and stakeholders, fostering a health care system that supports innovation and is responsive to evolving health care landscapes.

As a clinical leader you may be called on to ensure that the principles and policies related to DEIB are either developed, implemented, evaluated, and, when necessary, enforced. You may even be asked to work with an interdisciplinary team to establish a process for implementing a DEIB culture change in a health care organization.

DEIB represents a framework for creating a workplace and a community that values and respects individuals from a range of backgrounds and experiences. By prioritizing DEIB, clinical leaders and organizations can create a culture of inclusivity and belonging that leads to better employee morale, increased productivity and innovation, and improved health care outcomes for patients and communities. The main purpose of this chapter is to discuss evidence-based strategies that could help health care systems leaders design, implement, evaluate, and sustain efforts on advancing DEIB. We will provide an overview of the importance and the need to integrate DEIB in health care systems, outline the pivotal roles of nurses in clinical practice and academia in advancing and leading DEIB efforts, and discuss the challenges and benefits of making DEIB an important focus and priority of a health care system. Several exemplars that advance DEIB in practice and nursing education will also be included.

DEFINITIONS OF DIVERSITY, EQUITY, INCLUSION, AND BELONGING KEY TERMS AND CONCEPTS

To ensure that there is a shared understanding of the meanings of the key terms used in this chapter, there is a need to define terms that relate to DEIB. Defining these key terms at the outset will provide a foundation to prevent ambiguity and confusion, promote clear communication, spur effective collaborations, and support accountability among stakeholders.

- **Diversity** refers to the myriad of differences that exist among people, including but not limited to race, ethnicity, gender, sexual orientation, age, religion, and socioeconomic status. A diverse workplace or community includes individuals from a range of backgrounds and experiences (Moss & Phillips, 2020).
- **Inclusivity** refers to the practice of creating an environment where everyone feels valued and respected. An inclusive workplace or community welcomes diversity and makes everyone feel like they belong (Moss & Phillips, 2020).
- **Equity** is the concept of ensuring that everyone has access to the same opportunities and resources. In a workplace, equity means that all employees have an equal chance to succeed and advance, regardless of their race, gender, or other factors (National Academies of Sciences, Engineering, & Medicine, 2021).
- **Belonging** is the perception of being accepted and valued in a group or community. In a workplace, belonging means that employees feel like they are part of a team and that their contributions are appreciated (Moss & Phillips, 2020).

- **Social determinants of health** are conditions in the environment where people are born, live, learn, work, play, worship, and age that affect a wide range of health, functioning, and quality of life outcomes and risks. The primary domains include economic stability, education access, health care access, and neighborhood and social community (National Academies of Sciences, Engineering, & Medicine, 2021).
- **Implicit biases** are unconscious biases that can affect how we perceive and interact with others. They can be based on factors such as race, gender, age, and other personal characteristics. For example, a manager may unconsciously assume that a woman is less competent than a man in a particular role, even if there is no evidence to support this assumption (Moss & Phillips, 2020).
- **Stereotyping** is the act of assuming that individuals possess certain characteristics or abilities based on their membership in a particular group. For example, assuming that all Asian employees are good at math, or that all Black employees are athletic (Moss & Phillips, 2020).
- **Microaggressions** are subtle forms of discrimination that can be unintentional or intentional. They can take many forms, including comments, actions, or behaviors, and can be based on factors such as race, gender, sexuality, or disability. For example, a colleague making a comment about someone's accent or assuming that someone is not proficient in English because of their name (Moss & Phillips, 2020).
- **Harassment** is any behavior that creates a hostile or offensive work environment based on an individual's membership in a protected class. This can include sexual harassment, racial harassment, and other forms of discrimination (Organization of Nurse Leaders [ONL], 2022).
- **Systemic discrimination** refers to the ways in which organizations, policies, and practices can create barriers for individuals based on their membership in a particular group. This can include factors such as hiring practices, promotion policies, and pay equity (National Academies of Sciences, Engineering, & Medicine, 2021).
- Note: It's important to stress that bias and discrimination can take many forms and can be intentional or unintentional. Organizations should strive to create a culture of diversity, equity, and inclusion by addressing bias and discrimination in all its forms. This can

include providing training to employees and managers, establishing clear policies and procedures for addressing discrimination, and holding individuals accountable for their actions.

HEALTH SYSTEMS AND DIVERSITY, EQUITY, INCLUSION, AND BELONGING: AN OVERVIEW

The ability to embrace and recognize that diversity is essential for health systems, including nursing practice, has evolved through the years. From a patient and family perspective it has shown to positively impact outcomes and can contribute to enhancing their life experiences (Gill et al., 2018). From a workforce perspective it can help transform organizational culture for all employees regardless of their roles and positions. Creating a culture in large organizations takes time and leadership (Gill et al., 2018). Health systems strive to create safe and supportive spaces for employees and patients to have conversations and share experiences. Change begins when health systems leaders serve as role models and intentionally engage all stakeholders, including staff and patients, as partners in creating and sustaining a progressive DEIB culture.

DIVERSITY, EQUITY, INCLUSION, AND BELONGING AND THE WORKPLACE

There is a robust and growing body of evidence that supports the value and positive impact of DEIB efforts in the workplace. The literature revealed that proactive diversity strategies, such as policies, are essential to set expectations and requirements for an organization. When employees perceived practices advocating for diversity in their workplace, it was found that their sense of well-being improved regardless of minority or nonminority status. The literature also validates that successful growth of an organization that is attentive to DEIB efforts requires a commitment from executive leadership. This includes recruiting, retaining, developing, and supporting employees from underrepresented groups.

Further, creating policies and practices that foster self-value, belonging, and fairness while minimizing inequalities will help create an inclusive work environment. Leaders with an inclusive leadership style are essential for building relationships between staff members as well as motivating employee engagement with increased commitment for the organization's success. Finally, strategic initiatives implemented by organizational leaders can ensure staff buy-in to maintain a path of excellence through continuous learning opportunities within the health system.

Organizational strategic imperatives must begin with a focus on DEIB. Leaders should take time to assess if the organization's mission, vision, and values are inclusive of DEIB initiatives. Health systems leaders, including nursing leaders, have an important role in driving these initiatives forward and ensuring they become part of organizational strategy. Prestia (2023) suggests that organizations should make a conscious effort toward commitment, connection, and collaboration when it comes to their DEIB efforts—this then becomes the lens through which all policies, processes, and resources are aligned accordingly. To foster trust and enhance engagement in the workplace, employees need to feel valued by the organization and should have access to resources needed to contribute meaningfully. By ensuring organizational policies and processes that encourage inclusion, organizations can amplify trust and engagement outcomes among their staff and stakeholders.

A systematic review (Gomez & Bernet, 2019) of both medical and business research found that when a diversity-friendly environment was supported it serves as key in mitigating friction that occurs with organizational change. They also discuss how a DEIB culture in organizations can help improve quality patient care while at the same time have a positive impact on the organization's fiscal health. The review also shows that DEIB programs can lead to improvements, innovative initiatives, and better interdisciplinary team communication.

It is essential that health care systems are in tune with contemporary issues that impact the community they serve and where their staff practices. With the amount of civil unrest and social media outlets that can at times distort reality or sway public opinion, organizations must be prepared to guide staff and establish a culture where the employees can feel safe to express their opinions while still ensuring that they are delivering care that is focused on the needs of their community regardless of race, culture, creed, sexual orientation, ethnicity, gender, age, experience, or any other aspect of identity (American Nurses Association [ANA], 2021). Research has also shown that nurse retention is highly correlated with how nurses perceive their employer's commitment to DEIB values.

IMPACT OF A DIVERSITY, EQUITY, INCLUSION, AND BELONGING CULTURE ON POPULATION AND HEALTH CARE OUTCOMES

Health care systems cater to individuals from various ethnic and racial backgrounds necessitating the implementation of suitable systems and services to ensure the provision of high-quality and evidence-based healthcare. However, extensive research has shown that racial and ethnic minorities encounter unequal treatment when seeking health care services (National Academies of Sciences, Engineering, & Medicine, 2021). These disparities can arise from discriminatory practices by health care professionals and the system and the structure of health systems themselves, but can also be mitigated through intentional efforts of health care organizations. The factors that influence poor health care access and outcomes among minoritized individuals and groups include:

1. Discriminatory practices: Discrimination by health care practitioners is a significant factor that contributes to unequal treatment. Implicit biases, stereotypes, and prejudiced attitudes can influence medical decision making and interactions with patients, leading to disparities in diagnoses, treatment options, and overall quality of care (National Academies of Sciences, Engineering, & Medicine, 2021).
2. Structural and systemic factors: Structural and systemic barriers within health care systems can disproportionately affect racial and ethnic minorities. These barriers may include limited access to health care facilities, inadequate insurance coverage, socioeconomic disparities, language barriers, and cultural insensitivity in health care delivery. These factors can hinder individuals from receiving timely and appropriate care, leading to health inequities (National Academies of Sciences, Engineering, & Medicine, 2021).
3. Lack of cultural competence: Cultural competence, which refers to the ability of health care providers and organizations to understand and respond effectively to the unique cultural and linguistic needs of diverse populations, is often lacking. When health care professionals are not adequately trained or equipped to navigate cultural differences, misunderstandings can occur, leading to suboptimal care and diminished patient outcomes (Moss & Phillips, 2020).
4. Social determinants of health: Racial and ethnic minorities often experience higher rates of chronic diseases, poorer health outcomes, and lower socioeconomic status compared to their counterparts. These health disparities can be influenced by various social determinants of health, such as limited access to education, employment opportunities, safe housing, healthy food, and community resources. These underlying disparities can further exacerbate the unequal treatment experienced by racial and ethnic minorities in health care settings (National Academies of Sciences, Engineering, & Medicine, 2021).
5. Historical and intergenerational factors: Historical experiences of discrimination, racism, and marginalization have had long-lasting effects on minority communities. These experiences, along with intergenerational trauma, can result in distrust of the health care system and contribute to disparities in health care utilization and outcomes (National Academies of Sciences, Engineering, & Medicine, 2021).

Unequal access to healthcare and systemic and institutional barriers has significant effects on health outcomes of minoritized individuals and groups. These health and health care outcomes include:

1. Health disparities: Minoritized individuals and groups often experience higher rates of chronic diseases, poorer health outcomes, and shorter life expectancies compared to nonminoritized populations. These disparities are driven by limited access to quality health care services, delayed or inadequate treatment, and barriers to preventive care (National Academies of Sciences, Engineering, & Medicine, 2021).
2. Delayed diagnosis and treatment: Systemic and institutional barriers can lead to delayed diagnosis and treatment for minoritized individuals. Limited access to health care facilities, long wait times, and financial constraints can result in delayed health care seeking, leading to the progression of diseases and poorer prognosis (National Academies of Sciences, Engineering, & Medicine, 2021).
3. Higher disease burden: Minoritized populations often bear a disproportionate burden of certain

diseases and conditions, including cardiovascular diseases, diabetes, certain cancers, and mental health disorders. This can be attributed to a combination of genetic, socioeconomic, environmental, and healthcare-related factors (National Academies of Sciences, Engineering, & Medicine, 2021).

4. Health inequities: Unequal access to healthcare perpetuates existing health inequities. Minoritized individuals may face additional barriers related to socioeconomic status, language and cultural differences, and discriminatory practices, leading to disparities in health outcomes, health care utilization, and patient experiences (National Academies of Sciences, Engineering, & Medicine, 2021).

5. Decreased access to preventive care: Limited access to preventive care, such as screenings, vaccinations, and health promotion services, can result in higher rates of preventable illnesses and missed opportunities for early intervention. This contributes to a higher disease burden and poorer overall health outcomes (National Academies of Sciences, Engineering, & Medicine, 2021).

6. Increased health care costs: Inadequate access to healthcare and lack of preventive care can lead to the development of more severe health conditions over time. This, in turn, increases health care costs for minoritized individuals and the health care system. The burden of these costs can further exacerbate existing health disparities (National Academies of Sciences, Engineering, & Medicine, 2021).

7. Psychological and emotional impact: Systemic and institutional barriers to healthcare can have a detrimental psychological and emotional impact on minoritized individuals. Experiences of discrimination, stigma, and unequal treatment can lead to increased stress, anxiety, and mistrust toward the health care system, further hindering healthcare-seeking behavior (ANA, 2021).

NURSING'S PIVOTAL ROLE IN ADVANCING DIVERSITY, EQUITY, INCLUSION, AND BELONGING IN HEALTH CARE SYSTEMS

The notion that racial and ethnic diversity can contribute to reducing health care disparities and enhancing health care access and quality is widely acknowledged. Institutions highly value diversity as an essential principle, recognizing that diversifying the nursing workforce is crucial for promoting health equity. Further, *The Future of Nursing Report 2020–2030* calls for a new generation of nurse leaders who acknowledge the significance of diversity. This recognition is essential for effectively addressing the existing health inequities experienced by minority populations in our society today.

Nursing has the potential to be a leading force in reducing health inequities through increasing the racial and ethnic diversity of its workforce. This strategy is supported by strong evidence, demonstrating that cultural proficiency is important for all nurses to attain (Lyman et al., 2022). A diverse nursing workforce can bridge gaps in patient education, provide different cultural perspectives within nursing conversations, and return to their underrepresented communities (Foster-Smith et al., 2023; National Academies of Sciences, Engineering, & Medicine, 2021). The positive impact of this increased diversity extends beyond just health care access and delivery; it also affects educational opportunities, research initiatives, as well as clinical areas—creating an environment where everyone can benefit from improved care quality standards (Morrison et al., 2021).

Nurse leaders are positioned to help ensure from a macro level and a micro level that culture is assessed, and structural empowerment is encouraged to create a more diverse, equitable, and inclusive health care organization (Morrison et al., 2021). Nurse leaders will need to be strategic in their planning, development, and evaluation that will involve multiple disciplines and stakeholders. The strategy should be based on the mission, vision, and values for both the organization and their staff. By doing this it will help create environments where diversity and individualism thrive to help maximize talents, experiences, and perspectives that can help improve care (Lyman et al., 2022).

It is the responsibility of health care organizations to ensure an inclusive environment where nurses feel safe enough to discuss racism and discrimination openly and explore unconscious biases that can influence decisions in negative ways (ANA, 2021; American Psychological Association [APA], 2021). Additionally, organizations must take appropriate action when acts of overt or covert racism occur as part of systemic change needed for addressing health disparities in marginalized communities (ANA, 2021; APA, 2021). By creating a culture centered on DEIB, health care organizations will be better equipped to promote positive clinical environments while supporting the well-being of their staff members along with patient care outcomes overall (ANA, 2021; APA, 2021).

Health equity is considered as a key element needed to achieve optimum patient care and health and health care outcomes. Prestia (2023) discusses DEIB and how important it is for nurse leaders as they work to help transform their organizations and workforce. She discusses the need to address cultural humility, which is believed to be necessary to understanding DEIB. Leaders should be self-reflective and sensitive to unconscious bias that leads to exclusivity. She goes on to suggest that our nursing workforce should be a representative of humanity to ensure the overall health and well-being of people that we serve. To accomplish this, it requires intentionality through strategic thinking in our complex health care environment.

Foster-Smith and colleagues (2023) discuss how the time is now to transform our health care organizations to improve access, diversity, equity, inclusion, and belonging. As nurses and clinical leaders, it is our obligation to the future of nursing to ensure that there is a role for all of us in the DEIB journey to combat structural racism. Clinical leaders can impact change that drives health equity and improved health outcomes at the point of care. Nurses should also be encouraged to speak truth and bring clarity about the need and cause for DEIB. Advancing DEIB in the workplace requires a multifaceted approach that involves leaders, managers, and employees at all levels of the organization (Schmidt et al., 2017).

The literature also revealed that strategies to increase diversity in the health care workforce must begin early in nursing education (American Association of Colleges of Nursing [AACN], 2021). Socializing nursing students to DEIB prior to entering the workforce should be a priority. Being able to ensure that diverse voices are heard in nursing education is critical in helping develop a foundation that establishes a safe space as their practice develops and enculture them into the workplace (Brewington et al., 2023). The American Association of Colleges of Nursing (AACN, 2021) has strongly emphasized the importance of advancing efforts in DEIB to address persistent inequities in healthcare and associated educational programs. A systemic review process must be conducted to establish best practices surrounding DEIB, with curricula being systematically reexamined for inclusion of this content and results shared so changes can be made accordingly. Data assessments should also be collected from course materials that reflect DEIB and integrated throughout all curricula. Additional research is needed to help explore DEIB at all levels of nursing education to help ensure that contemporary evidence-based practices can be put in place to guide our evolving profession (Cary et al., 2020; Day & Beard, 2019; Sumo et al., 2021).

Furthermore, mission statements and strategic plans should include specific references to integrating DEIB content into their educational objectives; institutions must strive toward upholding these values while defining their position on such initiatives if they are truly dedicated to providing a comprehensive learning experience for all students. By increasing DEIB content within nursing curriculums, academic institutions can improve the quality and effectiveness of their programs, as well as better prepare nurses to effectively provide culturally competent care for an increasingly diverse population. (Sukhera & Watling, 2018). Furthermore, these efforts must be regularly evaluated to assess progress toward achieving greater diversity and inclusion at all levels of the institution's operations (Brown & Waller, 2022; National League for Nursing, 2017). See Box 28.1 for a curricular innovation (Ea et al., 2023) that integrates the social determinants of health in an undergraduate nursing program.

In addition, nursing school administrators must be intentional in their efforts to recruit, retain, and support a diverse student body (National Advisory Council on Nurse Education and Practice, 2019). Outreach tactics such as strategic recruitment, summer enrichment programs, holistic admission models, and enhanced curriculum with courses on health disparities and underserved populations are essential for creating a welcoming environment for graduates transitioning from academia into practice (National Academies of Sciences, Engineering, & Medicine, 2021).

BUILDING AND SUSTAINING A CULTURE OF DIVERSITY, EQUITY, INCLUSION, AND BELONGING IN THE WORKPLACE

Building and sustaining a culture of DEIB in health care systems require thoughtful planning. As with any major

> **BOX 28.1 Curriculum Innovation Integrating Social Determinants of Health**
>
> New York University Rory Meyers College of Nursing implemented a curricular innovation to address the nursing education's call to prepare nurses who can actively participate in addressing health disparities and inequities. This educational innovation revolved around the integration of Design Thinking principles into specific courses within its undergraduate program, spanning four semesters. Design Thinking, characterized by its human-centered approach to tackling problems, comprises five phases: Empathy, Problem Identification, Ideation, Prototyping, and Testing. Faculty members teaching in these courses adopted the Design Thinking framework as a pedagogical strategy, seamlessly weaving in crucial concepts related to the social determinants of health, social justice, and health equity.
>
> As an example, students taking the Community Health Nursing course in their final semester used the Design Thinking process to brainstorm innovative solutions throughout the semester to address public health challenges rooted in the social determinants of health. Students also had the opportunity to participate in a 3-hour long hackathon-style brainstorming session toward the end of the semester. Organized into groups, they were provided with essential tools like whiteboards, Post-it notes, and modeling clay, enabling them to create tangible prototypes representing their solutions derived during the hackathon. To cap off this brainstorming experience, students presented their work to both their peers and faculty at the conclusion of the semester.
>
> NYU Meyers's forward-thinking approach not only responds to the crucial need for nurses to address health disparities but also instills in its students the invaluable skills of empathy, innovative problem solving, and a deep commitment to promoting health equity and social justice as future leaders and innovators in healthcare.
>
> Data from Ea et al., 2023.

DIVERSITY, EQUITY, INCLUSION, AND BELONGING GUIDING FRAMEWORKS

A framework could serve as a road map, providing guidance, focus, strategy, stakeholder engagement, accountability, cultural integration, and long-term sustainability for DEIB initiatives. It ensures that efforts are purposeful, effective, and aligned with the organization's overall goals and values. Examples of these frameworks include:

1. The Cultural Competence Continuum: The Cultural Competence Continuum, developed by the National Center for Cultural Competence, provides a framework for assessing an organization's progression in cultural competence. It consists of six stages, ranging from cultural destructiveness to cultural proficiency. This framework helps evaluate the current state of cultural competence within the organization and identifies areas for improvement (Cross et al., 1989).
2. The Equity, Diversity, and Inclusion (EDI) Framework: The EDI Framework emphasizes the importance of equity, diversity, and inclusion in creating a fair and inclusive health care environment. It focuses on identifying and addressing systemic barriers and biases, fostering diversity within the workforce, and creating an inclusive culture that values and respects differences. This framework helps guide organizational policies, practices, and strategies to promote equitable and inclusive healthcare (APA, 2021).
3. The Plan-Do-Study-Act (PDSA) Cycle: The PDSA Cycle is a quality improvement framework that can be applied to DEIB efforts. It involves planning interventions, implementing them on a small scale, studying the outcomes, and acting on the findings to make iterative improvements. This framework allows for continuous learning, adaptation, and refinement of diversity and inclusion initiatives within the organization (Del Pino-Jones et al., 2021).
4. The Health Equity Framework: The Health Equity Framework focuses on addressing health disparities and promoting health equity. It involves assessing and addressing social determinants of health, promoting access to health care services, and incorporating equity considerations into policy and decision-making processes. This framework helps guide efforts to reduce health disparities and promote equitable health outcomes among diverse populations (Peterson et al., 2021).

change or shift in an organization, it takes strategy that should always begin with the key stakeholders and the health care system's mission and vision. It is also crucial that health care systems envision outcomes at the outset of the planning phase that are in alignment the organization's mission and vision to guide strategies and initiatives.

5. The Cultural Humility Model: The Cultural Humility Model emphasizes self-reflection, lifelong learning, and a commitment to understanding and respecting others' cultural perspectives. It encourages health care providers and organizations to approach cultural differences with humility, open-mindedness, and a willingness to learn from diverse communities. This framework promotes a culture of learning, growth, and continuous improvement within the organization (Robinson et al., 2021).

DESIGNING, IMPLEMENTING, EVALUATING, AND SUSTAINING DIVERSITY, EQUITY, INCLUSION, AND BELONGING PROGRAMS

Planning the design of DEIB programs is essential for aligning them with organizational goals, targeting interventions effectively, allocating resources appropriately, promoting an inclusive approach, enabling evaluation and continuous improvement, engaging stakeholders, and ensuring sustainability and long-term commitment. Overall, DEIB programs should be well defined with a focus on positive health care system outcomes, including workforce and patient and community outcomes (i.e., enhanced engagement, increased productivity, improved job satisfaction, increased talent pool, enhanced morale, increased trustworthiness, and community responsiveness). Below are some strategies that could guide the planning process:

1. Establish a diverse and inclusive task force: Form a diverse and inclusive task force or committee composed of representatives from different departments and levels within the organization. Ensure that the task force includes individuals from various racial, ethnic, gender, and cultural backgrounds. This task force will be responsible for guiding the program's design and implementation.
2. Assess the current state: Begin by conducting a comprehensive assessment of the organization's current state of diversity and inclusion. Evaluate workforce demographics, patient demographics, policies and procedures, cultural competence training, and any existing diversity and inclusion initiatives. Engage with stakeholders, including employees, patients, and community members, to gather their perspectives and understand their needs and expectations.
3. Conduct a gap analysis: Identify gaps and areas for improvement based on the assessment conducted in Step 1. Determine the specific areas where the organization needs to enhance diversity and inclusion efforts.
4. Conduct stakeholder engagement: Engage key stakeholders, such as employees, patients, community leaders, and advocacy groups, to gather their perspectives and input on diversity and inclusion initiatives. Prior to rolling out a DEIB program, focus groups or listening sessions can be conducted to ensure that frontline staff and leaders are able to express their needs, concerns, and expectations, and recommendations for improvement. Their input will help shape the program's strategies and ensure its relevance and effectiveness. Also, it is important to keep in mind that focus group leaders will need to be skilled and prepared to address questions that may not be answered immediately or have unrealistic expectations.
5. Set clear goals and objectives: Define specific, measurable, achievable, relevant, and time-bound goals and objectives for the diversity and inclusion program. Align these goals with the organization's mission, vision, and strategic priorities. Examples may include improving workforce diversity, enhancing cultural competence training, and reducing health disparities among underserved populations.
6. Develop an action plan: Based on the goals, objectives, gap analysis, and stakeholder input, create a detailed action plan that outlines the strategies, activities, and timelines for implementing the diversity and inclusion program. Include specific initiatives related to recruitment and retention, training and education, policy development, community partnerships, and measuring outcomes.
7. Implement initiatives: Begin implementing the identified initiatives outlined in the action plan. This may include initiatives such as targeted recruitment strategies to increase workforce diversity, cultural competence training for staff, establishing employee resource groups or affinity networks, and developing policies and practices that foster inclusivity and equity. For nurses and organizations that have a clinical ladder or professional advancement system, DEIB topics provide a perfect opportunity for the implementation of quality improvement, evidence-based practice, and research projects to help them meet the requirements. This will enable frontline

staff to address the needs of underrepresented people while at the same time helping with their professional development and build contemporary expertise. Projects can be encouraged that address DEIB either on the unit level or throughout the organization.

An example of implementing a unit-based clinical ladder project could include helping frontline nurses feel comfortable utilizing sexual orientation and gender identity (SOGI) language and terminology. Many of our patients entering our health care organizations may choose to identify as nonbinary. The compliance with staff asking SOGI questions may be lacking. This could be related to general knowledge or perhaps systems barriers such as processes in the electronic health record. The clinical nurses could review data, survey the staff, and determine the barriers, which perhaps are impacting the comfort of our patients and staff. This nurses with the assistance of clinical leaders can develop processes that help eliminate bias by asking all patients questions about their preferred pronoun preferences. Processes like this can be complex but can be very meaningful to ensure that structures and processes are in place for all to utilize based on the principles of DEIB.

1. Allocate resources: Identify the necessary resources, including financial, human, and technological, required for implementing the diversity and inclusion program. Ensure that these resources are allocated appropriately to support the initiatives and strategies.
2. Provide training and education: This should be a very thoughtful approach that will need to be planned over time with experts in education, including leveraging an academic practice partnership if available. Training and education programs would focus on topics that relate to enhancing cultural competence and humility, raising awareness of unconscious biases, and deepening their understanding of diverse cultures, identities, and health care disparities and health inequities. Opportunities for various teaching modalities should be offered as well as the ability to come together face to face to discuss cases and examples. Discussions on DEIB can be very personal to people, and this needs to be taken into consideration throughout the implementation of the project.
3. Monitor and evaluate progress: Establish metrics and mechanisms for monitoring and evaluating the program's progress and outcomes. Collect and analyze data related to workforce representation, patient satisfaction, health disparities, and other relevant measures. Regularly review the data, assess program effectiveness, and adjust as needed to ensure continuous improvement. There also is a need for policies, structures, and processes that allow proper communication about DEIB as well as safe channels for addressing or reporting inequality and racism in the workplace. This step is very important as it will help establish metrics that can be evaluated before and after implementation, which can purposefully help quantify the overall benefits of the program. Some examples of metrics that can be collected may include incident reports, corporate compliance complaints, recruitment and retention of staff, and exit interviews. Additionally, if there are opportunities, including DEIB in employee satisfaction surveys for comparison can also be helpful during the evaluation phase.
4. Foster accountability and communication: Establish clear lines of accountability for diversity and inclusion efforts within the organization. Assign responsibility to specific individuals or departments to oversee and champion the program. Ensure regular communication and transparency about program updates, achievements, and challenges to engage employees and stakeholders. This process should utilize various modes of communication such as internal newsletters, intranet sites, journal clubs, blogs, grand rounds, and lecture series; these modes can also be well received and represent the organization's commitment to creating safe spaces.
5. Sustain, evolve, and celebrate milestones and achievements: Diversity and inclusion efforts should be sustained and continuously improved over time. Foster a culture of inclusivity and diversity by integrating diversity and inclusion principles into organizational policies, performance evaluations, and leadership development programs. Seek feedback from employees and stakeholders to inform program evolution and respond to changing needs. This can be achieved by creating a steering committee that is made up of a variety of staff from all areas and levels that clearly have a passion and a good deal of understanding of the organization and DEIB. An example of a strategy to ensure that enculturation continues can include developing a DEIB mentoring program to help develop new leaders that will help with attrition and provide growth opportunities. Celebrate

milestones and achievements to maintain momentum and engagement.
6. Embrace feedback: As a nurse leader in any organization, it is important to listen to staff who may bring concerns to you related to DEIB. The first step is to acknowledge the concern or feeling being presented. Next is to discuss how the concern or feeling made the staff member feel. Last is to inform the staff of how you will address the concern and how you would follow through. As a leader a self-assessment of your comfort in discussing topics related to DEIB is paramount. Staff need to know you are engaged and that you are prepared and have confidence in discussing topics related to DEIB.

SPECIFIC STRATEGIES TO ADVANCE DIVERSITY, EQUITY, INCLUSION, AND BELONGING IN HEALTH CARE SYSTEMS

There are several strategies that organizations can use to implement DEIB initiatives and promote recruitment, retention, and advancement of underrepresented groups and support underrepresented patient populations. Here are some examples:

1. Recruitment: Organizations can implement several strategies to attract a diverse pool of candidates, such as using targeted job postings and advertising in publications or websites that are popular with underrepresented groups. They can also consider partnering with community organizations or attending job fairs that serve underrepresented populations. Additionally, organizations can review and revise their job descriptions and qualifications to remove any unintentional barriers that may discourage candidates from diverse backgrounds from applying. To ensure a multicultural workforce, it is essential for non-BIPOC (Black, Indigenous, People of Color) leaders to have access to curriculum that teaches them the management skills needed in this environment. This includes antiracism practices, managing raced-based conversations without "tip-toeing" behavior, communication triggers in a diverse environment and culture-based interpretations of valued organizational behaviors. Additionally, we must monitor and increase BIPOC hires from internships, fellowships, and workforce development programs as well as designate a DEIB officer who can oversee strategy related to diversity equity and inclusion efforts while serving as an employee resource.
2. Retention: Once a diverse workforce has been established, it is important to retain these employees. One effective strategy is to create an inclusive workplace culture that values and supports all employees. This can be achieved by implementing policies and practices that promote work–life balance, provide opportunities for professional development and advancement, and offer resources for mental health and well-being. Organizations can also conduct regular surveys and focus groups to gather feedback from employees on their experiences and identify areas for improvement.
3. Advancement: Organizations can promote advancement opportunities for underrepresented groups by establishing clear guidelines and pathways for promotion and career development. This can include offering mentorship and sponsorship programs, creating leadership training programs, and ensuring that underrepresented employees are represented in decision-making bodies and leadership positions.
4. Policies at the workplace: Organizations must have rules and procedures in place to ensure coherence, especially when it comes to a specific agenda. In nursing today, there is an urgent need for an accountability agenda that addresses BIPOC-specific issues. Without incorporating this reality into the policies, procedures, and practices that govern decision making, we are unable to make meaningful progress toward eliminating bias, discrimination, and racism from the profession. To address these issues effectively requires three key actions: (a) implementing operational definitions related to the issue, which are meaningful within each setting; (b) developing an organizational plan with buy-in from leadership staffs and employees, which include built-in accountability measures; and (c) establishing DEIB as a programmatic approach with its own line item in the organization's budget so as to ensure sustainability of this work.
5. Metrics and accountability: Organizations can establish metrics and goals related to DEIB initiatives and regularly track and report on their progress. This can help hold leaders and managers accountable and ensure that DEIB is a priority for the organization.

6. Cultural competence training: Provide comprehensive cultural competence training to health care providers and staff. Cultural competence has been recognized as one approach to tackle racial and ethnic health disparities in healthcare by delivering services that cater to clients' cultural, social, and communication requirements. This training should focus on increasing awareness of unconscious biases, developing cross-cultural communication skills, and promoting understanding of the unique needs and perspectives of diverse populations. Regular training sessions and workshops can ensure ongoing professional development in this area.
7. Language access services: Implement language access services, such as professional interpreters and translation services, to overcome language barriers. This will enable effective communication with individuals who have limited English proficiency and ensure they receive appropriate care and understand their treatment plans.
8. Community engagement and partnerships: Establish partnerships with community organizations, advocacy groups, and leaders from minoritized communities. Engage in community outreach programs to better understand the specific health care needs, concerns, and priorities of these populations. By involving them in decision-making processes and co-designing health care programs, we can tailor services to meet their unique requirements.
9. Health education and literacy: Develop culturally appropriate health education materials and programs that address the specific health challenges faced by minoritized communities. Focus on health literacy initiatives to empower individuals to make informed decisions about their health and navigate the health care system effectively.
10. Addressing social determinants of health: Collaborate with community stakeholders and policy makers to address the social determinants of health that disproportionately affect minoritized individuals and groups. This may involve advocating for policies that promote access to affordable housing, education, employment opportunities, nutritious food, and transportation.
11. Data collection and monitoring: Implement robust data collection systems to monitor and analyze health outcomes and disparities among different racial and ethnic groups. This will help identify areas of improvement, track progress, and inform evidence-based interventions to reduce disparities in health care delivery and outcomes.
12. Quality improvement initiatives: Implement quality improvement programs that specifically target health disparities and ensure that care delivery is equitable across all populations. Regularly assess and address gaps in care, measure outcomes, and implement evidence-based practices to improve the overall quality of health care services.

By implementing these strategies, organizations can create a more diverse, equitable, and inclusive workplace culture that values all employees and promotes the recruitment, retention, and advancement of underrepresented groups. See Table 28.1 for examples and best practices to advance DEIB in the workplace.

TABLE 28.1 Evidence-Based Exemplars and Best Practices to Advance DEIB in the Workplace	
Develop a diversity statement	This can be based on contemporary issues, nursing departments' core values, and a commitment to developing a diverse workforce with a final goal of establishing a culture in which all differences are valued and celebrated in a safe place.
Develop a DEIB community page	This can be accomplished through use of a hospital-based intranet system that can be updated to provide timely engaging information.
Develop a mentorship program for minorities in leadership position	A minority mentorship program can be developed and offered annually to help focus on minority leaders who aspire to attain senior nursing leadership positions. Each workshop can offer specific objectives and guest speakers.
Develop a DEIB newsletter	Newsletters can serve as a living document with information and resources to continue your commitment to promote DEIB.
Develop a learning series	A learning series can be developed that is either synchronous or asynchronous in order to ensure that all staff receives contemporary DEIB information. By utilizing a virtual format this will enable you to bring in national experts.

IMPLICATIONS FOR PRACTICE

Supporting DEIB in the workplace can have significant practice implications that benefit employees, the organization, and the populations and communities they serve. Here are some examples of the benefits of integrating a DEIB culture in the workplace:

1. Enhanced creativity and innovation: A diverse and inclusive workplace can bring together people with different perspectives, backgrounds, and experiences. This can lead to increased creativity and innovation as individuals approach challenges and opportunities from different angles. Diversity in the workplace can also encourage new ideas and perspectives. By encouraging employees to bring their unique experiences and ideas to the table, organizations can foster a culture of creativity and innovation (ONL, 2022).
2. Better decision making: A workplace that values diverse perspectives and creates a culture of inclusivity can lead to better decision making. This is because a diverse team can identify potential blind spots and develop more comprehensive solutions to problems (Coleman & Taylor, 2023).
3. Increased employee engagement: A workplace that prioritizes DEIB can foster a sense of belonging and create a positive work environment. This can lead to increased employee engagement, job satisfaction, and retention (ONL, 2022).
4. Better talent acquisition: Organizations that prioritize DEIB can attract a wider pool of talent from diverse backgrounds. This can lead to a more skilled and talented workforce that can help the organization achieve its goals (ONL, 2022).
5. Improved reputation: A workplace that values DEIB can create a positive reputation for the organization. This can lead to increased interest from potential customers, investors, and other stakeholders (Lyman et al., 2022).
6. Legal compliance: We have laws and regulations that support DEIB in the workplace. By complying with these regulations, organizations can avoid legal repercussions and create a more supportive and inclusive environment for employees (ONL, 2022).

Overall, supporting DEIB in the workplace can have numerous practice implications that benefit both employees and the organization. By creating a more inclusive and supportive environment, organizations can increase innovation, better decision making, and improve employee engagement and retention, ultimately leading to a more successful and thriving workplace culture.

SYNTHESIS

In conclusion we have made great strides in ensuring that DEIB is incorporated into everyday nursing practice. This chapter addressed the importance and implications of integrating a DEIB culture in the workplace. We presented clear definitions of key terms to ensure clarity, promote common understanding, raise awareness, guide decision making, and promote education and empowerment. We provided an overview of the role of nurses, especially nursing and health care system leaders, in influencing and steering the directions to align DEIB programs with organizational goals, provide and allocate resources, and be a role model promoting an inclusive approach and ensuring sustainability and long-term commitment to the DEIB culture. We also discussed recommendations on how to develop, implement, grow, and sustain a DEIB culture in the workplace. Several examples were presented that could be used as templates for health care systems to develop, grow, and sustain their own DEIB initiatives.

Overall, when nursing staff and leaders are actively involved in diversity and inclusivity efforts, health care systems benefit from improved cultural competence, patient satisfaction, access to care, communication, employee engagement, innovation, and community relationships. There is an opportunity to further explore the impact and influence of DEIB interventions on our workforce, patients, and communities that we serve. This is in line with the charge of leading professional organizations such as the Institute for Healthcare Improvement, National Institute for Nursing Research, the National Academy of Sciences (*The Future of Nursing Report 2020–2030*), and the American Nurses Credentialing Center, that strongly support a workplace that champions DEIB. As a clinical leader, you are in an ideal position to champion and promote this crucial work.

KEY POINTS

- By supporting DEIB in the workplace this can have significant practice implications that benefit employees, the organization, and the populations and communities they serve.
- By integrating DEIB into the culture this can improve employee engagement, create a sense of belonging and a positive work environment, and lead to increased employee engagement, job satisfaction, and retention.
- There are laws and regulations that support DEIB in the workplace, which can enable organizations to avoid legal repercussions and create a more supportive and inclusive environment for employees.
- By engaging in community outreach programs to better understand them in decision-making processes and co-designing health care programs, we can tailor services to meet their unique requirements.

REFERENCES

American Association of Colleges of Nursing (AACN). (2021). *Diversity, equity, and inclusion faculty tool kit*. https://www.aacnnursing.org/Portals/42/Diversity/Diversity-Tool-Kit.pdf.

American Nurses Association (ANA). (2021). *National commission to address racism in nursing. report series*. https://www.nursingworld.org/practice-policy/workforce/racism-in-nursing/national-commission-to-address-racism-in-nursing/commissions-foundational-report-on-racism--in-nursing/.

American Psychological Association (APA). (2021). *Equity, diversity, and inclusion framework*. https://www.apa.org/about/apa/equity-diversity-inclusion/framework.

Brewington, J., Phillips, B., & Godfrey, N. (2023). Professional identity in nursing: Adopting a systems approach regarding diversity, equity, and inclusion. *Nursing Education Perspectives*, 44(1), 70–71. https://doi.org/10.1097/01.NEP.0000000000001092.

Brown, J., & Waller, M. (2022). Enhancing diversity in nursing education: Implementing inclusive practices to create a bias-free learning environment. *Nursing Education Today*, 113. https://doi.org/10.1016/j.nedt.2022.105358.

Cary, M. P., Randolph, S. D., Broome, M. E., & Carter, B. M. (2020). Creating a culture that values diversity and inclusion: An action-oriented framework for schools of nursing. *Nursing Forum*, 55, 687–694. https://doi.org/10.1111/nuf.12485.

Coleman, L., & Taylor, E. (2023). The importance of diversity, equity, and inclusion for effective, ethical leadership. *Clinical Sports Medicine*, 42, 269–280. https://doi.org/10.1016/j.csm.2022.11.002.

Cross, T., Bazron, B., Dennis, K., & Isaacs, M. (1989). *Towards a culturally competent system of care, Vol. I*. Georgetown University Child Development Center, CASSP Technical Assistance Centre.

Day, L., & Beard, K. (2019). Meaningful inclusion of diverse voices: The case for culturally responsive teaching in nursing education. *Journal of Professional Nursing*, 35(4), 277–281. https://doi.org/10.1016/j.profnurs.2019.01.002.

Del Pino-Jones, A. D., Cervantes, L., Flores, S., Jones, C. D., Keach, J., Ngov, L. K., Schwartz, D. A., Wierman, M., Anstett, T., Bowden, K., Keniston, A., & Burden, M. (2021). Advancing diversity, equity, and inclusion in hospital medicine. *Journal of Hospital Medicine*, 16(4), 198–203. https://doi.org/10.12788/jhm.3574.

Ea, E., Vetter, M. J., Boyar, K., & Keating, S. (2023). Using design thinking to thread the social determinants of health in an undergraduate curriculum. *Nurse Educator*, 48(2), 114–115. https://doi.org/10.1097/NNE.0000000000001293.

Foster-Smith, R., Mitchell, N., & Bobo, M. (2023). Diversity, equity, inclusion, and belonging: A role for us all. *Nursing Management*, 54(5), 40–47. https://doi.org/10.1097/nmg.0000000000000015.

Gill, G. K., McNally, M. J., & Berman, V. (2018). Effective diversity, equity, and inclusion practices. *Healthcare Management Forum*, 31(5), 196–199. https://doi.org/10.1177/0840470418773785.

Gomez, L. E., & Bernet, P. (2019). Diversity improves performance and outcomes. *Journal of the National Medical Association*, 111(4), 383–392. https://doi.org/10.1016/j.jnma.2019.01.006.

Lyman, B., Parchment, J., & George, K. (2022). Diversity, equity, inclusion: Crucial for organizational learning and health equity. *Nurse Leader*, 20(2), 193–196. https://doi.org/10.1016/j.mnl.2021.10.012.

Morrison, V., Hauch, R., Perez, E., Bates, M., Sepe, P., & Dans, M. (2021). Diversity, equity, and inclusion in nursing: The pathway to excellence framework alignment. *Nursing Administration Quarterly*, 45(4), 311–323. https://doi.org/10.1097/NAQ.0000000000000494.

Moss, M., & Phillips, J. (2020). *Health equity and nursing: Achieving equity through policy, policy health, and interprofessional collaboration*. Springer Publishing Company.

National Academies of Sciences, Engineering, & Medicine. (2021). *The future of nursing 2020–2030: Charting a path to achieve health equity*. National Academies Press. https://doi.org/10.17226/25982.

National Advisory Council on Nurse Education and Practice (NACNEP), Health Resources and Services Administration (HRSA). (2019). Integration of social determinants of health in nursing education, practice, and research. *Sixteenth report to the Secretary of the U.S. Department of Health and Human Services and to Congress*. https://www.hrsa.gov/sites/default/files/hrsa/advisory-committees/nursing/reports/nacnep-2019-sixteenthreport.pdf.

National League for Nursing (NLN). (2017). *NLN diversity and inclusion toolkit*. https://www.nln.org/docs/default-Source/uploadedfiles/default-document-library/diversity-Toolkit.pdf?sfvrsn=178daf0d_0.

Organization of Nurse Leaders (ONL). (2022). *Nurses taking a stand: A tool kit for addressing racism in nursing and healthcare*. https://onl.memberclicks.net/assets/docs/DEIB/ONL-Tool-Kit-for-Addressing-Racism-in-Nursing-and-Healthcare.pdf.

Peterson, A., Charles, V., Yeung, D., & Coyle, K. (2021). The health equity framework: A science and justice-based model for public health researchers and practitioners. *Health Promotion and Practice*, 22(6), 741–746. https://doi.org/10.1177/1524839920950730.

Prestia, A. S. (2023). Leadership's role in assimilating DEI to improve health care. *Nurse Leader*. https://doi.org/10.1016/j.mnl.2022.12.016.

Robinson, D., Masters, C., & Ansari, A. (2021). The 5 Rs of cultural humility: A conceptual model for health care leaders. *The American Journal of Medicine*, 134(2), 161–163. https://doi.org/10.1016/j.amjmed.2020.09.029.

Schmidt, B., MacWilliams, B., & Neal-Boylan, L. (2017). Becoming inclusive: A code of conduct for inclusion and diversity. *Journal of Professional Nursing*, 33(2), 102–107. https://doi.org/10.1016/j.profnurs.2016.08.014.

Sukhera, J., & Watling, C. (2018). A framework for integrating implicit bias recommendations into health profession education. *Academic Medicine*, 93(1), 35–40. https://doi.org/10.1097/ACM.0000000000001819.

Sumo, J., Staffileno, B., Warner, K., Arrieta, M., & Salinas, I. (2021). The development of an online diversity and inclusion community: Promoting a culture of inclusion within a college of nursing. *Journal of Professional Nursing*, 37(1), 18–23. https://doi.org/10.1016/j.profnurs.2020.10.002.

APPENDIX A

AONL Nurse Leader Core Competencies

To access this Appendix, please scan the QR code with a mobile device.

Appendix B

IPEC Core Competencies for Interprofessional Collaborative Practice

To access this Appendix, please scan the QR code with a mobile device.

APPENDIX C

National Institute of Nursing Research 2022–2026 Strategic Plan

To access this Appendix, please scan the QR code with a mobile device.

D APPENDIX

Person-Centered Care

To access this Appendix, please scan the QR code with a mobile device.

GLOSSARY

Academic Practice Partnership A type of strategic relationship between educational and clinical practice settings, which can promote the mutual interests of both sides.

A priori Outcome predictions that are made before the measurement phase begins.

Absolute risk reduction The value that gives the reduction in risk in absolute terms. It is the difference between the observed risk in those who did and did not experience the event/disease.

Action Plan Is a written document developed by those leading implementation and other key stakeholders that outlines the objectives, actions, and responsibilities of individuals or groups necessary to implement the EBPs.

Active dissemination Real-time interaction with the intended audience to impart key messages or information. This type of dissemination is bidirectional communication, and multiple conversations are used to discuss EBPs and rationale for use.

After-only design This is a less frequently used and weaker design composed of two randomly assigned groups, but unlike the classic experimental design, neither group is pretested. The independent variable is manipulated for the experimental arm but not for the control group.

AGREE II tool A standardized tool and method for appraising clinical practice guidelines.

Altmetrics The nontraditional impact of a study, tracked by many publishers at the article level, may measure downloads, captures (bookmarks, favorites, watchers, and other indications a reader wants to return to an item), "mentions" in news outlets, blogs, tweets, and other social media.

Artificial intelligence A machine-based system that can, for a given set of human-defined objectives, make predictions, recommendations, or decisions influencing real or virtual environments.

Audit and feedback Ongoing auditing of performance indicators, aggregating data into reports, and discussing the findings with practitioners on a regular basis during the practice change.

Auditability Is a feature of establishing scientific rigor where the reader can follow the line of thinking used by the researcher in the development of thematic and the exhaustive description.

Background question Those questions that lead you to investigate information about a disease, a condition, or a treatment that is derived from a knowledge-focused trigger.

Benchmarking The process of comparing a practice's performance with an external standard.

Bias Any influencing factor that may affect a study's results.

Blinding Sometimes called masking, is the process of concealing from the researchers, recruiters, interventionists, and participants and/or data collectors what treatment the participants are receiving in the study.

Boolean connectors Search operators such as "AND," "OR," and "NOT" that define relationships among search terms to narrow or expand search results.

Bundles of Care A collection of interventions that may be applied to the management of a particular condition.

Burnout A syndrome conceptualized as resulting from chronic workplace stress that has not been successfully managed.

Case-control study Study designed to assess the association between an exposure (independent variable) and an outcome (dependent variable).

Case series Study that collects data from a consecutive sample of patients treated in a similar manner without a control group.

Case study Research is rooted in sociology and focuses on describing elements of an individual case.

Cause and effect diagrams Used to identify and treat the causes of performance problems.

Change champion Individual who takes a role in organizing and brokering change because of his or her advocacy and personal network relationships.

Citation management tools Tools, such as EndNote, Zotero, Mendeley, and RefWorks, among others, that are platforms for downloading citations from library catalogs, article databases, and websites to build a personal data/article repository.

Climate for evidence-based practice implementation Staff's shared perceptions of the practices, policies, procedures, and clinical behaviors that are rewarded, supported, and expected to facilitate effective implementation of evidence-based practices.

Clinical decision support Tools often designed in the form of algorithms that can help illustrate the compatibility of a new practice in the context of the organization.

Clinical meaningfulness The degree to which the differences and relationships reported in a study are relevant to nursing practice.

Clinical microsystems A quality improvement model developed specifically for healthcare. It is considered the building block of any health care system and is the smallest replicable unit in an organization.

Clinical practice guidelines Systematically developed statements or recommendations that link research and practice and provide an evidence-based best practice guide for clinicians.

Clinical question Forms the basis for searching the literature to identify supporting evidence from research to inform development or revision of clinical standards, protocols, and policies that guide professional nursing and interprofessional best practice.

Compassion fatigue The profound emotional and physical exhaustion that helping professionals/caregivers can develop over the course of their career.

Cohort study Study that collects data from the same group of participants.

Common cause variation Occurs at random and is considered a characteristic of the system.

Concealment A method of protecting the randomization process to make sure the group assignment is not readily known by anyone before the participant is assigned to a group.

Conduct of research The systematic investigation of a phenomenon to answer research questions or hypotheses that generate new knowledge and advance the state of the science.

Confidence interval Represents a range of values within which a given population parameter (e.g., a mean, test statistic, or effect size) may be expected to fall.

Confirmability Refers to confirmation of the researcher influence in interpreting data and evidence of bracketing their biases through journal writing.

CONSORT Diagram The abbreviation used for the Consolidated Standards of Reporting Trials. A CONSORT diagram often is required to report the enrollment of participants in a trial.

Constancy Sameness in methods and procedures of data collection.

Context Characteristics of the physical setting of implementation and the dynamic practice factors in which implementation processes occur.

Contextual barriers Challenges in the environment, health care system, clinical workflow, administrative, and patient care context that make engagement more difficult to accomplish.

Continuous data A variable that measures a degree of change or a difference on a range.

Control Measures that the researcher uses to hold the conditions of the study consistent.

Control chart Is used to track system performance over time, but it is a more sophisticated data tool than a run chart.

Control group The group in a study that receives a different or no intervention or treatment.

Controlled vocabulary An online thesaurus of terms that disambiguate and facilitate more precise retrieval using search terms.

Cost/benefit ratio Mathematic representation of the relationship of the cost of an activity to the benefit of its outcome.

Credibility Refers to the conscious effort to establish confidence in an accurate interpretation of the meaning of the data.

Critical appraisal A careful analysis of a study's methodology, results, and conclusions to assess the quality and validity of the study.

Cross-over design A repeated measures design in which participants serve as their own controls. Participants are randomized to one of two groups; one group initially receives the intervention, and the other group serves as the control.

Cross-sectional study Study design that assesses data at one point in time.

Data saturation Is determined by the researcher when no new information emerge from the informants.

Dependability Refers to whether the informants recognize the exhaustive description as their reality when the narrative is returned to them.

Dependent variable Outcome variable.

Descriptive statistics Statistics used to describe or summarize elements of the sample.

Design thinking A mindset and approach to problem-solving and innovation anchored around human-centered design.

Diagnosis A diagnosis question focuses on the establishment of the power of a test to differentiate between those with the disease or problem and those who do not experience the problem.

Dichotomous data A type of nominal data with only two levels that typically have no hierarchy.

Diffusion of Innovation Broad framework explaining the adoption of many types of innovations by various groups or populations.

Dissemination The act of widely spreading information or ideas to many individuals. In healthcare, dissemination is the purposeful distribution of information and intervention materials to a specific public health or clinical practice audience.

DMAIC Model Control is achieved by applying an improvement model.

Double blind Means that neither the participant nor the researcher knows to which arm the participant is assigned, that is, the intervention or the control arm of the study.

Effect size A measure of the degree to which the null hypothesis is false, that is, the treatment makes a significant difference.

Effectiveness When a study is designed to test an intervention under "real-world" conditions.

Efficacy When a study is designed to test an intervention under well-controlled conditions.

Emic Is the insiders' view of a culture.

Employee Assistance Program (EAP) Provides assessment, short-term counseling, referral, management consultation, and coaching services to employees in an organization.

Environmental scan Assessment of internal strengths and challenges for implementation of evidence-based practices. Environmental scans include the structure and function of the organization.

Ethnography Is associated with anthropology, the work of describing culture and the people of a particular culture.

Etic Is the outsider's view of a culture.

Evaluation A structured approach to evaluating the impact of evidence-based practices (EBPs) when implemented in practice. It includes collection and analysis of data from the practice setting to determine whether the EBPs should be retained, modified, or eliminated.

Evidence summary A short summary of available evidence that may provide presynthesized data as well as recommendations for research and clinical practice.

Evidence-based practice The conscientious and judicious use of current best evidence in conjunction with clinical expertise, patient values, and circumstances to guide health care decisions.

Exclusion criteria Specific factors or characteristics of potential research participants that should not be present when someone enrolls in a research study (e.g., poor health, pregnancy, moving soon).

Experimental arm The part of a randomized trial in which participants receive the investigational treatment or the new intervention.

Experimental group The group that receives the experimental treatment.

GLOSSARY

Exposure A harmful or beneficial condition that can affect the outcome of illness or health.

Extent of adoption Number of evidence-based practice users after implementation compared with the number before implementation.

External validity The degree to which findings can be generalized to other populations or environments.

Extraneous variable Variables that interfere with study and cannot be manipulated or controlled. Also called mediating variables.

Fail-safe number Uses an odds ratio to calculate the number of studies reporting no treatment effect that would need to be included in the analysis to reduce the pooled odds ratio to a nonsignificant value.

Fiscal outcomes Estimated health care costs that may be affected by implementing evidence-based practices. Fiscal measures can address cost savings, cost reductions, and cost benefit.

Fishbone diagrams Can be used proactively to prevent quality defects including errors and retrospectively to identify factors that potentially contributed to a quality defect or error that already has occurred.

Flowchart Depicts how a QI process works, detailing the sequence of steps from the beginning to the end of a process.

Forest plot A visual reporting diagram of the individual study odds ratios (ORs) and confidence intervals (CIs) and the pooled OR and CI for the combined studies, which illustrates the magnitude of the effect of the intervention.

Funnel plot A graph based on odds ratios that detects small study treatment effects.

Generalizability The extent to which a study's findings can be applied to a different population.

GRADE A standardized system for grading evidence.

Gray literature Fugitive, ephemeral, invisible, or unpublished, is unevaluated and not peer-reviewed.

Grounded theory Research is used to generate theories about clinical practice and understanding about many different aspects of healthcare.

Harm A harm question focuses on the potential harm of a symptom or group of symptoms, disorder, treatment, or intervention.

Health literacy An individual's ability to access, interpret, and understand qualitative data about his or her health (i.e., delivered without numbers, typically as words or pictures).

Health numeracy An individual's ability to access, interpret, and understand quantitative data about his or her health (i.e., delivered with numbers or portraying numbers).

Health policy The decisions, plans, and actions that are assumed by governments, organizations, and stakeholders to achieve population health, and safeguard access to quality healthcare services.

Heterophily Transfer of ideas between opposite or different groups where the individuals have different attributes (e.g., various levels of education or different organizational roles).

High reliability organization Organizations that consistently excel in quality and safety across all services maintained over long periods of time.

History Internal validity threat that refers to events outside the study that may affect the dependent variable.

Homogeneity Similarity of the sample's characteristics.

Homophily Transfer of ideas among groups of people who are similar (e.g., members of the same professional groups or specialty practices).

Hypothesis Is used in research studies to predict the outcome(s) of the study. A hypothesis is predictive in nature and typically used when significant knowledge already exists on the subject, which allows the prediction to be made.

Implementation Is the processes and strategies used to promote the uptake and use of EBPs by clinicians, consumers, and policy makers.

Implementation fidelity Measures the degree to which participants carry out the evidence-based practices as intended.

Implementation science Testing implementation interventions/strategies to improve uptake and use of evidence to improve patient outcomes and population health, as well as to clarify what implementation strategies work, for whom, in what settings, and why.

Independent variable The antecedent or variable that has the presumed effect on the dependent variable.

Inferential statistics Tests used to apply findings from a sample to a population.

Instrumentation Changes in the measurement of a variable that may account for changes in the obtained measurement.

Integrative review Critical appraisal of the literature in an area of interest that does not include a statistical analysis due to the limitations of the study designs or the heterogeneity of the designs and samples. A systematic approach using explicit criteria is often used.

Intent-to-treat method The statistical process of analyzing data according to randomized groups, exactly as it exists upon randomization (even if participants receive no or minimal exposure to the intervention).

Internal validity The degree to which one can infer that the experimental treatment, rather than another condition or variable, resulted in the outcome or observed effects.

Interval data A type of data where the values are numeric, there is a hierarchy to the data, and the distances between categories have consistent, set values with the same interpretation.

Intervening variable A variable that occurs during a study that affects the dependent variable.

Intervention dose An important component of intervention fidelity, is the amount of the "something" that is given to the study participants to create a change in the dependent variable(s).

Intervention fidelity Also called treatment fidelity, implementation fidelity, adherence to protocol. Process used to ensure that the research intervention was delivered exactly as planned; typically involves collecting data on how research staff were trained and the consistency with which the intervention was delivered and received by the participants.

Intervention studies Often called randomized controlled (clinical) trials and abbreviated as RCT, reflect the strongest design type for an individual study, located at Level II on the Evidence Hierarchy.

GLOSSARY

Knowledge-focused triggers Ideas that are generated when clinical teams or quality improvement committees read research studies, listen to scientific papers presented at professional conferences, or encounter practice guidelines published by federal organizations.

Leadership behaviors for evidence-based practice (EBP) implementation Enactment of behaviors by leaders that reflect the extent to which they support and foster EBP implementation.

Lean A quality improvement framework focused on eliminating waste from the production system by designing the most efficient and effective system.

Likelihood ratio Expresses the magnitude by which the probability of disease in a specific patient is modified by the result of a test.

Longitudinal study Also known as cohort, repeated measures, or prospective study.

Manipulation Means using a different dose of "something" in one group (the intervention arm) and not the other group (the control group).

Maturation Developmental, biological, physiological, or psychological processes within an individual as a function of time that are external to a study's events.

Mean The average of all the data in a set.

Meaning A meaning question focuses on the situation or processes related to how people experience, cope, or adapt to conditions, illnesses, or circumstances.

Measurement effects Administration of a pretest that affects the generalizability of a study's findings to other populations.

Median The value in a set that is closest to the middle of a range.

Meta-analysis A type of systematic review, combines the results of multiple studies in a specific area, quantitatively analyzes the findings as an aggregate, and presents a quantitative conclusion about the strength of the evidence provided by the group of studies and makes a recommendation about the applicability of the findings.

Metaliteracy An "ongoing adaptation to emerging technologies and an understanding of the critical thinking and reflection required to engage in these spaces."

Meta-synthesis Is a rigorous synthesis of a critical mass of qualitative research evidence that relates to answering a specific research question (sometimes call a meta-summary).

Mode The value that occurs most frequently in a data set.

Model for improvement Focuses on the aims, identifies measures to assess change, and specifies changes that will result in improvement.

Mortality Loss of participant.

Narrative review Review of the literature that includes studies that support an author's perspective and provides a broad background discussion in a focused area of interest. A systematic approach to searching for and appraising papers is often not used.

Negative predictive value The proportion of those with negative test results who truly do not have disease.

Nominal data A type of data that is not numeric and has no established hierarchy between values.

Nonparametric statistics Distribution-free statistical method used to analyze nominal and ordinal level data.

Null hypothesis A hypothesis that assumes there is no relationship between two variables.

Null value The value of no effect; in experimental study design it often means there is no difference in the outcomes between the experimental and control groups.

Numbers needed to treat The number of patients who need to be treated to get the desired outcome in one patient who would not have benefited otherwise.

Nursing scholarship Those activities that systematically advance the discipline of nursing by teaching, research, and practice through rigorous inquiry.

Nursing sensitive outcomes Specific patient outcomes that are influenced by nursing care.

Observational study A category of nonexperimental studies that constructs a picture of variables at one point or over a period of time. The variables are not manipulated or randomized as in a randomized clinical trial.

Odds ratio A numeric value that indicates the probability of an outcome occurring given exposure to a variable of interest. It compares the odds of the disease (or other phenomenon) occurring with those of the disease (or other phenomenon) not occurring when exposed to the variable of interest.

Opinion leader Individual who is able to informally influence others' ideas, attitudes, or overt behavior in a desired way.

Ordinal data A type of nonnumeric data that has an associated hierarchy but the distance between values may not be consistent and may have different interpretations.

Outcome The consequence of the exposure.

Outcome measures Measures projected to change as a result of evidence-based practice (EBP) implementation. They are used to evaluate whether implementation of the selected EBPs are resulting in improvements in health outcomes.

Outcomes The effect that the processes of care have on patients and populations.

Parametric statistics A method used to analyze data at the interval or ratio level. The parameters tested must be normally distributed in the population.

Passive dissemination A one-way communication or top-down process such as publishing or posting information with the expectation that the intended audience will access and use the information.

Patient activation The knowledge, confidence, and skills that a patient possesses and is willing to use to make decisions about his or her health.

Patient engagement A patient's knowledge, skills, ability, and willingness to manage his or her own health and care.

Patient portal A web-based platform that compiles various resources for patient engagement, such as decision-making aids, educational materials, and communication applications. It typically is connected to the Electronic Health Record used by providers to communicate health care data back to the patient.

Performance gap assessment The baseline practice performance that provides information about the state of current practices at the beginning of a practice change.

Person-Centered Care Integrated health care services delivered in a setting and manner that is responsive to individuals and their goals, values, and preferences, in a system that supports good provider–patient communication and empowers individuals receiving care and providers to make effective care plans together.

Phenomenology Is a science whose purpose is to describe particular phenomena, or the appearance of things, as lived experience.

GLOSSARY

PICOT Provides an effective format for developing focused and searchable clinical questions. PICOT is a tool to help you formulate the clinical question.

Pilot Trying an evidence-based practice for a period of time before full adoption.

Pilot study A small sample study conducted as a prelude to a larger scale study, often called the "parent study."

Plan-Do-Study-Act (PDSA) Improvement Cycles The improvement changes identified in the planning phase of the quality improvement process are tested using the PDSA improvement cycle, the last step in the quality improvement process.

Point-of-care tool Designed to aid decision support for clinicians by synthesizing evidence for common clinical problems, diseases, drugs, and therapies.

Population Health A interdisciplinary, customizable approach that allows health care organizations to connect practice to policy for changes to happen locally.

Positive predictive value The proportion of those with positive test results who truly have disease.

Power analysis A method of determining statistical power, the probability of correctly rejecting a null hypothesis.

Pragmatic trials Trials that evaluate the effectiveness of an intervention previously tested for efficacy in traditional experimental designs.

Prevalence Epidemiological term used to describe the number of people with a disease in a specified time period.

Primary source A book or article that contains original evidence.

PRISMA flowchart A graphical depiction of the process of identifying, screening, determining eligibility, and applying exclusion criteria during the process of creating an integrative or systematic review that can be very useful as a graphical depiction of your search.

Probability value (p value) A numeric value that helps determine whether the null hypothesis should be rejected or accepted.

Problem-focused triggers Those identified by staff through quality improvement, risk surveillance, benchmarking, and financial data or recurrent clinical problems.

Process measures Methods to evaluate staff's use of the evidence-based practices (EBPs) as detailed in the local EBP standard. They measure whether the EBPs demonstrated to benefit patients are being followed.

Processes of care The services and treatments patients receive.

Prognosis A prognosis question focuses on a patient's likely course for a disease state or factors that may alter a prognosis.

Public reporting Systems that compare treatment results, costs, and patient experiences.

Publication bias Misleading results as the set of published data may not be a representative sample of the overall evidence.

Purposive sampling Indicates that a sample is homogeneous and reflects the population being studied.

Qualitative research Is explanatory, descriptive, and inductive in nature and comprises methods that help us formulate an understanding of phenomena and their context answered by discovery-oriented research questions.

Quality healthcare Care that is safe, effective, patient-centered, timely, efficient, and equitable.

Quality improvement Uses data to monitor the outcomes of care processes and improvement methods to design and test changes to continuously improve the quality and safety of health care systems.

Quasi-experimental design A design located at Level III on the Evidence Hierarchy. Quasi-experimental designs differ from RCTs in that they lack either a comparison group or randomization and, as such, have a higher risk of bias.

Quick reference guides Guides that provide targeted, concise information designed to help practitioners perform specific tasks.

Randomization A sampling procedure in which each person has an equal chance of being selected to either the experimental or control group.

Randomized clinical trial Research study having at least two arms where the decision as to which arm the participant is assigned to is made by chance (usually computer-generated).

Range The lowest and highest values reported in a data set.

Rapid review Methodology that uses shorter time frames than for other evidence-based summaries. It provides a timely and valid view of evidence but sacrifices rigor. As such, RRs are both review and assessment and respond to urgent clinical and public health-related questions.

Rate of adoption Speed at which users begin to use new evidence-based practices.

Ratio data A type of data where the values are numeric and contain absolute zero (the complete absence of the variable), there is a hierarchy to the data, and the distances between categories have consistent, set values with the same interpretation.

Reactivity Distortion created when those who are being observed change their behavior because they know they are being observed.

Realist review Provides explanatory analysis aimed at discerning what works for whom, in what circumstances, and how. Sources can include theoretical, policy, and research literature that combine theoretical understanding with empirical evidence and focus on the context in which an intervention is applied, the mechanisms by which it works, and the outcomes it produces.

Receiver Operating Characteristics (ROC) curve A plot of the true positive rate against the false-positive rate for the different possible cutpoints of a diagnostic test.

Recognition Formal or informal action that recognizes staff for their efforts in implementing evidence-based practices. Examples include highlighting work in organizational publications; personal thank-you notes from leaders; highlighting the work at system-level quality improvement meetings; and nominating individuals or teams for practice excellence awards offered by the health system or professional organization.

Relative risk A numeric value that describes the probability of developing a disease when exposed to risk factor(s) compared with the probability of developing the disease when not exposed to risk factor(s).

Repeated measures study A study design in which data are collected from the same participants on multiple occasions.

Research The systematic investigation of a phenomenon to answer research questions or hypotheses that generate new knowledge and advance the state of the science.

Research question Addresses a gap or conflict in the literature. Tests a measurable relationship between the independent and dependent variable that is examined in the study.

Retrospective study A study that begins with an outcome (dependent variable) and examines its relationship to another variable (independent variable) that preceded it.

Review An evidence summary that synthesizes information from quantitative and qualitative research studies as well as theoretical and conceptual published and unpublished outputs.

Reward Form of monetary compensation such as a bonus payment, salary increase, or educational funds to be used at the discretion of the individual, team, or practice. For example, an individual or team who has been instrumental in implementing evidence-based practices may receive financial support to attend a regional or national conference to present their work.

Risk/benefit ratio Ratio of the risk of an action to its potential benefits. Risk–benefit analysis is analysis that seeks to quantify the risk and benefits.

Root cause analysis (RCA) Identify system design failures that caused errors.

Run chart A graphical data display that shows trends in a measure of interest; trends reveal what is occurring over time.

Scoping review A preliminary search and assessment of the potential size and scope of available research literature, including ongoing research. It aims to determine the value of undertaking a full systematic review.

Scoping search Identifies the existing evidence or a gap in research and informs the focus for developing a refined PICO question.

Search bias The skewed or insufficient retrieval of literature that results from a careless or incomplete search strategy or selection of the wrong database.

Secondary source Derived from or interpretation of primary sources.

Selection bias Internal validity threat that arises when pretreatment differences between the experimental and control group are present.

Sensitivity The ability of the instrument or test to predict a positive result when the phenomenon of interest is also positive or will occur.

Sensitivity analysis Used to examine the effect of studies that are "outliers."

Shared decision making A process by which patients and clinicians partner to make informed health decisions.

Shared decision-making aids Evidence-based documents or tools that portray health care options; give information about risks, benefits, and outcomes for the options; assist patients in clarifying their values; and incorporate clinical judgment and counseling.

Single blind Occurs when the participant does not know which intervention he or she is receiving. Solomon four-group design–A design with four groups (two experimental and two control). Two groups are identical to those used in the classic experimental design described earlier, plus two additional groups including an experimental after-group and a control after-group. Participants are randomly assigned to one of four groups before baseline data are collected. This design results in two groups that receive only a posttest rather than a pre- and posttest.

Six Sigma A quality improvement framework that emphasizes meeting customer requirements and eliminating errors or reworking with the goal of reducing process variation. Focuses on tightly controlling variations in production processes with the goal of reducing the number of defects using the DMAIC model.

Snowballing Following reference lists backward and following articles that cite an article following publication.

Social determinants of health The nonmedical factors that influence health outcomes.

Social system Context of a care delivery or practice setting where the evidence-based practices are being implemented.

Special cause variation Arises from a special situation that disrupts the causal system beyond what can be accounted for by random variation.

Specificity The ability of the instrument or test to predict a negative result when the phenomenon of interest is also negative or will not occur.

SQUIRE Guidelines Promote standardized guidelines for the publication and interpretation of applied research and used to evaluate QI projects.

Stakeholder A key individual or group of individuals who will be directly or indirectly affected by the implementation of the EBP.

Standard deviation A numeric measure of the variation or spread of values in a set of data.

Survey studies Provide information in areas where little is known, often ask broad questions, and generally have large sample sizes. Survey studies are also classified as descriptive, exploratory, or comparative.

Sustainability Occurs when a new practice becomes embedded into daily workflow.

Synthesis Critical appraisal of the overall strengths and weaknesses of the studies as a group to establish the state of the science for answering your PICO question and provide an evidence-based foundation on which to base practice and standards of care.

Systematic review A collection of research studies based on a clearly focused question that uses a clearly defined search strategy to locate and then assess relevant evidence for applicability to clinical practice.

Test for heterogeneity Sometimes referred to as the test of homogeneity, calculated to determine that the hypothesis that each study is measuring is similar across studies and for the same population.

Testing The effects of taking a pretest on a posttest that includes defining, measuring, analyzing, improving, and controlling processes.

Therapy A therapy question focuses on determining the effect of an intervention(s) on patient outcomes.

Total Quality Management/Continuous Quality Improvement A holistic management approach used to improve organizational performance. TQM/CQI tools and techniques are applied to specific performance problems in the form of improvement projects.

Transferability Focuses on whether the findings are applicable outside the study situation.

Translating Research into Practice Model Is a conceptual model to guide selection of implementation strategies for promoting adoption of EBPs. The model is derived from Roger's (2003) seminal work on diffusion of innovations.

Translation science Focuses on testing the implementation of interventions to improve uptake and use of evidence to improve patient outcomes, population health, and to clarify what implementation strategies work for whom, in what settings, and why.

Triple blind Occurs when the researcher, interventionist, and participants do not know which arm is receiving the experimental treatment versus the placebo.

Trustworthiness Refers to whether the participants recognize the experience as their own and whether adequate time has been allowed to fully understand the phenomenon.

Type I error When an instrument or test incorrectly predicts that a phenomenon of interest will occur.

Type II error When an instrument or test incorrectly predicts that a phenomenon of interest will not occur.

Users of EBPs Members of a practice setting who will be using and implementing the evidence-based practices. This may include nurses, physicians, respiratory therapists, and professionals from other disciplines.

Wellness Living optimally in the various dimensions and in a manner intended to maintain this positive state

INDEX

A

A priori, 181
AACN Essentials Domain 8: Core Competencies for Professional Nursing Education (2021), 360t–364t
AACR Cancer Disparities Progress Report, 170t
Absolute measures of risk, 186
Absorptive and Receptive Capacity Scale (ARCS), 265t
Abstract, peer review of, 324–326
Abstract submission, 323–324
ACA. See Affordable Care Act
Academic detailing, 248–249
Academic partners, 270
Academic-practice partnership (APP), 3, 7–18, 334–335, 338–339
  AACN/AONL guiding principles for, 9, 10t–11t
  action-oriented recommendations, 12f
  challenges, 8
  characteristics, 9–12
  history, 8–9
  mutual benefits of, 8
  operationalizing, 12–15
Accountable Care Organization (ACO), 205b
ACE Star Model of Knowledge Transformation, 45t
ACP. See American College of Physicians
Action plan, 236, 238b
Activation, patient, 281–282, 281f
Active dissemination, 318
Addressing social determinants of health, 427
Adequate sleep, 406
Adopter categories, 235t, 236b
Adoption, stages of, 234t
Advanced Cardiac Life Support (ACLS), guidelines for, 245
Advancement opportunities, 426

Advancing Research and Clinical Practice Through Close Collaboration Model, 44, 45t
Advocacy, 395
Affordable Care Act (ACA), 279–280
Agency for Healthcare Quality and Research, 26t–27t
Agency for Healthcare Research and Quality's (AHRQ) Hospital Survey, 167t
Aggregators, 66
AGREE instrument. See Appraisal of Guidelines Research and Evaluation (AGREE) instrument
AHRQ NPSD, 167t
Alerts and reminders, 372
Alert services, 66
Alma-Ata Declaration, 392
Alternative forms of scholarship, 311
Alternative Payment Models, 204, 224
American Association of Colleges of Nursing (AACN), 3
  APP guiding principles, 10t–11t
  Manatt report, 11t
American College of Physicians (ACP), 280
American Nurses Association, 168–169
American Nurses Credentialing Center (ANCC), 2, 21–25, 26t–27t, 365
  Magnet designation, 335–336
  Magnet Recognition model, 51
American Organization of Nurse Leaders (AONL), 9
  APP guiding principles, 10t–11t
American Recovery and Reinvestment Act of 2009, 371
AMSTAR-2 tool, 101
Analysis of variance (ANOVA) test, 185, 188
Analysis, sensitivity, 126
ANCC Magnet Standards for dissemination, 327, 328t
AND operator, 71
APN EBP Competency Scale, 265t

Application/practice scholarship, 309–310
Appraisal, critical, 40–42
  of CPGs, 123b, 136b, 137–139, 138b
  of evidence-based literature statistics, 185
  literature search, 75–76
  for observational studies, 113–115, 114t, 115b
  of qualitative research, 154t–155t
Appraisal of Guidelines Research and Evaluation (AGREE) instrument, 137
Appraisal of Guidelines Research and Evaluation II (AGREE II) instrument, 137, 138t
ARCS. See Absorptive and Receptive Capacity Scale
Area under ROC curve (AUROC), 192–193, 193f
  Braden Q versus Braden QD, 194f, 195t
  guide for interpretation, 194t
  of test with 100% sensitivity and specificity, 193f
  for worthless test, 194f
Area under the curve (AUC), 194
  Braden Q versus Braden QD, 195t
Artificial intelligence (AI), 348, 353, 373
ASAPBio, 65t
ASCVD risk calculator, 245
Attrition, 94–95
Auditability, of data, 152t
Audit and feedback, of evidence-based practice, 271–272, 272b
AUROC. See Area under ROC curve
Authenticity, of data, 151–153, 152t
Avocational interests, 408
Awareness tools, 66

B

Background questions, 68
Balint groups, 406–407
Bar chart, 216–217, 217f
Barriers to dissemination, 327

Note: Page numbers followed by "f" indicate figures, "t" indicate tables and "b" indicate boxes.

443

INDEX

Bell curve, 216–217
Belonging, 418
Benchmarking, 162–163, 203b, 204–205
Better decision making, 428
Better talent acquisition, 428
Bias
  defined, 82, 94–95
  publication, 124
Bibliographic records, 62
Big data, 373
Binary variables, 174
Birthweight, 385
Bivariate analysis, 188t
Blinding, 92
Blogs, 321
Boolean operators, 71, 72f
Bracketing, 153
Braden QD Scale, 194, 194f, 195t
Braden Q Scale, 194, 194f, 195t
Bundled Payments Initiative, 205b
Bundles of care, 23t–24t, 24–25
Burnout, 404

C

CAHPS Hospice, 163t–165t
Canadian Health Outcomes for Better Information and Care, 168–169
Cancer Disparities Progress Report, AACR, 170t
Capitation, 205b
Care Compare Website, 163t–165t
Care delivery, key EBP messages at point of, 245–246
Care Innovation and Transformation Program, 200–201
Care quality, 359–360
Case-control studies, 109–110, 110b, 382
Case series, 110–111
Case study, 148
CASP. See Critical Appraisal Skills Programme
Categorical data, 174
Catheter associated urinary tract infections (CAUTIs), 297
Cause and effect diagrams, 217–218, 218f
CAUTIs. See Catheter associated urinary tract infections
Centers for Disease Control and Prevention (CDC), 26t–27t

Centers for Medicare and Medicaid Services (CMS), 26t–27t, 65–66, 65t
  handwashing education, 161–162
  National Healthcare Safety Network, 167t
  Star Rating, 160, 163t–165t
  value-based programs, 26–27
CENTRAL, 66
Central limit theorem, in practice, 177–179, 178b
Central tendency, measures of, 176–177, 176t
Centre for Evidence-Based Medicine, 41t
Cerebral palsy (CP), 124
Champions, defined, 247–248
Change champions, 247–248
Change theory, 412
Chief nurse executive (CNE), 269
Chief nursing informatics officer (CNIO), 374
CINAHL. See Cumulative Index to Nursing and Allied Health Literature
Citation management software, 75, 75b
Cited reference searching, 73
Clinical analyst/nurse informaticist, 374
Clinical data registries, 373
Clinical decision support (CDS), 353
Clinical decision support systems (CDSS), 371
Clinical decision support tools, 245
  types of, 245
Clinical documentation, 372
Clinical leader, 396–397
  role of, in health care quality improvement, 200–201
Clinical meaningfulness, 181
Clinical Microsystems, 210t–211t
Clinical practice, 52
Clinical Practice Guidelines (CPGs), 131–134, 133b, 135b
  appraisal tools, 136b
  critical appraisal of, 137–139, 138b–139b
  definition of, 118
  implementation of, 134–137, 136b
  National Guideline Clearinghouse, 134, 135b
  selected databases for locating, 134b
  selected specialty databases, 134b

Clinical practice scholarship, 310
Clinical questions
  compelling, developing, 51–58
  definition of, 52–53
  and eligibility criteria, 66–68, 67b
  importance of, 53–54
  PICOT, 52
    case study, 56b
    formulation of, 54
    in observational studies, 106, 106t
    question components, 52b
    question formats, 53b
    in systematic review (SR), 118
    types of, 55
  of prognosis, 194–195
  versus research questions and hypotheses, 55–56
  sources of, 54–55
  types of, 54t, 55
Clinical scholarship, resources to support, 311t
Clinical teams, in systematic review, 118–119
Clinicaltrials.gov, 65t, 66
Clinical workflows, 365
CMS. See Centers for Medicare and Medicaid Services (CMS)
CMS Star Rating System, 160
CNE. See Chief nurse executive
Coalition building, 395
Code Lavender model, 407
Coefficient of determination, 186
Cohort studies, 108–109, 382
Collaboration, 336–337
Collaborative Practice Assessment instrument (CPAT), 167t
Combined models, 47–48
  Evidence-Based Practice Improvement Model, 47–48
  I3 Model, 47
Common cause variation, 215
Common sense, 411–412
Communicating narrative concerns entered by registered nurses (CONCERN), 353, 353b
Communication, defined, 246
Communication skills, 385–386
Community, 381
Community engagement, 395
Community engagement and partnerships, 427
Community partnerships, 385–386

INDEX

Comparative effectiveness research, 22t
Comparison group, 301
Comparison intervention, in PICOT, 52–53
Compassion fatigue, 404
Compassion satisfaction, 404
Compatibility, of EBP topics, 232t
Complexity, of EBP topics, 232t
Conceptual definition, 162
Conduct of research, 21, 239t
  comparison of EBP and, 23t–24t
  definition of, 21–25, 22t–24t, 25f
Confidence interval, 182, 183f–184f
Confirmability, of data, 152t
Confirmation, as stages of adoption, 234t
Consolidated Evidence for Reporting Trials (CONSORT), 121
Consolidated Framework for Implementation Research (CFIR), 46
CONSORT. *See* Consolidated Evidence for Reporting Trials
Constancy, 83
Construct validity, 95, 299
Consumer Assessment of Healthcare Providers and Systems (CAHPS) surveys, 163, 163t–165t
Contentment, 403–404
Content validity, 95, 299
Context assessment
  performing, 262b, 264–266
  in social system, 262, 265t
Context, definition of, 47
Contextual barriers, against person-centered care, 287–288
Continue learning, 349, 350t
Continuous variable, 175, 188
Control charts, trending variation in system performance with, 215–216, 215f–216f
Control, definition of, 82
Control groups, 82, 92
Control measures, 92
Convenience sampling, 150b
Convergent validity, 299
Core concepts, in database searches, 69
Correlation coefficient, Pearson's, 185–186
Cost-benefit analysis, 102
Council on Linkages Between Academia and Public Health Practice, 385, 386b

COVID-19
  academic-practice partnership and, 14–15
  mixed-methods research, 148
Covidence, 75, 75b
COVID-19 pandemic, 374, 392–393, 401–403, 410
  personal protective equipment, 387
  population health, 380, 386
CPGs. *See* Clinical Practice Guidelines
Credibility, of data, 150, 152t
Criterion validity, 299
Critical appraisal, 40–42
  of CPGs, 123b, 136b, 137–139, 138b
  of evidence-based literature statistics, 185
  literature search, 75–76
  for observational studies, 113–115, 114t, 115b
  of qualitative research, 154t–155t
Critical Appraisal Skills Programme, 41t
Critical appraisal tools, 40, 41t
Critical decision tree, 219, 220f
Critical Incident Stress Debriefing (CISD), 411–412
Critical thinking decision path
  measurement effects, 88, 88b
  reactive effects, 88
  selection effects, 85–88
  study's validity, potential threats to, 85b
Crossing the Quality Chasm, 199–200
Cross-sectional study, 105–106, 382
Cultivating growth, 403–404
Cultural competence
  lack of, 420
  training, 427
Cultural Competence Continuum, 423
Cultural Humility Model, 424
Culture of inquiry, 160
Cumulative incidence difference, risk, 187
Cumulative Index to Nursing and Allied Health Literature (CINAHL), 62t, 79

D

Data
  analysis and display of, 300–301
  in observational studies, 112–113, 113b

Data analysis
  in observational studies, 112–113
  in qualitative research, 150, 150b
Data analytics, 359–360
Database
  filters, 73
  health equity, 170t
  literature, 62–65, 62t
  managing and screening records, 75
  saving search strategies, 73–75
  techniques for searching, 68–73
    core search concepts and descriptive vocabulary, 69–70, 70f
    refining and revising, 73, 74f
    search query, structured, 70–73, 72f
    sensitivity and specificity, 68–69
  worker safety, 170t
Data collection, 384
Data collection and monitoring, 427
Data display, 301
Data extraction, 76–77, 78t
  in systematic review, 121
Data-Information-Knowledge-Wisdom (DIKW), 353, 353f, 366–367, 366f, 367t, 367b
Data integration, 371
Data mining, 370t
Data saturation, 145
Data sets, 384
Data sources, of evidence-based practices, 297–300, 300b
  adapting measures for practice, 299–300
  changing measurement during QI project, 298
Data use and evaluation, nursing informatics, 369–371, 370t, 371b
Decision, as stages of adoption, 234t
Decision-Making Algorithm, 118, 121f
Decision support tools, 372
Decreased access to preventive care, 421
Dedicated Education Unit (DEU), 13
Delayed diagnosis and treatment, 420
Deming, Edwards, 24
Department of Nursing Governance Structure, 264f
Dependability, of data, 150, 152t
Dependent variables, 82, 174
Descriptive statistics, 176–177, 176t

Design thinking (DT), 343–346, 347f, 351b
　in academic and clinical setting, 346–348
Desired Dementia Care Towards End of Life (DEDICATED), 111–112
Diagnostic test studies, statistics for, 189–194, 189b, 190t, 191f, 191b
Dichotomous data, 174
Diffusion, as quality strategy lever, 203
Diffusion of innovation (DOI), 243
Digital redlining checkpoint, 385
DIKW. *See* Data-Information-Knowledge-Wisdom (DIKW)
Discriminant validity, 299
Discriminatory practices, 420
Disease burden, 420–421
Dissemination, 338
Dissemination, of evidence-based practice projects, 317–332
　active, 318
　definition of, 317–318
　implementation science and, 321–323, 322t, 323f, 323b, 324t–325t
　intended audience in, 318
　objectives of, 318
　passive, 318
　peer review, 323–327
　principles of, 318
　social media methods in, 320–321
　strategies to overcome barriers to, 327–329
　　implications for practice settings, 329
　　outside of academic spaces, 328–329
　　synthesis of, 329
　traditional methods of, 319–320
　venues for, 319
Dissemination research, 22t
Dissemination venues, 319
DistillerSR, 75
Distribution-free statistical methods, 176
Divergent thinking, 352f
Diversity, 418
Diversity, equity, inclusion, and belonging (DEIB)
　best practices to advance, 427t
　building and sustaining, 422–423
　definitions of, 418–419

Diversity, equity, inclusion, and belonging (DEIB) *(Continued)*
　designing, implementing, evaluating, and sustaining, 424–426
　guiding frameworks, 423–424
　health systems and, 419
　implications for practice, 428
　nursing's pivotal role in, 421–422
　on population and health care outcomes, 420–421
　principles of, 417
　specific strategies, 426–427
　synthesis, 428
　and workplace, 419–420
DMAIC model, 44–45, 210t–211t
Dobbins's Framework for Dissemination and Utilization of Research, 45t
Doctorally prepared nurses
　academic-practice partnership influence, 338–339
　collaborative opportunities, 337b
　future opportunities for, 339–340
　history of, 334–335
　opportunities, 335–337
　research/evidence-based practice, 337
　scientific inquiry, 337–338
　synthesis, 340
Doctorate of education (EdD), 334t
Doctorate of nursing practice (DNP), 334t
Doctorate of philosophy (PhD), 334t
Doctor of Nursing Practice (DNP) programs, 2, 4
Documentation systems, of evidence-based practice, 272
Donabedian model, 161
Dynamed, 66
Dynamic Health, 65t, 66

E
Early adopters, 235t
Early career interventions, 409
Early majority, 235t
EBP assessment tools, 265t
EBP Competency Scale, 265t
EBPs. *See* Evidence-based practices
Education, 248, 397
　of nurses, 336
Educational outreach, 222, 248–249
Education and training, 372

Effectiveness, definition of, 93
Effect size, 126, 181
Efficacy, definition of, 93
EIDM. *See* Evidence-informed decision-making
80-20 Rule, 216–217
Electronic health record (EHR), 93, 287, 339, 359, 383–384
Eligibility criteria, PICOT question and, 67, 67t
EMBASE, 62t, 79
Emergency Department CAHPS, 163t–165t
Emic view, of ethnography, 147–148
Employee assistance program (EAP), 410–411
Employee engagement, 428
Employee engagement and satisfaction surveys, 165, 166t
Endemic, 381
Engagement, 404
Engagement principles, 345, 346b
Enhanced creativity and innovation, 428
Entry to practice, 409
Environmental factors, 397
Environmental scan, of evidence-based practice, 263–266
Epidemic, 381
Epidemiology, 381
Equity, 418
Equity, Diversity, and Inclusion (EDI) Framework, 423
Ethical considerations, for evidence-based practice, 236–240
Ethnography, 147–148
Etic view, of ethnography, 147–148
Evaluation
　definition of, 294
　for evidence-based practice, 294b, 304t
　　analysis and display of data of, 300–301
　　data sources, 297–300, 300b
　　guidelines for, 306b
　　methods for, 294–295
　　outcome measures of, 295–297, 296b, 305t
　　process measures of, 295, 295b, 305t
　　summary for key stakeholders, 301, 302f–303f
　　synthesis of, 301–302

Evidence
- appraising and synthesizing, 75–77, 77b, 78t
- assessing, principles of, 81–90
  - appraising, 88
  - data collection constancy in, 83
  - external validity in, 85–88
  - findings to practice, issues relating to maximizing applicability of, 81–83
  - homogenous sample in, 83
  - internal validity in, 85, 85b, 86t–87t
  - intervention fidelity in, 83–84, 84b
  - objectively conceptualized research question in, 83, 83b
- awareness tools, 66
- critical appraisal and synthesis of, 40–42
- definition of, 46
- discovering, 61–66
- finding, leveling, and grading, 38–40, 40t
- problem identification and nature of, 38
- production and communication of, 60, 61t
- quality of, 39, 40t
- searching the literature for, 59–80

EvidenceAlerts, 65t, 66

Evidence-based guidelines, 372

Evidence-based policy, 22t, 396

Evidence-Based Practice Improvement Model, 47–48

Evidence-based practices (EBPs), 19–36, 20b–21b, 25b, 143–144, 239t, 243, 333, 349, 352f, 359
- academic partners, 270
- audit and feedback, 271–272, 272b
- barriers and facilitators to implementation of, 254
- barriers to, 254–261
- call to action, 32–33
- case study of, 148
- climate, 263
- climate scale, 266
- conduct of research *versus*, 23t–24t
- culture of, 262–263
- data analysis, 150, 150b
- definition of terms in, 21–25, 22t–24t, 25f
- educational programs, 270

Evidence-based practices (EBPs) (Continued)
- engaging consumers in, 31–32, 32b
- environmental scan, 263–266
- ethical considerations for, 236–240
- ethnography of, 147–148
- evaluation of, 293, 294b, 304t
  - data sources, 297–300, 300b
- frameworks, 271
- grounded theory of, 147
- guidelines for, 306b
- historical overview of, 20–21
- impact of, 293–308
- implementation in, 229, 253
  - action plans with, 236, 238b
  - myths and realities of, 237t
  - principles of, 233–236
  - quality improvement as, 233
  - as stages of adoption, 234t
  - Translating Research into Practice Model for, 230, 230f
- key points, 33–34
- leader meetings, 270
- leadership implications for, 1–6
  - call to action, 3–4
  - opportunities, 2–3
  - scope of influence, 2
- meetings of, 268–270
- models of, 44, 45t
- national agenda for, 24–28, 26t–27t
- outcome measures of, 295–297, 296b, 305t
  - clinician outcome examples, 297
  - cost outcomes, 297, 297b
  - patient outcome examples, 296
- patient-centered, 277–292
  - challenges in post-COVID world, 288
  - clinical scenario in, 278, 278b
  - health literacy and numeracy, 282–283, 282b, 283f–284f, 286t
  - patient activation, 281–282, 281f
  - patient engagement and empowerment, 278–279
  - synthesis in, 288–289
- performance gap assessment of, 266
- phenomenology of, 147
- piloting change in, 270–271
- process measures of, 295, 295b, 305t
- projects, dissemination of, 317–332
  - active, 318

Evidence-based practices (EBPs) (Continued)
- definition of, 317–318
- implementation science and, 321–323, 322t, 323f, 323b, 324t–325t
- intended audience in, 318
- objectives of, 318
- passive, 318
- principles of, 318
- social media methods in, 320–321
- synthesis of, 329
- traditional methods of, 319–320
- venues for, 319
- qualitative methodologies in
  - key differences in, 149–150, 150b
  - and worldview, 145–147, 147b
- rationale for changing practice, 233b
- recommendations for action, 42–43
- social system in, 261–266
- statistics for, 173–198
  - comparing differences between groups, 185
  - data and design in, 174–176
  - descriptive statistics, 176–177, 176t
  - diagnostic test studies, 189–194, 189b, 190t, 191f, 191b
  - hypothesis testing and probability values, 180–182, 180t, 182t
  - implications for practice settings, 196
  - inferential statistics, 176–177
  - interventional study designs, 188–189
  - levels of measurement in, 174–176, 175t
  - literature statistics, 185
  - measuring relationships between variables, 185–186
  - meta-analysis, 195–196, 196f
  - normal distribution, 177, 178f
  - observational study designs, 189
  - odds ratios analysis, 187–188
  - prognosis articles, 194–195
  - risk reduction analysis, 186–187
  - synthesis, 196
  - test selection, 188–196
- steps of, 28, 28b, 29t–31t, 294b
- summary for key stakeholders, 301, 302f–303f
- synthesis of, 153–155, 240, 273, 301–302

Evidence-based practices (EBPs) *(Continued)*
  team, 28–31
  topic, 230–233, 231b–232b, 232t, 239t
  unit climate for, 266
  users of, 254, 261
Evidence-based project, clinical question in, 53–54
Evidence-based resources, 41t
Evidence hierarchy, 38, 39f
Evidence-informed decision making, 22t
Experimental designs, 91–93
Experimental groups, 82
Expertise and research, 395
Expert opinion, 60
Expert Recommendations for Implementing Change (ERIC), 254, 255t–258t
Exposure, in observational studies, 106
External benchmark, 162
External validity, 85–88, 96, 98t–100t, 152t
Extraction, data, 121
Extraneous variables, 83

F
Face validity, 299
Facilitation, definition of, 47
Facilitators and barriers, 254
Factorial designs, 94
Fagan nomogram, 191, 191f
Fail-Safe Number, 125
Fair and accountable systems, 408
False hits, 68
Feedback, as quality strategy lever, 201
Fidelity, 83, 95–96
Field tags, 71–73
Filters, database, 73
Financial benefits, of APP, 8
Fishbone diagram, 217, 218f
Five Whys method, 217
Flowcharting, 218, 219f
Food and Drug Administration Amendments Act, 124
Forest plot, 126, 128f, 195–196, 196f
Frameworks, evidence-based practice, 271
Funnel plot, 124–125, 125f

G
Gallup Q, 166t
Gemba Walk, 160–161
Generalizability, of data, 83, 152t
Global Health Observatory, 384
Google, 65
GoogleScholar, 65, 69–70
Government and legislative bodies in health policy, 394
GRADE system. *See* Grading of Recommendations Assessment, Development and Evaluation (GRADE) system
GRADE tool, 101
Grading evidence, 39–40
Grading of Recommendations Assessment, Development and Evaluation (GRADE) system, 39, 41t, 122
Graphs, 216–217, 217f
Grassroots advocacy, 395
Gravity Project, 384
Gray literature
  definition of, 61
  in systematic review, 121, 124
Grounded theory, 147
Group/team interventions, 406–407
Guidelines for the Prevention, Detection, Evaluation, and Management of High Blood Pressure in Adults, 135

H
Hands-on learning, 355
Handwashing education, 161–162
Happiness, 387
Harassment, 418
Hawthorne effect, 88
HCAHPS. *See* Hospital Consumer Assessment of Healthcare Providers and Systems
Health, 401
Health care access, 397
Healthcare Cost and Utilization Project (HCUP), 114–115
Health care costs, increased, 421
Healthcare Information and Management Systems Society (HIMSS), 365
Health care organizations, 310
Healthcare quality
  defined, 199–200
  improvement of
    accrediting organizations for, 204b
    benchmarking for, 203b, 204–205
    clinical leader's role in, 200–201
    evidence-based approaches for, 199–228, 204b, 214b, 216b, 224b
    national goals and strategies for, 201, 201b, 202t
    perspectives and models for, 205–211, 207b–208b, 209t–213t
    principles of, 210t–211t
    quality strategy levers for, 201–205, 202b–205b
    steps and tools for, 207b–208b, 211–224, 211b, 214t
  measurement of, 204, 206t
  six dimensions for, 200b
Health care statistics, 65–66
Health disparities, 420
Health education and literacy, 427
Health equity, 169, 385, 393
Health equity databases, 170t
Health Equity Framework, 423
Health Equity Research Guide, 170t
Health inequities, 421
Health information technology, as quality strategy lever, 203
Health literacy, 282–283
  assessing, 282b
  definition of, 282
  percentage of, 283f
  strategies to improve, 283–284, 285t–286t
Health numeracy, 282–283
  assessing, 282b
  definition of, 282
  percentage of, 284f
  strategies to improve, 283–284, 285t–286t
Health policy, 391
  addressing health disparities, 397–398
  advancing, into practice, 393–394
  harnessing evidence and research, 396
  impact on nursing practice, 395–396
  nurses impact at three levels of government, 394–395
  nursing's contribution in, 392–393

Health policy *(Continued)*
  overview of policy and, 391–392
  role of government and legislative bodies in, 394
  roles for clinical leaders in, 396–397
  synthesis, 398
Health systems
  and diversity, equity, inclusion, and belonging, 419
  embracing innovation, 354b
  strategic plans, 161
Healthy workforce, 401–402
Heterogeneity, test of, 126
Heterophily, 246
High-reliability organizing/organization, 206, 210t–211t
Histogram, 216–217
Historical and intergenerational factors, 420
History
  academic-practice partnership, 8–9
  threats to internal validity, 85, 86t–87t, 95
Home Health Care Consumer Assessment of Healthcare Providers and Systems (HHCAHPS), 26, 26t–27t, 163t–165t
Home Health Compare, 203b
Homogeneity, 83
Homophily, 246
Hospital-based patient complaints and grievances, 163, 163t–165t
Hospital CAHPS, 163t–165t
Hospital Care Compare, 167t
Hospital Compare, 203b
Hospital Consumer Assessment of Healthcare Providers and Systems (HCAHPS), 167t, 203b
Hospital Value-Based Purchasing Program, 204
Housing, 397
Humanity-centered approach, 344
Humanity-centered design thinking, 345f, 346
Hypotheses, 55–56
Hypothesis testing, 180–182

I
ICBS. *See* Implementation Citizenship Behavior Scale
ICS. *See* Implementation Climate Scale

IHI. *See* Institute for Healthcare Improvement
ILS. *See* Implementation Leadership Scale
I3 Model, 47
Implementation
  in evidence-based practice, 229
    action plans with, 236, 238b
    in evidence-based practice topic, 230–233, 231b–232b, 232t, 239t
    model of, 230, 230b
    myths and realities of, 237t
    principles of, 233–236
    quality improvement as, 233
    as stages of adoption, 234t
    Translating Research into Practice Model for, 230, 230f
  launching, 243–252, 244b, 246b, 248b
  strategies for, 253–276
    addressing characteristics of clinical topic, 244–246
    addressing communication, 246–249
    addressing social system/practice context, 261
    performance gap assessment of, 266
  sustainability of, 249
Implementation Citizenship Behavior Scale (ICBS), 265t
Implementation Climate Scale (ICS), 265t
Implementation fidelity, 330
Implementation Leadership Scale (ILS), 261, 261b, 265t
Implementation science (IS), 22t, 25, 43, 321–323, 322t
  Consolidated Framework for Implementation Research, 46
  definition of, 46
Implicit biases, 418
Improvement cycle, 222
In-Center Hemodialysis CAHPS, 163t–165t
Incidence rate difference, risk, 187
Inclusion/exclusion criteria, 66, 92
Inclusive teams, 345
Inclusivity, 418
Income and employment, 397
Independent variable, 83–84, 174

Indexing, 62–65
Inferential statistics, 176–177
Influence, 247–248
Informants, 247
Informatics, 359
Informatics and population health, 383–384
Innovation, 349
  definition, 343–344, 344b
  design thinking, 345–346, 347f
  in healthcare, 339
  methodology, 345–346
  as quality strategy lever, 203
  teams, 344–345
Innovators, 235t
Inspiration and motivation, 355
Institute for Healthcare Improvement (IHI), 26t–27t, 144, 161
Institute of Medicine (IOM), 144
Institutional repositories, 65, 65t
Instrumentation, threats to internal validity, 85, 86t–87t
Integrative reviews, 119t–120t, 128–129
Intellectual property, 355
Interdisciplinary relationships, 165–166, 167t
Internal benchmark, 162
Internal consistency, 298–299
Internal validity, 85, 86t–87t, 152t
  definition of, 94
  threats to, 94–96, 98t–100t
    measurement/statistical factors, 95
    person factors, 94–95
    situational factors, 95–96
International Clinical Trials Registry Platform (ICTRP), 65t, 66
Internet of Things (IoT), 373
Interoperability, 384
Interrater reliability, 298–299
Interval data, 174, 175t
Intervening variables, 84
Intervention
  in PICOT, 52–53
  targeting individuals, 405–406
Intervention fidelity, 82, 95–96
Intervention studies, 91–104. *See also* Randomized controlled trials
  factorial designs, 94
  pilot studies, 93–94
  pragmatic clinical trials, 94

Intervention studies *(Continued)*
　purpose of, 91
　research synthesis, 97–102
　　implementation factors, 102
　　scope of question, 97–100
　　selecting studies for inclusion, 100–101
　study designs, 188–189
　　experimental designs, 92–93
　　quasi-experimental design, 93
　synthesizing the studies, 101–102
　threats to validity, 94–97, 98t–100t
　　external validity, 96
　　internal validity, 94–96
　　statistical conclusions, 96–97
Introduction, Methods, Results, and Discussion (IMRAD), 323–324
IOM. *See* Institute of Medicine
Iowa Model of Evidence-Based Practice, 44, 45t
Issue of interest, in PICOT, 52–53

J
Johns Hopkins Nursing EBP Model, 44, 45t
Joint Commission, 204b
　for Accreditation of Healthcare Organizations, 26t–27t
Journal articles, 64–65
Journal clubs, 76b
JournalTOCs, 65t
Just culture, 408

K
Key stakeholders
　evaluation summary for, 301, 302f–303f
　meetings with, 269
Keywords, for database searches, 69, 71f
Knowledge, as stages of adoption, 234t
Knowledge Discovery in Databases (KDD), 370
Knowledge to action model (KTA) model, 45t
Knowledge transfer, 22t
Knowledge translation, 22t
KT+, 65t, 66
KTA model. *See* Knowledge to action (KTA) model

L
Laggards, 235t
Language access services, 427
Language barriers, in patient engagement, 287
Late majority, 235t
Law of the Few, 216–217
Leadership, 1–6, 335–336
　call to action, 3–4
　in evidence-based practice, 258–261
　opportunities, 2–3
　in population health, 386–387
　scope of influence, 2
Leadership behaviors, for evidence-based practice, 261
Lean, 210t–211t
Lean Six Sigma, 44–46
The Leapfrog Group, 203b
Learning, as quality strategy lever, 201–202
Learning management systems (LMSs), 365–366
Legal compliance, 428
Lexicomp, 65t, 66
Likelihood ratio (LR), 191
　changes affect probability of disease, 192t
　for chlamydia study data, 192f
　nomogram, 191f
　positive and negative, 191b
Limiters, database, 73
Linear regression, 186
Linking peers, 406–407
Lippincott Procedures and Advisor, 66
Literature
　databases, 62–65, 62t
　　indexing and metadata, 62–65
　　managing and screening records, 75
　　saving search strategies, 73–75
　　tools and repositories, 65–66, 65t
　gray, 61
Literature review, 66
Literature review screening tools, 75
Literature search flow diagrams, 75
Literature statistics, 185
Longitudinal study. *See* Cohort studies

M
Magnet-designated organizations, 312–313
Magnet Recognition Program, 312
MakerHealth, 355
Makerspace, 353–355
Manipulation, 92
Manuscript, peer review of, 326–327
Manuscript submission, 326
Mass media, 246–249
Maturation, threats to internal validity, 85, 86t–87t
Mayo Clinic framework, 403–404
Mayo High Performance Teamwork Scale (MHPTS), 167t
Mean, 176–177, 176t
Measurement
　effects, 88, 88b
　as quality strategy lever, 201, 202b
　standard setting groups for, 202b
Median, 176–177, 176t
Media sharing, 321
Medicare Access and CHIP Reauthorization Act (MACRA), 204
Medicare Advantage and Prescription Drug Plan CAHPS, 163t–165t
Meditation, 406
MEDLINE, 62t, 64–65, 79
MedRxiv, 65, 65t
Mental health issues, in health care workers, 409–410
Merit-Based Incentive Payment System (MIPS), 204, 206t
Meta-analysis, 102, 195
　definition of, 123–124
　protocol for, 124
　statistics common to, 195–196, 196f
　systematic review and, 119t, 122f
Metadata, 62–65
Meta-summary, 149
Meta-synthesis, 149, 149b
Methodist proficient assessment competency (MPAC), 267t
Metrics and accountability, 426
mHealth, 373
Microaggressions, 418
Microblogs, 321
Micromedex, 66
Mindfulness, 405–406
MIPS. *See* Merit-Based Incentive Payment System
Mixed-methods research, 101, 148–149, 148b
Mode, 176–177, 176t
Model for Improvement (MFI), 44

INDEX

The Model for Improvement, 218
Modified Index for Interdisciplinary Collaboration (MIIC), 167t
Monitoring and surveillance, 372
Mortality, threats to internal validity, 85, 86t–87t
Multiphase Optimization Strategy (MOST), 94
Multiple regression, 186

N

Narrative review, 101, 119t–120t
National Academies of Sciences, Engineering, and Medicine (NASEM), 347
National Center for Health Statistics, 65–66, 65t
National Comprehensive Cancer Network (NCCN), 134
National Council of State Boards of Nursing (NCSBN), 14–15
National Database of Nursing Quality Indicators (NDNQI), 159, 169t
National Guideline Clearinghouse (NGC), 134, 135b
National Healthcare Quality and Disparities Reports (NHQDR), 170t
National Institute of Nursing Research (NINR), 396
National Institutes of Health (NIH), 28
National Quality Forum (NQF), 26t–27t, 202b
National Quality Strategy, 201, 201b, 202t
Nationwide Adult Medicaid CAHPS, 163t–165t
NDNQI RN Survey with Practice Environment Scale, 165–166, 166t
Negative likelihood ratio (NLR), 191b, 192, 192t
Negative predictive value (NPV), 189–190, 189b
Neurodevelopmental therapy (NDT), 124
New York State Department of Health website, 163t–165t
NGC. See National Guideline Clearinghouse
Nightingale, Florence, 20, 200–201
Nominal data, 174, 175t
Nomogram, likelihood ratio, 191, 191f
Nonparametric statistics, 176, 179, 179b
Normal distribution, 177, 178f
NPV. See Negative predictive value
NQF. See National Quality Forum
NRC Health, 163t–165t
Null hypothesis, 180
Null value, 182
Nurse informaticist, roles of, 374–375, 374b–375b
Nurse Manager EBP Competency Scale, 265t
Nurse managers
  meetings with, 269–270
  of practice sites, 269–270
Nurses' Health Study (NHS), 109
Nurse wellness
  context for heightened attention to, 402–403
  frameworks, 403–404
  implications for practice settings, 411–413
  measures/indicators of, 404–405
  outcomes, 403–404
Nursing, 391
  evidence-based practice, 1–6, 19–36, 20b–21b, 25b
    call to action, 32–33
    conduct of research versus, 23t–24t
    definition of terms for, 21–25, 22t–24t, 25f
    engaging consumers in, 31–32, 32b
    historical overview of, 20–21
    national agenda for, 24–28, 26t–27t
    steps of, 28, 28b, 29t–31t
    team, 28–31
  innovation and technology, 352–353
  literature search, 59–80
  production and communication of evidence in, 60, 61t
Nursing Home Compare, 203b
Nursing informatics
  Data-Information-Knowledge-Wisdom, 366–367, 366f, 367t, 367b
  data use and evaluation, 369–371, 370t, 371b
  future of, 372–374
  historical background, 359–365
Nursing informatics (Continued)
  history in education, 365–366
  nursing support systems for decision making, 371–372, 372b
  principles of, 367–369
  reflections on knowledge application of, 375b
  roles of nurse informaticist, 374–375, 374b–375b
  scope and standards of practice, 367–369, 368t, 369b
  synthesis, 375
Nursing informatics project manager, 374
Nursing Leadership for EBP Scale, 265t
Nursing policy, 392
Nursing practice, 336–337
Nursing process versus design thinking method, 348f
Nursing Reference Center Plus, 66
Nursing scholarship, 309–310
  academic implications, 311
  future considerations, 313–314
  nursing implications, 312–313
  partnership implications, 313
  synthesis, 314
Nursing's contribution in health policy, 392–393
Nursing-sensitive indicators (NSIs), 166–169, 169t
Nursing support systems for decision making, 371–372
Nursing workforce, 8–9

O

Objectivity, of data, 152t
Observability, of EBP topics, 232t
Observational studies, 76, 105–116
  critically appraising, 113–115, 114t, 115b
  data and data analyses in, 112–113, 113b
  description of, 105–106
  designs, 189
  exposure in, 106
  outcome in, 106
  PICOT questions for, 106, 106t
  purpose of, 106–108, 107b
  structure of, 107f
  synthesis of, 115
  types of, 108–112, 112b

Observational studies *(Continued)*
   case-control studies, 109–110, 110b
   case series, 110–111
   cohort studies, 108–109
   survey studies, 111–112, 112b
Observational Teamwork Assessment for Surgery (OTAS), 167t
Observation period, 301
Odds ratio, 125, 188
OHSA-Ergonomics, 170t
One-tailed test, 181
OpenDOAR, 65t
Operational definitions, 162
Opinion leaders, 246–247
Oral Health Nursing Education and Practice (OHNEP) Program, 280
Oral Health Patient Facts, 280, 280b
Oral presentation, for disseminating evidence-based practice projects, 319–320, 320b
Ordinal data, 174, 175t
Organizational capacity, of evidence-based practice, 261–262
Organizational culture, 409–410
Organizational interventions, 407–411
Organizational Readiness for Implementation Change (ORIC) instrument, 265t
OR operator, 71
OSF Preprints, 65t
Outcome measures, 161–162
   in evidence-based practice, 295–297, 296b, 305t
   in observational studies, 106
   in PICOT, 53
Outcomes, 24
Outpatient and Ambulatory Surgery CAHPS, 163t–165t
Ownership, 247–248

P
Pandemic, 381
Parameter value, 176
Parametric statistics, 176–177, 180b
Pareto diagram, 216–217
Pareto principle, 216–217
Participative style, 247–248
Partnerships with local leaders, 395
Passive dissemination, 318
Patient activation, 281–282, 281f

Patient Activation Measure (PAM), 281–282, 281f
Patient and family advisory boards/committees, 163t–165t
Patient and family advisory council (PFAC), 163t–165t
Patient-centered care
   challenges in post-COVID world, 288
   individual barriers against, 287
   moving to person-centered care, 284–285
   strategies, 285t, 287
Patient-centered evidence-based practices, 277–292
   clinical scenario in, 278, 278b
   health literacy and numeracy, 282–283, 282b, 283f–284f, 286t
   patient activation, 281–282, 281f
   patient-centered care
      individual barriers against, 287
      strategies, 285t, 287
   patient engagement
      barriers against, 285t
      and empowerment, 278–279
      tools, development of, 280–281, 280b
   person-centered care, contextual barriers against, 287–288
   synthesis in, 288–289
Patient-Centered Outcomes Research Institute (PCORI), 279
Patient complaints and grievances, 163, 163t–165t
Patient decision support (PDS), 372
Patient engagement, 278–279
   barriers against, 285t
   tools, development of, 280–281, 280b
Patient engagement and empowerment, 278–279
Patient experience surveys, 163, 163t–165t
Patient family advisory councils (PFACs), 31–32
Patient population, in PICOT, 52
Patient portals, 285t
Patient-reported outcomes (PROs), 163
Patient safety, 166, 370
Pay for performance, 205b
Payment incentives, as quality strategy lever, 202–203, 205b

Pearson's correlation coefficient, 185–186
Peer review and dissemination, 323–327
   abstract submission, 323–324
   ANCC Magnet Standards for, 327, 328t
   manuscript submission, 326
   peer review of abstract, 324–326
   peer review of manuscript, 326–327
Peer-reviewed journals, 61
Peer to peer support, 406–407
Performance benchmarks, 159
   external benchmark, 162
   internal benchmark, 162
Performance gap assessment (PGA), 266
Personal health records (PHRs), 372–373
Personal protective equipment (PPE), 387
Person-centered care
   contextual barriers against, 287–288
   moving from patient-centered to, 284–285
Persuasion, as stages of adoption, 234t
Persuasiveness, 247–248
PGA. *See* Performance Gap Assessment
Phenomenology, 147
Physician quality reporting initiative, 203b
Picker, 163t–165t
PICOT questions, 52
   case study, 56b
   components of, 52b
   core concepts, in database searches, 69
   and eligibility criteria, 67, 67t
   formats of, 53b
   formulation of, 54
   in observational studies, 106, 106t, 107f
   search criteria and database search queries, 70f
   in systematic review, 118
   types of, 55
Piloting change, in evidence-based practice, 270–271
Pilot studies, 93–94
Plan-Do-Study-Act (PDSA), 44, 298
Plan-Do-Study-Act (PDSA) cycle, 222, 223f, 273, 423

INDEX

Plot
   forest, 126, 128f
   funnel, 124–125, 125f
POC tools. *See* Point-of-care (POC) tools
Point-of-care (POC) tools, 65t, 66
Policies, 391
   dissemination and implementation research, 22t
   at workplace, 426
Policy analysis, 393
Policy analysis and development, 395
Policy enactment, 394
Policy implementation, 394
Population health, 379
   competencies, 385
   data collection and data sets for, 384
   epidemiology of, 381–383
   essential skills in, 385–387
   history of, 380–381
   implications for practice, 387
   informatics and, 383–384
   leadership and systems thinking in, 386–387
   ongoing longitudinal studies in, 382t
Portal for Education and Advancement of Knowledge (PEAK), 366
Positive likelihood ratio, 191b, 192t
Positive predictive value (PPV), 189–190, 189b
Poster presentations, for disseminating evidence-based practice projects, 319, 319b
Power, 333–334
Power analysis, 96, 178–179
Power/interest matrix, 268
PPV. *See* Positive predictive value
Practice change
   evaluation of, 43
   implementation and dissemination of, 43
Practice context, implementation strategies to address, 261
Practice facilitation, 222
Pragmatic clinical trials, 94
Preferred Reporting Items for Systematic Reviews and Meta-Analyses (PRISMA), 121–122
Premature death, in United States, 383, 383f
Preprint repositories, 65, 65t
Press Ganey, 163t–165t

Prevalence difference, risk, 186–187
Prevalence, of disease, 189–190
Prevalence ratio, 187
Preventive Services Task Force, U.S., 26t–27t
Primary sources, of evidence, 60, 61t
PRISMA diagrams, 75
Proactive evidence-seeking approach, into clinical practice style, 54
Probability value (p-value), 180–182
Problem identification, 393
Processes of care, 24
Process measures, 161–162
   in evaluation of evidence-based practice, 24, 295, 295b, 305t
Professional endorsements, 348b
Professional networking, 321
Professional nursing associations, 395
Professional organizations, 394–395
Prognosis articles, statistics common to, 194–195
Program for International Assessment of Adult Competencies (PIAAC), 282
Promoting Action on Research Implementation in Health Services (PARIHS) model, 46–47
ProQuest Central, 62t
Prospective studies. *See* Cohort studies
Prototyping, 352f
Psychological and emotional impact, 421
Psychological health, 404
Psychological safety, 408
Psychology of Change framework, 260, 260f
Psychometrics, 298–299
PsycINFO, 62t, 79
Publication bias, 97–100, 124
Publications, for disseminating evidence-based practice projects, 320
Public health, 379
Public health emergencies, 384
Public reporting
   as quality strategy lever, 201, 203b
   systems for, 203b
PubMed, 62t, 64f, 71–73, 79
Punctuation, database searches, 71, 72f
Purposive sampling, 145, 150b

Q

QI. *See* Quality improvement
QI team, 298
Q Reviews, 163t–165t
Quadruple Aim Initiative, 144
Qualitative analysis, 174
Qualitative methodologies
   key differences in, 149–150, 150b
   worldview and, 145–147, 147b
Qualitative paradigm, 146
Qualitative research, 144b
   critical appraisal of, 154t–155t
   definition of, 143–144
   meta-synthesis, 149, 149b
   methodologies, 144
   methods to study transgender patient needs, 146f
   mixed-methods, 148–149, 148b
   process-related differences in, 151t
   versus quantitative studies, 145–146
   sampling in, 150b
   scientific rigor in, 150–153, 151t, 151b, 153b
Qualitative studies, 143–158
Quality and Safety Education for Nurses (QSEN), 2–3, 200–201
Quality assurance (QA) model, 206–211
Quality healthcare, 199–200
Quality improvement (QI), 21–24, 22t, 25f, 43, 144, 161, 200, 239t, 294, 359
   accrediting organizations for, 204b
   benchmarking for, 162–163, 203b, 204–205
   clinical leader's role in, 200–201
   data, 131–133
   employee engagement and satisfaction surveys, 165, 166t
   evidence-based approaches for, 199–228, 204b, 214b, 216b, 224b
   healthcare, in, 199–200, 200b
   health equity, 169, 170t
   implementation and, 239t
   interdisciplinary relationships, 165–166, 167t
   national goals and strategies for, 201, 201b, 202t
   nursing-sensitive indicators, 166–169, 169t
   patient safety, 166

Quality improvement (QI) (Continued)
  perspectives and models for, 205–211, 207b–208b, 209t–213t
  principles of, 210t–211t
  quality strategy levers for, 201–205, 202b–205b
  steps and tools for, 207b–208b, 211–224, 211b, 214t
    analysis in, 214–218
    assessment in, 214
    developing plan for, 218–219, 220f, 221t–222t
    summary of, 223f
    tests and implementation of, 222–224, 223f
  team for, leardership, 212–214
  voice of patient and family, 163, 163t–165t
  workforce safety, 169, 170t
Quality improvement initiatives, 427
Quality Improvement Minimum Quality Criteria Set (QI-MQCS), 219
Quality improvement models, 44–46
  Lean Six Sigma, 44–46
  Model for Improvement (MFI), 44
Quality of care, 8–9
Quality of evidence, 39, 40t
Quantitative analysis, 174
Quantitative research, 88
Quasi-experimental design, 91, 93, 93b
Quick reference guides, 244–246
Quick response (QR) code, 244–245

R
Randomization, 92
  to experimental groups and control groups, 82
Randomized controlled trials (RCTs), 91, 93b
  systematic reviews of, 118
Range, of data, 177
Rapid prototyping, 355
Rapid review, 119t–120t
Rate ratio, 187
Ratio data, 175, 175t
Raw data, 145
Rayyan, 75
RCTs. See Randomized controlled trials
Reach, Effectiveness, Adoption, Implementation, and Maintenance (RE-AIM) model, 46

Reactive effects, 88
Reactivity, defined, 88
Read by QxMD, 65t, 66
RE-AIM framework, 322–323, 323f, 324t
Realist review, 119t–120t
Received wisdom, 411–412
Receiver operating characteristics (ROC), 194t
Receiver operating characteristics (ROC) curve, 192–193, 193f
Recognition, of evidence-based practice, 272
Recruitment, 426
Refining, database searches, 73, 74f
Regional health information exchange (HIE), 373
Relative advantage, of EBP topics, 232t
Relative measures of risk, 187
Relative risk, 187
Reliability
  of data, 152t
  definition, 298–299
  interrater, 298–299
  test-retest, 298–299
Repeated measures study, 108
Research, 43
  conduct of
    definition of, 21–25, 22t–24t, 25f
    EBP versus, 23t–24t
  dissemination, 22t
  policy dissemination and implementation, 22t
  qualitative, 144b
    critical appraisal of, 154t–155t
    definition of, 143–144
    meta-synthesis, 149, 149b
    methods to study transgender patient needs, 146f
    process-related differences in, 151t
    sampling in, 150b
    scientific rigor in, 150–153, 151t, 151b, 153b
  quantitative, 88
  utilization, 20
Research evidence pyramid, 39–40
Research questions, 55–56
Resilience, 403–404
Respondent burden, 113–114
Retention, 426
Retrospective study, 108

Review, 117–118
  critically appraising systematic, 129–131, 132f
  integrative, 119t–120t, 128–129
  narrative, 119t–120t
  rapid, 119t–120t
  realist, 119t–120t
  scoping, 119t–120t
  types of, 118–131, 121f–122f, 121b, 123t, 125f, 126b, 127f–128f, 128b, 131b
Review article, in systematic review, 118
Reviewing, narrative, 101
Rewards, of evidence-based practice, 272
Risk difference (RD) calculations, 186
Risk of Bias Tool 2.0, 125–126, 127f
Risk ratio, 187
Risk reduction, 355
Risk reduction analysis, 186–187
ROC curve. See Receiver Operating Characteristics (ROC) curve
Root cause analyses, 217
Rule setting, 102
Run charts, trending variation in system performance with, 215–216, 215f–216f

S
Safe patient handling (SPH), 313
Safety, Communication, Operational Reliability, and Engagement (SCORE) survey, 166t
Saturation, 145
Scholarship of application, 309–310
Scholarship of discovery, 309–310
Scholarship of integration, 309–310
Scholarship of teaching, 309–310
Schwartz Center Rounds, 406–407
Scientific rigor, in qualitative research, 150–153, 151t, 151b, 153b
Scoping review, 119t–120t
Scoping searches, 68
Search string/search query, 70–73, 72f
Search tags, 71–73
Secondary sources, of evidence, 60, 61t
Selection bias, threats to internal validity, 85, 86t–87t
Selection effects, 85–88
Self-designating method, 247
Self-report, diagnostic tests, 190, 190t
Sensitive search, 68–69
Sensitivity analysis, 126

INDEX

Sensitivity, of test, 189, 190t
Sequential multiple assignment randomized trial (SMART) design, 94
Sexual orientation and gender identity (SOGI), 425
Shared decision making, 278–279
    aids, 279–280, 280b
    evidence to support, 279
Sigma Repository, 65, 65t
Six Sigma, 210t–211t
Skewness, 178, 179f
SMART design. *See* Sequential multiple assignment randomized trial (SMART) design
Snowballing, database searches, 73
Snowball sampling, 150b
Social and racial equity, 397
Social determinants of health (SDOH), 19–20, 203, 381, 385, 385f, 394, 397, 418, 420, 423b
    addressing, 427
Social media methods, in dissemination of evidence-based practice projects, 320–321
Social networking site, 321
Social Sciences Research Network (SSRN), 65, 65t
Social system
    environmental scan, 261b, 263–266
    in evidence-based practice, 261–266
    implementation strategies to address, 261
    leadership, 258–261
    organizational capacity of, 261–262
Sociometric method, 247
Special cause variation, 215, 215f
Specificity, of test, 189, 190t
Specific search, 68
Stakeholder mapping, 267–268, 268b
Stakeholders, 267–268
    evaluation summary for, 301, 302f–303f
    meetings, 268–270
        with key leadership stakeholders, 269
        nurse manager meetings, 269–270
        with other disciplines, 269
Standard deviation (SD), 177
Standards for Quality Improvement Reporting Excellence (SQUIRE), 320
Standards for Quality Improvement Reporting Excellence (SQUIRE 2.0) guidelines, 219, 221t–222t
Standards of practice, in evidence-based practice, 272
Star Rating System, CMS, 160, 163t–165t
Statistical conclusions, 96–97, 98t–100t
Statistical regression, 95
Statistics, 173–174
    for evidence-based practice, 173–198
        comparing differences between groups, 185
        data and design in, 174–176
        descriptive statistics, 176–177, 176t
        diagnostic test studies, 189–194, 189b, 190t, 191f, 191b
        hypothesis testing and probability values, 180–182, 180t, 182t
        implications for practice settings, 196
        inferential statistics, 176–177
        interventional study designs, 188–189
        levels of measurement in, 174–176, 175t
        literature statistics, 185
        measuring relationships between variables, 185–186
        meta-analysis, 195–196, 196f
        normal distribution, 177, 178f
        observational study designs, 189
        odds ratios analysis, 187–188
        prognosis articles, 194–195
        risk reduction analysis, 186–187
        synthesis, 196
        test selection, 188–196
    nonparametric, 176, 179, 179b
    parametric, 176–177, 180b
Stereotyping, 418
Stetler model, 45t
Strategic planning, 160–161
Strategy and policy development, 394
Strengthening the Reporting of Observational Studies in Epidemiology (STROBE), 121
Structural and systemic factors, 420
Structure, 24
Structured search query, 70–73, 72f
Structure measures, 161
Structure-Process-Outcome Framework, 206–211
Student assistance programs, 410–411
Student's *t* test, 185
Subject headings, 64–65
    identification, database searches, 69–70
Survey studies, 111–112, 112b
Sustainability, of EBP projects, 318
Sustainable Development Goals (SDGs), 380–381, 380f
Syndromic surveillance, 383–384
Synergy, 333
Synthesis table, 76, 78t
Systematic reviews, 117–142
    components, 123t
    critical appraisal tools, 123b
    critically appraising, 129–131, 132f
    definition of, 118
    intervention studies, 97–102
    versus literature review, 97
    meta-analysis and, 118, 119t, 122f
    types of, 119t
Systemic discrimination, 418
Systems thinking, in population health, 386–387

T

Table of evidence (TOE), 41, 42t, 76, 78t, 122
Team, 232–233
Team Climate Inventory (TCI), 167t
Team Emergency Assessment Measure (TEAM), 167t
Technical assistance, as quality strategy lever, 201–202
Technology, 359
Technology Informatics Guiding Education Reform (TIGER) Initiative, 367–369, 369t
Tester questions, 352b
Testing effects, 85
Testing, threats to internal validity, 86t–87t
Test of heterogeneity, 126
Test-retest reliability, 298–299
Therapy studies. *See* Randomized controlled trials
Total Quality Management/Continuous Quality Improvement (TQM/CQI), 210t–211t
Traditional problem solving *versus* design thinking, 349t

Training programs, 270
Transferability, of data, 150, 152t
Translating Research into Practice (TRIP) Model, 230, 230f, 243
Translational research, 22t
Translation, in patient engagement, 287
Translation science, 22t, 25, 244
Treatment fidelity, 95–96
Tree diagram, 217
Trialability, of EBP topics, 232t
Trial registries, 65–66
Trip (Turning Research Into Practice) database, 65t, 67
TRIP model. *See* Translating Research into Practice (TRIP) Model
Trustworthiness, of data, 150, 152t
Two-tailed test, 181
Type I error, 181
Type II error, 181

U

Unit climate, for EBP implementation, 266
University of California-San Diego (UCSD) Human Research Protections Program (HRPP), 239–240, 240b–241b
Unqualified search, 71–73
UpToDate, 65t, 66
User-centered approach, 344
Users, of evidence-based practice, 254, 261
U.S. Preventive Services Task Force, 26t–27t
Utrecht Work Engagement Scale, 166t

V

Validity, 299
Value-Based Health Care Purchasing, 205b
Value-based programs (VBPs), 26–27
Variables, 174
VBPs. *See* Value Based Programs
Vimeo, in dissemination of evidence-based practice projects, 321
Virtual reality (VR), 365
Vizient Clinical Database, 159
Vote counting, 101–102

W

Web of Science, 62t, 73
Well-being, 401
  interventions, 405–411
Wellness, 401, 403–404
  interventions, 405–411
Work Environment for EBP Scale, 265t
Worker safety databases, 170t
Worker Well-Being Questionnaire (NIOSH WellBQ), 405
Workforce development, as quality strategy lever, 203
Workforce health, 401–402
Workforce safety, 169
Work-life integration, 408–409
Workplace wellness programs, 405
World Bank Health Data, 65t
World Health Organization's International Clinical Trials Registry Platform (ICTRP), 65t, 66

Y

YouTube, in dissemination of evidence-based practice projects, 321